THE
COMPLETE
ENCYCLOPEDIA
OF
NATURAL HEALING

THE
COMPLETE
ENCYCLOPEDIA
OF
NATURAL HEALING

Gary Null, Ph.D.

Twin Streams
Kensington Publishing Corp.
http://www.kensingtonbooks.com

TWIN STREAMS BOOKS are published by

Kensington Publishing Corp.
850 Third Avenue
New York, NY 10022

All Kensington titles, imprints and distributed lines are available at special quantity discounts for bulk purchases for sales promotion, premiums, fund-raising, educational or institutional use.

Special book excerpts or customized printings can also be created to fit specific needs. For details, write or phone the office of the Kensington Special Sales Manager: Kensington Publishing Corp., 850 Third Avenue, New York, NY 10022, Attn. Special Sales Department. Phone: 1-800-221-2647.

Kensington and the K logo Reg. U.S. Pat. & TM Off.
Twin Streams and the TS logo are trademarks of Kensington Publishing Corp.

ISBN 0-7582-0211-3

First Kensington Hardcover Printing: March, 1998
First Kensington Trade Paperback Printing: September, 2000
10 9 8 7 6 5 4 3 2

Printed in the United States of America

ACKNOWLEDGMENTS

No book of this magnitude could ever be completed without the assistance of some outstanding and exceptionally gifted editors. As with previous books, I have relied upon Vicki Riba Koestler and Lois Zinn to help with editing and transcription. Additional thanks go to Lee Wigden, Caryn Warner, and Bruce Wilson.

Contents

Introduction   ix

I. Conditions   1

Aging   3
Alcoholism   17
Allergies   21
Alzheimer's Disease and Dementia   32
Anemia   39
Arthritis   44
Autism   55
AIDS   59
Back and Neck Pain   76
Breast Cancer   86
Breast Implant Reactions   93
Cancer   95
Candidiasis   112
Carpal Tunnel Syndrome   119
Cerebral Palsy   122
Cervical Dysplasia   124
Chronic Fatigue Syndrome   127
Chronic Pain   139
Cold and Canker Sores   152
Colds and Flu   154
Dental Disorders   162
Depression   170
Diabetes   177
Digestive Disorders   183
Dysmenorrhea   196

Ear Infections   201
Eating Disorders   205
Endometriosis   209
Environmental Illness   214
Eye Disorders   218
Fever   224
Fibroids and Uterine Bleeding   226
Foot and Leg Problems   231
Gallstones   242
Headaches   245
Heart Disease   253
Heatstroke   266
Hemorrhoids   268
Hepatitis   270
Herpes   273
High Cholesterol   278
Hypoglycemia   282
Hypothyroidism   286
Infertility   288
Learning Disorders   294
Lupus   298
Lyme Disease   301
Lymphedema   306
Menopause   310
Motion Sickness   317
Multiple Sclerosis   318
Obesity   321
Osteoporosis   327
Parasites   334
Parkinson's Disease   339
Periodontal Disease   342
Phobias   349
Pregnancy-Related Illnesses   355
Premenstrual Syndrome   363
Prostate Conditions   369
Respiratory Conditions   375
Sickle Cell Anemia   382
Sinusitis   383
Skin Cancer   386
Skin Conditions   389
Stroke   397
TMJ Dysfunction   401

Tinnitus   403
Toxic Shock Syndrome   405
Trauma   408
Urinary Tract Infections   411

II. Treatments and Patient Experiences   419

Acupuncture   421
Alexander Technique   427
Applied Kinesiology   429
Aromatherapy   432
Ayurvedic Medicine   433
Biofeedback   438
Biological Dentistry   440
Chelation Therapy   454
Chiropractic   463
Colon Therapy   474
Enzyme Therapy   483
Herbal Therapy   486
Homeopathy   488
Hypnotherapy   496
Massage Therapy   505
Nutritional Therapy   510
Oxygen Therapies   524
Qi Gong   535
Reconstructive Therapy   541
Reflexology   544
Reiki   546
Rolfing   549
Shiatsu   551
Tai Chi   553
Vitamin Drips   556

Patients Speak Out on Cancer Therapies That Work   561

Index   591

Introduction

Today, more than ever before, Americans by the tens of millions are seeking out alternative opinions on how diseases should be both treated and prevented. Why? Orthodox medicine just hasn't measured up to its billing as the be-all and end-all in health maintenance. Sure, traditional medicine does a superb job in certain crisis-oriented spheres; these include trauma and emergency medicine and acute health care, as in the areas of stroke treatment, organ transplants, intensive care, and burn treatment. But an objective review of overall care tells a different story. In the management of the chronic conditions besetting our society—heart disease, cancer, arthritis, mental illness, diabetes—the medical establishment has fallen short. Prevention isn't stressed to the extent that it should be. Drastic remedies, often resulting in iatrogenic (doctor- or hospital-induced) illnesses, are overused. It's because of this chronic-care situation that a book like this is needed.

This book is intended as a kind of second opinion for today's confused health care consumer. But it's not the sort of second opinion that most Americans are used to, the kind that's concerned with which beta blocker or antidepressant to take, or exactly how one's coronary bypass should be done. That's because it does no good to have a second, or even a third opinion, when all the opinion-givers are from the same school of thought. No, this, by contrast, is intended to be the type of second opinion that's like a breath of fresh air. The idea here is to look at things differently and to see how we can incorporate nature, and what's natural, into a new healing paradigm.

Of course I'm not your personal health care provider, so nothing here is going to be advocated specifically for your unique condition. But when you do get together with your health care professional to discuss options, every natural alternative will be here for you to refer to.

Finally, I also think it's important for anyone considering a treatment, whether alternative or mainstream, to hear what others who have undergone the treatment have to say about it. That's why patient experiences are part of this book. Read what patients have to say, about natural therapies that range from aromatherapy to vitamin drips, from chelation to qi gong. Their reports put a human face on these healing modalities, and the human aspect of health care is, after all, why the field matters.

I.

Conditions

Aging

Himalayan mountain people are famous for their longevity. It is common for the Hunzas to live 120 healthful years due to their intake of mineral-rich water, unpolluted air, and a diet rich in complex carbohydrates, as well as to their active, purposeful way of life. On Pitcairn Island, in the South Pacific, it's not unusual for residents past 70 to labor alongside 20-year-olds. Inhabitants credit their strength and vitality to a natural lifestyle and a menu consisting mostly of grains, fruits, and vegetables. In China, doctors have studied the secrets of rejuvenation for thousands of years, and have long known how to keep sex glands functioning well past the prime of life with herbs, acupuncture, and special exercises called tai chi and qi gong.

Americans have much to learn from these cultures. For the most part, we and the people of other Western nations have become fast-paced and out of step with nature. We manage on devitalized foods, and control failing body systems with multiple medications. In midlife, we stop exercising and lose lean muscle mass. As a result, bone density is lost and metabolism slows down, causing flabbiness and weakness, and setting the stage for osteoporosis. Most seniors are physically feeble, and some are mentally so, due to a lifetime of poor habits.

On the brighter side, scientists are teaching us why we age, and what we can do to slow down, and even reverse, the aging process. Through their efforts, we now know that aging begins at the cellular level with free radical damage, and that antioxidant vitamins, minerals, and enzymes can prevent such destruction. In addition, research confirms the value of natural regenerative remedies esteemed by the ancients, and new "smart drugs" that improve mental acuity.

As this information filters down to the general public, more and more people are attempting to turn back the clock by eating better, supplementing their diets, reducing stress, and increasing their exercise levels. Most important, attitudes are changing and people are seeing themselves as youthful at older ages. This is important because "thinking old" creates a physiological response in the body. When we picture ourselves losing strength and vitality with age, that is what occurs. Conversely, when we see time as a friend, we are apt to remain young and vibrant into our 50's, 60's, and beyond. In fact, with today's new knowledge and increasingly positive attitudes, extending our healthful years to equal those of the Hunzas does not seem an impossible goal.

To Fight Aging—Detoxify

The more toxic we are, the faster we age. Cosmetic changes, such as face-lifts and hair coloring, may temporarily help us appear younger, but to really regenerate we must detoxify, that is, clean ourselves up from the inside. The youthful appearance that results will be the natural byproduct of improved health.

Cleansing practices date back thousands of years. The Essenes, for example, filled gourds with clean river water, and used long reeds to wash "devils" out of their intestines. In the modern, polluted world, internal cleansing is especially important, for no matter how well we take care of ourselves, we still breathe in polluted air, bathe in polluted water, and take in all sorts of chemicals. Once these substances are absorbed, we never fully eliminate them unless we detoxify.

Some methods of detoxification focus on specific systems; others, such as juice fasting and chelation therapy, help the entire body at once.

Juice Fasting

Fasting can be likened to staying home to clean and repair the house. Going on a juice fast allows the digestive system to rest so that it can focus its attention on patching up all the areas that need healing. At the end of the process, everything works better and the skin takes on a healthy glow.

Fasting seems like an even better idea when you consider that, in this country, we generally take in from 10 to 20 percent more calories than our bodies need. In fact, most people can benefit from a one- to two-day fast of freshly squeezed juice, protein drinks, pure water, and herbal tea. Initially, it would be advisable to get clearance from a physician, one who understands the benefits of fasting. If you are taking medications, they should never be dispensed with before a doctor says it is safe to do so.

Here are a few guidelines: When making your juices, use organic produce whenever possible, as harmful chemicals found in tainted fruits and vegetables become more concentrated after juicing. That, obviously, is counterproductive when your object is internal cleansing. Drink about eight 10-ounce glasses of juice a day, and you'll be treating your whole body to a maximally usable supply of health-giving phytochemicals, antioxidant vitamins and minerals, chlorophyll, and enzymes.

To ensure digestibility, you should understand that the juices of dark green vegetables, such as spinach, arugula, parsley, and watercress, are very concentrated, and should be liberally diluted with more watery juices, such as those of cabbage, celery, or cucumber, or with aloe vera and mineral water. Also, to get the most physical and psychological benefit from juices, drink them slowly, consuming them as you would food, rather than water. Swallowing too fast cheats the mind of taste satisfaction and places unwanted stress on the kidneys and bladder. Finally, remember to come off a fast—especially a longer one—gradually. Eating too much is never a good idea, but it can be especially bad for the system after not eating.

Once these simple rules are learned, the fun of an all-juice diet begins. Alternating between carrot/apple, pineapple/sprout, and tomato/lemon with a dash of cayenne can keep the taste buds happy all day. Meanwhile, the body is getting vital nutrients to help it function at its best. Here are some beneficial fruits and vegetables from which to choose:

APPLE

Apple helps to correct skin and liver disorders. It has a laxative effect, and is a valuable aid to digestion and weight loss.

BEET

Drink beet juice to nourish the liver, one of the most important organs of the body, as it has hundreds of different functions. If your liver is functioning well, most likely everything else in your body will be, too.

CABBAGE

Cabbage is high in vitamin K, as well as cancer-fighting indoles. It is excellent for alleviating stomach ailments, especially when combined with comfrey.

CARROT

Carrot juice is high in the antioxidants, including beta carotene and vitamins A, C, and E. In addition, it is filled with health-giving minerals and antiaging enzymes. One caveat on carrot juice: Since it is high in natural sugar, this juice should be diluted with water, especially when there is a blood sugar imbalance.

CELERY

This one is moderately high in sodium, not the bad-for-you salt shaker kind, but the good, natural kind that promotes good cell chemistry.

MELON

Melon juices are wonderful kidney cleansers. And did you know that the rind provides a wide range of enzymes, minerals, and chlorophyll? Drink melon juice alone, not in combination with other fruits or vegetables.

PINEAPPLE

The juice of this fruit contains bromelain, which has an anti-inflammatory effect. This is especially good for alleviating arthritic symptoms.

Susan Lombardi, founder of the We Care Health Center, in Palm Springs, California, and author of *Ten Easy Steps for Complete Wellness,* recommends a combination of carrot, celery, cabbage, and beet juice, mixed in equal proportions, with a little cayenne for flavor and circulation. This mixture is taken throughout the day while fasting to promote healing in every corner of the body.

Sometimes a person feels temporarily unwell when fasting. This is called a healing crisis, and usually occurs around the third day. This is not necessarily a bad thing, but rather a sign that the body is releasing toxins and probably withdrawing from addictions, if you've been, for example, a habitual consumer of caffeine, sugar, or dairy foods. The best advice is to get plenty of rest and to drink lots of water during this time. After awhile, the discomfort will disappear, and the system will be newly recharged. Your health practitioner will give you more guidance on juice fasting.

Chelation Therapy

Chelation therapy has many benefits, all of which add up to a longer, healthier life. While no studies directly relate the treatment to increased life expectancy, several show it to favorably impact the four major causes of death in the United States: heart disease, cancer, cerebrovascular disease, and chronic obstructive lung disease.

During treatment, medical doctors administer a man-made amino acid, called EDTA, via intravenous drip. Once in the bloodstream, EDTA attaches itself to heavy metals, such as lead, cadmium, and mercury, and holds onto these toxic substances until they exit the body through the kidneys. Eliminating these substances prevents premature aging and disease.

In these polluted times, health professionals often recommend chelation therapy for many people over 30. As we get older the toxic metals from the environment, especially lead, build up in the skeleton. Even natural calcium can accumulate in the wrong places. Chelation therapy will take calcium out of the heart vessels and place it back into the long bones, thus preventing osteoporosis.

Another benefit of chelation is that it helps the brain work better. As artery blockages are removed, more blood flows to the brain and cognitive abilities improve. And when pathways are kept open, individuals are at lower risk for stroke.

Detoxification for Specific Systems

We have several organs for detoxification—the intestines, kidneys, liver, skin, and lungs. In addition, the lymph glands play a major role. Each area must work optimally to avoid overburdening other systems, and the following are some therapies beneficial to these organs:

INTESTINES

The average person carries around several pounds of impacted fecal matter on the intestinal walls, which can create constipation, emotional repression, and an environment conducive to bacteria and disease. To help with this problem, a detoxification drink can be made from ground flaxseeds, psyllium seeds, and bentonite, a liquid clay. This formula is excellent for colon cleansing because the clay absorbs toxins while the seeds expand in water and brush the intestines clean.

Another helpful technique is colonic irrigation. This therapy gently but thoroughly washes the intestines by infusing water into the large bowel in small amounts at steady intervals. Water travels the entire length of the colon. In the process, old encrustations of fecal matter are dislodged and swept away. Often this material has been attached to the bowel for many years, and is laden with millions of bacteria. Unless eliminated, this sets up the perfect environment for disease.

Colonic irrigation restores the colon to its natural shape and function so that food is better absorbed and eliminated, skin improves, and irritability, fatigue, and constipation disappear. A healthy colon means a healthy body.

KIDNEYS

The herbs dandelion leaf, echinacea, and corn silk are beneficial to the kidneys. Short fasts, during which apple juice is mixed with small amounts of parsley, also improve kidney health.

LIVER

Milk thistle protects liver function and helps this organ expel toxins. That, in turn, promotes health and youthfulness.

LUNGS

With each exhalation, waste products are removed from the system. And one of the best ways to improve lung capacity is through regular aerobic exercise. Of course, exercise has other age-defying benefits, in addition to its facilitating of lung function. It enables us to detoxify through our skin, as we sweat. It allows more blood to flow to tissues throughout the body, which keeps cells from dying prematurely. By oxygenating brain cells, exercise prevents or minimizes senility. And it improves metabolism, so that the body can easily maintain a normal weight. Finally, weight-bearing exercises, such as walking, jogging, and weight-lifting, enhance bone density, which helps prevent osteoporosis.

SKIN

Not only does our skin provide a protective covering, it also expels many toxins daily. But to do this job properly, the pores must not be clogged. One technique for ensuring this is skin brushing. Using a natural bristle brush or loofah, rub the skin all over in a circular motion, to get rid of dead skin that clogs up the pores. Always brush toward the heart, and never brush thin facial skin.

Taking a sauna is a good follow-up to dry skin brushing because sweat expels toxins through the now open pores. Beginners should keep the temperature at around 185 degrees Fahrenheit and start out slowly. There are different types of saunas, and the directions for each type should be followed.

LYMPHATIC SYSTEM

The job of the lymphatic system is to move disease-causing wastes out of the body. Cleansing herbs, such as burdock root, red clover, echinacea, dandelion, yellow dock, and garlic, can speed up a sluggish lymphatic system. Lymphatic massage and skin brushing also help.

Rebuilding

As we regain health through detoxification, the body becomes more responsive to therapies that rebuild the system, such as a healthy diet and vitamin/mineral supplements. Below are general recommendations for life-extending foods and nutrients. For more precise guidance, a holistic practitioner can make recommendations based on individual test results.

Tests are important because we do not age uniformly; rather, individual organs diminish in energy at different rates. One thing that Western medicine excels at is laboratory analysis, and a full spectrum of tests can determine which systems are out of balance, and thus causing premature aging. Tests can indicate, for instance, whether the adrenal glands are producing enough antiaging hormones, whether vitamins and minerals are being properly digested, and whether toxic metals are polluting the system. Findings may reveal that one person is anemic due to an iron deficiency, for example, while another is low in folic acid. Results help holistic health practitioners address the unique needs of their patients.

Once you begin a health regimen, subsequent testing shows how well recommendations are taking effect, and adjustments are made accordingly. Some nutrients can be dispensed with once the body starts producing more of its own, while others are needed on a continual basis. Thyroid supplements, for instance, are often needed by patients with low body temperatures until the system catches on, a few weeks later, and starts converting the hormone to a usable form on its own. Other nutrients, like vitamin C, leave the body rapidly and need to be taken several times each day.

Subjective measures of improvement must also be taken into account. This is done through observation of symptoms and appearance. If symptoms diminish and appearance improves over time, it is an indication that therapies are working. And as the body rejuvenates, a person will notice additional improvements, such as increased endurance, enhanced memory, and better body tone.

The Antiaging Diet

The foods we eat should keep us balanced—not too acid or alkaline. One way to keep our systems stable is to place a pH strip in a urine sample each morning. The ideal result should read in the range of 6.8. Deviations from that number mean that the foods eaten the day before were too acidic (downward deviations from 6.8) or too alkaline (upward). Acidic foods are especially harmful as they contribute to numerous diseases. Cutting down on these foods, and eating lots of fruits and vegetables instead, will support the body.

COMPLEX CARBOHYDRATES

An antiaging diet is high in complex carbohydrates, such as grains, legumes, fruits, vegetables, nuts, and seeds. Many are eaten raw or close to their natural state, and none are unnecessarily processed, or overcooked. Frying is minimized, although stir-frying is acceptable. Very little, if any, animal proteins are eaten, and fats are used sparingly. Only about 10 to 15 percent of calories should come from fat.

Complex carbohydrates help us in several ways. First, they are high in fiber, and can therefore prevent common afflictions associated with aging, such as constipation, hemorrhoids, intestinal diseases, ulcers, high blood pressure, colorectal cancer, and overall body toxemia. They are also rich in phytochemicals, antioxidant substances found in plants that help us prevent everything from cancer, arthritis, and heart disease, to wrinkles and age spots.

By eating diets centered on complex carbohydrates, we not only feel healthier, we look better. Most people tend to gain weight as they age because their metabolism slows down. Complex carbohydrates counter this problem because they are digested quickly. Thirty minutes after a meal of rice and vegetables, the body starts to burn up food at maximum speed, a process that continues for 2½ to 3 hours. Of course, this works best when foods are eaten without creamy or greasy sauces. But this does not mean that meals must be bland. Many cookbooks show how wholesome food can be healthfully spiced and dressed.

How can foods minimize wrinkling? Beta carotene, from carrots and other yellow/orange vegetables, enters the cell's outer membrane, and provides some protection against sun damage. This nutrient's cousin, lycopene, is twice as powerful. Lycopene is what gives the watermelon, tomato, and pink grapefruit their red color. According to studies, lycopene also enters the outer membrane of skin cells, and provides protection from ultraviolet damage while it is there.

GREEN FOODS

Greens are rich in chlorophyll, the ultimate blood purifier. Chlorophyll is known to cure various infections in the respiratory tract and can nullify the effects of various pollutants, such as second-hand smoke, diesel fuel, and coal dust. In addition, it can turn an acidic pH more alkaline. Then, food is better absorbed and antioxidants are able to effectively do their job of strengthening the immune system. This, in turn, is a key aspect of slowing the aging process.

For excellent sources of chlorophyll, think of barley grass and wheatgrass. These are high in superoxide dismutase (SOD), an antioxidant enzyme that scavenges free radicals from the body, and they're far richer in vitamins, minerals, amino acids, and trace elements than are most other vegetables.

SEA VEGETABLES AND ALGAE

They may not be household words, but you should know that the sea vegetables dulce, kelp, and nori are exceptionally high in minerals, particularly calcium, iodine, potassium, and magnesium, and in trace elements as well. Kelp can rebalance thyroid metabolism, resulting in successful weight management and the reversal of many conditions that are caused by a thyroid imbalance, including stomach and respiratory disorders.

Spirulina and chlorella are single-celled, waterborne algae that are rich in chlorophyll, vitamins, minerals, and amino acids. These foods help protect cells and boost energy levels. By building and strengthening at the cellular level, they protect against the effects of aging.

GARLIC AND ONIONS

These two are health superstars because they contain sulfur compounds that have an antiaging and anticancer effect.

WATER AND JUICE

Pure water is an essential part of a good diet, but most people don't get enough. This is important because suboptimal water intake can dehydrate the brain, causing symptoms of senility in the elderly. Eight 8-ounce glasses daily is a minimum requirement. In addition, fresh, enzyme-rich juices should be a regular part of the diet.

Antioxidant Supplements

By reducing free radical damage, antioxidants help us stay young, vital, and productive for as long as we live. Some antioxidants are naturally produced by the body, but to promote regeneration, we need to be taking additional ones in supplement form. Here is a list of nutrients we should be taking on a daily basis:

Vitamin A—1,000-3,000 IU per meal. Blood tests will determine whether or not a person is getting too much vitamin A, which can be toxic.

Beta Carotene—Up to 25,000 IU per meal. Beta carotene is a nontoxic precursor to vitamin A that helps slow down aging and lessens cancer risk.

Bioflavonoids—A minimum of 75 mg 3 times daily of grape seed extract, one of the most powerful antioxidant substances available.

Vitamin C—3,000-5,000 mg daily, in divided doses throughout the day. To fight disease, higher doses are given orally and intravenously. Vitamin C is a powerful immune system strengthener. When C is combined with vitamins A and E, as well as riboflavin and beta carotene, there is a lowered risk of cataracts and macular degeneration.

Vitamin E—400-800 IU per day, taken at the largest meal. Vitamin E is best in its natural form (as a mixed tocopherol or d-alpha tocopherol). Avoid synthetic vitamin E (dl-alpha).

Selenium—100 mcg per meal. Selenium is needed to produce glutathione peroxidase, an antioxidant enzyme that protects the body from free radical damage. It is also important in preventing cancer and cardiomegaly, an enlargement of the heart that causes premature aging and early death.

Zinc—30-50 mg daily. Zinc feeds over 100 enzyme systems in the brain, as well as various systems throughout the body. It is essential in the formation of stomach acid; without sufficient zinc, malabsorption syndrome occurs. Most older people are zinc-deficient.

NADH—2.5 mg per day. NADH, short for nicotinamide adenine dinucle-otide, is a potent antioxidant that is also called coenzyme Q1. Every living cell contains NADH, and in each one it plays a central role in energy production. Aging is associated with a loss of energy due to an increased incidence of cellular degeneration and death. NADH helps cells survive and thrive. It's recommended to counter memory loss, as well as in the treatment of Alzheimer's disease and other dementias, Parkinson's disease, and Huntington's chorea.

Minerals and Enzymes

Nina Anderson, author of *Over Fifty, Looking Thirty,* stresses the importance of minerals and enzymes as two key antiaging factors. Minerals are found in every part of us. They are in our tissues, blood, and bones. They assist in hormone production, as well as nerve transmission, and they balance our energy. Very little will work properly without them.

Getting the minerals we need keeps the body in balance, which is important because when we are unbalanced from a lack of essential minerals, the body tends to pick up harmful minerals, such as lead, aluminum, and mercury, in an attempt to compensate for the deficiency. Being balanced also lessens the incidence of degenerative diseases associated with aging, such as arthritis and osteoporosis. Arthritis begins when there is a shortage of calcium, magnesium, and electrolytes. Osteoporosis happens as a result of the body leaching minerals out of the bones when minerals are lacking in the blood.

Since a full spectrum of nutrients is no longer available from deficient soils, it is important to take mineral supplements. The best minerals to take are crystalloid. These are very fine, and so can permeate the cell wall and shore up the inside of the cell, keeping the cell round in shape by maintaining its osmotic pressure. This protects the cell against free radical damage.

Even more important are enzymes, catalysts that stimulate all cellular processes, essentially making everything happen. Unless enzymes function properly, vitamins and minerals cannot do their job. Before fat-soluble vitamins A, D, E, and K can be broken down, for example, they need the enzyme lipase. Otherwise, they are partially flushed out of the body. Abundant enzymes are found in raw foods, especially juices. But to increase enzyme levels further, they can be taken as supplements, and again, the crystalloid form is recommended.

Antioxidant enzymes are produced naturally by the body, and include superoxide dismutase (SOD), glutathione, and catalase. To keep enzyme production high, sufficient minerals are needed.

Herbs

Herbs help us resist disease by strengthening the immune system, so that it can ward off invaders of all types. They are an important part of any anti-aging protocol, and can be taken as capsules, powders, teas, or tinctures.

FO-TI TIENG

This is a blend of Chinese herbs that rejuvenate the endocrine system, keeping sex glands in top working condition well into one's years. This formula also revitalizes nerve cells and keeps the blood pure.

GARLIC

Garlic has multiple benefits and should be used by everyone. It protects the heart and liver and can prevent cancer. It is antiviral, antibacterial, anti-arthritic, and antiparasitic. By keeping the immune system strong, garlic helps the body fight off degenerative forces.

GINKGO BILOBA

The gingko leaf comes from the oldest species of tree on the planet. Its unique properties have allowed it to survive the natural hardships of the ages, and some say that these same traits may help people slow down their own aging process. Specifically, ginkgo is known to improve microcirculation, particularly in the brain. It may therefore be an excellent herb for those with Alzheimer's disease. And according to clinical research, subjects with this condition substantially improved recall when the herb was taken three times daily. Gingko will also address other common symptoms of aging related to poor circulation: headaches, vertigo, tinnitus, dizziness, coldness or numbness of the hands and feet, cramping, and reduced ability to walk distances.

GINSENG

The Chinese have revered ginseng for centuries, considering it an outstanding rejuvenator, aphrodisiac, and improver of most conditions. Its ability to help a variety of conditions may be due to the fact that ginseng is an adaptogen, meaning that it works with the body to correct imbalances. For instance, if blood pressure is too high, it helps bring it down; if it is too low, it pulls it up.

There are several types of ginseng on the market today, and it is important to note their differences. Korean (red) ginseng is very hot, and is said to be best suited for people with cold constitutions. The herb is also said to increase sexual fire, and, for that reason, is not recommended for people under 45. Chinese (white) ginseng is milder, and American ginseng is cool, and helpful for hot, or inflammatory, conditions. American ginseng supports digestion, adrenal function, and overall vitality.

GOTU KOLA

Elephants, animals known for their excellent memory and long life, browse on gotu kola. Similarly, people who ingest gotu kola can expect greater longevity, good memory, and mental alertness.

SARSAPARILLA

This herb contains phytoestrogens, plant compounds that resemble estrogen and act as precursors in the production of sex hormones by the adrenal glands and the ovaries or testes. These phytoestrogens also function as precursors in the adrenal glands' production of DHEA, one of our antiaging hormones.

Aromatherapy

Properly used, essential oils can help us overcome many physical and psychological conditions associated with aging. Often, they serve as a sensible alternative to medications, because unlike drugs, which distress the system with unwanted side effects, essential oils are natural substances that the body readily accepts. They benefit us on a physical level, and, at the same time, leave us feeling relaxed and uplifted.

Aromatherapist Shirley Price points out that none of us feel old until we fall sick, and that aromatherapy is one way to feel healthier, and, therefore, young again. She reminds us that when using aromatherapy, it is important to use pure oils from aromatic medicine markets whose distillers obtain organic plant materials from natural sources. She also recommends ordering oils by their Latin names, when possible, to make sure you don't purchase products with similar names whose effects are markedly different. Here are some conditions that commonly plague the elderly, and the essential oils that can alleviate them:

INSOMNIA

The essential oil universally used to help induce sleep is lavender *(Lavandula officinalis),* which can be vaporized, breathed in on a tissue, or added to a carrier lotion and massaged into the shoulders (about 12 drops per 4 fluid ounces). Other sleep-inducing essential oils are bergamot *(Citrus begamia),* marjoram *(Origanum majorana),* Roman chamomile *(Anthemis nobilis),* lemon *(Citrus limon),* and ylang ylang *Cananga odorata).*

INDIGESTION

Digestion difficulties can often be overcome by taking essential oils by mouth, but this should only be done under the supervision of a clinical aromatherapist. An essential oil tea can be made by adding one or two drops of a specified oil into a tea along with one tea bag. Caraway *(Carum carvi)* is an excellent choice, and can be taken together with bitter orange. Also beneficial to digestion is sweet fennel *(Foeniculum vulgare dulce),* which is powerful and should only be used in combination with other oils, under the guidance of an aromatherapist.

ARTHRITIS

Analgesic, anti-inflammatory oils help alleviate muscular pain and arthritis, and include coriander *(Coriandrum sativum)*, juniper *(Juniperus communis)*, rosemary *(Rosemarinus officinalis)*, and naoili *(Melaleuca viridiflora)*.

MEMORY LOSS

Rosemary *(Rosemarinus officinalis)* and peppermint *(Mentha piperita)* are gentle nervous system stimulants that are known to increase memory recall. Other good oils include frankincense, rose, and clary sage. Best effects are through inhalation, but these oils can also be added to bath water, or massaged into the scalp, hands, or feet.

Stress Reduction

Stress overtaxes the adrenal system, and is a major contributor to premature aging, degenerative disease, and early death. In these hurried times, we need to make a conscious effort to slow down and find satisfaction in life. Many methods help the mind overcome stress, including deep breathing, tai chi, yoga, meditation, qi gong, mantras, massage, reiki, and biofeedback.

One of these modalities, reiki, is a powerful tool toward this end. The term is Japanese for universal life force, and reiki, a form of therapeutic touch, works by amplifying and channeling this energy. This technique, like acupuncture, is centered on bodily meridians, or energy paths, and proponents extol its ability to release physical and emotional blockages, promote total relaxation, and enhance recovery from stress and injuries.

What to Avoid

Keeping young and healthy is a balancing act. We must stay away from or compensate for the myriad of factors that disturb our equilibrium, such as foods and chemicals that artificially stimulate energy and wear down the body (coffee, drugs, and cigarettes); alcohol, which accelerates brain cell deterioration; environmental toxins that compromise the immune system; and medicines that cover up symptoms, such as antacids, diuretics, or aspirin. It is equally important to let go of our preconceived notions of aging and, instead, stay active. Finally, we must remember not to let stress get the best of us.

Treatment Summary

Any method that removes the toxins that we accumulate every day will act to retard aging. Some detoxification methods are juice fasting, chelation therapy, colonic irrigation, exercise, skin brushing, saunas, and the use of herbs.

Laboratory tests can let us know which systems need boosting and thus which nutrients will be most helpful.

The antiaging diet is one that keeps our pH balanced. The best foods: fruits, vegetables, grains, legumes, nuts, and seeds.

Antioxidant supplements keep us young by slowing down free radical damage. These include vitamin A, beta carotene, bioflavonoids, vitamin C, vitamin E, selenium, zinc, and NADH.

Herbs important to an antiaging protocol include fo-ti-tieng, garlic, ginkgo biloba, ginseng, and gotu kola.

Essential oils may alleviate common conditions associated with aging, including insomnia, indigestion, arthritis, and memory loss.

Stress reduction is essential to slowing down the aging process, and preventing degenerative disease.

Alcoholism

Alcoholism wreaks havoc on mind, body, and spirit. The disease is a long, degenerative process, wherein a person gradually drinks more and more until he or she is addicted. It can be characterized by mental disturbances, cirrhosis of the liver, gastritis, nerve damage, and hallucinations. Stopping cold turkey, without nutritional support, can cause delirium tremens (a sudden, psychotic withdrawal that can result in death).

It is important to understand that alcoholism affects not just the alcoholic himself or herself, but that person's family, friends, coworkers, and employers. Those touched by alcoholism also include victims of drunk drivers. Ultimately, the country as a whole is affected by this massive problem, considering both the human and economic losses incurred.

One way of looking at the physiological aspects of alcoholism is to see it as a carbohydrate metabolism imbalance. Complementary physician Dr. Robert Atkins, of New York, explains that people crave alcohol for the sugar. In fact, many people who give up alcohol become sugarholics, or ''dry drunks,'' as they switch from alcohol to sugar. Orthomolecular physician Dr. Abram Hoffer stresses that nutrient deficiencies add to the problem. People do not eat healthfully and are low in essential nutrients, especially minerals, such as chromium, zinc, and manganese.

Treatment

Conventional alcoholism treatment programs combine drugs that make people sick when they take a drink, such as Antabuse, with counseling and other social supports. Many individuals do have success with Alcoholics Anonymous, especially with the addition of a good diet and supplemental support. The philosophy behind these modalities is that alcoholism is a lifelong disease that can be controlled, but never cured.

The Importance of Nutrition

A natural approach to treating alcoholism sees it as a correctable disease; in other words, through physical and emotional rebalancing a person can overcome the condition. Natural practitioners emphasize that good nutrition is key in combating alcoholism; they note that alcohol robs the system of nutrients, which causes free radical damage and degenerative disease. Heavy drinkers accelerate the process, but even moderate drinkers lose valuable vitamins and minerals. Therefore, anyone who drinks, or who is recovering from substance abuse and attempting to rebuild health, can benefit from a full spectrum of supplements. The ones listed here are particularly important:

VITAMIN B COMPLEX

B vitamins work together to restore integrity to the brain and nervous system. Certain members of the B family are especially important for alcoholics; these include vitamins B1, B2, B5, and B6. Pantothenic acid (B5) supports the adrenal glands and helps the body regulate its sugar metabolism.

ESSENTIAL FATTY ACIDS

Alcoholics tend to be deficient in these energy-providing substances, which can be taken in capsule form.

AMINO ACIDS

Two in particular—glutamine and L-methionine— are especially valuable for detoxifying the brain. And their effectiveness is boosted when they're combined with vitamins B6 and C. (Note: Glutamic acid should never be substituted for glutamine, as it does not have the same effect.)

TRACE MINERALS

Most people are deficient in trace minerals, a problem more prevalent today than it was in the past, because our agricultural soil is often depleted of these essential substances. Getting enough magnesium, manganese, chromium, and zinc is especially important for recovery from alcoholism.

VITAMIN C AND QUERCETIN

Vitamin C is a strong detoxification agent and healer, and its ability to heal is greatly enhanced by the addition of the bioflavonoid quercetin. High doses of intravenous vitamin C and other antioxdants can protect the liver and improve metabolism.

LECITHIN

Lecithin improves functioning of the brain and liver, two organs that alcohol users need to repair.

HERBS

In addition to nutrient supplements, herbs are valuable to the recovering alcoholic. Milk thistle, in particular, is important because it aids in repairing and rejuvenating the liver. The active ingredient in milk thistle is silymarin, shown in a recent double-blind study to have a liver-protective effect for those with cirrhosis. Valerian root can aid alcoholics in a different way. This is a nerve tonic that helps to heal the emotional stress and pain accompanying alcohol withdrawal. Siberian ginseng should also be remembered when alcoholism is a problem. This herb supports the liver, and has been shown to reduce the occurrence of people falling off the wagon after going through rehabilitation.

Homeopathy

According to scientific research, homeopathy can play a significant role in recovery from alcoholism. Studies reveal that patients given homeopathic medicines in chemical dependency programs retain significantly higher levels of abstinence for far longer periods of time after release than patients availing themselves of counseling, allopathic medication, and AA meetings without homeopathy. In fact, years later, most in the homeopathically treated group have not returned to drinking.

Part of the reason for homeopathy's success may lie in its ability to address individual needs. Just because two people are alcoholic does not mean that they are identical, and homeopathic remedies are individualized according to the types of symptoms a person manifests. For instance, the remedy called nux vomica is given to treat hangovers, and is considered appropriate for people who feel woozy or nauseous after drinking too much. Homeopaths prescribe nux vomica as a constitutional remedy for type A personalities—people who tend to be pushy, aggressive, and chilly, with constipation and liver problems.

Another homeopathic remedy given for alcoholism is sulphur. This one is for someone who sits and drinks brandy while reading or contemplating life. The type of patient for whom sulphur would be helpful is considered warm and sweaty, as opposed to the colder nux vomica candidate.

Treatment Summary

Conventional drug therapies are based on the premise that when people take these products, they will become sick after drinking, and thus break the habit.

Spiritual and social support can make a real difference. Alcoholics Anonymous is well known for helping alcoholics recover, and is especially effective when a person combines this therapy with a healthy diet and additional social support.

Supplements are vital. Vitamins and minerals for rebuilding a system damaged by alcohol include B complex vitamins, essential fatty acids, amino acids, trace minerals, and vitamin C.

Herbs to think of in connection with overcoming alcohol dependence are milk thistle, for healing a damaged liver; valerian root, to counter stress; and Siberian ginseng, which is associated with people remaining alcohol-free after rehabilitation.

Homeopathic treatments can be effective because they are tailored to individual needs.

Allergies

An allergy is the result of an overaggressive immune response to a substance that is inhaled or ingested, or that comes in contact with the skin. While one person can walk into a dusty room and have no reaction because her immune system cells (e.g., lymphocytes and phagocytes) are able to engulf or otherwise disable the antigens in the dust, another individual has an allergic response upon entering that same room because her immune system is not as efficient.

Allergies are so common that almost everyone has them to one degree or another. When we hear the word allergy, most of us think of classic, or fixed, allergies, such as hay fever or immediate reactions to certain foods. But we are less familiar with cyclic food allergies and chemical sensitivities. Different types of allergies are described below.

Hay Fever

About 37 million people suffer from this seasonal condition. During the spring and summer, people react to the germination of ragweed, which fills the air with microscopic particles. These substances enter the body and combine with immune cells known as immunoglobulins (specifically the type called IgE). Then they undergo chemical reactions, ending with the release of histamine. This causes an allergic response and a person experiences sneezing, itching, and an obstruction of the nose. If hay fever goes untreated, more serious problems, such as asthma, can develop.

Food Allergies

Sometimes a food allergy is obvious because it causes an immediate response after a food is ingested. For example, strawberries are eaten, and an individual breaks out in hives. This is a Type 1 or fixed allergic response because it occurs each time strawberries are eaten. Other food allergies are more difficult to diagnose as symptoms do not usually appear right after eating the offending substance, but rather hours or days later. Also, reactions may change with age, season, stress, and a host of other factors. Further, they can move from one organ system to another. Thus milk may cause an asthmatic response in a young child, and skin disruptions in the same person as an adolescent, for example.

These masked, or cyclic, allergies are responsible for most reactions. In fact, some reports indicate that as many as 90 percent of common complaints heard by general practitioners are related to food allergies, although they are often not understood as such by mainstream doctors. Seemingly unrelated allergy symptoms can include depression, headaches, joint pains, muscle pains, and abdominal complaints.

Food allergies can be linked to what is known as leaky gut syndrome. This is the result of a long history of insults to the gastrointestinal tract, to years of eating and drinking sugar, caffeine, refined foods, and other toxins. Leaky gut syndrome is also provoked by foods that are eaten repeatedly on a daily basis, such as wheat and milk products. After much abuse, the tiny openings of the semipermeable membrane in the small intestine expand, allowing large undigested food particles to pass through. These particles then settle in different parts of the body. If they lodge in the skin, they can then cause skin allergies. If they lodge in the brain, cerebral allergies result. In time, they can cause a host of diseases, including chronic fatigue syndrome, epilepsy, and attention deficit disorder. Instead of being nourished by food, the body is now harmed by it.

Chemical Sensitivity

Reactions can be brought on by substances in the environment, such as photocopy machines at work, dust and mold in the home, and pesticide residues on foods. Today, people are routinely exposed to thousands of such toxins. As a result, immunity may diminish and gradually disappear. The immune system reacts to one thing, then two, then more. Eventually, in the most extreme form of environmental illness, a person can become nonfunctional.

Allergy Tests

Type 1 allergies, the classic type, are IgE-mediated. IgE is an antibody, or immune cell, that binds to an irritant, such as a food or pollen. High IgE levels, which are detected by blood tests, are confirmation of Type 1 allergies. However, the type of blood test used does not generally identify cyclic food allergies.

Cyclic food allergies can be identified by both objective and subjective methods. Complementary physicians measure IgG food antibody levels or white blood cell reactions to antigens. Skin testing may also be done to check for reactions to foods, chemicals, pollens, dusts, molds, and other agents. Underlying problems, such as parasitic infections, candida, and the insufficient secretion of digestive enzymes may be identified and treated as well, because improvement in these areas may improve absorption and lessen reactivity to foods. In addition, patients answer questionnaires to help determine the cause and extent of the problem.

Applied kinesiology is another technique sometimes used as an allergy test. This diagnostic procedure has a patient place a food under the tongue while lowering an outstretched arm against the resistance of the doctor. Difficulty lowering the arm indicates that the food is causing weakness.

Allergies produce stimulating effects, followed by degenerative ones. Doctors rate severity on a scale of one to four. The first level of stimulation, in which a person remains relatively symptom-free, is called +1. The person is active, alert, and responsive, and behaves normally. At the +2 stage, a person becomes hyperactive, irritable, hungry, thirsty, tense, jittery, talkative, argumentative, and overly sensitive. With a +3 reaction, an individual becomes hypomanic, toxic, anxious, egocentric, aggressive, loquacious, clumsy, and apprehensive. An extreme +4 stimulation causes mania, excitement, agitation, and possibly convulsions.

At the degenerative end of the scale, a -1 reaction gives an allergic manifestation that might include a runny nose, hives, gas, diarrhea, frequent urination, or various eye and ear symptoms. At the -2 stage, there are systemic allergic reactions, such as tiredness, mild depression, swelling, pain, and cardiovascular effects. With a -3 reaction there are depression, disturbed mental processes, confusion, moodiness, and withdrawal. Finally, at the -4 stage, severe depression, and possibly paranoia or even suicide, can result.

Self-Diagnosis

There are several ways to check for food allergies on one's own. One is with the Coca test, based on Dr. Coca's observation that a person's pulse rate increases after eating a food to which he or she is allergic. The test consists of taking your pulse before eating, and every 30 minutes thereafter, for up to two hours. Normally, the average person's pulse is between 70 and 80 beats per minute. After eating a food to which one is allergic, however, the pulse can increase significantly, to a count that's 20, or even 40 beats above the normal level.

Another effective diagnostic measure that can be self-administered is the elimination test. Here, suspected allergy-producing foods are eliminated from the diet for four days. Every fifth day, one of the foods is added back in to see if an allergic reaction occurs. So if, for example, wheat is eliminated, on the fifth day a bowl of cracked wheat can be eaten. (Bread should not be used for this purpose because the person might be reacting to the yeast, sugar, or additives.)

Recording Symptoms

It is helpful to keep a food diary to isolate those chemicals and foods that make you ill. Ask yourself, Do I get bloated? Tired? Headaches? Even if symptoms are not immediate, write them down. If you are allergic to a food, patterns will begin to emerge. A wide array of symptoms can occur, depending upon which systems are most affected:

ADRENAL SYSTEM REACTIONS

Low energy or chronic fatigue is a common reaction, with immune dysfunction being at the most severe end of the spectrum. Another possibility is obesity, which can stem from a tendency to overeat in response to low glucose levels. A hypoglycemic person eats to raise the blood sugar and overcome inertia, and exercises too little because not enough energy is available.

CENTRAL NERVOUS SYSTEM REACTIONS

Brain allergies occur when molecules, breathed in or eaten, leave the blood and enter the brain. These foreign substances can interfere with enzymes, and lead to any number of reactions—diminished concentration, impaired thinking, spaciness, anxiety, headaches, aggressive or antisocial behavior, depression, rapid mood swings, insomnia, hallucinations, or episodic memory loss. Many children experience hyperactivity or fatigue from allergens. Even serious psychotic problems can result; it is estimated that for over 90 percent of schizophrenics, food or chemical intolerances are contributory factors to their conditions. Unfortunately, many allergic reactions, and many psychological problems compounded by allergic reactions, are mistaken for purely psychological problems.

SKIN PROBLEMS

Some people experience rashes, or skin redness, discoloration, roughness, or inflammation.

RESPIRATORY SYSTEM PROBLEMS

There may be wheezing or shortness of breath, asthma, or bronchitis.

CARDIOVASCULAR SYMPTOMS

These include heart pounding, rapid or skipped beats, flushing, pallor, tingling, redness or blueness of the hands, and faintness.

GASTROINTESTINAL SYMPTOMS

Numerous symptoms include dry mouth, burping, flatulence, bloating, canker sores, stinging tongue, diarrhea, constipation, nausea, abdominal pain, rectal itching, and indigestion.

OTHER PROBLEMS

Other annoying, uncomfortable symptoms are muscle aches and joint pain, ringing in the ears, and frequent urination.

Unless corrected, subclinical signs can turn into disease states. Most people mask their symptoms with medications instead of addressing the cause of the problem. They do not realize that seemingly diverse conditions, such as rheumatoid arthritis, osteoarthritis, asthma, migraines, irritable bowel syndrome, adult onset diabetes, and skin diseases, can have food and chemical allergies as an underlying cause.

Treatment

Detoxification

Most allergies can be traced to an impaired digestive system, the result of a toxic buildup within the intestines. Embarking on a cleansing program, then, is a first step in overcoming the problem, and can include the following.

BENTONITE CLAY

Bentonite clay has a negative charge and can therefore attract positively charged particles. Toxins are drawn to the clay and drawn out of the body. Bentonite clay is taken as a part of a drink; use one teaspoon in 10 ounces of water.

HYDROTHERAPY

A series of colonics and enemas cleanse and restore colon function. As a result, many allergic symptoms begin to clear up.

FASTING

A short watermelon and lemon fast is a great detoxifier, and will help eliminate allergies.

Detoxifying the home, schoolroom, and place of employment may be equally important, and you can work toward that end in numerous ways. The first step is to check the quality of indoor air, to find out what pollutants are being breathed in. It is not that expensive to hire professionals who will come in and measure contaminants.

Air can be vastly improved with a filtration system. Actually, units with three to four filtering systems are best. Those that filter down to a level of 3 microns are able to screen out most bacteria, mold, pollens, and animal danders. Placing a filter directly in a window and sealing the sides will limit the amount of pollutants coming into a room. (Many people mistakenly place air filters three to four feet away from a window, which prevents most incoming air from being drawn into the system.)

Plants are inexpensive natural air filters that can be extremely helpful. Spider plants will filter out toxins, including formaldehyde, and produce oxygen in return. Other helpful plants are Brazilian palms, wide-leaf wandering Jews, and marigolds.

Diet

A change of diet is often key in overcoming allergies. As mentioned earlier, suspect foods should be eliminated and gradually reintroduced to the diet to check for reactions. The most common allergy producers are sugar, wheat, dairy foods, beef, potatoes, shellfish, eggs, tomatoes, coffee, peanuts, soy, corn, yeast, and citrus fruit. Any other food that is eaten daily should be suspect as well.

The best menu for preventing allergies is the rotation diet. This involves eating different kinds of foods each day, and not repeating an item for four to seven days. Using grains as an example, if rice is eaten on Monday, you might use millet on Tuesday, wheat on Wednesday, and oats on Thursday, with rice eaten again no sooner than Friday. This type of diet keeps the body from overreacting to most foods, although some items will still need to be completely excluded. Milk, for example, may cause a reaction each time it is taken. But the majority of people can safely enjoy most foods with a rotation diet. Note that besides minimizing allergic reactions, a rotation diet provides the added benefit of ensuring that you consume a wide variety of nutrients.

Also, keep in mind that certain nutrients help build up immune response. Such nutrients can be obtained, first and foremost, from freshly squeezed juices, sprouts, grains, and legumes.

For mild allergies, a few changes in diet alone may be enough; but sometimes a doctor trained to see relationships between individuals and their surroundings, known as an environmental physician, may be needed to help get to the root of the problem.

Neutralization Immunotherapy

Neutralization immunotherapy is a way of provoking the body to produce antibodies against offending substances. Once an environmental physician, using blood and skin tests, discovers which foods, chemicals, pollens, etc., are causing allergies, allergy vaccines are administered. These are different from the classical allergist's treatment in which all patients are given equal amounts of antigens. Here, low doses of specific dilutions are tailor-made for each individual. When injections are given in small amounts, the body reacts by making antibodies against those allergens. Patients are retested until symptoms disappear. The method is highly effective.

Lifestyle Changes

Many of our daily routines involve the use of commercial products with artificial ingredients that can provoke sensitivities. Fortunately, many safe and inexpensive alternatives exist, such as the ones listed here:

Soaps without artificial scents and colors can be obtained in local health food stores.

Shaving cream can be made from a natural soap.

Shampoo can be made with Castile soap and olive or avocado oil. A tiny amount of sesame oil can be used as a conditioner.

Toothpaste can be inexpensively made with peppermint extract and baking soda.

Deodorant can be replaced with cornstarch.

Talcum powder should not be used as it may contain asbestos fibers. A good replacement for talc is cornstarch.

Moisturizer can be made from sesame oil, as it contains vitamin E.

Facial scrub can be made from vegetable oil, and applied with a soft loofah to remove dead epithelial cells.

Grease remover can be made from butter.

Room deodorizers can be made from lemon juice and vinegar, spritzed into the air. This will trap and kill many harmful bacteria. Also effective as a deodorizer is baking soda, which can be placed in a room and changed every six weeks. In addition, boiling peppermint oil will act as a deodorizer. An exhaust fan is useful as well.

Pesticides must be avoided and can be replaced naturally indoors and out. In the house, boric acid can be put down in a pencil-thin line—out of the reach of children and pets—at the baseboards and underneath places where there is moisture or paper, to get rid of roaches and ants. To prevent them from returning, simply apply a line of garlic powder, mixed with boric acid and Borax, around the perimeter of the room. In the garden, a product called Safer Insecticidal Soap can be used on fruits and vegetables. This nontoxic product is made from natural fatty acids and will kill most garden pests without harming beneficial bugs.

Cleansers made naturally are as effective as commercial brands and far less toxic. Glass cleaner can be made by adding three tablespoons of vinegar to one quart of water. Baking powder can be used in place of scouring powder as an abrasive cleaner in the bathroom and kitchen. And Borax mixed with water serves as an excellent all-purpose cleaner.

In the laundry, pure washing soda will remove residues of detergent from clothing, and clothes can then be rewashed using a mixture of washing soda and soap. One cup of vinegar added to the final rinse cycle will serve as a fabric softener, and leave no smell. In addition, some natural soaps and detergent can be obtained that are less chlorinated and less toxic than most commercial brands. Some good detergents are washing soda, Borax, and Bon Ami.

Dry cleaning should be avoided whenever possible. But when clothes must be dry cleaned, they should either be soaked in cold water afterwards to remove some of the chemicals or aired outside in the sun before wearing.

Supplements

Saturating the system with extra nutrients can be most helpful, especially when allergies are in full bloom. Exact requirements should be given by a complementary physician, but these general daily recommendations can serve as a guideline:

VITAMIN C

Taking 3,000 mg of vitamin C in divided doses throughout the day is excellent for reducing histamine levels in the blood. More can be taken when fighting off an allergy. Vitamin C detoxifies and strengthens the immune system, and helps overcome symptoms of withdrawal at the start of an allergen-free diet.

Vitamin C works best in combination with 100-200 mg of the bioflavonoid quercetin and 100-200 mg of pycnogenol. Quercetin increases the strength of mast cell membranes. Mast cells, part of our connective tissue, contain histamine, which can trigger allergic reactions. By strengthening their membranes with quercetin, one is preventing their bursting and hence preventing the release of histamine. The action of vitamin C and the bioflavonoids is further enhanced by the addition of other antioxidant nutrients, such as vitamin E, beta carotene, and selenium.

VITAMIN E

Among its many benefits, vitamin E strengthens the endocrine system, and by so doing, indirectly builds immunity. Vitamin E is especially important for women with allergies who are experiencing hormonal imbalances. A good natural source of E is soybean oil, which supplies the body with an unestrofied d-alpha tocopherol. People who have difficulty absorbing oil-based natural vitamin E can benefit from an easy-to-digest water-soluble form. Women with allergies and hormonal imbalances generally benefit from 600 IU a day. Men usually need 400. Vitamin E works well together with 100 mcg of the trace mineral selenium.

B COMPLEX

B vitamins work as a team to enhance immunity. Pantothenic acid (B5), pyridoxine (B6), and B12 are particularly effective in immune system rebalancing. B5 is especially important because it is a building block of cortisone, one of the basic defense mechanisms of allergic response.

MINERALS

The mineral zinc may help correct food allergies when the problem stems from undigested food particles that are the result of insufficient production of hydrochloric acid in the stomach. Another helpful mineral is calcium, in the form of 400-600 mg of calcium citrate or calcium chelate (increased to 1,000 mg during allergic response).

ESSENTIAL FATTY ACIDS AND GLA

Essential fatty acids found in one tablespoon of flaxseed oil or GLA found in 500 mg of borage, black currant seed, or evening primrose oil play a primary role in restoring immune function.

DIGESTIVE ENZYMES

Digestive enzymes help the stomach and pancreas break down large protein molecules so that they can be fully digested. This prevents large peptides from entering the bloodstream and setting off allergic responses.

Herbs

Herbs reduce allergy symptoms in a more gentle way than do most medications. Following are some that may prove helpful.

GARLIC

Garlic is the number one herb of all time, and it should be a frequent component of everyone's diet. Garlic builds immunity and also serves as a natural antiseptic agent.

ASTRAGALUS

Astragalus is one of the best-researched immune system stimulants now available. It works like echinacea, in that both herbs increase the number and activity of immune cells. However, astragalus concentrates on building the immune system, and unlike echinacea, it can be taken on a daily basis.

ECHINACEA

Echinacea boosts immune system activity and promotes fast recovery, especially when taken at the onset of symptoms. The most potent formulas have a peculiar tingling and numbing effect on the tongue. Since the body cannot sustain such high levels of activity without rest, echinacea should be used for short intervals at a time. In Europe, where echinacea is extensively used, people take the herb in a pattern of four days on and four days off.

GINSENG

The Chinese say that ginseng builds stamina and endurance by stabilizing the qi (pronounced "chee"), the life energy of the body. Another way of explaining ginseng's benefit is that it boosts the immune system.

WILD CHERRY BARK

This one helps hay fever and other allergies by healing irritated mucosal surfaces, including the lungs. It's also soothing to the skin.

MULLEIN LEAF

This herb protects the mucous surfaces, including the throat, esophagus, intestines, and lungs.

HOREHOUND

This affects respiration by dilating muscles.

Other good herbs for allergies include stinging nettle and capsicum.

What To Avoid

Allergies are exacerbated by stress; physical and psychological stressors should therefore be eliminated as much as possible. Stimulants in the form of caffeine, cigarettes, and recreational drugs are particularly bad. Nor should the same foods be eaten every day. Too much meat, sugar, and refined carbohydrates can lead to a state of acidosis. To neutralize an acidic system and stop an allergic response, a person can take baking soda, buffered vitamin C powder, or pantothenic acid in a glass of apple or pineapple juice.

Allergenic chemicals placed on the skin in the form of soaps, lotions, and shampoos, and those breathed in and found in the water should be minimized, and, when possible, eliminated, through the use of natural alternatives. ❧

Treatment Summary

Allergy sufferers often need to improve their digestive health. Recommended measures include a cleansing diet with the help of bentonite clay, hydrotherapy, and a short watermelon and lemon fast.

People are commonly allergic to one or more of the following: sugar, wheat, dairy, beef, peanuts, shellfish, eggs, tomatoes, coffee, peanuts, soy, corn, and yeast. An environmental physician can check for problem foods, which should be eliminated from the diet or eaten on a rotation basis, once every four to seven days.

With neutralization immunization therapy, injections of small amounts of specific allergens, tailor-made for an individual's needs, help the body develop antibodies to those substances.

Instead of using chemically-laced personal and home care products, we can lessen our allergic load by making or purchasing natural ones.

Cleansing the air with a filtration system and plants lessens the amount of inhaled contaminants.

Nutrients that give our immune system an extra boost include vitamin C, quercetin, pycnogenol, vitamin E, selenium, B-complex vitamins, zinc, essential fatty acids, and gamma linolenic acid.

Herbs that strengthen the immune system include garlic, astragalus, echinacea, ginseng, wild cherry bark, and horehound.

Alzheimer's Disease and Dementia

Approximately 2 million Americans are currently afflicted with some form of dementia, Alzheimer's disease being the most widely publicized form, due to its severity. Alzheimer's is a degenerative brain disease that manifests during the later years of life. It affects the hippocampus and cerebral cortex of the brain, where memory, language, and cognition are located, and is characterized by neurological damage and deterioration of the neurotransmitters, which are responsible for nerve communication. In addition, circulation in Alzheimer's patients can be impeded by up to 30 percent.

This condition, and other forms of dementia, develops when the neurons located in the front of the brain perish, resulting in diminished quantities of acetylcholine. Acetylcholine is the neurotransmitter responsible for fast reactions and muscular activity, and its absence can induce symptoms commonly associated with Alzheimer's, including difficulty communicating, memory loss, concentration problems, and reduced motor skills.

It should be noted that the symptoms of Creutzfeld-Jakob disease, which in cattle is known as mad cow disease, are sometimes mistaken for those of Alzheimer's. Creutzfeld-Jakob disease has a latency period of 30 years, which means that people who have eaten contaminated beef many years in the past may be infected without even knowing it, and may eventually experience symptoms almost identical to those of Alzheimer's. We should note too that a practice that has developed over the past 20 years in the meat industry does not bode well for beef-eaters' future health. Through a process called rendering, cattle parts that are not used by humans are actually being included in cattle feed. In effect, the cattle are forced to practice a type of cannibalism that propagates the spread of the disease.

Causes

One possible cause of Alzheimer's disease is atherosclerosis, a condition in which the diminished flow of blood within the body affects the brain and produces common Alzheimer's symptoms.

Also implicated in the onset of this condition is heavy-metal toxicity; in autopsies performed on victims of Alzheimer's, an accumulation of aluminum and mercury deposits is usually present in the areas of the brain affected by dementia. Unfortunately, toxic accumulations of metals, especially aluminum, have become quite prevalent in modern society, and our body can assimilate excessive quantities of aluminum without our knowing it. Also, despite the attempts of water treatment facilities to purify our water supply, the reservoirs from which we draw tap water continue to be besieged by various pollutants, including pesticides, bacteria, viruses, and aluminum. Since our bodies consist of over 70 percent water, this can obviously have health-compromising consequences. In addition to unfiltered tap water, aluminum deposition within the body can originate from aluminum cookware, antacids, deodorants, antidiarrheal preparations, buffered aspirin, and food additives.

Vitamin and mineral deficiencies constitute yet another potential cause of Alzheimer's disease, although the conventional medical community does not acknowledge this. But the fact is that the dominance of processed foods in the typical American diet has deprived us of essential nutrients required for proper brain functioning. Processed foods are often stripped of vital nutrients, which are replaced with processed sugars, such as fructose, corn sweetener, and corn syrup. Other unhealthy additives include trans fatty acids, such as partially hydrogenated vegetable oils. The bottom line is that deficiencies of essential nutrients can lead to a wide assortment of health problems, and facilitate the eventual onset of Alzheimer's.

Subclinical hypothyroidism is another factor that can contribute to the manifestation of symptoms, or compound a condition that already exists. Most doctors are dependent upon the results of blood tests in diagnosing thyroid problems, but sometimes hypothyroidism is not reflected in a blood test but may still be present, and contributing to a patient's dementia symptoms.

Treatment

Contrary to the beliefs of most mainstream doctors, safe, natural, nontoxic treatments for Alzheimer's disease and other types of dementia do exist. Research has demonstrated that these remedies can aid in preventing the onset of Alzheimer's or alleviating symptoms that have already developed. In past years, people allowed their loved ones to wither away before their eyes, citing aging as an uncontrollable force. While we cannot stop time, we can take action to prevent the later years of life from being characterized by rapid degeneration.

Nutrition and Supplements

As people age, their bodies become more susceptible to nutritional deficiencies, and a lifetime of deficiencies can encourage the development of degenerative disorders like Alzheimer's disease. The up side of this picture is that the cumulative effects of poor dietary habits can be avoided by improving dietary intake early in life.

As we've mentioned, the prevalence of processed and tainted foods in our society is a serious health risk factor for all of us. In order to obtain the nutrients our bodies need, we should try to consume an abundance of nonlabeled foods. Whole grains and fresh vegetables are especially healthful. And it is advisable to purchase organic foods, which are more likely than others to contain trace minerals that are vital to the brain, such as chromium, magnesium, selenium, and zinc.

If the Alzheimer's disease process has begun, there are a variety of nutritional programs that can be initiated to combat it. Since the severity of degeneration differs from one individual to the next, each patient should be evaluated by a qualified professional so that proper treatment can be prescribed. Advancing age hampers the body's ability to assimilate essential nutrients due to the diminished production of stomach acids within the digestive system. Deficiencies of vitamins B6, B12, and iron commonly develop during the later years, eventually causing symptomatic memory problems.

It is important for those with Alzheimer's disease to receive parenteral—i.e., injected or intravenous—supplements of vitamin B complex. Oral supplements are not usually as effective as internal supplements in reversing dementia symptoms because the necessary levels cannot be absorbed into the bloodstream through the intestines. Of course the dosage and procedure have to be supervised by a qualified medical practitioner.

Frequently unnoticed by the general public, the nutrient known as DMAE can augment the body's natural production of energy, enhance the sleeping cycle, and improve memory. Although this nutrient can be supplemented relatively safely, excessive consumption can result in the onset of insomnia, muscle tension, and mild headaches, so be sure to regulate dosages.

Daily consumption of coenzyme Q10, in quantities of 50 mg three times daily, can augment the supply of oxygen to the brain. This is useful in cases of Alzheimer's induced by atherosclerosis, where the blood supply to the brain is impeded and, consequently, the reduced oxygen supply can exacerbate cognitive deterioration.

Lecithin, which contains a substance known as choline, can enhance production of acetylcholine. Since deficiencies of this vital neurotransmitter have been correlated with the onset of Alzheimer's disease, one tablespoon of lecithin should be consumed daily with food. Lecithin also contains inositol, which can help alleviate anxiety by acting as a natural Valium minus this drug's adverse side effects.

Supplements of vitamin C are also crucial for older adults. One thousand milligrams of C should be taken three times daily, during mealtimes (vitamins are most easily assimilated into the system when they are taken with food).

Vitamin E has beneficial antioxidant properties and should be supplemented in quantities of 400 IU per day.

The mineral magnesium can relax the body by dilating the blood vessels and airways. Magnesium can aid in the treatment of circulatory and respiratory disorders, and so it's unfortunate that an overwhelming majority of the population does not receive an adequate amount of it in their diets. For maximum results, magnesium should be supplemented in the chelated form because the amino acid that it is paired with facilitates absorption into the blood. Between 500 to 1000 mg of magnesium should be consumed daily on an empty stomach, with 200 to 300 mg taken in the morning and the remainder taken before retiring for the evening. Since magnesium is a relaxing mineral, it can aid the sleep cycle. One possible side effect of this mineral is loose stool, so if this occurs, you should limit your dosage.

Many people who suffer from dementia have deficiencies of selenium and zinc. Supplements of selenium should be consumed in quantities of 200 mcg daily, while 40 to 50 mg of the chelated form of zinc, known as zinc picolinate, is recommended as well. One hundred milligrams of potassium should also be taken as a supplement on a daily basis.

Another nutrient that can aid in the battle with Alzheimer's disease is acetylcarnitine. This versatile nutrient is able to transport itself through the blood/brain barrier, and serves to stimulate and fortify the nerve cells within the brain. Acetylcarnitine directs fatty acids into the cell mitochondria, which are responsible for creating cell energy. Furthermore, it can act as an antioxidant and can supplement the neurotransmitter acetylcholine.

DHEA is a hormone produced by the adrenal glands, but production declines steadily with age. Clinical studies have indicated that the level of DHEA in a 60-year-old is only 10 percent of the amount in the average 20-year-old. DHEA supplementation during the later years can hinder the onset of an assortment of serious disorders, including heart disease, cancer, arthritis, and asthma. It can also aid our mental capabilities and alleviate stress. DHEA can be obtained in 5- to 25-mg form.

Flaxseed oil can provide the body with ample quantities of the essential fatty acid omega-3, which is transmuted into another fatty acid and ultimately provides nourishment for the cells in the brain. The recommended dosage of flaxseed oil is one tablespoon daily. Remember to keep flaxseed oil refrigerated and avoid cooking it, because heat can destroy its nutritional value.

Melatonin, which is manufactured naturally in the pineal gland, may need to be supplemented during the later years of life when natural production diminishes. Three mg taken prior to bedtime can help stabilize the sleeping cycle.

N-acetyl-cysteine has antioxidant properties that can promote healthy functioning of the brain, while phosphatidylserine enhances the ability of enzymes in membranes of nerve cells to relay messages in and out of the cells. This product can improve memory and learning capacity in older adults, and can ameliorate symptoms of depression. Phosphatidylserine is especially effective when paired with omega-3 fatty acid supplements.

Taurine is an antioxidant that protects the supply of magnesium and calcium within brain cells and enhances nerve cell functioning.

Tryptophane fosters comfortable sleep, which, in turn, enhances brain functioning.

Tyrosine and phenylalanine promote the production of dopamine within the brain, a vital compound responsible for regulating the operation of neurotransmitters.

Nicotinamide adenine dinucleotide, also known as NADH or coenzyme 1, is vital to the production of energy within the body due to its rich hydrogen content. Although NADH is a natural biological substance that should be present in all cells, older adults who suffer from Alzheimer's disease tend to lack up to 50 percent of the necessary amount of this chemical. When the body engages in rigorous activity, muscle and brain cells can contain up to 50 mcg of NADH per gram of tissue. An ample supply of NADH can allow the body to reap the benefits of an additional power source. Fortunately for Alzheimer's patients, risk-free supplements of coenzyme 1 are now available and can produce miraculous results. Studies have demonstrated that the administration of NADH supplements can halt further development of the disease, and can increase energy and improve functioning within 10 to 12 weeks. Unfortunately, the clinical effects of NADH last only for limited amounts of time.

SMART PILLS

Several pharmaceutical products currently on the market have illustrated their ability to aid brain functioning without causing harmful side effects. These are some that are worth looking into:

Depranil can protect neurons in the niagra striata, which is the portion of the brain commonly victimized by Parkinson's disease.

Hydergine can enhance the flow of oxygen to the brain, hence countering free radical damage and signs of aging. While the U.S. government allows prescriptions only in the form of 1-mg tablets, 4.5-mg tablets can be readily obtained via foreign mail order catalogs. The higher-potency tablets can substantially reduce memory loss when consumed twice daily.

The drug Lucidril aids in the elimination of toxic deposits in the brain that accrue throughout life. When the brain becomes overwhelmed with cellular debris, it ceases to function properly and senility sets in. After Lucidril drives out the hazardous buildup, the symptoms of aging can be reversed.

Although Piracetam is illegal within the U.S., it is widely available in 85 other nations. Piracetam performs similarly to Hydergine, in that it slows the destruction of brain cells by increasing the supply of oxygen to the brain. Furthermore, this versatile product promotes superconnecting, a process that increases the electric flow of information between the left and right hemispheres of the brain. According to clinical evidence, Alzheimer's patients who are treated with a combination of Piracetam and lecithin frequently experience remarkable memory recovery.

HERBAL TREATMENTS

Although the U.S. claims to lead the global community in medical technology, in some instances, we actually lag behind the times. As we discussed in the preceding section, some of the treatment modalities that have proven effective overseas are not being utilized to their full potential in our own country. A further example involves an herbal extract derived from the ginkgo biloba tree, used extensively throughout Europe for the past 20 years. This herbal remedy has produced remarkable results in the treatment of Alzheimer's and other age-related degenerative diseases, and consequently, has become the leading prescribed plant medicine in numerous countries. In fact, in France and Germany, ginkgo biloba currently ranks in the top five medications used overall. That's not the case here, where, unfortunately, the conventional medical community is generally ignorant of the vast assortment of herbs that possess medicinal capabilities. You have to journey to Europe, where herbal remedies have become an integral part of modern conventional medicine, to understand that the U.S. is not necessarily in the vanguard when it comes to knowledge about health.

Concerning ginkgo biloba, this herb is valuable because it can alleviate several dementia-related symptoms. First of all, ginkgo enhances the circulation to the central nervous system, which frequently becomes impeded in older adults. Furthermore, this herbal extract has a tendency to stabilize abnormal nerve communication in the brain. Within the U.S. pharmaceutical industry, a product known as Tacrin has enjoyed the status of being the only medication prescribed for the early stages of dementia. Interestingly, European studies comparing the effects of this product and ginkgo biloba have indicated that ginkgo extract is more effective in enhancing circulation and brain functioning.

Furthermore, ginkgo has potent antioxidant properties that are vital in protecting the cells of the central nervous system from free radical damage.

Elderly people who rely upon ginkgo to combat Alzheimer's disease or other forms of dementia should consume 240 mg daily divided into two or three doses throughout the day, while people who are just using ginkgo as part of their daily regimen should take only 120 mg.

The herb ginseng, especially Korean ginseng, has also demonstrated its capacity to curb the onset of psychological deterioration. In addition to aiding a patient's mental condition, ginseng can enhance adrenal functioning. Considering that many older adults suffer from deteriorated adrenal capacities, ginseng can provide a valuable supplement to ginkgo biloba extract.

Yet another herb that promotes healthy circulation to the brain is butcher's broom. Enhanced memory and clearer focus can be expected when two to four 425-mg capsules are taken daily.

What to Avoid

Unfortunately, most Americans indulge in an abundance of processed foods, foods stripped of vital nutrients. Vitamins and minerals that are crucial in preventing the onset of Alzheimer's disease and other forms of dementia are replaced by unhealthy additives. In order to avert nutritional deficiencies and harmful toxins, we need to limit our intake of salt, processed sugars, red meat, and trans fatty acids, and seek healthier sources of nourishment. It is also a good idea to completely avoid meats that are the product of animals supplied with rendered feed. In addition, it is important for elderly adults to avoid accumulations of hazardous metallic toxins within the body. So limiting use of aluminum-containing cookware, deodorants, antacids, and other preparations is prudent. And since our reservoirs often contain dangerous pollutants, charcoal block filters, which can effectively eliminate harmful toxins, should be installed on all sources of tap water used for drinking or cooking purposes.

Treatment Summary

Contrary to popular belief, Alzheimer's disease and other forms of dementia are not part of the normal aging process, and can be prevented or ameliorated by eating a nutritious, organic diet throughout one's life, by getting a nutritional evaluation to determine problems with assimilation, and by taking various supplements, herbs, and "smart pills."

The herb ginkgo biloba is noteworthy for its remarkable results in the treatment of Alzheimer's patients, and is used extensively in Europe for this purpose.

Anemia

Anemia is a medical condition characterized by a deficiency in the hemoglobin content of red blood cells. An insufficient amount of hemoglobin diminishes the ability of the blood to carry oxygen to the tissues and to remove carbon dioxide from the lungs. Anemia is a common affliction in the United States, which may seem surprising in light of the fact that so many foods are fortified with iron. However, iron deficiency is only one of several possible causes of the condition.

According to New York physician Dr. Dahlia Abraham, there are actually three major causes of anemia. First, acute or chronic blood loss could be responsible. Chronic blood loss can stem from a variety of conditions, including hemorrhoids, cancer, menstruation, and peptic ulcers. Another cause of anemia is excessive red blood cell destruction, that is, the condition that exists when the destruction of old cells exceeds the production of new ones. This condition can occur as a result of defective hemoglobin synthesis or trauma within the arteries. The final cause of anemia is a deficiency of vital nutrients, either iron, vitamin B12, or folic acid. This type of anemia—and specifically the iron-deficiency type—is the most common.

Getting enough iron is particularly important during the growth spurts of infancy and adolescence, while women may need additional supplements during pregnancy and lactation. Iron deficiency anemia is quite common in children under the age of two, and in teenagers. Children who eat nutritionally poor foods or do not include enough variety in their diets are the most at risk. Often, teenagers develop a habit of subsisting on junk foods, which do not satisfy their developmental needs. Sometimes supplements do not provide an adequate countermeasure because many people have difficulty absorbing iron due to a lack of hydrochloric acid, which allows the stomach to properly assimilate the mineral. Iron deficiency is especially common in elderly people, who do not produce the needed amounts of stomach acid, and in people who suffer from chronic diarrhea.

A deficiency in vitamin B12 is usually a result of defects in the absorption process. After food consumption, B12 is freed by hydrochloric acid and is bound to another chemical manufactured by the stomach, called intrinsic factor. The problem comes in when an individual does not secrete the necessary amounts of hydrochloric acid or intrinsic factor, because he or she may not then be able to properly absorb the B12 stored in food. Children brought up on strict vegetarian diets may experience B12 anemia if their parents do not offer supplements of the vitamin.

B12 anemia is often accompanied by folic acid anemia. One of the reasons folic acid is important is that it fosters healthy prenatal development: It aids in the prevention of birth defects, such as those of the neural tube, and is crucial for proper cell production in the growing fetus. Folic acid is easily consumed by heat; hence, diets that consist primarily of cooked foods, with few raw foods included, often result in this type of deficiency. In addition, young children may develop a folic acid deficiency if they are given goat's milk. (Although superior to cow's milk in many ways, goat's milk lacks folic acid.) Teenagers and adults who are vegetarians may also fall victim to this form of anemia if they do not carefully balance their diets. Finally, folic acid anemia can be induced by alcoholism, which completely drains the body of this nutrient, and by the consumption of certain prescription drugs, such as oral contraceptives and anticancer drugs.

An insufficient amount of protein in the body is yet another possible cause of anemia, as a deficiency in this nutrient may be responsible for a decrease in the body's red blood cell count. Actually, most people in the United States eat an excessive amount of protein, and therefore do not suffer from this condition. However, protein deficiency can affect those vegetarians whose diets consist of a multitude of refined foods and few or no whole grains, legumes, nuts, seeds, and soy products. Malabsorption syndrome is another possible cause of protein deficiency anemia, one that commonly affects older people who do not produce the necessary amount of protease, an enzyme that aids in the breakdown of protein. Although sufficient protein is being eaten, the lack of protease means that the system isn't getting it.

New York acupuncturist and educator Dr. Pat Gordon offers an Asian perspective on anemia in women. According to this philosophy, a woman's blood rises and falls in a cyclical fashion. Women can become anemic if they ignore the needs of their monthly cycle, especially during menstruation. In today's fast-paced world, though, many women claim that they simply cannot ignore their numerous commitments and rest while their body recuperates. In addition, Gordon explains, anemia can result from an incorrect approach to pregnancy. After the termination of pregnancy, whether it is a result of a miscarriage, induced abortion, or birth, women should let their bodies rest for at least a full month, regardless of other responsibilities. Plus after pregnancy termination, conception should be avoided for at least a year because the body needs to build up blood to sustain another pregnancy. If these guidelines are followed, women should be able to conceive healthy children and avoid anemia.

Symptoms associated with anemia include fatigue and weakness, headaches, irritability, dizziness, and sometimes gastrointestinal distress. In teenage girls, amenorrhea, or cessation of menstrual bleeding, is occasionally present. Children who are anemic are usually smaller in height and weight than other children. In older children and adults, B12 anemia may result in nerve damage, characterized by numbness or tingling in the hands or legs, depression, or confusion.

Treatment

Diet

Children should be encouraged to eat a wide variety of whole foods, especially leafy, green vegetables, and legumes. At approximately six months of age, parents should begin feeding their infants beets, broccoli, carrots, applesauce, blackberries, blueberries, and cherries. (Not all at once! New foods should be introduced to babies one at a time.) These foods are relatively hypoallergenic and rich in photochemicals and antioxidants.

Iron-rich vegetable juice can be made from a combination of beet juice, parsley, spinach, beet greens, and watercress. Green juices should be dispensed in small quantities, as a quarter of a cup daily can improve a child's condition in a short period. The juice should be diluted 50 percent with water or apple juice, and sipped slowly.

A vegetarian diet rich in vitamins includes sprouts, raisins, kale, prunes, parsley, watercress, dandelion greens, beets, and blackberries. Seaweeds, such as hijiki, wakame, and dulse, are also excellent nutritional sources, and can be added to soups and salads. Vegetarian sources of B12 include fermented soy products, such as soy sauce and tempeh, yogurt, cottage cheese, and eggs. Some sources of folic acid are legumes, orange juice, oatmeal, spinach, beets, broccoli, and Brussels sprouts. Protein should be part of everyone's daily consumption, especially if it is derived from vegetarian sources, such as grains, legumes, and soy milk. If meat is consumed, it is important that the animals were raised healthfully.

Supplementation

Supplementation to counter anemia makes sense only when it's keyed to the specific form of anemia that a person is suffering from, which is why you should be guided by a competent health professional. While iron remains a common recommendation, remember that some forms of anemia do not involve iron deficiency. In these cases, iron supplements are not appropriate and can become dangerous if taken in excess.

IRON

If a nursing child is iron-deficient, the mother should take a chelated form of the supplement so that her milk becomes enriched with the mineral. Typically, breast-fed babies do not develop an iron deficiency unless the mother suffers from the deficiency. A product known as Floradix, which can be found in most health food stores, offers a valuable source of iron. The liquid form of the product is recommended over the dry form.

BEE POLLEN

One ounce of bee pollen daily can serve as an additional combatant of iron-deficiency anemia.

B12

Vegetarians need to supplement their diet with B12 daily to prevent a deficiency. Although the condition takes three to four years to develop, it can become serious and potentially lead to nerve damage. Supplementing is especially important for pregnant mothers who expect to raise vegetarian children. Injections of B12 are useful for patients with pernicious anemia, the form that's more common in older people and caused by a deficiency of intrinsic factor needed to properly process the vitamin.

SPIRULINA

One teaspoon of spirulina provides the body with a useful amount of vitamin B12 and chlorophyll.

FOLIC ACID

Since folic acid is a vital nutrient for proper fetal development, pregnant women require 800 mcg of this nutrient daily, regardless of how good their regular diet is. Because it is water-soluble, excess folic acid in the body is simply washed out. Parents feeding their children goat's milk should add about 800 mcg of liquid folic acid to the milk.

ADDITIONAL SUPPLEMENTS

Sometimes supplements of hydrochloric acid and intrinsic factor need to be prescribed for people who lack these chemicals to aid in the nutrient absorption process.

Herbs

Dandelion root, gentian, and yellow dock are effective treatments for iron-deficiency anemia. Other useful herbs include alfalfa, parsley, burdock root, comfrey root, ginseng, red raspberry, and nettle leaves. Herbs can be taken separately or combined in capsules or tea. In addition, the Chinese herb dong quai contains phytoestrogens that aid women who become anemic as a result of heavy menstruation. The herb contains vitamins A, E, and B12, and can be taken most days of the month, until menstruation starts.

For people having difficulty absorbing B12, a combination of goldenseal, gentian, and wormwood powder taken in capsule form will help increase the level of hydrochloric acid, which will aid the stomach in digestion of the vitamin. This formula should be taken only on a temporary basis, for a couple of weeks at a time.

External Treatment

Alternating warm and cold water in showers, 30 minutes before or two hours after meals, and brushing the skin with a loofah when dry, can be useful as adjunctive measures in overcoming anemia. In addition, deep breathing exercises assist with the intake of oxygen and the elimination of carbon dioxide.

What to Avoid

Stay away from refined foods, salt, and too much meat. Also, caffeine and alcohol are detrimental to healthy blood and should be eliminated.

Treatment Summary

Before anemia is treated, its cause should be medically determined. Anemia stemming from nutritional problems can be due to a shortage of iron, vitamin B12, or folic acid. Iron-rich foods include green, leafy vegetables, legumes, and vegetable juices. Good sources of B12 (a nutrient especially important for pregnant women) are fermented foods, such as soy products, tempeh, and yogurt. Folic acid can be obtained from orange juice, oatmeal, spinach, and beets.

Good supplementary sources of iron include a product called Floradix, and bee pollen. B12 can be obtained from a B-complex vitamin, or from spirulina.

Sea vegetables, green vegetable juice, dandelion root, gentian, and yellow dock are herbs useful in countering iron deficiency.

Alternating hot and cold showers, skin brushing, and deep breathing exercises are useful supplementary treatments.

Arthritis

Forty million Americans experience the painful, crippling effects of arthritic diseases. Of that number, about 16 million have osteoarthritis and 7 million are afflicted with rheumatoid arthritis. Many others suffer from less common forms of the condition.

Osteoarthritis, the most common form of the disease, is the form that usually plagues older people or develops after overuse of the joints or an accident. This is an inflammatory condition affecting any of the 68 joints in the body. It occurs as the spongy cushioning at the end of the bones, known as cartilage, breaks down. Cartilage is encapsulated in a structure called the synovium. The synovium's function is to lubricate the area between the bones and to nourish cartilage. As cartilage wears away, it ceases to act as a shock absorber. Bones touch one another, resulting in stiffness, swelling, and painful friction.

Rheumatoid arthritis is more of a systemic disease than osteoarthritis. It is also characterized by painful, swollen joints, but differs from osteoarthritis in that the synovial membrane becomes inflamed and extra fluid leaks into the joints. The result is pain and swelling. Sometimes the whole body, not just the joints, is affected; early signs can include fatigue, weakness, mild fever, and anemia. Women between 20 and 50 are this condition's prime targets, although 25 percent of those affected are men. At times, onset is sudden and symptoms are severe; on other occasions, none manifest. At its worst, rheumatoid arthritis can be crippling.

Less common forms of arthritis include **gouty arthritis,** which occurs when excess uric acid crystallizes and settles into the joints and tissues. The condition affects mainly men, who experience pain and inflammation in the joints, accompanied by fever and chills. The disease can become crippling, and, if untreated, can lead to joint breakdown. **Psoriatic arthritis** is a form of rheumatoid arthritis that affects the bones, often occurring in the joints of the fingers or toes. **Juvenile rheumatoid arthritis** generally attacks the large joints of children, and may result in bone deformity. Ankylosing spondylitis is an inflammation of the vertebrae that causes back pain and stiffness, especially in young males.

Causes

Allergies

Arthritis is usually an allergic reaction to foods and substances in the environment. Generally, the foods people eat all the time are the ones to which they are allergic. Many people, for example, eat milk, beef, corn, or wheat just about daily. And many react to materials breathed in, such as dust, mold, or pollen. Since exposure is continual and invisible, and the effects are not always immediate, most people do not make the connection, and thus do not know to eliminate problem-causing substances.

Why do allergies in some people affect the joints while in others they affect the lungs, the stomach, or the skin? The reason has to do with genetic predisposition. Different people have different areas of weakness. So when the body becomes weak from an allergy, infection, yeast, or some other cause, the most vulnerable area is the one that suffers. Sometimes more than one system becomes affected at once. For example, after drinking milk, a person may experience both arthritis and asthma.

Environmental Toxicity

The body can weaken from continual exposures to poisonous substances in the environment, such as pesticides, artificial colorings and preservatives in foods, and chlorine and fluoride in water. These substances enter the bloodstream and cause autotoxemia, which leads to arthritic changes. An invisible enemy is electromagnetic radiation, which can deplete the system of energy. This creates an imbalance that can trigger an arthritic reaction.

Chronic Infections

A proliferation of pathogenic bacteria, viruses, yeast, or fungi can be a cofactor contributing to arthritis. Fats and carbohydrates ferment and create an environment that invites *Candida albicans,* unhealthy bacteria, and parasite growth. Some of the bacteria produce toxins that attack joints. The result is acute inflammation or a slow destruction of joint cartilage. Chronic infections are also the result of heavy metal poisoning, from lead, cadmium, and the mercury that leaches out of dental amalgams.

Symptoms

Symptoms of osteoarthritis increase as the disease progresses. In the beginning, there are no indications. The first sign to appear is usually joint pain, and it is commonly associated with exercising or the carrying of weighty items. Other signs may include inflexibility when getting out of bed in the morning, and when the weather is cold and damp. As the disease advances, swelling and inflammation of the joints may occur. If muscles are underused from a lack of exercise, there may be fatigue, loss of motion, and leg cramps.

The signs of rheumatoid arthritis also worsen gradually. At first there are vague feelings of ill health. Later, symptoms specific to the disease appear, such as joint pain, stiffness, swelling, and redness. Joints may become warm to the touch, and stiffness may follow periods of inactivity. Weakness and deterioration can eventually spread to the heart and lungs.

Treatment

Conventional Treatments

Orthodox medicine consistently maintains that arthritis is an incurable disease. Therapies are therefore geared toward alleviating symptoms only, not to stopping degenerative processes. Treatments can include rest, exercise, heat, surgery (including joint replacement), and rehabilitation. Mostly, though, conventional medical practice relies on various drugs.

Arthritis medications are primarily painkillers or anti-inflammatories, which can have serious side effects. Even aspirin, which is routinely given to patients in large doses on a constant basis, can be dangerous, resulting in dizziness, ringing in the ears, intestinal tract bleeding, kidney damage, and lowered immunity (aspirin destroys vitamin C).

As aspirin fails to work, nonsteroidal, anti-inflammatory medications, such as Motrin, are generally given in its place. Although less harmful than steroidal drugs containing cortisone, these produce many of the same side effects as aspirin, including gastrointestinal bleeding, peptic ulcers, ringing in the ears, and dizziness. In addition, there may be nausea, nervousness, and vomiting.

When nonsteroidals fail, drugs that contain cortisone, such as Prednisone, are given. These medications are notorious for their severe side effects. They interfere with the immune system directly, leaving a person defenseless against infections and other diseases, and making healing difficult.

Some rheumatologists give gold injections. At one time, this treatment fell out of favor because it was considered too dangerous, but unfortunately, more and more doctors are using it again. The intent with gold is to destroy the immune response. Doing so, however, can lead to massive infections.

These treatments totally miss the mark. Not only do they fail to get at the cause of arthritis, they are becoming increasingly expensive, invasive, and toxic.

Natural Treatments

Natural medicine reports much success in reversing arthritis because it addresses the cause of the problem, as opposed to just masking symptoms. The consumer should be aware that not all claims for natural arthritis treatments are valid, but that others do work, and can be scientifically validated. Some methods that can produce favorable results are described below:

THE ANTIARTHRITIS DIET

To prevent and combat arthritis, the types of foods that should be eaten most often are complex carbohydrates with lots of fresh fruits and vegetables. There should also be a small amount of high-quality proteins and fats. These foods are especially protective:

Foods rich in folic acid, such as lentils, split peas, barley, alfalfa, soy, and oats.

Garlic and onions; their high sulfur content stops inflammation.

Deep-sea cold-water fish, such as salmon, trout, tuna, sardines, and mackerel. These contain omega fatty acids that lubricate the joints. Olive oil, avocado, nuts, and seeds are good for their oils as well.

Soy products, such as tofu, tempeh, and miso. They are high in the amino acid methionine.

Foods that break apart and eliminate uric acid, such as dandelion greens, parsley, and alfalfa.

Plenty of pure drinking water, up to a gallon each day.

Juices from red, yellow, and green fruits and vegetables, six to eight times a day. This is the best way to get high amounts of phytochemicals. (Some recommended juices are listed later in this chapter.)

RECOMMENDING DIET BY BLOOD TYPE

There is evidence to the effect that a person's blood type determines the type of arthritis expressed, and the kind of treatment needed. This observation was first made by a naturopathic doctor, James D'Adamo, over 25 years ago. He noticed that people with type A blood usually developed puffiness, which could be termed rheumatoid arthritis, while those with type O blood were more prone to a granular or gritty type, associated with the more common osteoarthritis.

The first group responded better to a strictly vegetarian diet, while the second group tolerated lean animal proteins, but no dairy. People with type B or AB blood benefited from a more individualized approach. Today, this diagnostic and treatment strategy is employed by Dr. D'Adamo's son, Peter, in Greenwich, Connecticut.

JUICES

Fresh juices can make an important contribution to any antiarthritis program. Here are some recommendations:

Pineapple juice. The stem of the pineapple contains bromelain, which, when juiced, provides the body with important enzymes helpful against arthritis. This juice is better yet when some juiced alfalfa sprouts are added.

Potato juice. One raw potato can be juiced, diluted with water, and taken in the morning.

Combination vegetable juice. Aloe vera (from the bottle) can be mixed with organic red cabbage, cucumber, dandelion, celery, mint, apple, and carrot.

Star fruit juice. Juice from this sweet-tasting fruit can be blended with equal parts of pure water. Drinking this three times a day lessens or eliminates inflammatory joint pain.

Green juices are particularly healing, but are too strong to be taken straight. A good proportion is 2/3 green to 1/3 carrot or beet juice. Those just starting on a juice regimen may want to dilute their green juices with filtered water.

Cabbage juice. This is one of the best juices for helping arthritic patients. It can be mixed with carrot for flavor and aloe vera for better cleansing effects.

Chlorophyll combination. Two ounces of liquid chlorophyll can be mixed with diluted apple or carrot juice and taken daily.

Other good greens. These juices can be taken in any combination: celery, broccoli, zucchini, cucumber, kale, parsley, and spinach. Ginger root, apple, or carrot can be added for flavor and extra nutritional benefit.

HERBS

Many natural aids can be grown right in our own backyard. These are good ones to consider if you're concerned about arthritis:

Alfalfa—Alfalfa is rich in chlorophyll, making it an excellent blood purifier. By eliminating uric acid, it helps relieve joint pain. If you're taking this in tablet form, about 20 tablets can be taken each day for the first month; then decrease it to 6 to 10 a day.

Aloe vera—By cleansing the intestines, aloe vera rids the body of toxins that can cause arthritis.

Boneset—As its name implies, this herb can relieve aches and pain in the bones.

Boswellia—Many consider this botanical to be the best natural remedy for treating arthritis. In fact, its healing properties are recorded in Ayurvedic medical literature, dating back thousands of years. Boswellia works much like nonsteroidal anti-inflammatory compounds without the side effects. Additionally, it stimulates repair by increasing circulation to the joints.

Burdock root—This is a blood cleanser that is especially good for helping patients with gout.

Cayenne—This is a popular arthritis remedy used the world over. It can be taken internally in a capsule, as a tea, or as a tincture. And it can be used externally in liniments. If used as a spice, cayenne should be sprinkled on food after cooking to prevent irritation.

Comfrey—Comfrey promotes healing of the bones' fibrous coverings.

Devil's claw—One of the best herbs for helping joints. It removes deposits and helps eliminate uric acid from the body.

Nettles—Nettle leaves can be crushed and made into a poultice to stop rheumatic pain.

Prickly ash bark—Good for rheumatism and arthritis. As a blood purifier, it gets rid of deposits in the joints.

White willow bark—Nature's aspirin; alleviates joint pain.

Yucca—Research suggests that vaccines from yucca may be valuable for alleviating symptoms of rheumatoid arthritis.

SUPPLEMENTS

We have been told that nutrients do not make a difference in treating arthritis. In actuality, a large body of scientific literature demonstrates that they do. The fact is that arthritis patients can benefit from a full range of nutrients, with an emphasis on the ones listed below:

Antioxidant vitamins—Vitamins A, C, and E counter inflammation and stop free radical damage to joints. Among its many benefits, vitamin C is an essential nutrient for joint and cartilage repair, especially when taken in combination with glucosamine. Bowel tolerance doses can be taken daily, in divided amounts throughout the day. (Total daily dose may range from 2000 to 20,000 mg.) Generally, 400 IU of vitamin E and 50,000 IU of vitamin A or beta carotene each day help reduce arthritic pain. In cases of advanced arthritis, patients benefit from megadoses of these nutrients given intravenously.

Chondroitin sulfate—Chondroitin sulfate is a molecular cement that holds together cartilage, allowing collagen proteins to form actual tissue. It both prevents damage from arthritis and stimulates repair.

Cod liver oil—In generations past, this was a well-known remedy for arthritis. Although its popularity has declined, the remedy still works.

Gamma linoleic acid (GLA)—GLA is rich in prostaglandins that turn off pain and stop inflammation. It is contained in evening primrose, borage, and black currant oils. All forms are equally beneficial, but some are less expensive than others. Six capsules of evening primrose oil, or one capsule of borage oil, provide the needed 240 mg of GLA.

Glucosamine—This is one of the most important nutrients for repairing joint, cartilage, and tissue damage. It is sold as glucosamine sulfate and glucosamine hydrochloride, and both work equally well. Since glucosamine is a substance that each cell in the body naturally manufactures on its own, it is perfectly safe to use. Studies suggest 1500-2000 mg should be taken each day, divided into two or three doses.

Grape seed extract—Grape seed extract is rich in the antioxidant pycnogenol. It is known to strengthen collagen and support capillaries and veins.

Omega-3 fatty acids—These are anti-inflammatory, making them especially useful in the treatment of rheumatoid arthritis. Salmon oil is one good source. A vegetarian source is flaxseed oil, which is also rich in important omega-6 and omega-9 fatty acids, making it complete in polyunsaturated acids. Three capsules each day are generally recommended. If omega-3 fatty acids are taken as an oil, a tablespoon can be added to salads, but should not be cooked.

Minerals—Adequate supply and absorption of calcium, phosphorus, and magnesium are essential for the formation of healthy bone, while zinc and selenium are important for the immune system. Also, new findings suggest that 3-6 mg of boron may actually reverse symptoms of osteoarthritis. Other needed nutrients are potassium, copper, and manganese. It's important to note that the typical American diet does not contain adequate minerals, so eating it can eventually result in damage to the joints. A whole-foods diet, on the other hand, rich in raw fruits, vegetables, fresh juices, nuts, seeds, and grains, in combination with a multivitamin/mineral supplement, can make a positive difference.

Superoxide dismutase (SOD)—SOD should be taken on an empty stomach, with water, about a half hour before meals. This enhances energy, and reduces pain and inflammation. SOD's benefits are enhanced by the addition of vitamin E.

The B vitamins:

Niacinamide—This form of B3 helps both osteoarthritis and rheumatoid arthritis. For the best effect, 150-250 mg should be taken before a meal, three or four times daily. Effects are not immediate but result in a gradual reduction of symptoms and improved range of motion over time. Niacinamide is not to be confused with niacin, which is used for lowering cholesterol.

Pantothenic acid (vitamin B5)—This one is especially helpful for people with gout.

Other B vitamins—Include a B-complex supplement with approximately 150 mg of vitamin B6, 50 mg of B2, and 15-50 mg of B1.

ALLERGY TESTING FOR PROBLEM FOODS

Since allergic responses to foods are a major cause of arthritis, skin and blood allergy tests, administered by a complementary physician, can be of value in that they reveal problem foods and chemicals. The foods to which people are highly sensitive must be completely eliminated, at least for a while. Later, some of them can be returned to the diet. Foods that cause less of a reaction can be eaten infrequently, on a rotation diet, in which the same food is not eaten more than once every four to seven days. So, for example, if wheat is eaten on Monday, it is not eaten again until Friday at the earliest.

Sometimes, people are allergic to every food they eat. In these instances they are given low-dose allergy vaccines. Unlike typical allergy shots, where patients are uniformly given similar doses of a substance, these vaccines are prepared for the individual's unique requirements. Small doses of antigens are given to stimulate enzyme systems. Enzymes are particularly important as they help break down circulating immune complexes that lead to disease. With insufficient enzymes, these circulating immune complexes build up, enter the synovial membrane of a joint, and establish themselves there. The result is swelling, pain, and arthritis. When enzymes are active, food is metabolized and the body does not react to it as if it is a foreign substance. Then there is no inflammation and no disease.

DETOXIFICATION

Cleansing the body and the external environment are necessary to overcome arthritis. These are some methods to consider:

Chelation Therapy. Chelation, a treatment that gets rid of toxic heavy metals and plaque, is an adjunctive therapy that, by improving overall circulatory functioning, and lessening free radical damage, can lessen arthritic symptoms. This therapy is particularly good for alleviating the crippling effects of rheumatoid arthritis. Scientists hypothesize that the chelation drug EDTA has similar chemical properties to penicillamine, a drug rheumatologists use to treat the disease.

Colon Therapy. Many arthritic patients have constipation from an accumulation of toxins in the body. As a result, they have inflammation and suffer autotoxic reactions, in which the body reacts to the poisons. This can exacerbate any disease, including arthritis.

Colonic irrigation opens the digestive tract and thoroughly removes accumulated wastes, getting rid of harmful bacteria. A series of treatments leaves a person feeling lighter, cleaner, and more alive. When colon therapy is combined with an improved diet and supplementation, proper balance is restored. As a result, mobility increases and arthritis may even disappear.

BALANCED HORMONAL TREATMENT

This treatment was developed by Dr. Robert Liefman, a Canadian physician, who devoted his entire life to understanding the cause of arthritis, and who helped more than 30,000 individuals in his lifetime. After treatment, many were able to lead normal, pain-free lives.

Dr. Liefman and his associates began their research in the 1940s, when cortisone was being hailed as a miracle cure. It soon became apparent that the hormone produces dangerous side effects when used alone, but that it is less harmful when used concurrently with estrogens, and better still when testosterone is added. Dr. Liefman developed formulas consisting of various amounts of these three basic ingredients.

According to the proponents of this therapy, it is anti-inflammatory and healing, with minimal side effects, because the substances are in balance with each other. Effectiveness is enhanced further because it is adjusted to the individual needs of each patient, and used in conjunction with a healthy diet and an exercise program.

CHIROPRACTIC

Chiropractic care is a gentle, safe, noninvasive way to offer patients relief from osteoarthritis. During treatment, spinal adjustments are given to release nerve pressure. This allows nerve energy to flow properly. Circulation increases to the joints, enabling them to function better and to heal.

People not helped by this method are those in the advanced stages of the disease, where joints are fused together, causing nerve passageways to be blocked.

Chiropractic treatments increase range of motion, alleviate pain, and lengthen the spine, allowing the person to stand straighter and appear taller. Also, by encouraging proper posture, chiropractic treatments minimize pressure on the joints. (See chiropractic patient experiences in Treatments and Patient Experiences sections.)

HOMEOPATHIC REMEDIES

Homeopathic remedies for arthritis, like those for other ailments, are keyed to very specific conditions.

Rhus toxicodendron—For pain that worsens at night and in the morning on awakening. Pain is worse in cold, damp weather and before a storm. The person feels better with heat and motion.

Rhododendron—For joint pains that feel worse in the morning, before a storm or weather change, and in heavy winds. Symptoms are alleviated with heat and motion.

Calcarea carbonica—For pain that is worse in cold, damp weather, when there is exertion and motion, and when the limb is hanging downward.

Aconitum hapellus—For pain and inflammation, especially when the skin is hot and dry.

RECONSTRUCTIVE THERAPY

To stimulate the healing of ligaments, tendons, and cartilage, reconstructive therapy is sometimes used. Treatment involves low doses of nutritional substances that are injected into the ligaments. The substances vary according to the area being treated, but may include vitamin C, glutathione, shark cartilage, and glucosamine sulfate. As a result, ligaments become stronger, enabling them to support the vertebrae and joints with greater ease.

By correcting the root of the problem, symptoms naturally fade. Reconstructive therapy strengthens the structural foundation of the body, and pain dramatically disappears. (See reconstructive therapy patient experiences in Treatments and Patient Experiences sections.)

NEUROMUSCULAR THERAPY

Neuromuscular therapy uses touch to balance the muscular and nervous systems. The therapist improves skeletal alignment, thereby allowing energy to run freely throughout the joints. This is important because when energy is locked in place, blood and other fluids become stuck, and pain occurs. Arthritis can be a response to such stressors, according to neuromuscular therapist Sara Vogeler, who explains that postural distortion can cause pressure on the bones, which, in turn, can create stress and compression, causing the formation of bony spurs. A bony spur can aggravate surrounding soft tissue, and cause pain to travel to other parts of the body. Neuromuscular therapy helps to diminish pain by improving postural alignment and teaching correct ways of moving.

EXERCISE

An exercise routine is important for restoring mobility, function, and muscle mass. However, people should not push themselves beyond their limits. Pain is a warning signal to slow down, and people should wait until they are comfortable enough to engage in activities.

Walking is excellent for the total body and a good way for the novice to begin. It can improve circulation in the hands, knees, shoulders, and fingers, areas frequently affected by arthritis. Another type of exercise that benefits people of every age is yoga. Slow stretches lubricate joints and increase flexibility, while special breathing techniques expel toxins in the joints and muscles.

OTHER THERAPIES TO CONSIDER

A comprehensive program incorporates several modalities for complete healing. In addition to the approaches mentioned above, those suffering from arthritis might consider acupressure, acupuncture, aromatherapy, Ayurvedic medicine, Bach flower remedies, biological dentistry, hydrotherapy, light therapy, massage, meditation, oxygen therapy, ozone therapy, physical therapy, qi gong, tai chi, and vitamin drips. Combining a number of treatments is the best way to meet the unique needs of each patient.

What to Avoid

As mentioned previously, most any food, especially those eaten on an everyday basis, can cause an allergic response that produces arthritis. But certain foods and chemicals are common triggers. Highly acidic foods have been associated with the exacerbation of arthritis symptoms. Saturated fats found in meat, dairy, and fried foods, as well as alcohol and aspirin, produce prostaglandin-E2, which suppresses the immune system, causing inflammation and pain. Pork is one of the worst offenders, whether it is in the form of ham, bacon, or any food cooked in lard (a hidden ingredient in most restaurant foods).

A small percentage of people with arthritis need to avoid the nightshade family of vegetables: tomatoes, potatoes, eggplant, and bell peppers. You can tell if these foods affect you by staying away from them for 30 days and then eating all of them in one day. If you do not feel any worse after challenging yourself in this way, then you need not worry. If pain in the joints worsens, stay away from these foods.

Other substances to avoid include coffee and tobacco (both members of the nightshade family), caffeinated tea, sugar, and salt, as well as artificial colors, food additives, and preservatives. Carbonated drinks are high in phosphates, which change the mineral balance in the body. Margarine is unhealthful because of the partially hydrogenated trans fatty acids, which our bodies cannot digest. Overcooked and processed foods rob the body of essential nutrients and can pave the way for arthritis. Anti-inflammatory medications may appear helpful initially, but in the long term, they are destructive.

Another thing to avoid, for those with arthritis, is the prolonged immobility of a lengthy car or plane ride. To prevent the increased knee, ankle, or foot pain that can result from such a ride, travelers should try to exercise periodically during the trip, if this is at all possible.

See also: Allergies, Acupuncture, Chiropractic, Ozone Therapy, Reconstructive Therapy, Vitamin Drips

Autism

During the first month of life, newborns do not know that a world beyond themselves exists. As children grow, so do their interactions with the world. But in some instances, a child's ability to interact with the environment and people stays limited. This severe behavioral problem is known as autism.

Autistic children are extremely withdrawn and tend to live in their own fantasy worlds. They are often unable to express themselves verbally, and do not make eye contact. According to studies performed by the Autism Research Institute in San Diego, autistic children tend to have weak immune systems, which causes decreased resistance to infections, particularly upper respiratory and ear infections, as well as autoimmune problems.

Causes

Studies indicate that autism may be the result of adverse reactions to childhood vaccinations. Dr. Alan Cohen, an environmental physician from Connecticut, notes that high levels of autism and attention deficit disorder did not occur until the mandatory use of childhood vaccinations, and suggests that there may be a connection between certain vaccines and the onset of these conditions. According to Dr. Harris Coulter, author of *DPT: A Shot in the Dark*, the diphtheria/pertussis/tetanus vaccine plays a major role in the start of this problem. Medical journals document the fact that DPT can cause mild or severe encephalitis, which can then result in a variety of disorders, from autism to hyperactivity to severe mental retardation.

Hyperreactivity to vaccines can lead to immune system problems, causing some children to have increased sensitivity to infections. As a result, autistic children are commonly given repeated courses of antibiotics, which, in turn, cause a whole cascade of problems that ultimately exacerbate their condition.

Antibiotic overuse can lead to an inability to properly digest nutrients, known as malabsorption syndrome. What happens is that antibiotics destroy healthy bacteria in the gut, with a concomitant proliferation of yeast. The resulting imbalance can cause the digestive tract to become more permeable, allowing partially broken down proteins to leak into the bloodstream. Once in the blood, these foreign substances travel to the brain and secrete toxins. These cause inflammations that produce autism or other psychological disorders.

Many autistic children suffer from food allergies. Certain foods produce inflammatory compounds that travel to the brain and cause brain allergies, which are manifested as psychological disorders. Food allergies are actually easily tested for and treated; sadly, though, this is an area often neglected by mainstream medicine.

Autism can be related to biochemical abnormalities. Autistic children may be low in sulfur amino acids, which are needed by the liver for detoxification. When these amino acids are absent, the liver is unable to effectively purge harmful molecules taken in from the air, food, and water. As a result, poisonous substances reenter the bloodstream and circulate to the brain, where they can then cause behavioral, focusing, and memory problems.

Children with autism also tend to suffer from heavy metal toxicity. Hair analysis and other tests that detect this problem often show that autistic children have excessive amounts of antimony, aluminum, arsenic, lead, and cadmium. This may be related to the disordered sulfur chemistry, just mentioned, which prevents heavy metals from being excreted from the body. Supplying sulfur amino acids can sometimes eliminate this problem.

Autistic individuals tend as well to have vitamin and mineral deficiencies, particularly shortages of zinc, selenium, vitamin B6, and magnesium. Fortunately, it is easy to test for these problems and to correct them.

Sometimes autism is the result of subclinical hypothyroidism, a problem detected not by blood tests, but by temperature. If low body temperature is accompanied by cold hands and feet, dry skin, and memory and concentration problems, subclinical hypothyroidism may be at the root of the problem.

Treatment

Orthodox medicine approaches autism from a psychiatric perspective, and treats patients accordingly, with behavioral modification programs and medications. Although autism does manifest as a psychological disorder, the brain is a physical entity, whose functioning can be significantly improved through nutritional therapies. Environmental physicians—doctors who study the relationship between patients and their environment—see positive changes when nutritional protocols are followed. While exact recommendations should be made by a medical professional, and based on sound tests, some general guidelines can be offered.

Nutrition

Autistic children should be eating a variety of fresh foods that are free of additives and preservatives. A diet of organic food assures that what is eaten is pesticide-free. This is important for anyone, but especially for these children who have difficulty eliminating toxins.

In addition, autistic children are often low in vitamin B6 and magnesium, two nutrients that, when given as supplements, can produce vast improvements. Several studies show that between 30 and 40 percent of autistic children respond to B6 replacement.

The herb ginkgo biloba is good for anyone who needs to enhance brain functioning because it strengthens circulation to the brain. Ginkgo's effects are further amplified by the addition of coenzyme Q10, an enzyme that gets more oxygen to all parts of the body, particularly the brain. Dimethyl glycine, an over-the-counter vitamin-like compound that is taken sublingually, has a similar effect. Bee pollen can be wonderful for improving focus, if the child is not allergic to bee stings. It is especially high in B vitamins, which are essential for good mental health. Vitamin E with selenium aids circulation, as do choline and inositol. Moreover, vitamin C, an effective free radical scavenger, builds the immune system and improves circulation. Research suggests that the amino acid L-glutamine is helpful for anyone with mental and emotional problems. Autistic children can benefit from papaya and pineapple enzymes to a degree when there are digestive problems related to a difficulty in breaking down protein. Autism caused by subclinical hypothyroidism can be corrected with a natural thyroid medicine, available by prescription, called Armour Thyroid, while garlic, citrus seed extract, and caprylic acid can help keep down the growth of yeast. For the latter problem, nontoxic antifungal medications, such as Nystatin or Diflucan, can also be of benefit.

Most autistic children can benefit from a multivitamin and from essential fatty acids, found in flaxseed oil or fish oil. It is important to remember that children need smaller doses of nutrients than do adults. Exact amounts depend on the age and size of the child, and supplement intake should be prescribed and monitored by a health practitioner, but here we can offer general ranges for daily doses:

Vitamin B6—50 to 200 mg, although some physicians prescribe more
Magnesium—200 to 300 mg
Zinc picolinate—20 to 40 mg
Selenium—100 to 200 mcg
Calcium—200 to 500 mg
Vitamin E—200 to 800 IU

What to Avoid

Pollutants, and food additives and preservatives, should be avoided as much as possible. Foods containing yeast and mold should also be avoided in the diet of the autistic child because yeast overgrowth in the intestinal tract can lead to worsening of the condition. Autistic children must also stay away from any foods that provoke brain allergies. Often there is a sensitivity to gluten, found in grains, and to casein, the main protein component of milk and milk products. Other common foods that produce allergies include corn, soy products, eggs, tomatoes, beef, and peanuts. The specific foods responsible for causing reactions can be detected through food allergy tests.

Treatment Summary

Eating organically grown fresh foods is especially important for the autistic child, so that chemicals added to foods will not set off unwanted brain reactions.

Nutrients that can improve brain function include vitamin B6, magnesium, the herb ginkgo biloba, coenzyme Q10, dimethyl glycine, bee pollen, and the amino acid L-glutamine.

See also: Allergies

Acquired Immune Deficiency Syndrome

There is disagreement over what causes AIDS, how to treat it, and whether or not the condition is curable. The accepted viewpoint is that the human immunodeficiency, or HIV, virus causes AIDS. While this may be one factor, the belief that HIV alone is responsible for the massive deterioration that characterizes AIDS is a gross oversimplification. After years of research, there is no solid scientific evidence supporting this virus-as-sole-cause theory. Rather, the virus may be a cofactor, with other factors necessary before a person becomes ill.

AIDS is officially defined by the Centers for Disease Control as the presence of HIV with the manifestation of one or more of a list of over two dozen previously known diseases. So, for example, tuberculosis with HIV is AIDS; without it, it is still tuberculosis. Other diseases on the list are Kaposi's sarcoma, progressive multifocal leukoencephalopathy, disseminated cytomegalovirus, pneumonia, and candidiasis.

Nagging questions persist about the HIV=AIDS concept. For one, why are some people with AIDS symptoms actually HIV-negative? And if AIDS is spread by bodily fluids, why has it not spread to the general population, and why has it not reached epidemic proportions? The fact is that most research outside of the HIV=AIDS paradigm suggests that AIDS can occur only after the immune system is worn down. This can be caused by long-term drug use—either intravenous or oral, and either recreational or prescription; by hepatitis; or by malnutrition. Also excessive sexual activity can weaken the immune system, and sexually transmitted diseases, acquired before the individual was exposed to HIV, may contribute to immune system breakdown as well. Additionally, multiple infections place an increased burden on the immune system. Yeasts, molds, fungi, and a variety of viruses can play a part. Unfortunately, the all too common treatment for infections—antibiotics—suppresses the immune system further.

Symptoms

Initial symptoms can include extreme fatigue, night sweats, fever, chills, swollen lymph glands, swollen spleen, loss of appetite, weight loss, severe diarrhea, and depression. As AIDS progresses and the immune system weakens, the body becomes receptive to opportunistic infections. A form of pneumonia (pneumocystis carinii) and a rare cancer (Kaposi's syndrome) are commonly contracted. Other forms of cancer associated with the condition include non-Hodgkin's lymphoma and Burkitt's syndrome. A swelling of the lining of the spine (meningitis) or the brain (encephalitis) may also occur.

Treatment

Up until recently, HIV or AIDS were considered tantamount to a death sentence. The conventional treatment has relied on powerful drugs given in the hope of slowing the progression of the disease. The trouble is, such drugs add toxins to an already weakened immune system. Researchers now seem hopeful that new drug combinations can keep the disease under control, and this approach does seem to be helping some patients. At this point, though, no one knows the long-term effects of these drugs.

What we do know is that long-term survivors do not rely totally on pharmaceuticals. Many do not take drugs at all. They alter their diets and lifestyles to maximize the health-giving elements in each. Plus they make positive affirmations about the future.

Under the guidance of a holistically trained physician, AIDS patients should incorporate multiple healing modalities that stimulate the immune system to a healthy state of activity. Different remedies may be needed at different times, and individuals need to be flexible in their approach. The therapies listed here are immune-enhancing, antibacterial, antiviral, antimicrobial, and nontoxic or minimally toxic.

Diet

Everyone needs a good diet, but when people have severely weakened immune systems, high-quality nutrition becomes essential. This means eating organic vegetarian (or mostly vegetarian) foods, and drinking lots of filtered water.

Complex carbohydrates should be the mainstay of the diet. Unlike simple sugars, these foods are close to their natural form when eaten, and work to strengthen the immune system. There are plenty of whole grains from which to choose, including brown rice, wheat berries, barley, millet, whole oats, amaranth, quinoa, and bulgur wheat.

Vegetables are rich in several important antioxidants, including beta carotene, vitamin C, vitamin E, and selenium, which work together as a team to fight free radical damage. Six to eight cups of various types of vegetables should be eaten daily. Good sources of vitamin C, as well as calcium, are kale, collards, and broccoli. Squash, almonds, and carrots are high in beta carotene, while wheat germ and nuts are good sources of vitamin E. Because these foods are high in fiber, they stimulate the immune-enhancing cells of our intestinal lining, and cleanse the colon of toxins. Fiber helps prevent intestinal infections as well.

Raw foods are good sources of enzymes, but should not be eaten if there is a problem with diarrhea. Be sure to get your produce cleaned off before eating it. A good way to wash foods is with food-grade hydrogen peroxide from the pharmacy.

Easily digestible proteins are something you should look for. Think in terms of vegetable proteins and sprouts. Fermented food products, such as tempeh or miso, are also easy to digest. A cup of miso soup can be eaten daily.

To keep calorie consumption up, eat avocado, nut butters, almonds, and sunflower seeds.

Small quantities of fat are important, but these should come from high-quality sources. A tablespoon of unrefined olive oil can be added to salads. Flaxseed oil and fatty fish, like salmon, are also excellent. Remember that oils need refrigeration to prevent rancidity.

Oriental mushrooms, like shiitake and maitake, boost the immune system. Shiitake mushrooms contain lentinan, a substance that stimulates the body's interferon and helps to fight viruses. Soups and teas can be made from these mushrooms and taken daily.

Garlic is another valuable food. It contains allicin, a potent antibacterial and antiviral agent. When garlic is cooked, allicin is lost, so try to take this herb raw or in capsules. Garlic also contains protein, vitamins A and C, thiamin, calcium, potassium, copper, and selenium. Note that garlic can be juiced along with your other vegetables.

Sea vegetables, which include dulse, kombu, nori, and wakame, contain trace minerals that are no longer found in foods grown on land. Studies show that dulse destroys heavy metals and removes radiation from the body.

An important part of a health-maximizing diet is juicing. Freshly made juice supplies concentrated nutrients and plenty of raw enzymes, which help the body digest foods, making their nutrients available to our cells. Juices also contain an abundance of antioxidants.

A small amount of greens can be juiced together with carrot, beet, garlic, or apple. Greens should be rotated; your choices can include cabbage, kale, broccoli, mustard, collard and dandelion greens, Swiss chard, spinach, watercress, parsley, and wheatgrass. All of these are high in chlorophyll, which is antibacterial and a good energy provider. People with digestion problems should start off slowly, diluting a glass of juice with a glass of water. Gradually, they can build up to 4 to 6 glasses of juice a day. A holistic health practitioner can provide individualized guidance on juicing and other aspects of diet.

AIDS researcher, Mark Konlee, offers this juice recipe for building the immune system, flushing the liver and the lymphatic system, getting nutrients, and increasing energy: Wash a whole undyed lemon, cut it in quarters, blend in a blender. Add one cup of water and one tablespoon cold-pressed, extra virgin organic olive oil. The drink can be sweetened with a few tablespoons of orange juice. Blend. Strain and drink juice. Taking this drink once a day, Konlee reports, can raise T-cell counts, decrease viral load, and improve lymphatic drainage.

Supplements

AIDS patients need large doses of immune-building nutrients, both orally and intravenously. Particularly important are antioxidants, which provide essential protection from free radical damage. Vitamin C, beta carotene, vitamin E, and selenium, four star nutrients of the antioxidant group, work best as a team to clean up the system and resist infections.

VITAMIN C

AIDS patients need considerable amounts of C, between 10 and 200 grams daily, oral and intravenous, to build immunity and protect against secondary infections. Such high dosages make intravenous administration a necessity. In addition, vitamin C should be taken orally; a buffered form of the nutrient protects the stomach. Ester C polyascorbate is the most easily assimilated form of vitamin C and is recommended for people suffering from chronic illnesses. For those with Kaposi's lesions, applying a topical paste is quite healing.

Vitamin C stimulates white blood cell activity, causing cells to surround viruses, and place them in vacuoles, so that superoxide dismutase and other substances in the body can fill the space, killing the viruses.

Research supports vitamin C's ability to inhibit the replication of HIV and other pathogenic microorganisms commonly found in HIV-positive individuals, including Rous sarcoma virus, Epstein-Barr virus, and cytomegalovirus. This is accomplished in several ways. Vitamin C decreases viral production, increases the immune system cells called monocytes, which fight viruses, and stimulates interferon, a natural antiviral, antibacterial substance produced by the immune system.

The power of intravenous vitamin C drips is further enhanced with the addition of antibiotic and immune-enhancing herbs such as garlic, chaparral, red clover, pau d'arco, echinacea, goldenseal, lobelia, ginger, astragalus, ganoderma, and licorice root.

VITAMIN B6

This vitamin, recommended in dosages of 100 mg daily, is important for building up red blood cells and activating natural killer cells. Deficiencies in B6 have been related to suppressed natural killer cell activity.

BETA CAROTENE

Studies show that beta carotene increases T-cell numbers, which protects against infections. Beta carotene is converted by the body into vitamin A, and is safer in large doses than vitamin A.

BIOFLAVONOIDS

These enhance the absorption of vitamin C, and they are found together in nature.

BUTYRIC ACID

This nutrient helps cellular repair, and is especially good in treating lymphomas and leukemia.

CITRUS SEED EXTRACTS

Extracts from oranges, grapefruits, lemons, and limes are credited with enormous antimicrobial activity. They are broad-spectrum, nontoxic antibiotics, with antifungal, antibacterial, and antiviral properties. Citrus seed extracts can fight off a wide variety of infections, including E. coli, intestinal protozoa, fungi, and viruses.

In addition, they can kill over 30 types of yeast, including *Candida albicans*. At the same time, citrus seed extracts do not interfere with healthful bacteria that are needed to rebalance the system.

A final benefit of these extracts, sold in powder and liquid form, is that a few drops added to water can be used to clean bacteria from fruits and vegetables.

DIOXYCHLOR

Dioxychlor is an antiviral, antibacterial, antifungal, and antiparasitic agent. More research needs to be done, but in the test tube, this substance disarms HIV as well as cytomegalovirus, herpes, and other infectious organisms. In fact, any pathogenic virus moving from one point to another comes under attack. Dioxychlor can be administered intravenously, orally, or topically as a gel.

EGG LIPIDS (AL-721)

AL-721, a formula made from two active phospholipids found in egg yolk, is an adjunctive therapy for the containment of HIV and other viruses. The substance was first developed at the Weitzmann Institute of Science in Israel by a team of scientists, led by Meier Shinitsky. They found this formula effective in treating memory loss, and impaired immune function, and in easing the withdrawal effects from alcohol and drug addiction.

AL-721 was also found to prevent human T cells from becoming infected by HIV. It is thought to work by removing cholesterol from the envelope surrounding the virus, and in the process rendering it ineffective. Egg lipids have none of the toxicity problems found in drugs such as AZT.

ESSENTIAL FATTY ACIDS

Essential fatty acids contain GLA, which is converted by the body into prostaglandin-E1. This helps stimulate T-lymphocyte function and has a direct inhibitory effect on the replication of the HIV virus.

GLUTATHIONE PEROXIDASE

This protective antioxidant is produced by the body naturally, and found to be deficient in AIDS patients. Intravenous glutathione protects the organs and blood cells against damage, especially when used in conjunction with selenium, vitamin C, and vitamin E. Sometimes N-acetyl-cysteine, which is converted by the system into glutathione, is given in its place.

INTESTINAL FLORA

Lactobacillus acidophilus, lactobacillus bulgarigus, and bifido bacteria are healthful bacteria that many people lose after taking antibiotics. These flora strengthen the body's infection-fighting power by generating more lympho-cytes.

SHARK CARTILAGE

According to research, shark cartilage may be useful in the treatment of AIDS, cancer, arthritis, and a variety of other degenerative diseases. It may be particularly effective in stopping Kaposi's sarcoma.

The idea behind the use of shark cartilage is that the skeleton of the shark contains a great amount of anti-angiogenesis factor. Angiogenesis refers to formation of the local capillary network that sustains a tumor. When that production is stopped, there is no network of blood vessels to feed the tumor. The tumor stops growing and spreading. It may even begin to shrink and disappear.

VITAMIN B6

This is important because it stimulates white blood cells in the bone marrow and stimulates immunoglobulins, proteins created by white cells that latch onto viruses, bacteria, parasites, and food allergy antigens. Immunoglobulins lock up these substances, which helps the body get rid of them.

Herbs

Traditional Chinese medicine holds that the terrain is more important than the germ attacking it. A healthy person easily resists foreign invaders, while a weak one is susceptible to most everything. Based on this philosophy, certain plants have been used for thousands of years as a fundamental part of Chinese medicine to strengthen the immune system. Now, mainstream Western medicine is getting interested in herbs, opening its eyes to what Oriental, Native American, and other types of herbs can offer.

Up until now, herbal therapy has been based on empirical evidence, but the recent challenge of AIDS and other modern-day diseases has generated scientific interest in the field. Experimenters ask if herbs can help to overcome dreaded diseases, and if so, how?

Research does scientifically confirm the value of plant medicines, both alone and in conjunction with other therapies. For example, double-blind studies show that AIDS patients who are given Chinese herbs and AZT consistently do better than patients given placebos in place of the botanicals. Other studies report remission from cancer when astragalus is given alone.

Dr. R.S. Chang, Professor of Medical Microbiology and Immunology at the University of California School of Medicine, has listed Chinese herbs according to their specific actions on the immune system. Ethnobiologist Dr. James Duke has done the same, looking at herbs the world over. Some of the herbs that keep coming up again and again on such lists are astragalus, panax ginseng, ganoderma, and ligustrum. Herbs that increase the number of T-lymphocytes, according to Chang, are:

    Panax ginseng
    Ganoderma lucidum
    Coriolius versicolor
    Lentinus edodes
    Phaseolus vulgaris
    Atractylodes macrocephala
    Coix lachryma-jobi
    Polygonatum sibiricum
    Asparagus cochinchinensis
    Ligustrum lucidum
    Epimedium grandiflorum

Duke lists as promoting phagocytosis:

Aconitum	Cynanchum	Matricaria
Adina	Datura	Mentha
Allium	Dioscorea	Morus
Althaea	Dyera	Myroxylum
Angelica	Echinacea	Oldenlandia
Aralia	Eleuthero	Panax
Aristolochia	Epimedium	Persea
Astragalus	Eucommia	Petiveria
Atractylodes	Eupatorium	Phytolacca
Aucoumea	Forsythia	Pistacia
Boswellia	Ganoderma	Platycodon
Byrsonima	Glycine	Polyporus
Canarium	Glycyrrhiza	Psoralea
Cephaelis	Hedyotis	Rehmannia
Chrysanthemum	Houttuynia	Scutellaria
Clastanthus	Indigofera	Stephania
Codonopsis	Lentinus	Styrax
Commiphora	Ligusticum	Tussilago
Coptis	Lonicera	Uncaria
Curculigo	Manilkara	Vinca

Many of the plants that appear to be most useful belong to a category of herbs known as adaptogens. These work through a wide variety of actions to help create homeostasis or biological balance. So, for example, if the blood pressure is too high, adaptogens help the body lower it; if it is too low, the body responds by raising it. Adaptogens help normalize the system regardless of the pathology.

Studies demonstrate that adaptogenic plants are especially good at stimulating the body's own natural immune functions. For example, they have been shown to increase CD4 counts, interferon production, macrophage activity, and natural killer cell action. Adaptogens are often combined for a more potent synergistic effect. An example is astragalus and legustrum; the combination is more effective than either plant used alone.

These herbs may be helpful in an AIDS treatment protocol:

ASTRAGALUS
Astragalus membranaceous root has been used medicinally in China for centuries, and, indeed, modern scientific research shows the herb to possess powerful immune-strengthening properties. Of particular note is its ability to

foster normal immune response in cancer and AIDS patients, to correct T-cell deficiency, and to promote antiviral action.

Astragalus increases interferon production as well as phagocytosis, allowing the body to consume more pathogenic microorganisms. It also decreases tumor cell growth and lessens the suppression of the immune system caused by drugs, making it a good adjunctive therapy.

When combined with legustrum, astragalus is even more potent, and is especially good at increasing the activity of spleen cells. These two herbs are sold in combination in extract and capsule form. They can also be bought whole in Chinatown, then crushed, and then simmered in a small amount of water for several hours. The Chinese prepare herbs in this way and consume them daily.

GINSENG

Both Siberian and panax ginseng boost the immune system by increasing the number and activity of natural killer cells. These herbs work to prevent liver toxicity and are anticarcinogenic. Ginseng is best taken as an extract or a tea.

BITTER MELON

This vegetable has been popular in China, Indonesia, and the Philippines for centuries, and recently has been proven effective against HIV activity, in laboratory studies. Some AIDS patients who use the juice report substantial improvement. It reduces night sweats, helps with weight gain, and stops viral replication.

CATERPILLAR FUNGUS

This Chinese tonic has been used by people recovering from illness since ancient times. Its positive effects include strengthening of the kidneys, clearing of the lungs, and fortification of the bone marrow, an essential part of the immune system. Caterpillar fungus also inhibits bacterial and fungal infections. It is currently being used in combination with other herbs to treat malignant tumors, anemia, asthma, and most recently, AIDS.

OSHA ROOT AND LEPTOTANIA

These plants are native to the American West and an integral part of Native American medicine. Although scientific studies of their beneficial effects on the immune system have yet to be conducted, empirical evidence with viral diseases strongly suggests their use in a protocol for viral diseases.

Other plant remedies that are not characterized as adaptogens should be considered in a treatment protocol for HIV and AIDS. While there is no one magic bullet against the syndrome, combining several of these nonspecific immune enhancers can make a positive difference:

ALOE VERA

Even though aloe vera is over 99 percent water, it is a nutritionally dense substance, with over 200 active ingredients. Aloe vera contains 17 amino acids, as well as the minerals calcium, copper, iron, phosphorus, potassium, and zinc. It supplies live enzymes and essential fatty acids, which are needed for good health. Additionally, it has substances that stimulate phagocytosis, the process by which white blood cells work to destroy invading organisms.

Not all brands of aloe vera are qualitatively equal. Heat-processing destroys vital nutrients. Look for brands that cold-process the whole leaf, for maximum benefit.

CARNIVORA (VENUS FLY TRAP)

Carnivora has been proven effective against cancer, AIDS, and other chronic pathologies. According to studies, unless the immune system has been damaged by radiation and chemotherapy, many cancers will diminish, or go into remission, with its use.

Carnivora works by building the immune components of the blood. It increases the numbers of B cells, T cells, lymphocytes, granulocytes, monocytes, phagocytes, and other solid components of the immune system. Additionally, it excites inactive blood elements to begin functioning again. The immune system can then mobilize against disease-producing pathogens. They begin to attack and devour cancer cells, much like carnivora swallows and digests flies.

American laws prevent carnivora from being shipped to doctors, but the product can be mailed directly to consumers, who can then hand-deliver it to doctors. Severely compromised AIDS patients may need a two- or three-hour infusion five days a week for three to four months. As an individual improves, the treatment can be given intramuscularly, three times a week, for about two years. Carnivora can be acquired from the manufacturer, Edgar Fischer, Manager, Carnivora-Forschungs-GmBH, Postfach 8, Lobensteiner Strasse 3, D-8646 Nordhalben, Germany.

ECHINACEA

Echinacea stimulates immune cell production and activity, as well as levels of interferon and interleuken-2. The herb is usually sold as a tincture, and the best brands produce a strong tingling and numbing sensation on the tongue.

Research shows benefits to be short-term. Echinacea boosts the immune system to high levels of activity, but to do this continuously would be too much for the body. For this reason, it is best to take the extract for up to four days, and then to rest an equal length of time before starting again.

CAT'S CLAW

This rain forest herb is useful in treating numerous conditions, and may be especially important for stimulating immune system activity.

LICORICE ROOT (GLYCYRRHIZIN)

Licorice is a powerful detoxifying agent. Research shows it to inhibit the replication of HIV, with no toxicity to normal cells having been noted.

PHYLLANTHIUS (LIFE PLANT)

Traditionally used in Oriental medicine, phyllanthius is new to this country, where it is now being researched for its antiretroviral and anti-HIV activity.

ST. JOHN'S WORT

This is a common weed that is now being studied by AIDS activists because it seems to help prevent infection of T cells by making it more difficult for what we are calling the AIDS virus to get into the cells.

Homeopathy

Homeopathy works on emotional, mental, and physical levels. Treating the whole person is particularly important in AIDS and other diseases deemed incurable by allopathic medicine, as the shock of the diagnosis often triggers an emotional state that worsens the physical state of the patient.

According to classical homeopath Kevin Korins of New York City, one appropriate remedy should be chosen for each patient on an individualized basis. As symptoms change, and lessen with time, so should the remedy. When using homeopathic remedies, Korins advises, avoid mints, perfumes, and coffee. These medicines should be taken 20 minutes before eating.

IGNATIA

The person is silent, brooding, with changeable moods. There is a lot of sighing and sobbing and a great despair of being cured.

GELSEMIUM

Symptoms include listlessness and apathy. The person has a dread of being alone and wants to be with people. There is an apathy regarding the illness. Diarrhea accompanies bad news.

ARSENICUM ALBUM

For fear of dying. The person has a restless mental state, almost to the point of panic. There are periodic fevers.

THUJA

This person has a high sex drive and a history of sexually transmitted conditions, such as discharges, gonorrhea, genital warts, and herpes. There is rapid exhaustion with emaciation. The individual has fixed ideas. Often there are feelings of weakness and a feeling that one is weaker and sicker than the physical condition would warrant.

MERCURIUS

The person has a history of syphilis. Fevers and night sweats occur without amelioration. Any type of weather aggravates this person, who never feels comfortable. There are also tendencies to have swollen glands, sore throats, sores in the mouth, and thrush. Mentally, the person is paranoid, especially in the advanced stages.

ARSENICUM IODADUM

Symptoms for which this remedy is prescribed are similar to Arsenicum album, except that the person feels warmer and better in the cold. There is also a tendency to get swollen glands and periodic fevers.

IODADUM

This remedy is indicated when there is sudden emaciation with swollen glands. Despite loss of weight, there is a great appetite. Restlessness is a characteristic here.

PHOSPHORIC ACID

The person is extremely exhausted, feeling apathetic and ready to give up the fight. There is a sadness regarding the future, without fear and anxiety about death.

Thinking may be scattered.

MEDORRHINUM

Acute diseases manifest as discharges, such as bladder infections and prostatitis. There is restlessness; the person does not sleep well at night.

SYPHILINUM

The person has a lot of pain and suffering, with a great fear of not recovering. The person may have tried arsenicum first, and found that it did not really help. An extreme fear of germs is associated with this one.

PYROGENIUM

This is a remedy for septic fevers. The whole body aches and there is great restlessness from the fever. Pyrogenium is also associated with offensive odors, such as bad breath. There are sores that don't heal, and the person can go into a septic state.

BAPTISIA

Symptoms here are similar to those associated with Pyrogenium, but are less severe.

CARSINONIMA

This may help when Kaposi's sarcoma is present.

Ozone Therapy

This is one of the most important therapies for patients with AIDS or HIV to consider. During treatment, small amounts of medical ozone are introduced into the bloodstream to kill harmful microbes. The therapy activates the immune system to increase CD4 (T4) cells, and has been shown to change the HIV status of some patients from positive to negative.

HIV reversal is no small matter. Nathaniel Altman, author of *Oxygen Healing Therapies* (Health Arts Press), explains: "When I was in Cuba, I interviewed one of the chemists doing research on the subject. She said if a person infected with HIV receives ozone before it gets into the lymphatic and bone systems, HIV can be killed and stopped right on the spot."

Ozone therapy can stop intractable diarrhea, prevent the development of new opportunistic infections, and improve blood circulation, which allows more life-giving oxygen to reach tissues. It is often given in conjunction with vitamin C to enable patients to better tolerate it. When properly administered, there are no adverse side effects.

Various protocols have been developed for treating AIDS patients with ozone. An anonymous doctor (practicing in a state where ozone users are not safe from prosecution) recommends 12 treatments on 12 consecutive days. He cites dramatic improvement in patients. "Virtually all the people I have treated—and I have treated over 170—have improved their condition within days," he reports. This doctor strongly believes that for AIDS, ozone is the most important modality of all because it removes infections.

Aqueous Penicillin Treatment

According to Dr. Michael Culbert, megadoses of aqueous penicillin, as part of a total AIDS treatment program, have had highly positive effects. Culbert, who treats AIDS patients in his Mexican clinic utilizing an eclectic treatment approach, reports that advanced AIDS patients with cryptococcal meningitis, toxoplasmosis, and advanced PCP, respond favorably to a combination of aqueous penicillin, vitamin C and dioxychlor within a matter of days. This implies, Culbert asserts, that AIDS, in part, may actually be stage IV neurosyphilis, which can be managed by an unpatented old drug. Dr. Culbert can be reached at 1-800-227-4458.

Other Approaches

Naltrexone is a prescription drug that can triple killer cell activity. This inexpensive medication has been used for nine years, and no side effects have become evident in that time. Another promising and low-cost treatment, called DNCB, is a topical agent that promotes natural killer cells.

A totally different kind of approach is found in live cell therapy. This modality has been used for almost half a century in Europe and is just now being investigated in the United States for its remarkable ability to repair cells. The fetal cells of an animal are injected into a patient. The body takes in this embryonic material, and absorbs it through the macrophages. The living material develops receptor sites, which direct the immune system to take this fresh material to any matching tissue, e.g., spleen to spleen, heart to heart, thymus to thymus.

In terminal end-stage AIDS, live cell therapy may not be indicated because it may enhance cancers and other pathogens in the patient. But for patients in the early stages, with mild symptoms, this therapy may enhance their chances for survival, especially when it is accompanied by detoxification.

Yet another totally different treatment approach is urine therapy. It may sound strange, but it's not new: The practice of drinking urine is a 4,000-year-old one, recorded in Indian Ayurvedic scriptures. Today proponents of the practice claim that urine therapy is successful in the treatment of AIDS and cancer, and that there are no side effects.

Dr. Revici's Therapy

Dr. Emanuel Revici, of New York, treats people with advanced stages of pneumocystic carinii pneumonia, Kaposi's sarcoma, massive thrush, and opportunistic infections. Patients report that his nontoxic protocol results in objective and subjective measures of success; laboratory tests reveal vastly improved T-counts, and the patients feel significantly better, as they explain:

MARY

I have been HIV-positive for a very long time, probably longer than I realize. It first appeared on a test about six years ago . . . I was on methadone, a recovering addict. I never developed AIDS symptoms, but the media saying that HIV causes AIDS, over and over, made me afraid that I was going to die. I was very depressed.

My T cells dropped, and my doctor suggested AZT. But I was frightened to take it . . . [Then I} . . . started seeing Dr. Revici, which I have been doing for the past two years. I have had no deterioration at all in my condition, and I feel wonderful.

WALLACE

I am a hemophiliac and I take blood products. As I understand it, that's how I became infected. In August 1988, I was diagnosed as being HIV-positive. I had a T4 count of about 400. Then I had it checked again, and it was around 300. I was feeling good except for a prickly feeling, some kind of myopathy.

I started seeing Dr. Revici, and have been with him ever since. Dr. Revici put me on medication. The treatments were nontoxic, so I never felt any side effects. About two or three weeks later, I began feeling better, and I have been feeling great ever since. I feel very confident in what I am doing because my blood cell count has gone up. In fact, the numbers have doubled. That gives me great mental stability. I really do feel well, and I haven't had any problems.

I see another doctor for my hemophilia who tries to convince me to go on AZT and who advises me against what I am doing. He was quite surprised when I showed him my T-cell results, but oddly enough, he never asked me much about it.

JIM

I have been seeing Dr. Revici for about eight months now. He seems to have maintained my T cells; they haven't gone up or down for the past eight months. Overall, I feel terrific. I am very active, and able to exercise and work. I am not fatigued and I actually feel wonderful.

RENE

I am a 32-year-old male from LaFayette, Louisiana. I am HIV-infected. I went into the hospital with toxoplasmosis, [an] illness that plagues HIV-infected people. I heard about Dr. Revici from a doctor down here. When I went to see him, my T-cell count was at 12. Now it's up to 44. Dr. Revici said he would cure me of the toxoplasmosis and he did. Now they're working on the HIV infection.

I feel that Dr. Revici has helped my condition immensely. I have a lot of energy and I have not been plagued by any illnesses since seeing him.

JANET

I was diagnosed about two years ago with HIV, which I contracted from my husband, an intravenous drug user. I went to Dr. Revici because I wasn't feeling that good. My T cells were 200. Dr. Revici told me I had a good chance.

Since I have been seeing him, he has had me on different medications. Right now my T cells have skyrocketed to 763, and I couldn't feel better. I do a lot of jogging and other exercises. I take vitamins and I have a very good, high spirit. Dr. Revici has made a great difference in my life. I would recommend him highly. Anyone who wants to live should go and see him.

What To Avoid

Stay away from anything that weakens the immune system, including drugs, stress, excess sexual activity, and poor food choices, such as white flour, refined salt, margarine, and sugar. Studies show that sugar suppresses antibody activity for hours after consumption, which means that eating sugar regularly compromises immune health. In particular, studies show that sugar paralyzes the phagocytic activity of immune cells, so that these cells become unable to surround and destroy viruses and bacteria. Large amounts of sugar are also associated with thrush. Note that sugar is disguised in many foods as sucrose, fructose, maltose, corn syrup, and dextrose; all of these forms are detrimental to good health. There should be no caffeine, alcohol, or cigarettes used either. If animal proteins are in the diet, they must be used sparingly. These carry residues of antibiotics and steroids, which weaken the immune system.

Dairy products, especially commercial milk, can be irritating and should be avoided by the person with a weakened immune system.

Treatment Summary

It is important to remember that there are long-term AIDS survivors, and that a variety of holistic approaches exist that can be undertaken with the help of a health care professional.

The AIDS patient must be particularly careful about diet, choosing healthful, life-promoting foods, with a concentration on complex carbohydrates. Organic, whole foods should be chosen over processed foods. Of special value are fresh juices, sea vegetables, Oriental mushrooms, and garlic.

Herbs exist the world over for strengthening the immune system. Of particular note for AIDS are astragalus, especially when combined with legustrum; ginseng; and bitter melon. Echinacea, cat's claw, and other herbs are also beneficial.

Homeopathic AIDS remedies can be prescribed according to symptoms.

Large doses of intravenous and oral supplements are usually required. Antioxidant nutrients are particularly important.

Ozone therapy is one of the best modalities for reversing and overcoming AIDS, when used in conjunction with other treatments.

Live cell therapy is an approach to repairing cells that is widely used in Europe and now being investigated in the U.S.

Other approaches include treatment with dioxychlor, shark cartilage, and aqueous penicillin.

Dr. Emanuel Revici has had good results with his nontoxic AIDS treatment protocol.

Back and Neck Pain

Our prehistoric ancestors' switch from quadrupedism to an upright, two-legged posture was a great achievement. Unfortunately, this advance had a price attached: It heralded the beginning of human back and neck pain. Studies have shown that even ancient civilizations, such as the Egyptians, were plagued by these pains; in fact, they devised forms of spinal manipulative therapy using their hands and other parts of the body as levers. Today, approximately 80 percent of all people will experience back pain at some point during their lives. While neck pain is not quite as common as back pain, the two together are responsible for millions of lost work hours and billions of dollars of lost earnings, not to mention untold human unhappiness.

Back ailments are especially problematic in the industrialized nations of the world, where people have lost touch with natural ways of working and using their bodies and are thus more prone to overexertion and injury. Backaches become a recurring affliction in over half the people who have them, and at present there are over a million people in the U.S. who have been disabled by back pain. One study revealed that, yearly, there are approximately 19 million patients who visit doctors with this complaint.

Who is the typical back pain patient? Most people with back discomfort are age 30 or older. And people who are overweight, especially in the abdominal region, are more likely than their slimmer counterparts to be afflicted with lower back pain because of the greater amount of pressure and strain being placed upon this region. If there is a variance in the length of a person's legs, with one leg being 1/2 or 3/4 of an inch shorter than the other, there is often an imbalance, or mechanical dysfunction, in the person's gait and distribution of weight, which can lead to back pain. Other causes of back pain can be spinal curvature, as well as poor muscle tone in the lower back and abdominal regions. Finally, a major characteristic associated with the onset of back pain is the presence of unusually high stress, which can be caused by anxiety, tension, fatigue, or depression.

The workplace is often not a back-friendly place. Over half of back-related injuries are caused by the lifting of equipment or products on the job. Vibration of factory equipment tends to traumatize the spinal cord, while driving can severely aggravate lower back pain. Industrial workers who engage in prolonged bending, twisting, heavy manual labor, and repetitive processes are prime candidates for backaches. For both blue collar and white collar employees, the maintenance of continuously static postures at the workplace is yet another cause of back pain. And for both, stress related to dissatisfaction with working conditions can contribute to the physical pain.

Back injuries can have lasting financial and psychological effects on workers, in that employees who miss work for prolonged periods as a result of backaches often do not have a job to return to. Furthermore, studies have shown that, of disabled workers who are out more than three months, those with back problem suffer more from emotional distress than do those forced to stay out as a result of injury to the extremities. Some employers, who stand to lose millions of dollars in disability payments and lost hours, have instituted "back schools" at the workplace to teach their employees how to properly bend, lift, and stand.

Symptoms

Back and neck pain can vary widely in severity, ranging from mild sensation to excruciating suffering that warrants immediate medical attention. Usually, the appearance of certain symptoms requires medical attention. A burning or tingling sensation, or numbness in the arms, back, or legs accompanying back pain warrants a visit to a medical practitioner. Also, increasing severity of pain in the back or neck, or a lack of improvement in your condition despite the application of self-help remedies, is an indication that professional advice should be sought. The concomitant appearance of a fever, with or without a headache, is yet another indicator, as is complete immobilization.

The Importance of Seeking Treatment

When the proper therapy or combination of therapies is used, back pain patients can usually experience significant improvement in their physical condition. As there are an infinite number of possible ways to injure your back, so there is not one single treatment approach that can be applied to everyone. However, one can say that, generally, a patient's lifestyle needs to be looked into when he or she is being treated for back pain, because this often reveals why the problem has arisen in the first place.

Many times people, especially men, ignore back problems until they are in severe pain, and only then seek medical attention. This is not the model to follow. If the patient deals with the problem at its onset, extraordinary pain will probably never develop. And while studies have been conducted indicating that people with backaches are capable of recovering on their own after several months, these reports neglect the fact that people who recover are likely to experience recurrences of greater severity at a later time. In addition, people who initially recover as a result of exercise and then discontinue their exercise programs can also experience severe recurrences. It is important to note too that a lack of symptoms does not necessarily signify that the underlying condition no longer poses a threat. In short, evidence indicates that people who follow medical advice recover more quickly and suffer from fewer recurrences.

Professional Assistance

There are numerous people one can consult when suffering from back pain, but only some are capable of offering suitable treatment. Most individuals who seek professional help initiate their treatment with a medical doctor, such as an orthopedic surgeon, but eventually turn to nonmedical practitioners after experiencing unsatisfactory results. This is usually due to the medical establishment's failure to acknowledge exercise as an alternative treatment, or stress as a possible cause of the pain.

Orthopedic doctors, who specialize in injuries related to the muscles, joints, bones, tendons, and ligaments, are often inexperienced with conservative methods of treatment and are sometimes too willing to engage in unnecessary surgery. The problem is that surgery has limited long-range benefits and is completely unnecessary for many lower back pain sufferers. When confronted with pain caused by a factor that does not show up on an x-ray, an orthopedist will generally refer the patient to another professional. If you are going to an orthopedic specialist for advice on back pain, it is recommended that you see one who does not reflexively advocate surgery or prolonged reliance on prescription drugs.

Internists and general practitioners are generally more versatile than orthopedists in their approach to helping patients cope with back pain. They're more apt to delve into their patients' lifestyles and exercise habits, and more willing to initiate a wide variety of treatments that do not involve dependence on prescriptions. Internists often have a close relationship with their patients and are truly interested in helping them solve their problems. Also, an internist or general practitioner may be more open than an orthopedist to making a referral to an alternative practitioner, such as an acupuncturist.

Neurosurgeons rely on surgery and drug prescriptions to alleviate back pain, but the surgical alternative should be resorted to only when all others have failed. If a neurosurgeon suggests an operation as a back pain cure, it's a good idea to get several other opinions, both from other neurosurgeons and from doctors in other fields. When making a decision on surgery versus alternative methods of coping with the pain, one must factor in the risks of the surgery and the difficulty of rehabilitation. **Neurologists** should also be approached with caution because of their dependence on prescription drugs, such as antidepressants and antipsychotics, which can have adverse side effects.

Physiatrists, who specialize in rehabilitative medicine, are dedicated to helping their patients discover the cause of their pain. They generally investigate all aspects of their patients' lives until they find the source of pain, are quite responsive to the needs of their patients, and do not rely heavily on drugs. What they do is develop special treatment programs for their patients, which may involve a variety of techniques such as hydrotherapy, ice, exercise, heat, and even manipulation. Unfortunately, there are fewer than 2000 physiatrists in the entire U.S.

Acupuncturists can be quite helpful in alleviating back pain, and they provide virtually risk-free care. Because acupuncture is not a part of orthodox Western medicine, many Americans are reluctant to try it, but those who have are often impressed with the results.

Rheumatologists' specialty is treating pain that is a result of arthritis. Back pain with a gynecological basis can sometimes be treated by an **obstetrician** or **gynecologist,** but their expertise in regard to general pain is also quite limited. **Sports medicine specialists** have achieved some short-term success with athletes suffering from chronic pain, but generally, they are not recommended for long-term relief.

Chiropractors have enjoyed widespread success in treating back pain and, consequently, have become the primary source for nonmedicinal care in this area. Chiropractors treat approximately 60 million patients annually, which is about three times the number seen by regular physicians. Their therapy consists mainly of a variety of manipulative reflex techniques, from low-force and low-velocity manipulation to powerful and deep manipulation, depending on the needs of the individual. Evidence has indicated that gentle manipulation of the spine contributes to the release of endorphins, which are opiates produced by the body that help it cope with pain, including spinal pain caused by disc disease. Also, chiropractors often use nutrition as part of their treatment, because patients' eating habits can be directly connected to their strength and ability to recover. Clinical evidence reveals that patients who are malnourished will not effectively respond to manipulation.

Chiropractors can be expected to study the lifestyles of their patients, as this often reveals the cause of pain. They usually design exercise programs for their patients, which is crucial for maintaining relief over the long term. Drug therapy, on the other hand, they generally regard as useless in the treatment of lower back pain, feeling that it can even be dangerous.

Physical therapists are helpful in treating an assortment of back problems, but they can only treat after they receive consent from a licensed medical doctor. In addition to exercise and education, their healing arsenal includes electrical muscle stimulation, ultrasound, and trancutaneous electrical nerve stimulation (TENS). Physical therapists are qualified in aiding patients who suffer from weak or tight muscles and can correctly evaluate posture and sleeping position. Sometimes, they offer at-home service for patients who are in serious pain.

A nonmedical method of coping with back pain is participation in yoga, exercises that use the strengthening and stretching of muscles, ligaments, and tendons crucial to long-term rehabilitation. Despite yoga's helpfulness in alleviating back pain, inexperienced participants should be warned that engaging in yoga while experiencing pain can complicate back problems further. People interested in yoga should find a qualified instructor; the personal touch here is much superior to an instructional video.

Although **massage therapists** trained in Swedish massage may offer immediate relief and pleasure, they usually are not trained to offer self-care advice, and do not provide the long-term rehabilitation program that is essential. **Shiatsu,** a 20th-century Japanese massage technique that is something like acupuncture without the needles, can be used in the treatment of minimal lower back pain, but is too complex to try on your own. Relatively controversial is the technique called **Rolfing,** which involves using fingertips, knuckles, and elbows to deeply probe the muscles in order to relieve them from tightness, adhesions, and malfunctions. The **Alexander technique,** which was devised by 19th-century actor Frederick Mathias Alexander, is based on the philosophy that back pain is a result of misusing the body. This abuse may be caused by physical elements, such as standing or moving incorrectly, or by emotional factors such as stress. The Alexander technique can be a useful treatment for maintaining rehabilitation, but initial treatment by another trained professional is suggested.

Self-Help

When suffering from back pain, you should use ice during the initial 24 to 48 hours, applying it, wrapped in a towel if this is most comfortable, for 20-minute periods. Heat should not be used during this initial period because it will irritate the inflammation, but it can be used after the first 48 hours of pain. Sometimes you can vary your treatment with four minutes of a hot compress followed by one minute of cold.

After your back has recovered, do not immediately resume exercise. Many times people engage in full range of motion (ROM) exercises immediately and continue to do so even after feeling recurrences of pain. If you feel pain while performing ROM exercises, this signifies that you are not ready to do these exercises and should regress to an easier form that does not cause pain.

Nevertheless, do remember that regular exercise should serve as the basis for a proper self-help regimen. If you exercise consistently your body will be able to recover more quickly from an injury and there will be less chance of a recurrence. After receiving care—and your initial exercise go-ahead—from a health care professional, it is important to maintain your rehabilitation by adhering to an exercise program that suits your needs. Exercise that creates bodily aggravation should be immediately discontinued, and warm-up and cool-down exercises should be integral parts of your routine. Strenuous exercise immediately after you awaken is not recommended because your body lacks nutritional sustenance and your muscles are not prepared for any type of vigorous action at that particular time. Your routine should consist of a careful balance of light exercise, such as biking or swimming, and more difficult exercises. If you are lifting any type of heavy weight, forward bending—a common irritant of back problems—should not be practiced.

Before commencing your regular exercise, it is imperative to stretch smoothly and gently, avoiding jerky motions. Muscles need to be warmed up before they engage in rigorous activity, and a proper warm-up routine will enable the muscles to effectively respond to the body's increasing demands. Some people need more time to warm up than others, but in general, each stretching exercise should last at least 15 to 20 seconds.

When stretching the muscles, ligaments, and tendons, concentrate on the movements your body is making and be alert to any subtle twinges of pain. Be aware too that when stretching tight muscles, you shouldn't overexert your body by stretching past the point of joint resistance, as this will only cause discomfort later. Stretching can be quite therapeutic, but only if you are aware of the signals your body is giving you. Feelings of pain, fatigue, or stiffness should provide an instant cue to stop what you are doing. Some popular stretches include trunk rotations, extension lifts, cat stretches, elbow props, pelvic swings, hip rolls, knee-to-chest rocking exercises, back leg swings, and hand and knee exercises.

Stretching properly can provide a multitude of advantages for the body. First of all, it can improve the body's full range of motion (ROM) because the muscles loosen up and become increasingly more mobile. As you become proficient in stretching, the amount of pain associated with the body's movement will decrease as a result of increased circulation throughout the muscles. The muscles will begin to pump additional blood, causing improvements in your pulse rate, blood pressure, and overall strength. Stretching also contributes to the detoxification of the body because it increases venous drainage.

Once you've stretched, beneficial exercises include brisk walking while swinging the arms and breathing deeply, skipping or jumping rope, swimming, and bicycling. All of these exercises help to improve circulation, which is important for the healing process. Since a strong abdominal region is vital to increasing back strength, pushups and knee pushups, which strengthen both the upper body muscles and abdomen, are also advantageous. People with a history of back ailments should start out doing three to five repetitions of each exercise and work their way up to doing ten. But if pain is experienced during the performance of an exercise, the exercise should be discontinued immediately. Remember not to strain your body, and do not hesitate to seek professional advice if a pain persists.

According to chiropractor Dr. Allen Pressman, athletic activities can be divided into three categories as a guide for back and neck patients. The first group, low-risk activities, includes water aerobics, ballroom dancing, cycling, horseback riding, ice skating, basketball, the martial arts, skiing (without the falling aspect), soccer, swimming, and yoga. Medium-risk activities are badminton, baseball, jogging, sailing, squash, racquetball, tennis, volleyball, and wrestling. Some medium-risk activities, notes Pressman, should be considered high-risk for people with especially injury-prone backs or necks. The high-risk category includes such activities as aerobics, ballet, football, gymnastics, rowing, track and field, diving, weight training, and surfing. Activities in this final group should be avoided by people with back or neck problems, or should be performed under close supervision. Aerobics and jazzercise are quite popular, and they can be a lot of fun, but they often involve bending, twisting, and jerky motions, which can aggravate an injured back. So if you want to move on to these advanced forms of exercise, be sure to build up your fitness level at an easier low-impact level.

A final caveat concerning your exercise regimen: Rest, as well as movement, is an integral part of it. In order to fully reap the benefits of stretching and exercise, the body requires rest and relaxation after its workout to allow time for the muscles to repair themselves and grow.

To Prevent Reinjury

To prevent reinjury to your back, there are several guidelines people who partake in athletic activities should obey. First, don't overtrain, because this can cause the body to behave as if it were in a constant state of stress. Eventually this stress will become too difficult for the body to handle, and an injury will result. The definition of overtraining, of course, varies from individual to individual, with people in better shape able to sustain more vigorous activity. People who have had a history of back problems should beware of participating in contact sports, as this type of activity is notorious for provoking reinjury. And remember to avoid fatigue, which will hamper your ability to correctly perform your stretches and exercise.

Eating a healthy diet is an important factor in avoiding reinjury; it also enables the body to heal quickly from back or neck pain. A nutritious diet with the correct amount of calories will prevent infection and the loss of muscle, and note that people who become involved in difficult training routines sometimes need to increase their caloric intake by up to 200 percent. A proper diet consists of at least 50 to 60 percent complex carbohydrates, such as fruits and vegetables, potatoes, pasta, and rice, and requires few or no simple carbohydrates, such as sugar. Those who suffer from injuries will need to increase the percentage of protein in their diet to approximately 18 to 20 percent.

Be aware of your nutrient status. Deficiencies of iron, zinc, and other antioxidants should be avoided because an insufficient intake of these nutrients can impair the body's ability to heal, cause a breakdown of connective tissue, and prolong the inflammation period. It's a good idea to take 25,000 IU of vitamin A and 30 mg of zinc per day to aid in tissue repair. In general, 50 mg of B-complex vitamins daily is recommended, and a minimum of 1000 to 2000 mg of vitamin C can be especially helpful for healing back injuries. When taking C, remember to apportion your intake so that you are not taking more than 1000 mg (1 g) at a time. Calcium and magnesium in a 1-to-1 ratio, and 10 to 50 mg per day of manganese are additional nutrients that can aid the healing process.

Reinjury frequently occurs as a result of a person's inability to correctly perform a particular exercise or stretch. Many people like to watch television while exercising, which causes them to be distracted and prevents them from concentrating on the body's movement. During the healing process it is imperative to be wary of exercises that have caused or might aggravate an injury. Allow ample time for the body to readjust to your exercise regimen. It is also important to wear the proper attire while training. Sneakers that do not fit right do more than hurt the feet; they can cause a multitude of injuries to different parts of the body, especially the joints. Clothing that is too tight will prevent proper movement, in addition to not allowing sweat to evaporate.

Avoiding Back and Neck Pain

Preventing a back or neck injury from occurring in the first place is preferable to having to deal with one once it happens. First, be aware of proper lifting technique. Although the act of lifting may seem quite simple, improperly done it causes an astounding number of injuries. The correct method involves bending the knees and using the quadriceps and hamstring muscles in your legs to support the weight of the object. Thus, the lower back is spared strain.

Second, to minimize the chance of neck and back problems, see if you can reduce the amount of prolonged stress in your life. If reducing your stress level is out of the question, try to find outlets to cope with the stress, so it will not have physically adverse effects. Also, correct posture is vital to averting back and neck pain, so try to refrain from slouching and slumping. People who suspect that they have a posture problem should have their posture evaluated by a trained professional, such as a chiropractor. And since a significant portion of back injuries are caused by foot or ankle problems, people involved in athletic activities such as running or walking should wear footwear that provides adequate support. Also, women should be wary of continual use of high heels.

When working out at the gym or at home, be sure that your clothes are loose-fitting. When walking with a briefcase or gym bag, do not overload it, and shift the bag from one side of the body to the other periodically to avoid a weight imbalance. An overweight body places a tremendous amount of strain on the lower back region, causing eventual pain and suffering, so keeping trim is a good back-preserving strategy.

If you're sitting or driving for long periods, support your back with a rolled-up towel or other supportive material. In addition, avoid sitting in uncomfortable chairs or chairs that are too soft, and make sure that your wallet is not causing an imbalance in your posture. It is important to shift your weight frequently, because continuously sitting on the same place can lead to injury. Finally, avoid crossing your legs for extended periods; instead, maintain a straight posture with your feet flat on the ground. People who have had back problems in the past should try not to sit for more than a half hour without getting up to stretch.

When you are about to stand up from a seated position you can follow a simple procedure that will prevent you from irritating your bad back. First, push yourself gently to the edge of your seat, with one foot placed carefully in front of the other. Remember to use the quadriceps and hamstrings in your legs to lift yourself, refrain from leaning forward, and keep a vertical center of gravity when rising.

Driving can easily aggravate an injured back, so when you are experiencing back pain you should try to stay away from your automobile. If you do have to drive, bring your seat as close to the steering wheel as possible, allowing the knees to rise above the hips. After 30 minutes of driving you should pull over to the side of the road and allow your body some time to stretch. At break time, passengers suffering from back pain should lay down on the back seat, bend their knees, and try to relax their body.

When purchasing a mattress, back pain sufferers should stay away from extra-firm ones as well as from overly soft mattresses and waterbeds. A medium-firm mattress is your best bet. In the morning, you should move your body to one side of the bed, shift onto your side, pull your knees upward, drop your feet carefully to the ground, sit up slowly, and finally, stand up using the proper technique previously described. Be sure to avoid bending at the waist when rising, as this can be detrimental to an injured back.

Treatment Summary

People who follow medical advice recover more quickly from back pain and have fewer recurrences.

Surgery should be used only after other methods of dealing with back pain have failed.

In addition to mainstream medical practitioners, acupuncturists and chiropractors can offer significant help to those suffering from back and neck pain.

The Alexander technique may be useful in maintaining rehabilitation after an injury.

First aid measures taken immediately after an injury can prevent inflammation, and reduce pain.

To prevent reinjury, athletes need to remember to rest, not to overtrain, and to perform stretches correctly.

Eating a nutritious diet speeds up the healing process.

Breast Cancer

While in 1950 only one in 20 women suffered from breast cancer, today this figure has risen to one in eight. Although the medical establishment has recommended early diagnosis via periodic breast examinations and mammograms, less stress has been placed on possible causes of the disease and preventive measures. Yet it's these last areas of understanding that hold the most promise.

Causes

A family history of breast cancer does put one at higher risk for the disease. But there's so very much more that comes in to play. Medical evidence indicates that prolonged exposure to the female sex hormone estrogen as a result of either an early onset of menstruation or a late menopause increases the chance for acquisition of breast cancer. In addition, women who have not had children or have not breast-fed are at higher risk of developing breast cancer, implying that the female sex hormone progesterone can serve as a preventive agent. Estrogen and progesterone are usually equally balanced, but when the amount of estrogen increases or the amount of progesterone decreases, an imbalance, known as estrogen dominance, is created. Increased levels of estrogen are associated with a high alcohol intake, being overweight, and consuming a lot of fatty foods. Also, people who eat large quantities of meat are more susceptible to breast cancer due to the estrogen-stimulating hormones that are frequently used to improve the texture of meat products.

A diet that is high in fat has other adverse effects upon the body. One is that when a person consumes a large amount of fatty food the membranes of body cells can become damaged by the fat. After this occurs, the cell can either die and eventually be replaced by another cell, or it can attempt to repair the damage that has been done. During the latter process it is possible for the damaged cell to transform itself into a cancer cell while attempting to fix itself.

The liver, which is responsible for the elimination of estrogen and other hazardous materials, is often overwhelmed by the abundance of toxic substances that find their way into the human body each day. Problems with the breakdown of estrogen by the liver can also be compounded by the presence of excessive amounts of sugar or alcohol.

The presence of foreign chemicals in the body known as xenoestrogens can be troublesome. While forms of xenoestrogen that are derived from plant foods can have positive effects on the body, forms that originate from synthetic materials such as fuel, pesticides, or plastics have proved to be carcinogenic.

Another possible cause of breast cancer is a dysfunction in the lymphatic system, which is responsible for the drainage of toxic substances from the tissues. The lymphatic system is essential to the body's immune system and aids in the removal of the xenoestrogens that can accumulate in the fatty tissue of the breast. The flow of lymphatic fluid, which carries the body's toxins and waste products away from the cells, is not analogous to that of blood, as it can be interrupted by muscle contraction and external force. It is important to note that an excessively constrictive bra can be a cause of lymphatic blockage, and that, eventually, the accumulation of harmful materials within the breast can lead to cancer. Studies have indicated that wearing a bra for more than 12 hours a day is correlated with an increased incidence of breast cancer; therefore, it is advisable to limit the wearing of a bra as much as possible and to beware of bras that may constrict the flow of waste products from the breast.

The absorption of excessive amounts of radiation, such as medical x-rays, can be a causal factor in breast cancer. Years ago doctors were ignorant of the dangers of radiation because the manifestation of harmful side effects can take decades. Consequently, the amount of ''rads'' a patient received was not a cause for concern, and many treatment procedures, such as fluoroscopic examinations, exposed patients to excessive radiation numerous times a year. Excessive exposure to harmful rays can lead to chromosomal damage, and eventually, to various forms of cancer. Dr. John Gofman of the University of California at Berkeley, who investigated the correlation between x-rays and breast cancer, has asserted that up to 90 percent of all cases of breast cancer can be attributed to overexposure to x-rays. It is true that during the past few decades radiological facilities have been forced to lower their dosages dramatically, but there is still substantial room for improvement. Dr. Gofman feels that pressure should be applied to the medical community to further reduce dosages. And he recommends that people alert themselves to the potential dangers of medical x-rays and insist that when they receive an x-ray, a low dosage is administered.

Studies have demonstrated that excessive absorption of electromagnetic radiation, which can be emitted from common household objects like televisions, digital clocks, and microwave ovens, contributes to the development of breast cancer in men and women by preventing the production of melatonin in the pineal gland during the sleeping cycle. Numerous tests have been conducted in this field, including one that revealed a cancer rate directly proportional to the use of electric blankets.

Some studies have also shown that the performance of a mastectomy during the first phase of the menstrual cycle can increase the possibility of a recurrence of breast cancer. During the first half of the menstrual cycle, only estrogen is produced, and when a mastectomy is done at this time the small quantity of cancer cells left behind may have their growth enhanced by the estrogen. On the other hand, mastectomies performed after the first half of the menstrual cycle have been more successful. The recurrence rate is halved due to the presence of progesterone, which enables the cells to differentiate.

Other factors that are contributory to breast cancer are use of alcohol and tobacco products. Nicotine is the second largest cause of breast cancer (after elevated estrogen levels due to dietary and environmental factors). And the consumption of only two to three alcoholic beverages a week increases breast cancer risk significantly.

Symptoms

Early symptoms of breast cancer are thickening of the breast, a lump, and dimpling of the skin. The person may experience pain, ulcers, nipple discharge, and swollen lymph glands under the arm at a later time.

After the manifestation of any of these symptoms, you should immediately seek professional assistance. When a diagnosis of breast cancer is confirmed, there are several facts that one should be aware of. First, the survival rate is dependent on whether or not the cancer has spread to the regional lymph nodes, on the size of the cancerous region within the breast, on how fast-growing the tumor is, and finally, on whether or not the cancer has spread to other parts of the body. During the initial, very localized, stage of breast cancer known as stage 0, the 5-year survival rate is approximately 90 percent. If the cancer has spread to the lymph nodes above the collarbone or to other vital organs (stage 4), the 5-year survival rate is only 10 percent. This is why early diagnosis is stressed.

Treatments

The mainstream medical establishment often prescribes mastectomy, radiation, and chemotherapy to treat breast cancer, an approach that has been described as a slash and burn strategy. This approach may be in for a reappraisal with the recent insight by the medical world that breast cancer is actually three different diseases, with indistinct boundaries, rather than one. In other words, only some breast cancers fit the image of a disease that is fast-growing and fast-spreading. Two other categories of this condition exist, the slowest-growing of which may never spread or be life-threatening at all. With this realization comes the idea that giving everyone with breast cancer chemotherapy may be unnecessary. Considering the harmful effects of chemotherapy, the belated nature of this realization is disturbing, to say the least.

A bottom line in understanding breast cancer remains that lifestyle as an important factor should never be ignored. Consider that women in our country suffer from one of the highest breast cancer rates in the world, while women in Japan have one of the lowest. The message here is that some cases of breast cancer can be avoided if we make needed changes, adopting some of the ways of Asian culture. Studies have shown that the consumption of cleansing herbs; lessened levels of stress, alcohol, and tobacco intake; enforcement of stringent pollution laws; and lower levels of dangerous radiation are factors that work to the advantage of women in Asian countries.

Diet and Supplements

One of the most important steps to take in preventing breast cancer is to avoid a diet that is high in animal fat while at the same time increasing consumption of fruits, vegetables, beans, and whole grains. The abundance of fiber in vegetarian diets helps the colon dispose of unnecessary estrogen, while the low fiber and high iron content of beef and processed foods can damage cells and encourage the spread of cancer. In addition, some foods, such as lima beans, soy beans, and other soy products, seem to have medicinal capabilities because of the presence of isoflavones and phytoestrogens, or plant estrogens. These substances actually curb the activity of the excess estrogen in the body's tissues. Phytoestrogens can also be found in other vegetables and in fruits, along with useful amounts of nonsoluble fiber, beta carotene, and selenium. Flaxseeds and certain types of fish, including salmon, tuna, sardines, mackerel, and herring, contain omega-3 fatty acids, which have an anticancer effect. The consumption of broccoli, cauliflower, Brussels sprouts, and other cruciferous vegetables is also recommended to combat cancer. The daily addition of acidophilus and approximately an ounce of wheat fiber to the diet can further enhance the colon's ability to eliminate estrogen. An adequate amount of wheat fiber can be obtained by taking two tablespoons of raw wheat bran per day. Finally, evidence has shown that reishi, shiitake, and maitake mushrooms can serve as formidable opponents of cancer cells.

Supplements of vitamin D can protect the body from breast cancer, especially if you are deficient in phosphorus, but do not exceed 400 IU per day without medical supervision. Medical evidence has indicated that the prevention of breast cancer may also be related to consuming the proper ratio of calcium to phosphorous. The optimal ratio is 1.5:1, but most people have a greater phosphorus intake because of the presence of meat in their diets. Although meat products contain calcium, the phosphorus content can push the calcium out of the tissues and into the bloodstream, where it eventually lodges in the walls of the arteries and in the joints.

Damage to the tissues of the breast can be avoided with a proper intake of antioxidants. Many doctors are currently recommending the following important nutrients to prevent the onset of breast cancer: between 10,000 and 25,000 units of beta carotene, 100 mg of coenzyme Q10, the mineral germanium, DMG (dimethyl glycine), two capsules of garlic three times a day, 400 IU of vitamin E, and up to 10,000 mg of vitamin C taken as divided doses throughout the day. Other doctors have stressed that the body requires the proper amounts of calcium, magnesium, selenium, chromium, alpha linolenic acid, and molybdenum, all of which can be supplemented if a deficiency develops. Borage, evening primrose, and black currant seed oils contain a cancer-fighting agent known as gamma linoleic acid. In addition, in order for the bodily protein SOD to function correctly and prevent oxidation damage in the cells, we must avoid deficiencies of zinc, copper, and manganese. A nutritionally oriented physician can help you decide which nutrients are most important for you, and in what amounts.

Herbs

Numerous herbs are protective against breast cancer. The Venus fly trap has become quite popular in Europe. On this side of the Atlantic, the native American herbal formula called Essiac is used to prevent cancer and treat cancer that is already present. Cat's claw, an herb used by Peruvian Indians, is another known cancer combatant. Xiao Yao Wan, a Chinese combination of digestive herbs that people take to improve circulation, build blood, and treat fibroids, is often used to combat breast cancer as well. Astragalus can aid in preventing and treating breast cancer by enhancing the immune system, and is especially useful for people undergoing chemotherapy who need to regain strength. One teaspoon of the herb should be added to purified water and consumed once or twice daily. Other herbal solutions for avoiding breast cancer use echinacea, pau d'arco, sassafras, red clover, and burdock, which improve the immune system and purify the blood. Studies have also shown that extracts of mistletoe can be of use for immunity enhancement.

Detoxification

Activities that detoxify the body can further reduce the chance of acquiring breast cancer. For instance, aerobic exercise assists in lymphatic drainage and induces sweating, which is a natural way for the body to rid itself of waste products. And exercise has in fact been shown by studies to be correlated with a lowered breast cancer risk. The removal of hazardous waste products by the lymphatic system can be aided by manual lymphatic drainage, which involves a light massage that stimulates the lymph nodes and enables them to properly dispose of waste. As mentioned earlier, the blockage of the lymph fluid in the breast, which can occur after the performance of a mastectomy, allows potentially dangerous substances to collect in the breast, eventually leading to cancer.

Immuno-Augmentative Therapy

The restoration of the immune system can enable a patient to successfully control cancer without a need for toxic chemical treatments. Immuno-Augmentative Therapy attempts to accomplish this using noninvasive treatment, and caters to the unique needs of each individual by studying the contents of the patient's blood and correcting factors that may contribute to cancer. This method of therapy, devised during the 1950's by Dr. Lawrence Burton and his associates, has been successfully used with numerous breast cancer patients, and is performed outside the United States in Freeport's (Bahamas) Immunology Research Center, by Dr. Burton's successor, Dr. John Clement.

Psychoneuroimmunology

A new branch of science, known as psychoneuroimmunology, studies the integration of thoughts, emotions, and physical reactions at the cellular level. When a person feels depressed for extended periods of time, this state of mind can have an adverse effect on the body's ability to fight off disease and to heal itself. On the other hand, positive emotions can aid in maintaining or regaining physical health.

According to Dr. Carl Simonton, director of the Simonton Cancer Center in California, women who are diagnosed with breast cancer should work to overcome the stereotypes associated with cancer. Women in this position are often under the impression that their cancer can easily overwhelm and destroy their health, and that their bodies will be severely victimized by harsh treatments. If a person has this defeatist attitude, then her body will read these signals and act accordingly. It is important for patients to evaluate their thoughts about the disease, the treatment, and their chances of recovery, and to remain confident.

One way to improve one's psychological and physical health, and to lessen one's chance of breast cancer, is through meditation. Studies report this fact, and give the explanation that women who meditate have more melatonin in their blood than women who do not. This is the case because the pineal gland, which secretes melatonin, is sensitive to psychological processes, and in turn, is important because melatonin is known to inhibit estrogen, and breast cancer is associated with higher levels of estrogen in the body.

What to Avoid

There are a multitude of precautions we can take to prevent breast cancer. First of all, it is utterly foolish to abuse tobacco and alcohol products, as medical evidence has linked these directly to various forms of cancer, including breast cancer. Furthermore, we know that estrogen is a risk factor, so fatty food, which increase levels of this hormone, are to be avoided. Also, consider that an excessively fatty diet can induce free radical production, resulting in the damage of healthy cells and their eventual conversion to cancerous cells. Be especially careful to curtail processed meat products, margarine, and other saturated fats. Beware too of excessive intake of hot, spicy foods, oily foods, foods high in sugar, and stimulants such as coffee, tea, and recreational narcotics. Another precaution we can take is to avoid unnecessary exposure to X-rays and other forms of radiation. And remember to try to limit your use of bras to less than 12 hours per day, and do not purchase a constrictive bra that may impede lymphatic drainage. Finally, be aware of the quality of the water that you consume, as many urban and suburban water supplies require filtration of fluoride and chlorine.

Treatment Summary

There is a proven correlation between high-fat diets and breast cancer. Conversely, populations that eat more fruit, vegetables, and legumes, with an emphasis on soy products, have lower incidences of the disease.

Extra protection from breast cancer can be obtained with vitamin C, vitamin D, a proper ratio of calcium to phosphorus (higher in the former), and antioxidant nutrients.

Herbs provide extra protection from breast cancer; especially noteworthy are the Venus fly trap, the herbal formula Essiac, cat's claw, astragalus, and pau d'arco.

Aerobic exercise and manual lymphatic drainage rid the body of stored-up wastes that can otherwise lead to cancer.

Some people have success with Immuno-Augmentative Therapy, a nontoxic, noninvasive approach to treatment.

The new field of psychoneuroimmunotherapy stresses positive emotions and meditation as health and healing promoters.

Breast Implant Reactions

Are breast implants safe? The answer is that anything placed within the body has a good chance of poisoning it. Silicone is not compatible with human body tissue, and will cause everything from mild irritation, fatigue, and depression to severe pain. Such silicone reactions show up as abnormal immunological responses on blood tests. In time, breasts that were once soft and supple turn into hard lumps, and well-shaped ones become grotesquely deformed. Even so-called safe saline implants are contained within a silicone sack. Pieces of silicone mix with tissue, even when the capsule remains intact.

Women usually shun the idea of implant removal, fearing that their breasts will look worse than before. Their surgeons tell them that their breasts are too stretched out for corrective surgery. Indeed, it is true that up until recently, most operations resulted in gross breast deformity.

Treatment

Obviously prevention—not having implants put in in the first place—is the best course to take. But in a society that judges women by their appearance, actresses, models, and even average young women often feel pressured into getting implants, especially when they are not warned of the potential dangers.

Breast Conservation Surgery

Fortunately, there is a new procedure for removing breast implants without ruining a woman's appearance. Dr. Vicki Hufnagel has pioneered a surgical technique using an argon beam to remove implants without having the breasts cave in. The beam sprays heat to the area and is able to shrink tissue without burning the body. The technique also restores the healthy growth of breast tissue. Hufnagel reports great success and spends much of her time educating doctors on this method.

If you have implants, it is best to have them removed. Use a doctor with a high success rate; speak with that doctor's former patients. And whether or not you decide to have the implants removed, it is important to report any problems from breast implants to the Food and Drug Administration. This will help other women in the future.

Treatment Summary

With everything we know today about the dangers associated with breast implants, the best course of action is to avoid getting them.

A new surgical technique uses an argon beam to remove breast implants without causing a deformity.

Cancer

Cancer refers to a group of diseases in which cells deviate from the usual controls that regulate cellular growth and reproduction. They begin to multiply more rapidly than is normal, invading and destroying other body cells. Cancerous cells can spread, or metastasize, from their primary site to other parts of the body through the bloodstream and lymphatic system.

The most common form of cancer is the carcinoma. This is a tumor that originates in the skin, in the epithelial tissue that lines the body, or in glandular tissue, such as the breast or prostate gland. Another type of cancer is the sarcoma, affecting connective and supportive tissue, such as bone, muscle, cartilage, and fat. Melanomas are a type of skin cancer; lymphomas affect the lymphatic system; and leukemias are cancers of the blood-forming organs.

Causes

Cancer is largely attributable to the cumulative impact of toxins on our systems. External factors, such as polluted air, water, and food, play a major role, as do microscopic pathogens in our internal environment, such as parasites, fungi, bacteria, viruses, and toxic chemicals, including heavy metals. Genetic tendencies and immunological weakness come into play, and psychological factors are also believed to affect the incidence and course of cancer.

Lifestyle Factors

Over half of all cancers have been linked to lifestyle factors, with some estimates as high as 70 percent. Prime among these factors is the altered state of our nutrition. More than 60 percent of all women's cancers and 40 percent of men's have been attributed to nutritional losses incurred as a result of modern farming and food industry practices.

Before the 1940s, most food was organically grown. Then, the widespread introduction of pesticides, fertilizers, antibiotics, and mono-crop farming changed the face of agriculture forever, and with it, the health of consumers. These changes were coupled with the increased promotion of processed foods designed for long shelf-life and addictive tastes, but filled with empty calories. Today, chemically grown and denatured foods and drugs are the norm; these include such poisons as processed meats, caffeinated tea and coffee, soft drinks, liquor, tobacco, meat, white sugar, white flour, and margarine.

Modern diets create a state of chronic toxicity and slow down the organs of elimination: the bowels, kidneys, liver, lungs, and skin. Poisons eventually accumulate around the weakest organs and set the stage for the development of cancer. Three ways an inadequate diet harms the system are through nutrient depletion, free radical damage, and a shift in pH levels.

Nutrient depletion may be the result of gross deficiencies of certain nutrients over long periods of time. An analogy can be drawn between the body's nutrient supply and a reservoir of water. Ideally, a reservoir should be full and able to trickle over slightly. When levels are lower, people can still fish and boat quite comfortably. But at a certain point, the water is too low for these activities. The same is true in terms of a person's nutrient reservoir. It can be significantly reduced without producing any symptoms, but once it reaches a certain level of depletion, the disease process begins.

The average American diet lacks sufficient nutrients to keep the reservoir full. A healthful diet is high in potassium and low in sodium, for example, but processed foods reverse this ratio. People need only between 600 and 700 mg of sodium a day, but one fast-food meal supplies them with over 5000. Also missing from the average diet are enough essential fatty acids, such as omega-3 and gamma linoleic acid (GLA), found in deep-sea fish and unsaturated oils such as flaxseed oil. Instead, people get an excess of arachidonic acid from too many animal proteins. This combination of factors sets the stage for the development of cancer.

Modern farming practices may make agribusiness more efficient, but they have depleted essential trace elements from our soils. A lack of selenium, zinc, chromium, and magnesium in foods grown today has been implicated in increased incidences of cancer. Without these protective nutrients, free radical damage goes unchecked in our systems, and abnormal cell reproduction can lead to cancer.

Genetic Predisposition

Heredity plays a role, albeit a limited one, in determining who gets cancer. Researchers have shown that some people are more prone to the disease than others because their cancer-causing genes, known as oncogenes, are more readily triggered.

It should be stressed that while a genetic tendency predisposes a person to a condition, it does not mean that the condition will necessarily be manifested. Educating oneself about factors that increase the likelihood of cancer can lead to lifestyle decisions that decrease the chance of cancer's appearance. While rules of good health are universally applicable, a person genetically predisposed to cancer would be especially wise to abstain from smoking, to eat a whole-foods diet supplemented with anticancer nutrients, and to learn to deal with anger constructively.

The Psychological Connection

Experts in the study of mind/body connections, a field known as psychoneuroimmunology, find that depression, hopelessness, a perceived lack of closeness to parents, and an inability to cope with life are associated with increased cancer risk. Some researchers even talk about a type C personality. They describe this cancer-prone type as someone who feels that he or she is living the life that others have dictated for her, rather than the life she would like to be living. Emotions are suppressed and anger is held inside. Of course this is a generalization, and should not be used as a fatalistic explanation of cancer, or as a way of blaming the victim.

Symptoms

The American Cancer Society states that people who treat the disease early have a better chance of survival. Their list of seven early warning signs in adults includes a change in bowel or bladder habits, unusual bleeding or discharge, a thickening or lump in the breast or elsewhere, an obvious change in a wart or mole, a nagging cough or hoarseness, a sore throat that does not heal, and indigestion or difficulty swallowing. For children, indications are marked change in bowel or bladder habits, nausea and vomiting for no apparent reason, bloody discharge and failure to stop bleeding, swelling, lumps, or masses anywhere in the body, unexplained stumbling, a generally rundown condition, and pains or persistent crying for no apparent reason.

Treatment

The Conventional Approach: Chemotherapy

A patient is diagnosed with cancer, and told that chemotherapy is his or her only hope of survival. Frightened and confused, the individual places full confidence in the doctor's expertise, and undergoes a costly therapy that can produce side effects worse than the cancer itself. The hope is that the ends will justify the means as the tumor shrinks and disappears, never to return.

What the patient does not realize is that, in most instances, his assumptions are not based on sound studies supporting chemotherapy's effectiveness.

Historically, chemotherapy has helped patients overcome a small number of cancers only. It has prolonged the life of children and young adults with rare cancers, such as childhood leukemia and later-stage Hodgkin's disease. Some effectiveness has also been seen in certain common cancers, such as ovarian cancer in women and testicular cancer in men, as well as Duke's C, a form of colon cancer that has spread to regional muscles and lymph nodes. In small-cell lung cancer, life can be extended from several weeks to several months. But outside of these instances, there is no proof that chemotherapy increases life expectancy.

Chemotherapy's use far exceeds its proven effectiveness. The number of cancer patients cured by chemotherapy is in the range of 2 to 5 percent, but about 50 percent receive this treatment. The logical question to ask would be, if chemotherapy has such a low rate of success, why is it used so often? Dr. Ralph Moss, author of *Questioning Chemotherapy,* explains that most people confuse decreased tumor size with disappearance of disease. The association appears logical, but no proof exists to support the connection.

First developed from a U.S. Army poison gas program during World War II, chemotherapy was used after some initial trials showed it to diminish tumor size, without attention to whether or not patients actually improved. This blind spot has continued to the present day, where randomized clinical studies report success when tumors shrink. Since tumor shrinkage is not the same as increased life expectancy, such studies are worthless. The few researchers who have actually assessed chemotherapy's effectiveness report no correlation between tumor shrinkage and patient survival for all but the few cancers mentioned previously. Technically speaking, then, chemotherapy cannot be considered a proven treatment.

Interestingly, alternative therapies are criticized for not demonstrating patient success according to scientific standards. But why are conventional therapies exempt from the same rigorous requirements expected of alternative treatments? The answer appears to be economics. While the cost of natural protocols is usually nominal, chemotherapy treatments can run into the six figures. Bone marrow transplants, for example, which combine high doses of chemotherapy and radiation, cost an average of $150,000. While the patient may not benefit from chemotherapy, the drug company investor surely does. From a business point of view, chemotherapy is a profitable commodity, and so the more people who use it the better.

The cold facts are difficult for the average person to accept, especially in light of the enormous human suffering from cancer. The facts are especially difficult for the newly diagnosed cancer patient to fathom because the individual wants to believe that doctors represent a trustworthy medical establishment whose motives are pure and noble. But what we want to believe and what is true are two separate entities. We must understand the reality of the situation so that we can best help ourselves and others.

Alternative Approaches to Prevention and Treatment

For well over 50 years, billions of dollars have been poured into cancer research. Commensurate results haven't been forthcoming, though. Today, one in three people get the disease, and by the year 2000, it is predicted that two out of five individuals will be affected.

To reverse the trend will require taking an entirely new approach to research and treatment. Instead of continuing to view cancer as a single disease in need of a single cure, cancer must be addressed as a complex phenomenon, since multiple factors are involved. As oncologist Dr. Michael Williams, chief medical officer of the Cancer Treatment Centers of America, explains, the reductionist, scientific model of testing A versus B will not get to the root of the problem. Rather, attention needs to be focused on environmental, nutritional, and body/mind considerations.

Unbeknownst to the general public, there are several noninvasive cancer protocols outside of the mainstream medical approach that have excellent track records for curing patients well beyond the orthodox definition of cure: five years. Many patients given up on by the orthodox medical community are alive and well 10, 15, and 20 years after diagnosis. The therapies of Drs. Revici, Gerson, Burzynski, and Burton, and firsthand accounts of recoveries are described in the Cancer Therapies section. Here, we look at ways to support the immune system for cancer prevention and treatment.

DIET

Eating an organic, whole-foods diet and drinking plenty of pure water ensures us valuable nutrients and keeps the bloodstream pure so that cancer is unlikely to develop. If cancer is already there, these foods give the body the best support for overcoming the condition and preventing recurrence. The following foods are particularly important for their cancer-fighting properties:

Alkaline Foods. Eating alkaline foods balances the pH of the blood, which, in turn, inhibits the proliferation of cancer cells. Alkaline foods keep the blood pH in its ideal range of between 7.2 and 7.4, which is important for the prevention and treatment of cancer.

Ideally, the diet should consist of 80 percent alkaline-forming foods, such as those available from many raw fruits and vegetables, as well as nuts, seeds, grains, and legumes. Among recommended alkaline-forming fruits are berries, apples, apricots, avocados, bananas, currants, dates, figs, grapes, grapefruit, kiwis, lemons, limes, mangoes, melons, nectarines, olives, oranges, papayas, peaches, pears, persimmons, pineapple, quince, raisins, raspberries, strawberries, tangerines, and watermelon. Lemons—contrary to what you might think—and melons are the most alkaline-forming foods. A good idea is to eat some melon first thing in the morning, and then to wait 20 to 30 minutes before eating other foods.

Among the recommended vegetables are artichokes, asparagus, sprouts, beets, broccoli, Brussels sprouts, cabbage, carrots, cauliflower, celery, collards, corn, cucumbers, eggplant, endive, ginger, horseradish, kale, kelp, seaweeds, mustard greens, okra, onions, parsley, bell peppers, potatoes, pumpkin, radishes, spinach, squash, tomatoes, watercress, and yams.

In addition, there are a variety of whole grains, seeds, and nuts from which to choose. Alkaline-forming beans include green beans, limas, peas, soybean products, and string beans. Grains such as rice, quinoa, amaranth, barley, and oats are good. The most alkaline-producing nuts and seeds are almonds, chestnuts, coconuts, and pignolias. Seeds, such as alfalfa, chia, radish, and sesame, are excellent, especially sprouted.

Cruciferous Vegetables. Vegetables in the cruciferous family—kale, mustard greens, collards, broccoli, cabbage, cauliflower, and Brussels sprouts—contain compounds called indoles that act as detoxifying agents. Indoles are believed to remove cancer-causing substances from the body.

Fiber. This isn't a food itself, but it's an important component of grains, fruits, and vegetables; it's actually the structural support of these plants, and we need it for its ability to facilitate the transit of foods through our system. Unfortunately, fiber is often lost when food is processed. The typical American diet includes about five grams of fiber each day, which is not nearly enough for cancer prevention. Studies show that 30 grams a day significantly reduce the risk of colorectal cancer. Good sources of fiber are fruits, vegetables, and whole grains. Initially, increasing the fiber in your diet may create gas and abdominal discomfort, but this problem usually clears up.

Olive Oil. Olive oil is composed of monounsaturated fatty acids, which studies show have a protective effect against breast cancer, especially in postmenopausal women. Olive oil should be used in moderation and eaten raw for maximum benefit. One tablespoon of extra virgin, cold-pressed olive oil can be added to salads.

Flaxseed Oil. One to two tablespoons of flaxseed oil daily may be protective against cancer.

Primrose, Borage, and Black Currant Oils. These provide gamma linolenic acid, an omega-6 fatty acid important as a cancer preventive.

Green Foods. Wheatgrass, barley grass, alfalfa, blue-green algae, chlorella, and spirulina are rich in blood-purifying chlorophyll and important nutrients for detoxifying the system and rejuvenating the organs. Chlorophyll has strong antimutation factors.

Soybean Products. Soybeans, soy milk, tofu, miso, and tempeh contain phytoestrogens that help prevent many forms of cancer. Indeed, Japanese women, who eat soy on a daily basis, have the lowest incidence of breast cancer in the world. Because soy products are high in protein, they make excellent replacements for meat.

Juices. Freshly squeezed juices provide valuable enzymes and antioxidant nutrients that are easily digestible. One of the most potent juices for liver detoxification is blueberry juice, while cabbage juice prevents stomach and colorectal cancer. Carrot juice is valuable for its high beta carotene and vitamin A content, but should be watered down as it is also high in sugar, and can adversely affect blood sugar. Adding a teaspoon of vitamin C to juices makes them into a real preventive tonic.

Green Tea. The Chinese, who have low incidences of cancer, routinely drink this beverage instead of coffee. Green tea counters the effects of radiation, keeps the pH of the blood balanced, and is high in antioxidants. The substances called polyphenolic catechins found in green tea are actually stronger than vitamin E in fighting free radicals.

Mushrooms. Several mushrooms have extraordinary healing properties. The maitake mushroom kills cancer cells by enhancing the activity of T-helper cells. Scientific studies report this food's effectiveness in controlling cancers of the breast, lung, and prostate, and in minimizing the side effects of chemotherapy. Shiitake and reishi mushrooms, also called ganoderma mushrooms, exhibit anticancer properties as well, and are used by Orientals to enhance longevity. Animal research done in Japan showed a highly significant rate of tumor elimination in animals fed extracts of maitake, shiitake, and reishi mushrooms.

Enoki mushrooms are the long, thin mushrooms grown in an area of Japan known to have the lowest incidence of cancer in the country.

Macrobiotic Foods. Proponents of macrobiotic eating claim that cancer patients following this approach lead longer and better-quality lives. In several instances, patients deemed incurable have reported full recoveries. Success may be due to high levels of antioxidant nutrients and low amounts of fat. In fact, the total percentage of calories from fat in macrobiotic diets is approximately 10-12 percent, a 30-percent drop from the average American diet. Best results with the macrobiotic diet are seen with endocrine-related cancers, such as cancer of the breast, prostate, pancreas, uterus, and ovaries. This is because, with these cancers, too many fat cells produce or synthesize estrogen and androgen hormones that contribute to the disease; reducing the amount of dietary fat lessens hormone production.

Seaweed. Chinese medicine recognizes the value of seaweed for treating cancers as it softens hardened tumors.

ANTIOXIDANT SUPPLEMENTS

The value of antioxidants, particularly beta carotene; vitamins A, C, and E; flavonoids; selenium; glutathione; superoxide dismutase; coenzyme Q10; and grape seeds cannot be overestimated in disease fighting and prevention. Antioxidants attack free radicals before they do irrevocable damage. Many clinical studies confirm their protective effects, while other research shows that antioxidants increase a patient's tolerance of chemotherapy and radiation.

Vitamin C. Vitamin C is the prime nutrient when it comes to overall support of the immune system. When fighting cancer, large quantities are required both orally and intravenously. Orally, bowel-tolerance levels are recommended: that is, one should take an amount that almost causes diarrhea. (Most people can tolerate up to 12 grams daily of vitamin C, dividing this dose throughout the day.) But for best results, intravenous vitamin C drips are needed as well. Research indicates that this method supplies the greatest healing effects because more of the vitamin can be easily tolerated. Patients are often given between 50 and 100 grams of intravenous vitamin C, which is an excellent jump-start to any health protocol. This treatment relieves pain and nausea, often making painkilling drugs unnecessary. High doses of intravenous vitamins C and A are associated with long-term survival of a variety of cancers, even after they have metastasized.

Vitamin A. Vitamin A reduces infections and tumors, and is especially noteworthy for its ability to clear the lungs of smoke and other pollutants. Emulsified vitamin A comes from fish oil and is easy to digest. Vitamin A also comes from nonanimal sources, such as lemon grass, wheatgrass, and carrots. Since vitamin A is fat-soluble and not excreted by the body, excessive intake can be dangerous. But huge quantities of vitamin A (about 100,000 IU taken daily for three years) are needed for this to happen. Four thousand to 7000 units of vitamin A, from supplemental and food sources, are recommended daily—less if beta carotene is taken.

Beta Carotene. The liver converts beta carotene to vitamin A as needed, making it a safe source of the vitamin, especially for women of child-bearing years, as no fetal problems are associated with it. (Note: People with liver problems may be unable to convert beta carotene into vitamin A.) In addition, beta carotene itself stimulates T-helper cells, which prevent the development of cancer, and studies have in fact shown that the substance protects against lung and colon cancer. Fifty thousand IU taken daily may prevent cancer in cigarette smokers. For general purposes, 20,000 to 30,000 IU of beta carotene is extremely helpful.

Flavonoids. Bright colors in fresh fruits and vegetables are usually indicative of flavonoids, phytochemicals (or plant chemicals) that are efficient free-radical scavengers. Citrin, hesperidin, quercetin, and rutin are names of some of these disease-fighting substances.

Vitamin E. Much like vitamin C, E prevents cancer by preventing free radical damage, and activating immune system cells against tumors and infections. In clinical studies, 400-1200 IU daily have been shown to help patients with breast or cervical cancer. Vitamin E works especially well when taken in conjunction with 200 micrograms of selenium.

Selenium. This trace element, which is involved in DNA metabolism and the health of cell membranes, can play a part in both cancer prevention and treatment.

Glutathione Peroxidase. Glutathione is found in every cell of our bodies, where it plays a major role in defending our systems. Studies show that low levels of glutathione increase the risk for cancer, AIDS, and chronic fatigue syndrome. To stimulate glutathione production, L-glutathione and N-acetyl-cysteine (NAC, a precursor of glutathione) should be taken.

Superoxide Dismutase and Catalase. Much like glutathione, these antioxidants are front-line defenses against free radical damage, and are especially protective of the heart, brain, lungs, kidney, and liver.

Coenzyme Q10. Coenzyme Q10 works in conjunction with other enzymes in the body to optimize energy. Specifically, Q10 improves oxygen utilization, acts as a stimulus to the immune system, and serves as an antioxidant. According to studies, its concurrent use with the chemotherapeutic agent Adriamycin prevents the latter from harming the heart.

Grape Seed Extract. Grape seeds contain pycnogenol, a powerful disease-fighting antioxidant. Pycnogenol, among its various age-retardant capabilities, slows cell mutation.

ADDITIONAL SUPPLEMENTS

DHEA. Although DHEA is naturally produced in our bodies, we tend to produce less of this important hormone as we age. This decrease is connected to a number of degenerative conditions, including cancer. Taking DHEA has been shown to reverse many illnesses.

Melatonin. The pineal gland, located in the brain, produces this hormone, which is not only vital in regulating sleep cycles, as most of us have heard by now, but is immune-enhancing as well. As with DHEA, levels of melatonin decrease as we age, so supplementation can be helpful. Melatonin increases the activity of our T-helper cells, and aids our natural killer cells in getting rid of tumors. Supplements seem to extend the life, and the quality of life, of patients with inoperable brain tumors and metastatic gastric, colon, and breast cancer, as well as advanced endocrine tumors.

Enzymes. Enzymes, which are catalysts for all life processes, are found in abundant supply in raw fruits and vegetables. Studies show that enzymes modulate inflammation, and that they may have a direct effect on controlling soft tissue cancers.

Enzymes increase the action of antibodies against circulating immune complexes, which can otherwise build up and become cancerous. Antibodies look like upside-down brooms split apart. Antigens stick to the ends of these brooms, which allows macrophages to chew them up, break them down, and expel them from the system.

Types of enzymes needed by cancer patients include trypsin, tyrotrypsin, pancreatin, bromelain (from pineapple), papain (from papaya), amylase, and lipase. The bioflavonoid rutin may be of additional benefit when combined with these enzymes.

Folic Acid. This vitamin is especially helpful for patients with a history of breast cancer, cervical dysplasia, and smoking. For smokers, it cuts down on the adverse effects of nicotine on the lungs.

N-Acetyl-Cysteine. N-acetyl-cysteine, or NAC, reduces free radical damage in the body and helps metabolize carcinogens. This immunity-enhancer also helps prevent bladder hemorrhage from cancer drugs.

Shark Cartilage. When tumors begin to form, they establish their own blood vessels. Shark cartilage contains anti-angiogenesis factor, a protein that inhibits the growth of these new blood vessels. As a result, small masses never enlarge and the immune system has an easier time destroying them.

Shark Liver Oil. Shark liver oil contains alkyl glycerols, substances that have antitumor effects. Studies show that when alkyl glycerols are given to women with uterine cancer prior to radium and x-ray therapy, the damage from these treatments is reduced.

Thymus Glandulars. Animal thymus glandulars support the ability of the human thymus gland to produce T-lymphocytes, which are important for healthy immunological function.

Zinc. Zinc provides the body with a wide range of immune system functions. It supports the T and B cells in fighting infection and producing antibodies, and works to promote healing and reduce infection.

Chromium. This mineral acts like a hormone in the body in that it helps to regulate our levels of blood sugar. When blood sugar is normalized, immune function, and hence cancer resistance, is improved, which is why chromium supplements may be helpful in the prevention and treatment of cancer.

Genistein. Along with daidsein, genistein is a phytoestrogen from legumes that has antioxidant, anti-"bad" estrogen, and antitumor properties.

HERBS

Herbs can help the immune system in three ways. They can stimulate immune defense reactions, suppress immune overreaction, and stimulate specific functions for short periods of time. The following herbs have multiple benefits, and are particularly noteworthy for their anticancer properties.

Aloe Vera. Aloe vera is antiseptic, antimicrobial, and anti-inflammatory. It supplies the system with amino acids and minerals, such as calcium, copper, iron, phosphorus, potassium, and zinc. Aloe vera contains live enzymes, including amylase, lactic dehydrogenase, and lipase, as well as the essential fatty acids needed for optimum health. Its role in treating tumors, research shows, is due to its ability to stimulate phagocytic activity.

Astragalus. Although new to the West, astragalus is a time-honored Chinese remedy. In fact, Oriental medical literature from 4000 years ago says astragalus has the ability to strengthen resistance to disease. Modern scientific research confirms these claims, demonstrating that cells damaged by cancer and radiation are stimulated to full function with the introduction of this herb. Astragalus is considered a life energy or qi (pronounced ''chee'') tonic that strengthens vitality, and increases white blood cell and phagocytic activity. It is safe to take on a daily basis, making it an ideal preventive tonic.

Ginkgo Biloba. This antioxidant herb, long used by the Chinese, works to counter a substance in the body called platelet activation factor, or PAF, which may act to encourage tumor growth. By interfering with PAF, ginkgo may fight cancer.

Echinacea. When taken for short periods, echinacea revs up the immune system, stimulating the production and mobilization of white blood cells. It also stimulates cells in the lymphatic system, as well as important immune compounds, including interferon and tumor necrosis factor.

Garlic. There are numerous advantages to taking garlic, including anti-cancer benefits. Garlic makes cancer more recognizable to the immune system and interferes with the beginnings of tumor development. In addition, it stimulates immunity against formed tumor cells. The National Cancer Institute recognizes a connection between garlic, onions, and related plants and a lower incidence of stomach cancer.

Ginger. Ginger will alleviate nausea associated with chemotherapy. It can be taken as a tea, or a small (½-1-inch) cube can be added to 10 ounces of juice.

Turmeric. Part of the ginger family, and an ingredient of curry powder, turmeric, or its main active component, curcumin, is a powerful antioxidant that seems to work against skin cancer.

Ginseng. Studies associate the use of ginseng with lower incidences of all forms of cancer. It contains ingredients called saponins that encourage macrophage and natural killer cell activity.

Lentinan. This extract of the shiitake mushroom acts as an immune modulator and can help reduce the side effects of chemotherapy. Peer-reviewed journals report that lentinan also helps colorectal, stomach, and breast cancers.

Red Clover. Red clover checks free radical damage and protects DNA, which, in turn, helps to prevent mutations.

Essiac. Taken in tea form, Essiac is an herbal formula that has been used for years to fight cancer. Among its immune-enhancing ingredients are burdock, Indian rhubarb, sheep sorrel, and slippery elm.

Hoxsey Herbs. Lymphoma and skin cancer have responded well to treatment with this herbal formula, which contains red clover, buckthorn bark, stillingia root, barberry bark, chaparral, licorice root, cascara amarga, and prickly ash bark, along with potassium iodide.

Other anticancer herbs to consider include African cayenne, bilberry, bloodroot, comfrey, dandelion root, goldenseal, pau d'arco, and suma. Goldenseal should be taken for short periods of time, and not taken during pregnancy.

OZONE

Not to be confused with atmospheric ozone, medical ozone is pure and concentrated, and has unique healing properties. Unfortunately, medical use of this nontoxic molecule is legal in only a few of our states, although Europeans and Cubans have been benefiting from ozone treatments for years.

Ozone is used both prophylactically and as a treatment for a wide variety of diseases, including cancer. An antineoplastic substance (one that inhibits the growth of tumors), ozone stimulates the production of white blood cells and increases production of alpha interferon, interleukin-2, and tumor necrosis factor. It has also been found to enhance the action of various antitumor drugs.

According to the naturopathic physician Dr. Stanley Beyerle, prostate cancer patients often respond quite well to ozone treatment if the cancer is left encapsulated (that is, not biopsied). Other types of cancer that Beyerle has seen major improvements with, using ozone, are tonsillar, throat, ovarian, colon, and breast cancer.

One mode of delivery of medical ozone is autohemotherapy, in which a portion of the patient's blood is mixed, outside the body, with a dose of ozone/oxygen, and then reintroduced into the circulation. Other methods used are rectal insufflation and drinking ozonated water.

OTHER TREATMENTS

Individualized Vaccines. When some of a patient's own cancer cells are combined in a laboratory with some of his or her white blood cells, it's now possible—experimentally, and in certain cases—to create a personalized vaccine that works to stimulate the patient's immune system to destroy the cancer.

Dramatic results have been seen in Europe with this new approach. The extent of its applicability still has to be determined.

Coley's Toxins. This is another, older, vaccine approach to cancer. Dr. William Coley, who practiced in the early part of this century, found that certain inactivated bacteria could be given to patients to energize their immune systems against cancer. It was as if, by first fighting against the weaker opponent, the bacteria, the body built up its defenses and became more able to fight the cancer. Research has shown this treatment to be of significant value, although a perceived drawback is the fever that develops shortly after the vaccine is given. This, explain proponents of Coley's treatment, is actually a sign that the vaccine is working, and should not be suppressed.

714X. Nitrogen-rich camphor and organic salts are used to make this substance, which is given to render the immune system more efficient in its combat against cancer cells. Results of 714X treatment, which usually consists of a series of injections into the lymph nodes of the groin, include tumor shrinkage, weight gain, a lessening of pain, and extended survival time. People receiving this treatment are cautioned not to take vitamins E or B12 at the same time as 714X treatment, lest they counter its effects.

Interferon. This natural protein, or lymphokine, is produced by our bodies in response to foreign substances.

Pancreatic Enzymes. These are a type of proteolytic, or protein-degrading enzymes that are useful in digesting the protein coating of cancer cells. This is important because it's a necessary step before the cancer cells are destroyed by the body's immune cells. What's more, pancreatic enzymes can stimulate anticancer factors in the blood, i.e., natural killer cells, T cells, and tumor necrosis factor.

Hydrazine Sulfate. This experimental treatment shows promise as it helps cancer patients regain lost weight. It seems to improve appetite and feelings of well-being, and may help to shrink tumors.

Ukrain. The plant celandine is combined with thiophosphoric acid to create ukrain, a substance used by so-called terminal cancer patients to block tumor growth and rev up their immune systems.

Indosin. Indosin, a nonsteroidal medication, acts to slow the growth of tumors.

Carnivora. A treatment for skin cancer, carnivora is a mixture of the juice of the Venus fly trap, alcohol, and purified water. This preparation, applied topically, stimulates T-helper cells.

Iscador. This is a mistletoe derivative given by injection. It's not at present approved for sale in this country, but it has been shown effective in the treatment of breast, cervical, bladder, bronchial, ovarian, and skin cancers.

Larch Arabinogalactan. This is a substance derived from the Western larch tree. It's used in the form of a powder called Larix, or Ara-6, which stimulates immune cell activity and raises patients' energy levels.

PSYCHOLOGICAL FACTORS

It's been theorized, as mentioned earlier, that people who tend to suppress anger are more prone to cancer than are others. While learning how to release emotions in a constructive way is important for everyone, those concerned with or confronted by cancer may want to pay particular attention to this issue. Part of what's involved here is addressing one's own personal needs, as opposed to living according to other people's expectations.

Also, for those being treated for cancer, creative imagery used in conjunction with standard counseling can be an important adjunct to physical treatments. Dr. Carl Simonton, medical director of the Simonton Cancer Center in California, and coauthor of *Getting Well Again* and *The Healing Journey,* has written extensively on this. Focusing on what is right with an individual and helping the person get in touch with goals, aspirations, creativity, and purpose, provides a sense of connection and a will to live that enhances inherent healing mechanisms.

What to Avoid

Unfortunately, our food, water, and surroundings are tainted with thousands of carcinogenic substances, making it impossible to avoid contact with every one of them. Until the time comes when the health of citizens is taken seriously by governments, the best we can do is to educate ourselves and become advocates for change. These are some foods, drugs, and chemicals associated with increased incidences of cancer:

Meat

Meat should be avoided, and this is especially true of meat from animals raised on factory farms, because these animals are given high levels of hormones. Estrogenic compounds are routinely injected into commercially raised animals to fatten them up. Once eaten, these hormones are stored in gonadal tissue, whether it be ovarian, testicular, or prostatic, where they overstimulate the body's own hormones, and lead to cancer. If you must eat meat, small quantities of meat from animals raised naturally is a safer alternative. Also, removing the fat from meat gets rid of some estrogen.

Dairy Products

Dairy products contain large amounts of estrogen. One reason Japanese women do not get breast cancer as frequently as American women do may be that milk is not a staple in the Japanese diet. Dairy products also contain the chlorine-based pollutant dioxin. A recent Environmental Protection Agency report on dioxin concludes that common levels of exposure may threaten human health by causing cancer, as well as fetal, immune-related, and reproductive problems. Adverse reactions can occur at very low concentrations, and minute quantities found in food are implicated. Anywhere from 4 to 12 percent of a person's lifetime accumulation of dioxin could come from breast-feeding during the first year of life. The largest sources of human exposure are generally milk, animal fat, fish, and eggs. Over the past few years, the banning of PCPs and 245T herbicide and other highly toxic compounds has resulted in a lowering of dioxin in the environment and in people's bodies.

Antibiotics

Antibiotics are not just overprescribed for us, they are routinely injected into livestock and thus become part of the food we eat. These drugs adversely affect the immune system by diminishing white blood cells needed to fight disease.

Pesticides

In the 1960's, science writer Rachel Carson alerted the world to the life-destroying properties of pesticides in her highly acclaimed book *Silent Spring.* Sadly, the world has not heeded her warning and is paying dearly for it.

Recent studies associate indoor and outdoor pesticide use with sharp increases in childhood cancer, particularly soft tissue carcinoma, a cancer originating in bone and connective tissue. Common pesticide ingredients, such as chlordane, heptachlor, Diazinon, and chlorpyrifos are also associated with lymphomas, brain tumors, and non-Hodgkin's lymphoma.

Other research links a threefold increase in leukemia to pest-strip exposure. The active ingredient, dichlorvos, is specifically associated with leukemia in adult males and in babies born to mothers exposed to the substance during the last trimester of pregnancy.

Tobacco

Everyone knows that smoking is a prime cause of the most prevalent form of cancer, lung cancer. And more people are becoming alerted to the dangers of second-hand smoke. Studies now confirm that 17 percent of lung cancers occur in people exposed to second-hand smoke between the ages of three and 50, but who have never smoked themselves. Cervical cancer is also associated with the inhalation of second-hand smoke. Chewing tobacco is not a good alternative to smoking, though; it can lead to mouth cancer.

Alcohol

While two to three alcoholic beverages weekly is considered moderate drinking in some circles, this amount has been associated with a fourfold increase in breast cancer. (One drink is considered one 12-ounce can of beer, 4 ounces of wine, or 1½ ounces of whisky.)

Radiation

X-rays should be taken only when absolutely necessary, as even low levels are implicated in cancer. In addition, radiation from overexposure to sunlight can cause skin cancer. A hole in the ozone is believed responsible for the increasing incidence of melanoma, and thus sunscreens, sunglasses, and hats are wise precautions.

Electromagnetic Radiation (EMR)

According to studies, people living close to high-tension wires are more apt to develop leukemia and breast cancer than is the general population. Low-level emissions of electromagnetic radiation from these wires over long periods of time are responsible. Electrical workers have an especially high incidence of leukemia.

In the home, EMR comes from various appliances, such as microwave ovens, electric blankets, and digital clocks. It is therefore important to unplug these items before going to sleep if they face the bed, even when they are behind a wall.

Promiscuity

Women who engage in sexual intercourse before age 16, especially with uncircumcised partners, have higher than usual rates of cervical cancer. Penile cancer is the equivalent condition in promiscuous uncircumcised men.

Hormone Replacement Therapy

This popular prescription is offered to postmenopausal women by medical professionals who commend it as a way of reducing osteoporosis and cardiovascular disease. What they fail to emphasize is the relationship between hormone replacement therapy and an increased risk of cancers of the breast and uterus.

Oral Contraceptives

Birth control pills deplete anticancer vitamins and minerals, and are associated with an increased incidence of breast cancer. If oral contraceptives are used, additional supplements are needed to make up for the losses.

Denatured Foods

Sugar, salt, processed foods, cured or smoked foods, fatty foods, hydrogenated oils, food additives, pickled foods, foods cured in salt, and caffeine
should be avoided. A high-protein diet, and foods high in cholesterol, are also
linked to cancer.

Treatment Summary

Cancer is a complex phenomenon, necessitating attention to environment,
nutrition, and body/mind considerations, rather than a search for a single
cure.

A diet containing vegetarian, organic whole foods and lots of pure water
provides valuable nutrients and keeps the bloodstream pure, both important
factors in the prevention and treatment of cancer.

The anticancer diet contains alkaline foods, cruciferous vegetables, fiber,
flaxseed oil, olive oil, green foods, green tea, fresh juices, seaweeds, and soybean
products.

Antioxidant supplements prevent cells from becoming cancerous and can
increase a patient's tolerance for chemotherapy and radiation; vitamins C and
A are especially important as they are associated with long-term survival of
cancer patients.

While many herbs stimulate appropriate immune response against cancer,
astragalus is particularly powerful for that purpose and can be safely taken on
a daily basis.

Ozone therapy inhibits the growth of tumors, stimulates the production of
white blood cells, and increases the production of natural cancer-fighting
agents.

Creative imagery, in addition to standard counseling, can be an important
adjunct to physical treatment.

See also: Breast Cancer, Cervical Dysplasia, Prostate Cancer, Skin Cancer,
Treatments and Patient Experiences

Candidiasis

Candidiasis is a disorder caused by an overgrowth of the yeast *Candida albicans* within the body. Given that yeast resides in the skin, mouth, genital tract, and gastrointestinal tract, it can affect almost every organ. It is important to note that a certain level of candida yeast is a useful, natural part of the human system, helping to balance normal body function. However, when there is an abnormal increase in the amount of yeast, it can secrete a large volume of toxins into the body, which may weaken the immune system.

Once this happens, a self-perpetuating cycle can develop. The longer the yeast is in the system, the weaker the immune system becomes. The weaker the immune system, the higher the tolerance it has to the yeast itself. This allows the yeast colonies to continue to propagate, releasing more toxins and further impairing the immune system. The result, as described by Dr. Marjorie Siebert of New York, is a variety of conditions at different levels of severity and discomfort, experienced by over 60 million Americans each year. Candidiasis occurs in both males and females, although it is more prevalent among females, given their more complex anatomical structure.

Causes

Oral antibiotics are a common cause of increased yeast production. While fighting harmful bacteria, they also kill off much of the normal bacteria in the system as well. Dr. Siebert submits that since yeast has a different biochemical structure than bacteria, it is not affected by the antibiotics. Therefore, when these medicines destroy bacteria, the yeast is left with more room to spread and food upon which to grow. This is a significant point because as the candida yeast may manifest itself in various conditions, antibiotics are often used for symptomatic relief of those conditions. The antibiotics then allow the candida to reproduce elsewhere, causing recurring infections and other maladies.

There are certain physical conditions that make it easier for candida to spread. Pregnancy and menopause create an environment in which estrogen levels vary greatly from the norm, and this may cause a higher rate of infection. And, in general, women are more susceptible at the end of each month's menstrual flow. Diabetes can also lead to increased risk for candidiasis. Other factors that weaken the immune system and create the perfect environment for candida overgrowth are stress, and a diet containing large amounts of sweets and processed foods. Oral contraceptives can further promote yeast growth.

Symptoms

Since candida can cause multiple systemic illnesses, a whole gamut of symptoms, ranging from the general to those affecting specific areas, are possible. These include low energy and fatigue, irritability, anxiety, fear, depression, "brain fog," memory loss, headaches, lightheadedness, muscle and joint pain (arthritis), sensitivity to chemicals, poor circulation, resulting in consistently cold hands and feet, urinary tract infections, rectal itching, white coating on the tongue or esophagus (thrush), heart palpitations, and irregular pulse.

Symptoms that show up in the digestive tract include gas, bloating, periodic constipation and diarrhea, indigestion, and intestinal cramps.

In the respiratory tract, problems caused by candida range from chronic post-nasal drip and coughs to sore throats, colds, and asthma.

The skin can be affected too, with eczema, itching, rashes, acne, and fungal infections.

A variety of gynecological symptoms are possible with candida, the most common one being a vaginal yeast infection characterized by itching, redness, irritation, and a cheesy, white discharge.

Treatment

Rectifying immediate and local symptoms is relatively easy. There are many nonprescription corrective measures that can be used, including natural remedies. However, treating local infections does not address the root of the problem, and the overall condition really should be treated, so that yeast-related maladies don't continue to occur.

Currently there is no test that can precisely conclude whether a person has a yeast-related illness or not. However, some tests are considered helpful indicators. A stool study will show whether a person has an abnormally high amount of yeast, given that the intestines serve as a repository for yeast growth. A skin test may also suggest a yeast-related allergy. For vaginal infections, an analysis of the discharge may help to ascertain the presence of a yeast infection.

However, since these tests are not completely accurate and will zero in only on a local infection, natural, nondrug remedies that are mild to the system can be tested to see if they alleviate a variety of symptoms.

Diet

A person's approach to food is important, as it can either inhibit or accelerate yeast-related problems. In using dietary strategies as a treatment for candida overgrowth, a restricted diet should be followed for several weeks. Actually, this diet can be followed for an indeterminate amount of time, and foods can also be added back eventually. This should be done in a gradual, one-at-a-time manner, to determine a specific food's effect. If symptoms recur after a particular food is reintroduced, that food should then be avoided.

The main thing to remember as you follow an anti-candida diet is to exclude sugar. The idea is to guard against the continued growth of yeast and to fortify the immune system, and since sugar is a main food source for yeast, and does not benefit the immune system, it has to be eliminated. Don't just ban granulated sugar, though; also be on guard against honey, corn and maple syrup, fruit, maltose, artificial sweeteners, fructose, cornstarch, sodas, and lactose (a milk sugar found in dairy products).

A second rule of thumb: Follow a yeast-free diet in order to deter further yeast-induced maladies. Eliminate fermented, or yeast- and mold-containing products such as breads, including muffins, cake, cookies, and other refined carbohydrates; fruit, including fruit juice and dried fruit; cheese; vinegar; pickled and smoked foods; alcohol; mushrooms; tomato sauce (unless it's prepared with fresh tomatoes); nuts; and food products containing monosodium glutamate and hydrolyzed vegetable protein.

Eat natural, healthy foods. These include whole grains (brown rice, millet, amaranth, quinoa, and barley), fresh vegetables; tofu; miso; plain yogurt; lean meats; fresh fish; and eggs from free-range hens. Yeast growth may also be averted by using small amounts of organic extra virgin olive oil.

Supplements

In addition to diet, natural supplements can be used to specifically target yeast-induced illnesses.

Special flora can be taken in order to build up the beneficial bacteria in the system, which will then decrease the yeast. It can be consumed as a powder or as a part of sugar-free yogurt.

Antifungal, anti-yeast agents can be used to rid the body of excess yeast. These include nonprescription supplements such as citrus seed extract, Kyolic garlic, caprylic acid, and berberine. Prescription remedies such as Nystatin can also be helpful.

Homeopathic candida extract, given in injection form, can help to overturn the immune suppression through introduction of the yeast itself.

In the case of vaginal yeast infections, garlic suppositories are often effective.

To improve total body health and sustain balanced nutrition overall, multivitamin/mineral supplements are recommended. These will help to increase immune function and deter continued yeast-related infections. They should be yeast-free natural formulas containing zinc, magnesium, vitamins A and B6, folic acid, iron, essential fatty acids, and trace minerals. The following specific supplements may also be tested to see if they are effective:

ESSENTIAL FATTY ACIDS

3,000 mg of evening primrose, borage, or black currant seed oil daily in three even doses, or one tablespoon of organic flaxseed oil. (Flaxseed oil should never be cooked, and should be kept refrigerated.)

VITAMIN C

Recommended dosage is 3,000-15,000 mg daily in three even portions to fight infection.

B COMPLEX

Used to alleviate stress, the recommended dosage is 50-100 mg with each meal.

CHLOROPHYLL

This can help by cleaning the intestines and filtering the blood. Six 8-ounce glasses vegetable juice recommended.

Herbs

Herbs can also be instrumental in inhibiting yeast, particularly in the digestive system. There are several that may prove helpful.

GARLIC

One of the star herbal performers, garlic is exceptional for warding off infections. It can be ingested raw, lightly cooked, or in capsule form.

BLACK WALNUT TINCTURE

This can be added to water; the recommended dosage is 30 drops three times daily.

PAU D'ARCO

This is an herb that combines immune-enhancing and antifungal properties. According to medical writer Kenneth Jones, author of *Pau d'arco: The Immune Power from the Rain Forest,* there are two possible ways that the herb may work to help overcome candidiasis. One is by stimulating the immune system cells known as macrophages to devour *Candida albicans.* The other is a possible direct antibiotic action against the bacterium *Staphylococcus aureus,* which works in conjunction with *Candida albicans* to produce more serious debilitation. Three to four cups of pau d'arco tea can be taken daily.

OREGON GRAPE AND GERMAN CHAMOMILE

These herbs, made into teas, are beneficial to the immune system. Aloe vera, rosemary, ginger, alfalfa, red clover, goldenseal, barberry, and fennel also have this effect.

DIGESTIVE HARMONY

This is an Oriental bitter herb combination that works as an anti-yeast agent systemically.

HERBASTATIN

This gets rid of yeast caused by mucus.

YUDAIWAN

A Chinese treatment, yudaiwan helps to eliminate cheesy vaginal discharges.

KU SHEN

This Oriental herb is used in a wash to cleanse the vagina.

Homeopathy

While homeopathic formulas are chosen according to the symptoms that manifest, they do more than just suppress particular symptoms; they arouse the body's own healing capacity. These particular formulas may activate recovery responses in individuals with candida:

Pulsatilla may be indicated where there is a thick, creamy, yellow or green vaginal discharge. The woman feels weepy and craves sympathy.

Silica should be used when the vulva or vagina itch and are sensitive to touch, with a thin or curdly discharge.

Kreosotum is for severe symptoms. There are heavy discharges, profuse burning, a foul odor, violent itching, and a burning and swelling of the labia. Discharges may be yellow and watery.

Hepera sulph is used for symptoms that resemble those associated with silica, but they are more chronic. There is an itching of the vagina, especially after intercourse, and an odor similar to that of old cheese. Both hepera sulph and silica can be used to treat sores or cysts, especially Bartholin cysts.

Colon Therapy

According to colon therapist Tova Finman-Nahman of New York, colon therapy will help to produce clean internal surroundings and calm an irritated colon. Further, in combination with colonics, psyllium can be taken orally. This moisturizes impacted stool in the colon, which further aids cleansing. Finman-Nahman suggests that a person may take as many colonics in a series as necessary in order to get candida under control.

Tea Tree Oil

Tea tree oil, an antifungal, anti-yeast, and antiviral agent, can be used to treat vaginal yeast infections. One tablespoon of it mixed with a pint of water, and used in a douche, will help to abolish yeast infections. This can be followed with the insertion of acidophilus tablets or capsules into the vagina to re-establish appropriate vaginal bacteria.

Everyday Habits

Incorporating good habits into one's daily routine is an important way of guarding against yeast infections. Overall, stress needs to be minimized, since it can lead to impairment of the immune system. Other particular lifestyle strategies that work, specifically, to decrease the incidence of vaginal yeast infections, are as follows: Allow air to circulate in the genital area by wearing cotton crotch underwear and avoiding pantyhose and tight clothing; keep anal bacteria from entering the vagina by wiping from front to back; and avoid "feminine hygiene" sprays and powders which can cause irritation. Also, you should understand that douching is not necessary, as a healthy vagina is naturally clean.

Treatment Summary

Diet either inhibits or accelerates yeast-related problems. Three dietary anti-yeast strategies are: excluding sugar; eliminating fermented or yeast- and mold-containing products; and eating only natural, health-giving foods.

Supplements can either specifically target yeast-induced illnesses or help sustain balanced overall nutrition. The following are recommended: appropriate flora; antifungal, anti-yeast agents; multivitamin/mineral supplements; and chlorophyll.

Herbs that aid in expelling yeast from the system include garlic, black walnut tincture, pau d'arco, aloe vera, rosemary, ginger, alfalfa, red clover, goldenseal, barberry, fennel, the formula Digestive Harmony, Herbastatin, Yudaiwan, and Ku shen.

Homeopathic remedies that may activate a healing response in individuals with candidiasis include pulsatilla, silica, kreosotum, and hepera sulph. Also, homeopathic candida extract is sometimes used.

Colon therapy can aid in getting candida under control.

Tea tree oil can be used to eliminate vaginal yeast infections. Also effective are garlic suppositories.

Habits to develop, to guard against yeast infections, are: minimize stress, wear clothes that allow air to circulate in the genital area, employ good bathroom hygiene, and avoid products that produce irritation.

Carpal Tunnel Syndrome

Repetitive trauma disorders, of which carpal tunnel syndrome is one, constitute the most frequent type of work-related illness in the U.S. today. With the increasing use of computers, we're hearing more and more about CTS, and it's important to understand what it is and how to prevent it.

Carpal tunnel syndrome stems from pressure to the middle nerve in the channel in the wrist that houses nerves and tendons. It can occur after many years of work involving repetitive use of the hands, as on a computer keyboard, or it can occur more suddenly, after a blow or swelling. CTS can also be brought on by rheumatoid arthritis, and sometimes the fluid retention of pregnancy is a contributory factor.

The syndrome is characterized by pain in the wrist and hand, especially when the thumb is bent toward the palm. Sensations include a burning, tingling, or aching that may spread to the forearm and shoulder. Pain may be persistent or intermittent, and is frequently experienced at night. When the condition is severe, the muscles of the hand stop functioning, and may waste away from lack of use.

Treatment

Orthodox medical treatment for CTS includes drug therapy and surgery. But there are other approaches that can be tried. One is pressure point therapy, a self-administered treatment that has the advantages of being safe and easy to learn. Surprisingly, most of the pressure points for treating carpal tunnel syndrome are not in the hand or wrist itself, but by the elbow.

Try this. Place the index finger two inches below the crease of the elbow. Press this spot for 10 to 15 seconds. If carpal tunnel syndrome is present, this spot will feel quite tender at first, but relaxed at the end of the treatment.

Reconstructive therapy is another approach that syndrome patients have had success with. Performed by osteopathic physicians, who specialize in musculoskeletal disorders, this therapy involves injection of a saline solution into muscle/ligament groups, to stimulate the formation of new blood vessels. With new blood vessel formation in the ligaments, a variety of nutrients, vitamins, and growth factors that enhance tissue repair and growth can be delivered.

Prevention

The best way to combat carpal tunnel syndrome and other repetitive strain injuries is not to get them in the first place. Susan Fulton is a New York City journalist who sustained computer-related injuries and went on to develop prevention training. She delineates four physical factors in the workplace that can contribute to the development of CTS: repetitive activity, awkward positions, static posture, and excessive force. Emphasizing first that no two people are going to react to these the same way, and at the same rate, she goes on to outline steps people can take to counteract them.

First, take breaks from repetitive work, and vary your tasks. For instance, phone calls can be an opportunity to move away from the computer. Or try computer "take-a-break" software programs.

Rearrange your work area and furniture with an eye to minimizing sharp angles in your joints that will pinch and irritate internal tissue. Ask yourself these questions about your desk posture: Are my hands angled up from my wrists when I type? If so, try raising yourself or lowering the key surface. Am I hunching my shoulders down because the table's too low? Make appropriate adjustments. Am I pinching the phone handset between ear and shoulder? Use a headset. Am I pushing my head forward to see the monitor? Move it closer and lower it. Am I reaching for a phone that's too far away, stressing my shoulder? Move the phone closer.

A good idea to keep in mind during the workday is to stretch and move around as much as possible. Fulton notes that sitting in one position actually takes work in that your muscles have to hold you in place. They get tight and less supple in the process.

Using less force in your work is a concept that might not come to mind if you're an office worker. But try holding the pencil less tightly. At the computer, don't squeeze the mouse and pound the keys. The idea, Fulton says, is to work your body less, but accomplish the same thing. Be aware of the tension you routinely have in your work life and how it affects you.

Treatment Summary

Pressure point therapy, which can be self-administered, can alleviate carpal tunnel symptoms.

Reconstructive therapy, administered by osteopathic physicians, stimulates new blood vessel growth, so that healing nutrients can reach the area.

Prevention of repetitive strain injuries starts with understanding the ergonomic risk factors: repetitive activity, awkward positions, static posture, and excessive force.

To protect yourself from CTS and related problems, rearrange your work space, vary tasks and take breaks, stretch and move when possible, and monitor your work habits for excess muscle tension.

Cerebral Palsy

Cerebral palsy is a broad term used to describe brain-related motor problems. Injury to the cerebrum, occurring at birth or soon afterwards, results in a muscle/nerve dysfunction which is manifested as a lifelong paralysis of one or more parts of the body.

Causes

Usually cerebral palsy is associated with a lack of oxygen during birth, a premature birth, or low birth weight. Low birth weight is related to premature delivery; for this reason, mothers who experience early contractions may be placed on medications to prolong their pregnancy. In recent years, it's been shown that low birth weight is related to the expectant mother smoking or taking drugs. There is an especially high risk of cerebral palsy in drug-addicted mothers.

Symptoms

Symptoms range in severity, from a mild paralysis of the extremities on one side of the body, to an extreme loss of muscle control, speech, and vision. Hearing disorders and mental retardation can occur as well. Signs of abnormal breathing, sucking, and swallowing may be noticeable at birth or soon afterwards, although they are sometimes overlooked for several months. Later, the child's gross and fine motor development will be spastic and slow to develop. Delayed walking and acquisition of bowel and bladder habits may be present, as well as overly strong reflexes, slurred speech, and slow movements of the face.

Treatment

The success of treatment depends on when the diagnosis is made and on the severity of disorder. The earlier the problem is identified and treated, the greater the effect of the treatment. Orthodox treatment programs may consist of exercise, braces, corrective surgery, and drugs that relax muscles and prevent seizures. As a result of therapy, many patients lead independent lives; those severely affected often improve to the point of being able to learn activities of daily living.

In addition to conventional treatment, the patient with cerebral palsy can be helped by herbs. Many herbal teas nourish the muscles and nerves with valuable minerals and enzymes. When highly diluted, they become gentle enough for infants and children. Some herbs act as antioxidants; they help to fight the free radicals that are prevalent in this condition. These include rosemary, ginkgo biloba, and ginger. In addition to being an antioxidant, ginger improves circulation to the extremities. Other herbs to consider are yellow dock, watercress, and milk thistle. It is important to work with a knowledgeable health practitioner, especially when treating children.

What To Avoid

Expectant mothers should stay away from drugs and cigarettes. They should also be careful to avoid exposures to pesticides, as the chemicals breathed in enter the placenta, where they can harm the muscles and nerves of the developing fetus.

Cervical Dysplasia

Cervical dysplasia is an abnormal growth of cervical tissue. It is caused by the sexually transmitted human papilloma virus (HPV), the same virus responsible for cervicitis, genital warts, and cervical cancer. These conditions are detected with a Pap smear.

The term cervical dysplasia actually refers to a progression that occurs over time. The condition may change from warty tissue to mild dysplasia, to moderate dysplasia, to severe dysplasia, to carcinoma in situ, and then invasive cancer.

The conventional medical approach typically does nothing for mild dysplasia and genital warts. The attitude is usually one of "Let's see if the body takes care of itself." In the later stages, the preferred conventional treatment uses an electrical wire to cut out abnormal tissue. In advanced disease states, a hysterectomy may be the only way to save a woman's life.

But much can be done to avoid cervical problems. Prevention is always the best policy, and it is particularly so with this condition. Women should understand that cervical dysplasia, genital warts, and cervical cancer are sexually transmitted diseases that can be eliminated with safe sex, and improved by healthy lifestyle. Also, if you take birth control pills, it is advisable to take folic acid and vitamin C. Be sure to have a yearly Pap smear to detect the condition early. Statistics show that the longer a woman waits between Pap smears, the higher her chances of getting cervical dysplasia and cervical cancer.

Diagnosis

Before treatment, it is essential to get fully diagnosed to determine the stage of the illness. If a woman has an abnormal Pap smear, her partner needs to be examined by a urologist for warty tissue. Otherwise, they will be passing the virus back and forth and reinfecting each other. Diagnosis by a licensed, well-trained, alternative practitioner will determine if a woman is a candidate for natural treatments only, or whether she needs to integrate these approaches with conventional methods.

Naturopathic Treatments

Women with cervical dysplasia often have excellent results using naturopathic approaches. Dr. Tori Hudson of Portland, Oregon, notes, "In the results of a research study that I conducted at the College of Naturopathic Medicine, we had 43 cases of all degrees of cervical dysplasia. Through my treatment protocol, 38 of the 43 reverted to normal, 3 partially improved, and 2 had no change, meaning they didn't get better and they didn't get worse." Dr. Hudson's protocol consists of three types of treatment: systemic, local, and constitutional. An overview of her therapy is outlined below:

Systemic Treatment

> Beta carotene
> Vitamin C
> Folic acid
> Immunity-enhancing herbal formulation

Local Treatment

> Vitamin A suppositories
> Herbal suppositories

Constitutional Treatment

> Dietary changes
> Use of condoms
> Avoidance of smoking

A diet that optimizes immunity is low in fat and high in whole grains, vegetables, and fruits. Immune-system inhibitors such as coffee, sugar, alcohol, and fat are omitted.

At the end of three months of treatment, it is very important to follow up with a health practitioner, and to obtain another Pap smear. Sometimes a biopsy is also needed.

What to Avoid

Cervical dysplasia increases with sexual activity at an early age; women who have intercourse young are more vulnerable because of the nature of the cervical cells at that time. Smoking is another factor in acquiring cervical dysplasia. If you smoke and are exposed to the virus, you are more likely to develop dysplasia and cervical cancer. Nicotine actually lodges in the tissue of the cervix. Then, when exposed to the virus, the DNA can become abnormal. Smoking may also cause genital warts to become cancerous. A deficiency in folic acid is associated with acquiring cervical dysplasia. Oral contraceptive use is known to reduce folic acid in the body.

Treatment Summary

Preventive measures include safe sex, regular Pap smears, and a healthy lifestyle, with no smoking. Also, if you take oral contraceptives, you should take folic acid and vitamin C.

A multifaceted naturopathic approach will often reverse cervical dysplasia.

Chronic Fatigue Syndrome

Everyone experiences fatigue from time to time, but when exhaustion perseveres for extended periods, it's called chronic fatigue syndrome (CFS). During recent years chronic fatigue has become an increasingly prevalent condition, although conservative elements of the medical establishment continue to question its legitimacy as a distinct syndrome. In fact, federal health agencies, which are appropriated large sums of money to study and treat emerging infectious diseases, have virtually ignored this burgeoning problem.

The condition first became prevalent during the 1980's, when clusters of CFS cases were reported in various parts of the country. In 1988, the Centers for Disease Control finally acknowledged the existence of the condition, designating the term "chronic fatigue syndrome" to describe a constant state of exhaustion. Since then, conservative estimates have put the number of Americans affected at 2 million. A study performed at Harvard University concluded that 3 out of every 1000 people in the U.S. suffer from the syndrome.

Although it is not a fatal disease, chronic fatigue syndrome can be devastating to those who live with it. Most CFS sufferers are young, previously seemingly healthy individuals. (While chronic fatigue affects a broad spectrum of people with regard to age, national origin, and sex, recent studies have indicated that a significant percentage of sufferers are in their mid-30's, while the ratio of women to men who are affected is approximately two to one.) Since symptoms of the syndrome tend to be more felt than visible, CFS can be quite frustrating for people experiencing it, who have to convince family members, friends, employers, and doctors that a problem truly exists.

The U.S. is not alone in facing this health problem, as nations throughout the world have reported increased incidence of the condition during the past few years. In Japan, the condition is labeled low natural killer syndrome, or LNKS, while in Great Britain chronic fatigue has been dubbed myalgic encephalomyelitis. Chronic fatigue has become common in several other countries, including Canada, Australia, and Holland, where a variety of support groups have been established to help people cope with the condition.

Causes

Research has correlated the onset of chronic fatigue to a breakdown in the immune system that permits viral or bacterial infections—such as Epstein-Barr, herpes, cytomegalovirus, mycoplasma, or candida—to gain ascendancy in the body. When immune system function falters, the body is left susceptible to previously present but previously untroublesome organisms, and to overgrowth of friendly organisms. Chronic muscle dysfunction can be involved; fibromyalgia, which sometimes accompanies CFS, is a painful musculoskeletal disease characterized by the thickening and tightening of muscle fibers.

In the majority of cases, chronic fatigue isn't something that hits a person out of the blue, but is, rather, the result of years of bodily assault in the form of poor health habits. During those years the person proabably suffered from general fatigue a good deal of the time, but she or he may have considered that normal, as many high-powered, ever-on-the-go Americans do. Years of chronic stress, with its concomitant adrenal overload, often precede the onset of CFS. A person may go along for decades never really relaxing, gulping down coffee and sugary snacks, smoking cigarettes, eating fatty and processed foods, taking excessive antibiotics, and indulging in other unhealthy habits, without thinking that she is paying much of a price beyond a low energy level. Weakened immunity may not show up at this point. But then a major stress introduced into the person's life can tip the balance in favor of previously dormant viruses within the body. The result—chronic fatigue, which may seem like it struck from out of nowhere but was actually the result of a way of life. This is not to blame the victim, but to say that there are often complex underlying cofactors, besides microorganisms, involved in this condition.

An occupational group that has a high level of chronic fatigue syndrome is flight attendants. People with this job constantly have their systems assaulted: Their workplace is one of contained and contaminated air, pressure changes, atmospheric radiation, and high stress, not to mention less than ideal food. It's no wonder that flight attendants tend to age prematurely, and to experience CFS more than the general population does.

Some scientists have attributed the onset of chronic fatigue to the administration of vaccinations. Epstein-Barr virus, which has a tendency to enhance rapid cell division, is sometimes amalgamated with other viruses during the vaccine manufacture process; consequently, once the vaccines are dispensed, acquisition of chronic fatigue may be facilitated. Another theory suggests that the implementation of childhood and infant vaccination programs can contribute to the development of CFS by artificially reducing the quantity of uncommitted immune cells within the system. When the body's supply of uncommitted immune cells is committed to fight specific infections within the body, their ability to counteract new challenges is compromised. During the early years, the body encounters a myriad of these challenges; hence, some doctors have begun to question the wisdom of early childhood inoculation programs. Although more extensive research on this hypothesis is needed, preliminary examination of numerous CFS patients has revealed that many suffer from a deficiency of these uncommitted immune cells.

Several members of the scientific community have reinforced the argument against vaccinations by establishing a correlation between Gulf War syndrome, which is predominantly characterized by chronic fatigue, and the vaccination program carried out by the military during the Persian Gulf War. Although the federal government denies this, doctors have implicated the administration of multiple inoculations as a partial cause of Gulf War syndrome, asserting that it was responsible for immune system debilitation in numerous servicemen and women. Also, chemical and biological warfare agents—some newly engineered—that our Gulf War troops came in contact with, as well as highly toxic pollutants such as those from burning oil wells, made our Gulf service people prime candidates for CFS.

General Fatigue

When a person initially experiences fatigue it is important to identify the cause, as most cases of exhaustion are brought on by factors other than viral infections. Viral-induced fatigue is usually accompanied by an assortment of other typical viral symptoms, while with general fatigue these additional symptoms are absent. General fatigue is frequently prompted by exposure to excessive stress, or by sleeping disorders. Insomnia, often worsened by stress, can have a serious effect on the body, which is deprived of proper rest time and will inevitably experience fatigue. Sleep disorders can be quite frustrating and debilitating for their victims; therefore it is important to control them before they take their toll on the body.

General fatigue is often caused by poor dietary habits, which can include a lack of calories. And although most Americans tend to consume a more than adequate supply of calories, often the calories taken in lack nutritional value. Studies have revealed that people who have an excessive intake of sugar and other simple carbohydrates, eating, for instance, a lot of pastries and white bread, will usually experience some degree of fatigue. A typical pattern is fatigue that hits in the mid- to late morning, after a short-lived caffeine-and-donut-induced energy surge has dropped away, then again right after a heavier than necessary lunch, and then again in the late afternoon or early evening. A poor diet often prompts the onset of hypoglycemia, a condition characterized by a disturbance of blood sugar patterns and insulin production. And hypoglycemia frequently induces fatigue subsequent to mealtime, when the oversecretion of insulin adversely affects the central nervous system.

Another common cause of fatigue is hypothyroidism, or low thyroid function. Hypothyroidism, which can also cause constipation, weight gain, dry skin, and menstrual irregularities, can cause fatigue even when it's of marginal severity. Unfortunately, doctors often fail to diagnose it and consequently mistakenly attribute the patient's fatigue to other factors, such as depression or poor dietary habits.

A significant cause of general fatigue is caffeine withdrawal. Since millions of Americans have caffeine addictions, caffeine-related fatigue is a common problem. When a person accustomed to large quantities of caffeine suddenly limits his or her intake, the result will be fatigue, probably accompanied by a headache. Eliminating dependence upon coffee and other caffeinated products is crucial to maintaining health and avoiding debilitating bouts with fatigue.

Symptoms of Chronic Fatigue Syndrome

Ordinary fatigue comes and goes, and people can function with it. But the predominant symptom of chronic fatigue syndrome is overwhelming, unrelenting exhaustion. The severity of chronic fatigue is unrivaled by the typical degree of exhaustion that one encounters after hard work or athletic competition. Victims of chronic fatigue often experience difficulty when trying to rise from a lying position, and eventually they may have no desire to get up at all and will remain in bed indefinitely. Unfortunately, chronic fatigue tends to plague its victims for years at a time and can completely alter even the most active person's daily routine. Sometimes the onset of CFS occurs suddenly, while in other cases its manifestation is gradual.

In addition to incapacitating fatigue, an abundance of secondary symptoms are associated with CFS. The early stages of the syndrome are frequently characterized by acute flu-like symptoms, while depression, irritability, headaches, low-grade fever, sharp muscle pain and weakness, swollen glands, sore throats, and diarrhea commonly manifest later. In addition, chronic fatigue is often accompanied by cognitive impairment, characterized by memory loss, confusion, and difficulty concentrating. Sometimes the patient will be unable to recall even the most simple details of everyday life, such as his or her name or the reason he went into another room. Another common attribute of CFS patients is an inability to cope with emotional or physical stress. Sleep disturbances are also quite prevalent among chronic fatigue patients; many feel as if their energy level is not being replenished overnight. Often the person will be unable to fall asleep, while at other times sleep will be frequently interrupted by nightmares. Additional symptoms commonly associated with CFS include numbness or tingling sensations, moodiness, ringing in the ears, rashes, and impotence.

Treatment

Prior to initiating a holistic treatment regimen, it is important for a doctor to examine the chronic fatigue sufferer in order to assess the severity of the situation and to determine possible causes. Often patients will undergo a variety of tests designed to ascertain the presence of any food allergies that may have fostered the debilitation, or the existence of a thyroid, pituitary, or adrenal dysfunction.

Diet

People suffering from chronic fatigue, and from less severe fatigue as well, should incorporate an abundance of complex carbohydrates into their diets, because these are used slowly by the digestive system, and consequently provide a good, steady source of energy for the body to use. Whole grains, as well as vegetables, fruits, nuts, and seeds, are good sources of complex carbohydrates.

In addition, juices, especially juices containing dark vegetables, such as collards and dandelion, are essential for the chronic fatigue victim because they provide an ample supply of immune-system-boosting enzymes. These green, chlorophyll-rich juices should be taken liberally—six 10-ounce glasses per day are not too much. Aloe vera can be a valuable component of these juices, as well as celery and cucumber, and lemon. Purification and stimulation of the spleen and lymphatic system can be enhanced by consuming fresh dandelions, sprouts, asparagus, mustard greens, radishes, and cruciferous vegetables, such as broccoli and cauliflower. Sea vegetables, including kombu, wakame, hijiki, arame, and dulse, are beneficial for the maintenance of bone marrow and the thymus gland.

People with CFS should incorporate high-quality protein derived from vegetarian sources into their diets. Some good examples of vegetarian sources of protein include tofu, tempeh, fortified soy milk, and legumes. Since fish contain a rich supply of omega-3 fatty acids, small quantities of fresh fish may also be advantageous, but be sure that the fish that you consume are obtained from an unpolluted source and are not submerged into chlorine during preparation. If you eat animal protein, consumption of this type of food should not exceed eight ounces daily. Also, keep in mind that since many animals raised in factory farm conditions are exposed to harmful hormones and pesticides, organic supplies of animal protein are recommended.

There is an immune-enhancing soup created by the Chinese that can help weakened individuals regain energy. The recipe consists of a mixture of a whole astragalus root with onions, garlic, ginger, and either organic poultry, fish, tofu, or tempeh. Brown rice and fresh green vegetables can also be added. After the soup reaches the boiling point, it should be allowed to simmer. Finally, miso is added to further boost nutrition, and enhance flavor.

Proper maintenance of the immune system can be helped along by drinking a sufficient amount of purified water. During the colder months, unsweetened herbal tea, such as echinacea tea, can provide additional benefit. Since cold liquids tend to shock CFS patients, warm ones are preferable.

It is important for people with hypoglycemic-induced fatigue to alter their diets, incorporating high-fiber, protein-containing complex carbohydrates, such as oatmeal, into their meals, and consuming nutritious snacks during the mid-morning and afternoon. Complex carbohydrates and high-protein (from fish and vegetable sources) diets can also be useful in combating fatigue resulting from caffeine withdrawal.

Supplements

There are a variety of nutritional supplements that can aid proper functioning of the immune system. Since many CFS victims suffer from deficiencies of magnesium, chromium, zinc, and other nutrients, a multivitamin, multimineral supplement can make a real contribution to recovery.

People with chronic fatigue should try to consume between 5000 and 20,000 mg of vitamin C daily, as C is crucial for proper functioning of the immune system and thymus gland. Since this beneficial antioxidant tends to be discharged from the body during excretion, distributing the dose over the course of a day is a wise way to go about taking it. Higher dosages of vitamin C can be administered through intravenous drips under the supervision of a physician. Intravenous supplements have proven to be quite successful in the treatment of chronic fatigue syndrome. Often 150,000 to 200,000 mg of vitamin C is dispensed intravenously, while the patient continues to consume quantities of oral supplements to bowel tolerance. (These high IV dosages of therapeutic vitamin C are gradually built up to—and then stepped down from—over the course of many weeks, with medical monitoring; they're not suddenly foisted upon the body.)

Vitamin E, another useful antioxidant, should be supplemented in quantities of 400 to 800 units per day, while 100 mg of vitamin B complex should be consumed three times daily. Vitamin B3, also known as niacinamide, is useful in amending blood sugar abnormalities, while B6 tends to shelter the thymus gland from free radical damage.

Zinc picolinate can substantially augment the body's supply of zinc when it's taken in quantities of 35-50 mg daily. The picolinate element of the supplement aids in transporting this vital element into the cell. But be sure not to take excessive quantities of zinc, as amounts over 100 mg have been found to have an adverse effect on the immune system.

Chromium supplements, in either the GTF form or the chromium picolinate form, enable the body's supply of insulin to carry blood sugar into the cells.

The mineral magnesium is also crucial to the production of energy; unfortunately, it's one that is overlooked by many adults. Magnesium can be found in 300 different enzyme systems, and it aids in the synthesis of ATP, an all-important compound manufactured at the cellular level that serves as the energy currency of the body. Often, women who are supplementing calcium to combat osteoporosis neglect to consume equal quantities of magnesium, and consequently suffer from fatigue. Unfortunately the presence of a magnesium deficiency is difficult to ascertain, as standard blood tests fail to take into account actual mineral levels within the cells.

NADH, commonly known as coenzyme 1, is a relatively new therapy that has demonstrated an ability to alleviate chronic fatigue without harmful side effects. Coenzyme 1 is a natural substance that can be found in every cell within the human body; it's essential in the production of bodily energy. Supplementing it on a daily basis can naturally augment the energy supply. The amino acid tyrosine also enhances the production of energy by aiding functioning of the neurotransmitters. Tyrosine is not recommended, though, for those suffering from melanoma or schizophrenia.

Coenzyme Q10, which works within mitochondria (our cells' powerhouses), acts as an energy stimulant and can be effectively supplemented in quantities of 75 to 300 mg per day, while the amino acid glutamine can further increase energy.

Herbal Remedies

Although there are a variety of herbal remedies that can be useful in combating fatigue, consumption of herbs should be supervised by a qualified professional who can determine which are best for your unique needs. Some medicinal herbs are not ideal for general use, in that they can induce adverse side effects if used inappropriately. Others are safer to use on a daily basis. Adaptogenic herbs, which are mild tonics, fall into this second category, and can be useful in alleviating fatigue because they enable the body to naturally create more energy. Examples of popular adaptogenic herbs include astragalus, panax ginseng, Siberian ginseng, lonicera, and glycyrrhiza, also known as licorice root.

The herb astragalus has been researched thoroughly and is available from an abundance of sources. Studies have revealed that astragalus is quite effective in enhancing immune function and can be used to treat a wide variety of illnesses, ranging from the common cold to cancer. Instead of directly attacking infectious organisms, astragalus aids the body by fortifying the existing immune system. This useful herb can be taken on a daily basis, and is especially effective when paired with the Chinese herb legustrum.

Tulip poplar bark, which Western cultures have borrowed from traditional Native American medicine, is yet another energy stimulant.

Originally used by the Chinese, Siberian ginseng and panax ginseng effectively stabilize the level of energy within the body by heightening vitality during the day and promoting relaxation at night. Furthermore, ginseng strengthens the immune system by increasing the quantity and performance of disease-fighting cells. The recommended dosage of Siberian ginseng is 200 to 300 mg per day, while the suggested dosage of panax is slightly less. Ginseng can be consumed either as a tea or as an extract.

The herb echinacea can increase the number of immune cells and promote increased cell functioning, when taken three to four days out of the week. Echinacea is widely available in tincture form or as a tea. High-quality sources of the herb can be identified by their tendency to create a tingling sensation and a numbing effect on the tongue.

Fresh oats are a nervous system rejuvenator, used to counter chronic fatigue syndrome. In addition, fresh oats can quell recreational drug, cigarette, and coffee withdrawal symptoms. Remember, though, that fresh oats should not be confused with rolled or quick oats, as they possess their own distinct qualities and benefits.

Garlic is yet another immunosupportive substance that can be used to combat the body's susceptibility to infectious organisms. It aids the immune system by promoting activity of the body's natural killer cells, which are used to eliminate infectious viruses and tumor cells. When garlic is taken in tablet form, two capsules should be consumed with every meal.

Popularized by the Chinese and Japanese, ganoderma, also known as reishi mushroom, is a general energy stimulant that also possesses cancer-fighting abilities. It is particularly effective when used along with astragalus and legustrum.

Licorice root aids in arousing adrenal energy, has powerful antiviral qualities, and is useful in cleansing the blood and liver, while cayenne pepper is useful in eliminating mucus and purifying the blood.

A fungus commonly used by Asians, poria cocos, is used to purify the blood and can aid in increasing stamina. Usnea and lomacium have antiviral characteristics and have also demonstrated their ability to quell chronic fatigue.

Finally, stinging nettle and common burdock root have proven useful in fortifying the immune system.

Homeopathic Remedies

In addition to medicinal herbs, a wide range of homeopathic remedies are available to help alleviate chronic fatigue. Some of these are listed below, along with the types of symptoms—and types of patients—they are considered effective for.

Anacardium is prescribed by homeopathic practitioners for chronic fatigue with brain fog, forgetfulness, and fixed ideas.

Arsenicum album is a remedy for exhaustion accompanied by anxiety. The person may fear death and disease, and feel despair over lack of recovery. There may be burning symptoms in the stomach as well as hay fever, and thin, watery, excretions. Other symptoms include weight loss, shortness of breath with exertion, and dry, rough, scaly skin. The patient has great thirst and tends to crave ice cold water.

Baryta carbonica is prescribed for people with a slow mental grasp. There is a lot of confusion and difficulty learning, and there may be chronically enlarged tonsils. These people tend to get colds easily.

Gelsenium is for extreme tiredness and muscular soreness, even with very little exertion. The patient wants to remain in bed all the time. Eyelids droop heavily and blurred or double vision is common. A band-like headache may occur and there is fever without thirst.

Kali phosphoricum is considered useful for anxiety, fear, and brain fog. The person can't recall names or words and has other problems with memory.

Lycopodium is for brain fog, with weak memory, confused thoughts, dyslexia, an inability to find the right words, and indecisiveness. There are also abdominal symptoms, with noisy flatulence, especially after eating; bloating, excessive hunger, and desire for sweets.

Muriaticum acid is a homeopathic remedy designed specifically to extinguish fatigue with physical origins. Usually, the physical fatigue victim is emotionally and mentally healthy, but the body is simply unable to function properly and constant bed rest is necessitated. If the patient does not receive immediate attention the fatigue can extend to the person's mental capabilities. This particular homeopathic remedy is used to combat fatigue that commonly accompanies chronic diarrhea, gastrointestinal disorders, such as chronic colitis or liver dysfunction, and the HIV virus.

Nux vomica helps with impaired liver function, especially when liver damage was due to toxins, such as drugs, chemicals, meats, and fats. It is also for the patient with irritable bowel syndromes, and constipation alternating with diarrhea.

Phosphoric acid is quite helpful in alleviating fatigue induced by extraordinary emotional events, such as a difficult divorce, a bad relationship, or an accident. In these cases the patient typically becomes withdrawn from others, stays in bed for long periods, refuses to eat, avoids talking, and, in general, seems to be frozen at all times. In addition, this remedy is prescribed to alleviate fatigue brought on by too much sexual activity, as well as fatigue associated with cancer, drug abuse, or mononucleosis.

Ticitum acid is commonly used by homeopaths to treat fatigue induced by mental exhaustion, a state that has become prevalent in many professionals due to overwork. Indications of mental fatigue include an inability to perform even the most simple functions, general confusion, and difficulty with the elements of everyday life.

Exercise

Although it doesn't come naturally, chronic fatigue patients should push themselves to exercise, as incorporating a regular aerobic exercise program can produce remarkable results in terms of boosting the body's energy level. A sustained, repetitive, total body activity aids functioning of the adrenal glands and helps release stress. Ideally, an exercise routine should be performed for 20 to 30 minutes, five days a week, although a patient with severe fatigue will obviously have to build up to this level. Actually, the diminished strength of a chronic fatigue patient can be dramatically enhanced by participating in relatively gentle exercises. For instance, walking in a swimming pool, gradually building up to a power-walking level of exertion, is quite beneficial.

Outdoor exercises are especially advantageous, as they allow the patient to assimilate fresh air into the system. Walking on cold winter days can be quite invigorating, but remember to bundle up! Tai chi, qi gong, and yoga are also recommended for chronic fatigue patients because of their salutary effects on the endocrine and immune systems.

Relaxation

Studies have shown that a significant percentage of chronic fatigue patients have encountered an inordinate amount of stress in their lives. Prolonged exposure to intense stress can debilitate the immune system, and indeed contribute to the onset of CFS. That's why people suffering from chronic fatigue may benefit from engaging in meditation as a way of calming the mind and eliminating stress. Twenty minutes, twice a day, is the meditation schedule often recommended. Engaging in breathing exercises and being generally cognizant of breathing patterns during everyday activities can also be beneficial in eliminating anxiety. Other relaxation techniques that may be helpful are creative dance and yoga. Focusing on the positive aspects of life and nurturing an optimistic outlook will reduce the effects of stress upon the body and aid the individual in coping with and improving his or her condition.

Detoxification

Victims of chronic fatigue syndrome have usually accumulated poisonous waste products within their bodies; hence, it is important to detoxify the system regularly for one to two months. The detoxification protocol can include colonics, which should be performed once a month for three months; and enemas, performed once a week. Furthermore, wheatgrass and other green juices can cleanse the blood, while bitters can aid in eliminating bodily impurities and stimulating liver and kidney function. The detoxification process should also incorporate lymphatic stimulation, which can be achieved with acupuncture or massage.

Pressure Point Therapy

Pressure point therapy is another approach that has proven helpful in treating some CFS patients. Pressure points for increasing energy are situated primarily in the chest region. The first point can be located by placing the hand on the notch above the chest in the throat region. Do not press here, but instead slide your fingers approximately two inches below the notch. Once you have reached this lower point, press for 10 to 15 seconds.

Another pressure point is located one inch directly below the first. While these points may appear tender at first, applying firm pressure can alleviate sensitivity and tension. This particular method of pressure point therapy is also quite useful in quelling fatigue induced by jet lag.

What to Avoid

Chronic and general fatigue can be compounded by a variety of factors, and prime among these are poor dietary habits. Foods that should be avoided include coffee and other caffeinated products, dairy products, meat, and refined foods. In addition, stress can contribute to the onset of fatigue, so stress reduction is recommended. Also, since vaccinations have been implicated as a potential causal factor in CFS, it is advisable to seek out information on alternatives to vaccines and to weigh the risks and benefits before getting them.

Summary

Prior to following a holistic treatment regimen, the chronic fatigue sufferer should be tested by a doctor for specific causes of the condition, such as food allergies, hypothyroidism, or adrenal dysfunction.

The diet should contain complex carbohydrates, as these foods provide energy slowly and steadily; enzymes from raw juices stimulate the immune system to health; protein from vegetarian sources and unpolluted fish is advantageous.

Herbs stimulate the immune system and enhance energy.

A multiple-vitamin/mineral supplement should be included, as many chronic fatigue sufferers have nutritional deficiencies.

Vitamin C is needed throughout the day, and is particularly beneficial when taken intravenously under a physician's supervision.

A wide range of homeopathic remedies can help counter chronic fatigue.

Regular exercise will augment the body's natural energy supply.

Relaxation techniques can reduce stress levels, thereby benefiting the immune system.

Detoxification is essential for the elimination of poisonous waste products that slow down body systems, contributing to chronic fatigue.

Stimulation of pressure points is a technique for releasing energy.

Chronic Pain

Constant or long-term pain is a widespread problem. If we listen to the mass media, the painkillers manufactured by large pharmaceutical companies are the way we should seek relief. But there are alternatives to these products, and Americans who suffer from chronic pain would do well to stop obeying the commands of their television sets. Although running to the medicine chest and swallowing a few over-the-counter or prescription pills may provide immediate comfort by eliminating the perception of pain by the brain, underlying causes are not addressed, and overall health has not been improved in any way. By contrast, a wide variety of natural treatment modalities exist that can aid the body in coping with chronic pain at a more fundamental level.

Causes

Pain is a signal that something is wrong with the body. It may be triggered by a myriad of factors, ranging from diseases, such as rheumatoid arthritis and cancer, to injuries from exercise or accidents, to food allergies, which can, for example, provoke migraines. While the causes of pain are many, the mechanisms used by the body to produce pain are similar. When the body experiences pain, a nerve impulse travels from the injured site up through the spinal cord, and to the brain. At this point the brain reacts by registering the pain in our consciousness.

When the body experiences pain, inflammation usually results. Inflammation is characterized by swelling, redness, heat, and pain, and if left untreated, partial or complete loss of function of the affected area. During inflammation, protease, an enzyme that aids in the assimilation of protein, is liberated in the injured region, initiating a chain reaction that compounds the problem. Small particles of protein, known as bradykinins, are also released and interact with the nerve receptors, resulting in the perception of pain. In addition, the bradykinins summon the immune cells to the region and widen the blood vessels.

Treatment

Nutrition

One of the most effective methods of combating chronic pain is saturation. This can be effectively achieved by consuming eight 6- to 8-ounce glasses of water per day. For the elderly, this is especially important, as recent medical research reveals that dehydration can play a major role in the onset of chronic pain due to the spinal discs drying out. Note that when the body feels sensations of thirst, partial dehydration has already occurred. Therefore, we should try to quench the body's need for liquid prior to actually feeling it.

In addition to water, organic fruits and vegetables, and certain juices create an acid/base balance within the body, which is important for diminishing pain. Excess acidity encourages the stimulation of peripheral nerves and increases our perception of pain. By alkalinizing the body, this type of stimulation can be prevented. Furthermore, juices derived from plant sources provide abundant sources of phytochemicals and antioxidant vitamins, minerals, and enzymes.

The acidity of the body can have a profound effect upon health. According to Dr. Emanuel Revici, a renowned health educator and researcher who has dedicated a great portion of his life to devising treatments for pain, pain sensations can be substantially alleviated by altering our dietary habits. In his research, Dr. Revici succeeded in eliminating severe pancreatic cancer pain by raising the pH level in his patients. While an excess of acidic foods can contribute to the accumulation of hazardous waste products within the system, recent studies of the average American diet have revealed that 80 percent of our dietary intake is acidic, while only 20 percent is alkaline. In a healthy diet these figures should be reversed. Some good examples of alkaline foods are soybeans, potatoes, melons, and lemons: These foods aid the body in eliminating harmful accumulations. It is important to note that beneficial forms of acid do exist and can be derived from coconuts, Brazil nuts, filberts, macadamians, pecans, and walnuts. And although a variety of beans—black beans, adzuki beans, chick peas, kidney beans, lentils, mung beans, navy beans, red beans, white beans, and pintos—register on the acidic (low) side of the pH scale, they too can be considered healthy acids. The same principle applies to oats, rice, and whole wheat. Negative acids generally register extremely low on the pH scale, meaning that they are highly acidic. Red meat falls into this category. If the bulk of your dietary intake lies on the acidic side of the pH scale, you should neutralize your body by concentrating on more alkaline foods.

Supplements

Our body can block the sensation of pain with endorphins, which are natural proteins manufactured by the pituitary gland in the brain. Endorphins are an effective alternative to typical conventional treatments and, fortunately, their production within the brain can be facilitated with a nutritional approach.

DL-PHENYLALANINE (DLPA)

The substance DLPA can be part of this approach. This essential fatty acid is crucial in preventing the breakdown of endorphins by enzymes in the brain. These enzymes are secreted by the brain to prevent the body from becoming addicted to its own endorphins. By slowing down this process, the body will experience reduced amounts of pain. Studies indicate that 4 grams of DLPA administered a half hour before a tooth extraction can reduce pain by up to 50 percent. DLPA has also been shown to be quite effective in alleviating chronic lower back pain. It is important to remember that this product will not completely eliminate all pain; however, it can increase the pain threshold significantly in most individuals and can serve as a safe, natural alternative to conventional painkillers. The generally recommended dosage is 500 mg, three or four times per day, to substantially reduce the perception of pain.

B VITAMINS

Clinical evidence indicates that injections of B vitamins, especially B1 (thiamin) and B12, can ameliorate severe pain induced by headaches, arthritis, and dental surgery. Deficiencies of vitamin B12, which are often responsible for the onset of neuropathies, can be eliminated with intramuscular injections. Patients can receive injections of 1 mg in their doctors' offices, and symptoms of neuropathy will disappear within several days. Many times blood tests do not provide adequate evidence that a B12 deficiency exists, and consequently, the patient is told that intramuscular injections are not needed. However, it is important to realize that there is not a direct correlation between the amount of B12 in the blood and that within the nerve cells. An injection of B12 is completely safe and can produce dramatic results.

VITAMIN C

Vitamin C will alleviate the problem of sensitive gums, and recent clinical evidence reveals that most patients with this problem benefit from taking vitamin C supplements to bowel tolerance, the point just before experiencing diarrhea. These patients receive help even after they have exhausted all other alternatives, including painkillers, nonsteroidals, and even cortisone. While some people can only tolerate 10 grams per day, others are able to absorb 50 grams of vitamin C. On average, the tolerable oral dosage is 20 grams. Much higher doses can be taken intravenously, and can provide substantial pain relief.

PROTEASE

As mentioned earlier, proteolytic enzymes cause inflammation after injury and, thus, pain. By halting the production of protease, the effects of inflammation can be reduced. But since the healing process and inflammation are linked, it's not advisable to eliminate inflammation altogether. Doing so may inhibit the body's ability to heal itself. Basically, the objective with protease supplements is to obtain a limited amount of inflammation that will not hinder the healing process.

In the past, studies have correlated the injection of protease with allergic reactions, but oral supplements are now recommended, and have the ability to promote healing and expedite the inflammation period. The enzymes are eventually assimilated into the bloodstream, where they are transported to injured areas and aid the body's natural protease. Protease supplements have established their effectiveness in ameliorating sports-related injuries, bruises, episiotomies, tooth extractions, sunburn, and sciatica in a large number of clinical studies. Supplements of protease can accelerate the healing process and diminish the severity of pain by up to 50 percent. If you normally take a week to recuperate from an injury, your recovery time can be reduced to three days.

Unlike typical painkillers, such as aspirin, proteolytic enzymes do not completely block out all pain. This is actually a positive effect because the inflammation that manages to develop stimulates the body's natural healing agents. Although a large body of medical research has substantiated the role of protease in the healing process, the public is still by and large unaware of its potential benefits. The reason is that nonsteroidal anti-inflammatory medications, such as ibuprofen, appeared on the marketplace at the same time that protease supplements were first being accepted. Unfortunately, the painkillers assumed a dominant role in the medical market because, although they did not aid the body in naturally healing its wounds, products like ibuprofen could provide total relief, while protease supplements could only ensure partial pain alleviation.

People interested in natural protease supplements should follow several basic guidelines. First, protease should be consumed on an empty stomach, in order to prevent digestion by our other natural enzymes. In addition, it is advisable to take supplements three to four times daily. They should be consumed before meals and before retiring for the night. Furthermore, it is important to purchase a product with high potency. Sometimes this is difficult because the information on package labels can be extremely vague. Also, the potency of protease can deteriorate with time, rendering year-old packages completely useless.

Protease supplements can be obtained from most health food stores in a variety of products. One example is bromelain, which is derived from pineapple, while another common source is papain, which originates from papayas. Animal sources of protease are found in trypsin/chymotrypsin. Since the potency of protease supplements is characterized by inconsistency, you should select a product with the highest possible protease content. If this particular product is ineffective, try another package or a completely different product.

Herbal Remedies

Following are some of the many herbs that can be used to treat pain from common sources. Remember, though, that before initiating herbal therapy, it is a good idea to seek professional supervision. A trained herbalist can provide the necessary expertise and assistance.

FOR MENSTRUAL PAIN

The most common treatment for menstrual cramps is dong quai, although a mixture of other remedies can also be used. Herbalist Christopher Trahan recommends a tincture of equal quantities of angelica sinensis, viburnum opulus, and the Chinese herb corydalis for treating severe cramps. The muscle-relaxant American wild yam, also known as dioscorea, is incorporated into the tincture, along with a small amount of black haw, also known as viburnum. Additional herbs that can be included in an anti-cramps mixture are Chinese cinnamon, wild ginger, and cassia. If taken as a tincture, the herbs listed above are taken in a dosage of 15 to 30 drops every half hour, during acute pain. These herbs can also be brewed as a tea.

FOR PREMENSTRUAL SYNDROME

Premenstrual problems can be treated by dong quai, as well as by the American herb dandelion root. The latter is especially versatile because it can direct other medicinal herbs to injured tissue within the body. The Chinese herbs bupleurum, cyperus, and melia are said to enhance the energy flow and to be particularly good for alleviating pain in the breast region. Salvia, which is the Chinese version of sage, is said to enhance qi, or life energy, and can be used to treat the heart and chest area.

FOR HEADACHES

The American herbs valerian and skullcap are commonly used to treat painful headaches. The two herbs can be quite effective when taken together. A tincture of the two, consisting of 15 to 30 drops, or several capsules of each herb, can be taken. Be aware, however, that although valerian can be useful in reducing pain, nervous conditions, and insomnia, this herb can have some adverse side effects, such as overheating and heart palpitations. Skullcap, by contrast, is a relatively safe herb and can successfully eliminate head pain. It can be used by people who suffer from Parkinson's disease, twitching, and tremors.

The herb feverfew is used to effectively combat the onset of migraine headaches by altering blood vessel functioning and cellular magnesium transfer. (Headaches induced by stressful situations or muscle tension cannot be treated with this particular herb, only true migraines.) Wild ginger can be used to alleviate head pain, while the versatile dong quai soothes muscle tissue. After a workout, dong quai can be taken along with either ginger or mint. Only small amounts of ginger should be taken at a time, though, and one should be especially careful on hot days, because ginger has a warming effect. Mint, on the other hand, is cooling.

White willow bark can be useful in alleviating headache pain. Aspirin, a product that most of us are familiar with, is actually a derivative of an ingredient in white willow bark, salicylic acid. Natural sources of this compound, though, are safer than the synthetic versions prevalent in most stores because their potency is lower. Several grams of white willow bark are required to obtain an aspirin-like effect.

FOR STOMACH PAIN

Mint is used for stomach pain and is often paired with either slippery elm or licorice root. Also, the Chinese herb corydalis can be applied to a wide variety of pains, including uterine and stomach pain. For stomach pain, as for other types, a health care professional should be consulted.

FOR URINARY TRACT INFECTIONS

Pain from urinary tract infections is typically treated with herbs that contain the alkaloid berberine. Sometimes goldenseal is appropriate, but Oregon grape *root* is used more often due to its potent concentration. Another herb commonly used is barberry bark. The Chinese herb coptis, which resembles goldenseal, is extraordinarily potent and can be used as an antibiotic or antiseptic. Since coptis is so powerful, the soothing effects of marshmallow are frequently employed after its consumption.

FOR GENERAL PAIN

Kava kava, which can found on Fiji and several other South Pacific islands, is especially effective in combating chronic pain because of its ability to bind to nerve receptor sites and numb the brain's perception of pain. The effects of kava kava mimic those of drugs, without the addictive element. This relatively safe herb can also promote relaxation and reduce anxiety.

Additional herbs that can aid the treatment of chronic pain include wood betony and rosemary. Wood betony, which has been used for centuries by folk healers, can also serve as a sedative and a carminative, and is a useful remedy for diarrhea and severe cases of gout. Rosemary, which many know as a culinary herb, has strong analgesic qualities and is particularly beneficial when used as a massage oil for muscle aches or headaches. Rosemary oil is commonly paired with a diffusing agent, usually either almond or olive oil.

The herb blue vervain contains anti-inflammatory and analgesic properties, and finally, curcumin, which is a bright yellow compound derived from tumeric and curry, is another nutritional substance that can be used to treat pain. Like the drug indomethacin, curcumin reduces the inflammation of arthritis and other conditions. But curcumin does not induce adverse side effects, such as the burning of stomach lining holes and the joint deterioration frequently associated with indomethacin. The recommended dosage of curcumin is 1200 mg daily.

Exercise

People who are experiencing extremely severe pain are obviously not candidates for a regular exercise program. In many instances, however, moderate exercise can be quite beneficial in the pain treatment process. When a person engages in exercise, endorphins, which act as natural opiates, are released by the body. This is why professional athletes are often able to continue partaking in athletic events after they are injured. In these situations, sensations of pain are not experienced during participation due to the constant release of endorphins. It is only after the event is finished that the pain is felt.

In addition to the release of endorphins, moderate exercise promotes the release of natural cortisone. Also, since pain and discomfort are frequently accompanied by excessive anxiety, the stress-relieving aspect of exercise can be quite beneficial. Furthermore, exercise can normalize sleep patterns and enhance self-confidence, both of which can be useful in the treatment of pain. Moderate exercise includes activities like brisk walking, biking, and swimming. The idea is to choose something pleasurable that one can look forward to doing, and stick with.

There are a variety of stretches and exercises that can aid in the healing process and alleviate a number of painful disorders:

FOR SCIATICA

People suffering from acute sciatic pain, which is characterized by numbness or tingling in the thigh, buttocks, calf, toe, or groin, should lie on their back and carefully pull their knee toward their chest. This activity can alleviate symptoms of sciatic pain by opening the lower lumbar discs. In addition, treatment for sciatic pain can be performed by laying on one's side and assuming the fetal position.

FOR NECK PAIN

Habitual poor posture while sitting at a desk or computer, and sleeping on one's stomach, commonly result in neck tension and eventual pain. A stretch that can be performed to alleviate these problems involves gentle rotation of the head and holding it in place in each direction.

Remember that a sedentary lifestyle can result in the onset of chronic neck, back, and leg pain. It is important to take a short break every hour to stretch the muscles and reduce susceptibility to chronic pain.

FOR ARTHRITIS

Studies have indicated that arthritis, which can involve the increasing proximity of spinal-column bones and eventual pinching of the nerves, can be effectively combated with regular stretching, exercise, and chiropractic adjustments. Swimming for 30 to 40 minutes, three or four times a week, can be particularly advantageous. Injury to arthritic joints is prevented by the buoyancy of the water.

FOR LEG PAIN

Chronic pain in the legs can be treated by placing the injured leg on a chair and bending forward from the waist. This exercise will enable the patient to stretch out the muscles of the legs. While performing this exercise, one should remember to stretch using the waist and avoid using the lower back. Next, the patient should attempt to bend over while in a seated position. These stretches are especially useful for people who are constantly seated at a computer or desk.

Chiropractic Care

Studies have demonstrated that chiropractic care is a most effective means of treating chronic pain, especially when it involves the lower back region and arthritis. Chiropractors are able to alleviate pain by eliminating subluxations, or pinched nerves. They work through manipulation of the spinal column, eschewing drugs and surgery. Some are involved with nutrition.

Home Remedies

Severe headaches and neck tension can be combated by placing a few tennis balls in a sock and positioning the "package" at the base of the neck. After one remains in this position for approximately 20 minutes, the neck muscles tend to relax, thus eliminating the neck pain and any accompanying headaches. Often, headaches that occur during neck pain are caused by compression in the cervical spine that is alleviated with the technique.

For muscle spasms, ice can be applied to the affected area for 10 to 15 minutes, and then removed for an hour. This procedure should be repeated several times. Ice works for muscle spasms because it limits the signals being sent to the brain, hence, decreasing pain awareness.

Psychological Health

People who experience chronic pain are often plagued by bouts of depression. This can be extremely detrimental to the recovery process because negative emotions can actually expedite the onset of adverse symptoms. Then, pain and depression can become a vicious cycle. The other side of the coin is that people can improve their psychological outlook and, consequently, aid the healing process, by engaging in relaxation and meditation, or by increasing the flow of endorphins through exercise. Depression can also be lifted through nutritional protocols. Doctors who tailor such programs to a patient's specific needs are known as orthomolecular physicians. By avoiding depression, when possible, and having a positive outlook, we can contribute to the treatment of chronic pain by allowing the brain to secrete chemicals that actually aid the healing process.

Acupuncture

The Chinese concept of qi (pronounced "chee") pertains to the flow of energy within our bodies that is responsible for life. In general, qi can be described as the sum of all physiological processes, metabolism, and consciousness. According to Chinese beliefs, clinical disorders can be explained by a deficiency of qi, while pain is commonly a product of blocked qi. Thus, chronic pain often necessitates eliminating blockage and strengthening the qi, which can be achieved with acupuncture. The therapy involves placing extremely thin needles into the skin along a series of lines, called meridians. These facilitate ionic transfer and encourage the generation of cellular energy.

Acupuncture is used in a wide variety of situations. It can serve as an analgesic, a sedative, and a muscle-relaxant. It can improve immune functioning, increase circulation, and strengthen the lymphatic system. In addition, acupuncture can promote production of dopamine within the brain, improve our psychological state, and aid motor recovery after an injury.

Frequently muscle strains and sprains can lead to the onset of chronic pain. Even if the injury occurred several years back, the body can enter a vicious cycle of pain. The muscle tone in the injured region can become imbalanced and muscle spasms can manifest. Acupuncture can aid the body in defeating chronic symptoms by acting as an anti-inflammatory agent.

Finally, acupuncture can be used to treat joint injuries that elude the tools of modern science, including orthopedic examinations and MRI's. Numerous cases have been documented in which acupuncture has remedied an "untraceable" condition.

Following the traditions of Chinese medicine, a qualified acupuncturist does not merely block pain, but instead, treats the overall structure of the body. The Chinese believe that a single symptom cannot develop by itself; it must be accompanied by a wider variety of problems, and hence the entire system needs to be treated. Furthermore, when treating a patient, the person's entire medical history is taken into consideration by the acupuncturist. Although it is difficult for most medical professionals and patients in the West to accept, the concept of balancing the qi within the body can produce dramatic results in the treatment of chronic pain.

Biofeedback

Biofeedback uses scientific instruments to help patients determine for themselves when their body is stressed and when it is relaxed. Biofeedback instruments register an aspect of physiology, such as muscle tension, fingertip temperature, or brain waves. When the body experiences anger or fear, for example, our extremities drop in temperature. Irregular breathing often results from stress.

The idea behind biofeedback is that people can learn to relax by altering their body processes. Breathing patterns can be analyzed and then altered, to create a calmer state. Muscle tension can be lessened, reducing pain. The highly advanced equipment that is employed can measure even the most subtle body changes.

A wide variety of pain-oriented problems can be effectively treated with biofeedback, including neck and shoulder pain, muscle strains, and extremity pain. In addition, biofeedback can be used to remedy chronic tension headaches. For patients seeking treatment for headaches, the initial visit to a biofeedback specialist will consist of a stress analysis test to determine stress tolerance. Also, the specialist may request a detailed medical history, in order to ascertain the presence of any conditions that may exacerbate the headache. After the preliminary information is obtained, the biofeedback equipment is attached to the patient. There are several devices that can aid in evaluating a headache patient, including instruments that measure muscle tension and nervous perspiration. The patient sits in front of the output monitors, and watches as the instruments read electrical signals from the skin surface. Then the specialist instructs the patient to close his or her eyes. After observing the patient's ability to relax, the specialist tries to recreate a stressful event that occurred in the past. The biofeedback instruments measure any variations in perspiration, muscle tension, and breathing patterns. Learning to change these is the next step.

Numerous biofeedback sessions are required to measure a patient's progress. A key element to biofeedback therapy involves a patient's personal commitment to practicing relaxation techniques at home.

Magnetic Healing

It's not a generally recognized therapy, but proponents of magnetic healing are convinced of this modality's efficacy, and explain that magnets are helpful in overcoming pain because they repolarize the cells of the body. This allows more nutrition and oxygen into the cells, and greater amounts of toxins out.

When pain is systemic, magnetic bed pads are used, with the idea of bathing the whole body overnight in a beneficial magnetic field. This is to oxygenate all the cells. In addition, a 2- x 4-inch, or 4- x 6-inch magnet, placed above the headboard, is used to bathe the pineal gland, which is a small but powerful gland in the center of the head. Among other things, the pineal gland is responsible for melatonin production, which helps us get restorative sleep.

Magnets can also be placed on the site of the pain. During the day, magnets can be wrapped over an affected area. Another method sometimes advocated is to use 2- x 5-inch bar magnets or Neodymium round magnets. These are very powerful magnets, and it is recommended that they be worn for short periods of time, approximately 30 minutes a day.

Some words of caution: Do not sleep on a magnetic bed pad for more then 8 to 10 hours a night. Also, those practiced in this area explain that the body should touch the north, or negative side, of the magnet, as this produces healing effects. The southern pole, or positive side, is said to have the opposite effect, exacerbating pain and disease.

Therapeutic Touch

Therapeutic touch is a method of healing that involves the conscious transfer of energy from the hands of the healer to the body of the client. The technique is an ancient one; in fact it is documented in cave drawings. In the 1970's, therapeutic touch was reintroduced by Dr. Dolores Krieger, a professor of nursing at New York University.

This modality can help a variety of conditions, particularly those involving pain and anxiety. This approach can help alleviate chronic pain because it relaxes the person, and helps the movement of energy.

During a session, the practitioner centers his or her body, mind, and emotions. Then the hands are placed two to four inches from the body of the client, and the entire body is scanned for energy imbalances. Basic cues are tingling, pressure, static, heat, and cold. Treatment is carried out administering the law of opposites. In other words, if heat is picked up, the practitioner might balance that energy by sending cool energy, and visualizing the color blue. Conversely, if cold energy is picked up, the practitioner might send a warm energy to that part of the body, and visualize the color yellow. Other techniques, practitioners explain, involve pulling out static and congested energy from the body, and "aura brushing," which cleanses the aura and places negative energy that is pulled off into the ground. The therapeutic touch practitioner uses calm, rhythmic movements from head to toe, with the aim of clearing all imbalances.

What to Avoid

As discussed earlier, the pH level of the body can be directly correlated with general health. Studies have shown that people with an exceedingly acidic diet are more likely to suffer from pain. When searching for a protein source it is important to avoid heavy proteins, such as red meat, because they are extremely acidic. Additional acid-forming foods include gelatin, vinegar, mayonnaise, mustard, table salt, soy sauce, and ketchup. Sugar, alcohol, coffee, carbonated sodas, and even black tea are acidic, and consequently, should not be consumed in excess. Although moderate consumption of some acidic foods is acceptable, the typical American diet significantly surpasses the moderate threshold.

People also need to beware of invisible, but detrimental, electromagnetic fields that come at us from constant exposure to computers, digital clocks, microwave ovens, and electric power lines. These aberrant fields can throw our systems out of balance.

Treatment Summary

Saturating the body with water may prevent pain caused by the drying out of spinal discs. An alkaline diet of mostly fruits, vegetables, and fresh juices prevents the stimulation of peripheral nerves that causes pain sensations.

Endorphins, proteins naturally produced by the body, help us feel good and are enhanced by certain nutrients, particularly DLPA.

The B vitamins have an analgesic effect, and vitamin C alleviates gum sensitivity.

Taking protease orally will speed up recovery from injuries and diminish the severity of pain.

Numerous herbs have pain-relieving properties specific to different conditions. Examples are dong quai for menstrual cramps, feverfew for migraines, and white willow bark for regular headaches.

A moderate exercise program will produce endorphins to help alleviate pain.

The practice of chiropractic care can correct problems that are at the root of chronic pain, especially when they relate to the spine and nerves.

Working to overcome the depression that often accompanies chronic pain may speed up the healing process.

Acupuncture, a time-honored Chinese system of healing, alleviates pain by releasing blockages to energy flows throughout the body.

In biofeedback, scientific instruments are used to teach people how to relax, and thus minimize their sensations of pain.

Magnets can be effective against pain, some find, by correcting polarity imbalances at the cellular level.

Therapeutic touch, which involves the transfer of energy from practitioner to patient, can relieve pain and anxiety.

Cold and Canker Sores

Cold sores, also known as fever blisters, are caused by the herpes simplex virus (HSV1). The virus lodges in the nervous system, and occasionally manifests in short-lived, but painful, fluid-filled blisters on the skin and mucous membranes, particularly around the mouth and nose. *Canker sores* are similar, and can be brought on by the herpes virus as well as by allergies, anemia, or poor intestinal flora. Some women experience canker sores with hormonal changes.

Cold and canker sores reflect a weakened immune system. When exhaustion or stress set in, the virus expresses itself. This is one more reason why it is important to keep the immune system functioning optimally at all times.

Treatment

Ice is an external treatment that can relieve swelling and pain during an outbreak. But much more can be done internally, with supplements and herbs.

Supplements

Beneficial bacteria, such as those found in yogurt or lactobacillus and acidophilus supplements, promote digestive processes necessary for the maintenance of a healthy immune system. Zinc gluconate, vitamin C, bee propolis, and beta carotene provide further immune support. Between 4,000 and 10,000 mg of vitamin C will treat an inflammation of the nerve endings, and works especially well with the bioflavonoid quercetin. The amino acid L-lysine can effectively quell an outbreak. At least 500 mg are needed, two to four times a day. B vitamins counteract biochemical stress, and therefore are good as preventive medicine. One good source of B vitamins is bee pollen, unless there is an allergy to bee stings. Other good sources are green algae and the bioflavonoid pycnogenol. And taking pycnogenol daily (60 mg) has the side benefit of keeping the skin healthy and young. Vitamin A is healing to the skin as well, and preventive against infections. Another important nutrient is coenzyme Q10, which provides oxygen to the tissues, helping them to heal.

Herbs

There is an abundance of herbs that support the immune system before or during an outbreak. Echinacea, goldenseal, and chaparral are especially effective at stopping symptoms from worsening when they first begin to manifest. Cayenne has lots of immune-enhancing vitamin C, and relieves pain and itching when taken internally or applied externally in a cream. Clinical research confirms that aloe vera is as effective as orthodox medicine in combating herpes in tissue cultures, with no side effects. Red clover blossoms and burdock root cleanse the blood and are good to take as a tea. Garlic is gentle to the system and can be taken daily as a preventive or during an attack. Chewing on licorice root can also be of benefit. Health food stores sell many of these herbs in salves, which quickly soothe skin inflammations. Some combinations to look for contain goldenseal, comfrey, bee propolis, aloe vera, and vitamin E.

What to Avoid

Cold and canker sores usually surface when stress appears. While this cannot always be avoided, it is important to note what situations create stress and to address those issues. Stress can also be minimized through relaxation techniques, such as meditation, or biofeedback. Foods that stress the system should be avoided in general, and especially during an outbreak. Sugar and caffeine should not be used. Also, acidic foods, such as meat, tomatoes, and oranges, can be problematic.

Treatment Summary

External application of ice is helpful.

Various nutrients and plant remedies will boost the immune system to aid healing, relieve inflammation and pain, and even prevent cold and canker sores from appearing in the first place.

See also: Herpes

Colds and Flu

People sometimes confuse colds and the flu. The latter is characterized by a swift, severe onset, prostration, high temperature, chills, extreme fatigue, sore throat, and a severe, hacking cough. A cold, on the other hand, has a slow onset and is not always accompanied by high fever. Symptoms tend to be localized in the upper respiratory tract, and include hoarseness, stuffiness, watery eyes, runny nose, sneezing, listlessness, mild fatigue, some chest discomfort, and generally a sore or burning throat.

While colds and influenza (the flu) are contagious, whether or not one gets sick is not merely a matter of exposure. Individuals with weak immune systems seem to catch every new bug going around and to stay ill longer, while those with strong defenses remain healthy. Also, there's a psychological element associated with the frequency with which people get colds. Studies show that people who experience high levels of anger, tension, and frustration are four times as likely to develop colds as people with easygoing attitudes.

Treatment

Most doctors dispense antibiotics at the first sign of a cold or flu, to fight for the body. But the body has a remarkable fighting capacity of its own that can be enhanced through natural means. Here are some ideas.

Diet

People who get lots of colds during the winter should cut down on acidic foods, and eat more fruits and vegetables. These foods are high in antioxidants, which give the body the tools it needs to fight off colds on its own.

Once you have a cold, it's a good idea to cut down on or get rid of the gluten in your diet, as well as dairy foods, meat, sugar, and refined carbohydrates, and to focus instead on plant foods high in antioxidants, phytochemicals, and chlorophyll. Juices are particularly recommended; if at all possible, these should be freshly made from organic vegetables and fruits.

Herbs

These are some of nature's remedies for fighting colds and the flu:

ASTRAGALUS

The Chinese have been using astragalus for thousands of years for immune-system strengthening. Studies have proven that this herb can reduce the frequency and duration of colds and the flu by boosting the immune system rather than by killing viruses directly. Astragalus can be taken as an extract, or the root can be added to soups.

ECHINACEA

Taking echinacea at the first sign of a cold or flu often results in the disappearance of all symptoms the very next morning. This extract of the purple coneflower was well appreciated by Native Americans and was used by early American doctors before the widespread use of drugs.

Now echinacea is enjoying a well-deserved renaissance, and is once again America's top herb. The reason is simple: It works. This is how. Echinacea revs up the immune system at the cellular level. First, it stimulates the bone marrow to increase phagocyte production. Then it facilitates the release of these phagocytes into the bloodstream and lymphatic system. Once there, these fighter cells seek out and destroy cold- and flu-causing microorganisms with a greater than normal intensity.

Since heightened immunity can last for only a short period, echinacea should be used for no longer than four days. If the need for it continues, the immune system should rest for another four days before the herb is employed once again.

GOLDENSEAL

Goldenseal has powerful antiseptic qualities, enabling it to destroy a number of microorganisms, including parasites, bacteria, and viruses. It has a soothing effect on mucous linings, and is therefore an excellent remedy for sore throats.

Formulas that combine goldenseal with echinacea are especially good for treating colds in progress, as well as influenza affecting the respiratory area. Like echinacea, goldenseal should be taken for short stretches of time only.

GINGER

Ginger is an excellent bronchial decongestant. As an expectorant, it helps clear out mucus from the bronchi due to chest colds. And unlike the foregoing herbs, ginger can be taken every day. It can be grated and taken as a tea, used in powder form, or taken in liquid extract form. One squirt of ginger extract into the mouth will clear the bronchi in a few minutes' time. This is also an excellent stomach remedy that counteracts nausea and alleviates the symptoms of stomach flu.

GREEN TEA

Green tea has great cleansing properties and should be taken throughout the day for influenza.

SLIPPERY ELM

To soothe a scratchy, tired, or sore throat, or help stop a dry cough, slippery elm can be taken as a lozenge, tea, or tincture. To make the tea, pour a pint of boiled water over one ounce of powdered bark, stir, and simmer for 15 minutes.

COMBINATION REMEDY FOR COLDS AND SORE THROATS

One teaspoon of bee propolis in a homeopathic solution is combined with extracts of red clover and licorice root. Ten drops of colloidal silver are added. Gargling with this formula and then swallowing it, every four hours, can help knock out local bacterial and viral infections in the throat and trachea.

OTHER COLD-FIGHTING HERBS

These herbs, taken as teas, tinctures, or capsules, also help prevent or stop colds: elderflower, elecampagne, eyebright, sage, peppermint, wood betony, angelica, yarrow, gentian, hyssop, masterwort, sarsaparilla, saw palmetto berries, horehound, usnea, and lomacium.

Cold- and Flu-Fighting Nutrients

Keep the following nutrients in mind when cold season comes.

VITAMIN C

If you find yourself craving grapefruits and oranges when you're sick, think of this as the body's call for extra vitamin C. Among its many functions, this nutrient strengthens the immune system, accelerating its ability to combat harmful substances. Bowel tolerance doses can be taken orally (this is the amount taken just before getting diarrhea), and more can be taken without this effect when administered intravenously.

BIOFLAVONOIDS

These water-soluble substances enhance vitamin C's protection of cells against viral and bacterial invasion. That's why bioflavonoids and C are always found together in nature. Excellent food sources of bioflavonoids include grapes, rose hips, prunes, oranges, lemon juice, cherries, black currants, plums, parsley, cabbage, apricots, peppers, papaya, cantaloupe, tomatoes, broccoli, and blackberries, as well as the inside white parts of grapefruits.

GAMMA-LINOLEIC ACID (GLA)

The GLA found in evening primrose oil, black currant seed oil, and borage oil helps relieve fever and muscle soreness associated with the flu. It has an anti-inflammatory effect and reduces sensitivity to pain.

Rest

In our busy—some would say overly workaholic—society, we lose sight of the fact that an important natural remedy for colds and flu is rest. People used to know this, and it's only common sense that you shouldn't keep the body going at full throttle when it's beset by an infection. Yet there's a trend these days for employees to drag themselves into work when they have the flu or a bad cold. This is unfortunate, not just for the person suffering, but for other workers, who now become infected.

When a cold or the flu has gotten you down, **lie** down, if this is at all possible. Don't try to keep up with a strenuous workout routine. Take the day off from work or school if you can, get under the covers with a good book and a supply of fresh juice nearby, and give yourself a physical and mental stress break. You'll be giving your immune system its best fighting chance.

Granted, some jobs—primary caregiver of young children, for one—don't lend themselves to days off, but perhaps you can arrange for temporary help. Don't be a cold or flu martyr if you don't have to be; you don't want your symptoms to worsen. Besides, everyone deserves a sick day once in a while!

Homeopathy

In deciding which remedy to use, the homeopathic physician analyzes several factors, including the speed of onset of symptoms, sensation, how the patient looks, and his or her mental state. These are some common cold and flu remedies and their keynote symptoms.

FOR THE EARLY STAGES OF A COLD:

Aconite or Aconitum napellus. This is for the first stages of a cold or flu that appears suddenly. It is worse in dry heat and cold wind and often appears when the weather first turns chilly and people turn on the heat, causing the air to get very dry. The coldness outside combined with the dryness inside causes the sudden onset of a cold and fever. This remedy is often prescribed for robust people, as well as those who eat meat. Three 30c pellets, under the tongue, are often all that is needed to get a cold or the flu to disappear just as quickly as it materialized.

Belladonna. This remedy is for serious symptoms of colds, the flu, infections, and sore throats, that suddenly appear. If it does not take effect within a few hours, professional help should be sought.

Ferrum phosphoricum. This formula is prescribed for people with weak immune systems who tend to drag, but whose actual cold and flu symptoms never fully manifest. Symptoms are vague, but uncomfortable. There might be a slight earache, a clear, runny nose, a mild sore throat, or a low-grade fever. The person tends to be anemic. Three pellets are placed under the tongue every few hours when discomfort first appears.

FOR COLDS IN MID-STAGE:

Allium cepa. People are given allium cepa when their eyes are watery and clear but their nose is red and irritated. Other symptoms include violent multiple sneezes and burning nasal discharge. A person feels worse in a warm room, and better in the fresh air. A good way to remember allium cepa is to think of the red onion from which it is derived. Onions make the eyes tear and this remedy is for watery eyes.

Euphrasia. Symptoms are similar to indications for allium cepa. There is a lot of sneezing. Eyes and nose have watery discharge, but here, eyes are red and swollen, not clear.

Natrum muriaticum. The person has a thick, clear, fluid discharge that resembles raw egg whites. Lips are dry and cracked, with cold sores on the inside or outside of the mouth. Often the person catches a cold after suffering grief.

FOR ADVANCED COLDS:

Arsenicum album. This is for a cold or flu in its late stages with symptoms that include burning eyes and sinuses; irritation in the nose, causing sneezing; extreme chill; restlessness; weakness; fever; and exhaustion. If a cough develops, it can sink into the chest and develop into bronchitis. The person feels worse at night and better in fresh air.

Mercurius vivus. Here the cold is already advanced and the immune system is weakened. There is a sore throat that feels worse with swallowing, as well as sneezing, nasal discharge, foul-smelling breath, bad cough, profuse saliva, and night sweats.

Hepar sulph. This mineral remedy helps deep colds and the flu when these turn into infections and sinusitis. The person may have tried antibiotic treatments, which did not help. The person is very chilly, and there is often mucus in the lungs with a thick, yellow discharge. The emotional portrait is of a person who is extremely irritable and explosive, even toward people who try to help him or her. This is because the nervous system has become affected by the infection.

FOR THE FLU:

Eupatorium perfoliatum. This remedy is made from the herb boneset, and as its name implies, it is for a flu with achiness in the limbs, muscles, and bones, especially the long bones of the legs. The person has recurring fever with chill, preceded by thirst.

Nux vomica. This one is important for stomach flu. The picture here is of someone who is very chilly but who feels better in the open air. The person is worse after eating and has a dry, tickling feeling in the nose and throat. Emotionally, there is extreme irritability. But the main feeling here is, "If I could throw up or have a bowel movement, I would feel better." This remedy often helps the person to let go and feel much better.

Gelsemium. This remedy is often indicated for acute flu. A key symptom for this remedy is fever with absence of thirst.

FOR COUGHS:

Antimonium tartaricum. This is important for people who have very loose, rattling sounds in their chest during or after a cold. The cough is moist and the person coughs to expel mucus but finds that it remains. This remedy helps the type of cough that elderly people get in winter, the type that lasts all season. As with the other remedies, if this one does not help, it is advisable to consult with a health professional.

Dulcamara. Dulcamara is needed for coughs that get worse when weather begins to turn cold and damp. It is also for coughs that come on after the feet get wet. A typical time to take dulcamara is in the autumn.

Rhumex crispus. This is for a dry, hacking cough that remains after a cold, particularly when the person keeps losing his or her voice. Typically, it is worse in the evening and upon arising in the morning. It also worsens when the weather changes from cold to warm or vice versa.

Ignatia. The cold and cough for which ignatia is prescribed follow an emotional upset. The cough is tickling and irritating, and the person can cough until exhaustion.

FOR BLOCKED SINUSES:

Kali bichromicum. This remedy is for people who exhibit thick green or yellow mucus. There is pain at the root of the nose, in between the eyes. There can also be pain in small spots in the face, which feel better when pressed.

Pulsatilla. Here the mucus can be blown out easily. These people usually feel better in fresh air with movement. The cold is worse in the evening or at night.

Reflexology

Reflexology is the application of pressure to the feet in order to promote healing in other parts of the body. The idea is to work specific points on the feet that are said to correspond to these other problem areas. While reflexology is not in and of itself curative, it can allow energy that was previously blocked to reinvigorate the body, and in that way it can be part of an overall healing program.

Generally, for a cold, reflexologists say that the main area of focus is the toes, as they represent the head and throat. The very top of the toes corresponds to the brain, while the bottom of the toes corresponds to the face, eyes, sinuses, eustacian tubes, jaw, and throat. Another connection that reflexologists cite is the part on the foot that meets the toes, and the nerves in the spine. An additional important area to work is the ball of the foot, said to correspond to the chest/lung area.

Aromatherapy

Inhaling the volatile oils of eucalyptus and thyme can relieve lung congestion in that the oils act as expectorants, helping us to cough up mucus and pollution. Other helpful oils include garlic, lemon, pine, rosemary, lavender, peppermint, and hyssop. Aromatherapist Valerie Cooksley, author of *Aromatherapy: A Lifetime Guide to Healing with Essential Oils,* describes how to do this, through steam inhalation: Add the oil to a ceramic or glass bowl of water that is hot, but not boiling. Then close your eyes, and hold your head about 8 inches from the bowl with a tent made from a towel over your head. Inhale slowly and deeply for 5 to 10 minutes. The process can be repeated 2 or 3 times a day, when needed.

Aromatic baths with essential oils can be helpful too. Lavender, geranium, and hyssop are recommended for this purpose. Be sure to use a carrier, such as Epsom salt, sea salt, honey, or cream. Otherwise, the oils will just float to the top.

As a preventive measure, mists of essential oils can be sprayed into our living quarters to kill harmful bacteria in the air. Oils with antiseptic qualities include lemon, orange, bergamot, citronella, eucalyptus, juniper, lemon grass, peppermint, pine, rosemary, sandalwood, and tea tree oil.

Treatment Summary

Alkaline fruits and vegetables are rich in nutrients that help the body fight off colds and the flu.

Herbs have immune-enhancing properties, especially when taken at the first sign of a cold or flu.

Vitamin C, bioflavonoids, and GLA strengthen the immune system, thus helping us counteract colds and the flu.

Getting enough rest is an important strategy in fighting off these illnesses.

Homeopathic remedies for alleviating colds and flu are given according to symptoms and stage of illness.

Applying pressure to points on the feet can speed up recovery.

Inhaling essential oils can help clear up congestion, and when sprayed into the air, mists of these oils have a germ-deactivating effect.

See also: Fever

Dental Disorders

Going to the dentist is often considered an unpleasant experience. Most people associate the dentist's office with pain, jarring sounds and medical devices that contribute to patient anxiety just by virtue of their appearance. Of course, much of this apprehension is due to the many common dental problems a person will probably experience at some point in life, such as cavities, root canal problems, and gum disease.

What many people do not know is that these conditions, which are commonly viewed simply as uncomfortable, anxiety-producing annoyances, can actually lead to a variety of infections in the body. The potentially harmful consequences are little known because conventional dentistry treats the mouth as if it is separate from the rest of the body; the assumption is that once the problem is corrected there is no further cause for concern. Biological or holistic dentistry, on the other hand, supports the view that infections of the teeth, gums, and other areas in the mouth can spread bacteria, viruses, and other toxins. This can depress the immune system, which, in turn, can lead to disease.

Teeth contain tubules, and these can harbor billions of germs. These microorganisms can then spread to infect the lymph, blood, and nerve networks to activate severe illnesses anywhere in the body, including the heart, kidneys, joints, endocrine system, nervous system, and brain. Biological dentists therefore devote part of their attention to eliminating toxic dental materials, ensuring that infections do not emerge or remain in areas where they often go unnoticed, and minimizing other stresses to the immune system. Of course, they also deal with common dental ailments.

Common Problems

Cavities

Most people experience tooth decay, which begins as small holes in the teeth. When a cavity occurs, it is important to get it filled, as decay progresses and can get larger, leading to more severe loss of tooth structure. However, the substances used as fillings for cavities can be harmful. The most common type of filling, which has been used for over 150 years, is the silver amalgam filling. What many people do not know is that it contains a large percentage of mercury, which is a material known to be more toxic than lead. It is believed that vapors from the mercury in fillings are released at low levels and can enter the body through inhalation. The material can also be ingested, as tiny portions of the metal may dislodge.

Periodontal Disease

The first stage of periodontal, or gum, disease is gingivitis, which is an inflammation of the gum tissue due to bacterial infection. If left unattended for a long time, gingivitis can evolve into a more serious form of periodontal disease called periodontitis. In this condition, the bone underneath the gum begins to dissolve. Not only can this cause pain and eventual tooth loss, it has the capability of spreading bacterial infection to the rest of the body.

Cavitations

These are chronic infections within the jawbone. This condition is generally a result of diseased tissue or infected bone which are left after teeth have been removed. Circulation is then impeded and proper healing cannot take place. This situation can be corrected by cleaning the lesion.

Bruxism

This is the condition popularly known as grinding the teeth. It is not uncommon, and it occurs most often at night. The reason this condition is a cause for concern is that when people grind their teeth, it places abnormal pressures on the teeth and on surrounding areas. This can create an environment that leads to more serious dental problems, such as toothaches, periodontal disease, and infections.

Causes

Poor diet and lack of proper nutrients constitute a major reason for tooth decay, infection, and bruxism. All the refined foods in today's American diet, particularly sugar, fuel bacteria, and our resistance to the bacteria is at the same time lowered by the sugar, so they are able to grow and spread. Hidden food allergies, which increase chances of infection, can also be a problem.

Stress is another cause of dental disorders. It affects our bodies in a few ways. It can overactivate the adrenal glands, which allows for too much calcium in the bloodstream. That calcium is taken from bones, causing them to be weakened and damaged. Stress can also negatively impact upon the immune system, lowering resistance to overall infection and disease.

There are also lifestyle considerations, oral habits, and environmental factors that will contribute to an increased amount of bacteria in the mouth. These include smoking, chewing tobacco, heavy metal contamination, swallowing incorrectly, biting lips or nails, breathing through the mouth, thumb sucking, chewing gum, poorly fitting bridges, crowns (caps), and chemicals such as pesticides and drugs. The teeth may also be filled with toxic metals and other dental materials which are poisonous. Other factors in dental health include the resistance level of the individual (if it's low, infection can take hold more easily), and skeletal deformities, either congenital or due to trauma, which can necessitate dental work. In addition, electrogalvinism, electrical currents created by dissimilar metals in dental fillings and on different teeth, can create health problems.

Symptoms

When dental problems extend their effects to other parts of the body, they do so by contributing to such conditions as high blood pressure, chronic fatigue, heart problems, epilepsy, multiple sclerosis, brain tumors, arthritis, some forms of cancer (e.g., osteosarcoma and thyroid cancer), vision impairment, and pain in the face, head, or joints.

The major signs of advanced cavities are pain and extreme sensitivity to heat and cold, since the nerve is more exposed. When fillings are too old, material will get worn and change shape. Teeth can break causing fillings to fall out. Then food can wedge in the hole causing constant irritation.

Bacterial infection in the gums is characterized by bleeding, puffy gums, gum erosion at the base of the tooth, and bad breath. When gum infection advances to a more serious stage, it can be marked by bone loss in addition to gum loss, toothache, loose teeth, and nerve sensitivity.

Cavitations may cause no symptoms or, at the other extreme, severe discomfort. This can manifest as chronic facial pain, persistent pain in the eyes, and distress in other areas of the body.

Treatment

The Conventional Approach

DRILLING

This is usually an accepted part of several procedures used to correct a wide variety of dental problems. While drilling is helpful in removing decay, patients should be aware that it can also cause a variety of difficulties. For instance, if a drill is used improperly or at too high a speed, it can cause trauma to the tooth, resulting in inflammation and infection. As in all areas of health care, it is important to choose your dentist carefully, seeking someone recommended by satisfied patients.

ROOT CANAL THERAPY

This is a procedure performed to salvage a badly damaged tooth where the nerve is affected. In the root canal process, the dentist will remove the contents from the pulp chamber (nerve and other debris), and then seal the root canal space. One problem with root canal therapy is that thousands of tubules can harbor bacteria. Doing the root canal does not remove bacteria from these tubules. Further, since antibacterial drugs cannot eliminate the bacteria from the tubules in the root of the tooth, these bacteria can eventually discharge toxins into the bloodstream.

FLUORIDATION

Fluoride has generally been considered beneficial for preventing tooth decay. It is contained in toothpastes and in some communities' tap water. The problem is, though, that fluoride is actually a toxic chemical. Studies have shown that areas using fluoridated drinking water have a higher percentage of hip fracture and cancer cases among their populations than do neighborhoods with non-fluoridated water. In addition, research shows no difference in decay rates between children who consume fluoridated water and those who do not.

Prevention

We've all heard it, but it bears repeating: The best treatment for dental problems is prevention. And this starts with a good dietary foundation. To maintain a healthy mouth, make sure your meals are centered on whole fresh foods, and include a high-protein breakfast. Products rich in calcium, such as milk, cheese, yogurt, and green, leafy vegetables, will help to produce strong teeth. Raw fruits and vegetables are particularly important because of their ability to enhance enzyme functioning.

SUPPLEMENTS AND HERBS

Vitamins E, A, and D are beneficial to healthy teeth and gums overall, and vitamin C (500 mg 4 times daily) is important for gum health and will help fight plaque. In order to properly fortify the bone, which is the foundation of the teeth, the following are suggested: silica and zinc to ensure adequate bone formation; manganese to maintain the ligaments that surround the teeth;

and magnesium and calcium, which are crucial to ensuring the strength of the bones. Essential fatty acids, including EPA and DHA, are also beneficial because they facilitate the transport of calcium and magnesium through the cell membrane. Other recommended supplements include bioflavonoids, coenzyme Q10 (100 mg per day) to aid in cellular respiration, garlic and chlorella to neutralize and eliminate some of the contaminating heavy metals and strengthen the immune system, and GLA, which enhances prostaglandin production and possesses anti-inflammatory abilities.

PROPER DENTAL HYGIENE

Tooth brushing should be made a part of any daily routine. And one should not forget to include the tongue in the brushing routine. The tongue houses germs that can cause dental problems, and rinses are not generally effective against these bacteria. It is recommended that a person brush gently with baking soda as it is a germ-fighter.

Additionally, flossing should be performed on a regular basis since this technique can get to the plaque between teeth where brushing can't. One should also remember that regular professional cleanings in a dental office are imperative since they can better remove the hardened material around the teeth. The dentist can also check to see if there are any emerging problems in order to prevent their worsening.

Biological Dentistry

If a problem already exists, there are many treatments that can be considered. In the case of cavities, both conventional dentists and holistic, or biological, dentists will agree that fillings need to be placed. However, given the potentially harmful effects of the silver amalgam filling, it is important to discuss the other options available with the dentist. Biological dentistry will ensure that the patient receives the type of filling that is best suited to his or her needs. The dentist will test the patient for biocompatibility of the materials that are to be used. Often, people have several types of metals in their mouth, from fillings, crowns, and other dental work. Dissimilar metals in the mouth can block energy and incite illnesses in the body. Therefore, ensuring that the metals in the mouth are compatible is an important practice that most conventional dentists do not perform.

With regard to infection and inflammation, conventional dentistry will tend to focus on cleaning and removing the bacteria and their source. The affected tooth may be removed so that infection doesn't persist and negatively impact the immune system. While these surgical treatments are often necessary, the holistic dentist also stresses consideration of natural solutions, either in addition to or instead of conventional treatments. The relation of the mouth to the rest of the body is a main tenet of biological dentistry.

Homeopathic Dental Remedies

ACONITE

A dosage of 30-200c can be given to a person for an abrupt rush of intense pain (commonly due to cold air). Aconite can also be used for panic, fright, and general restlessness.

APIS MELLIFICA

This remedy helps decrease inflammation after injection, and is usually given in 30c potency three times a day.

ARNICA

This can be used after trauma in general, particularly where there is bleeding. Specifically, it is a good remedy for drilling. The recommended potency for arnica is 30c.

ARSENICA ALBUM

This is used in doses of 6 to 30c for delicate, bleeding gums or a toothache that is alleviated by warm water.

BELLADONNA

This is prescribed for early dental abscess characterized by redness and irritation in dosages of 30-200c. It is also beneficial for the pain associated with bruxism.

CALENDULA

This topical solution can be used as a general disinfectant to heal injuries and reduce pain. (However, it should not be applied where an infection exits on broken skin, to guard against closing the wound before the infection has had time to drain.) It can also be used as a mouthwash.

COFFEA CRUDA

This has a tranquilizing effect and is often used for a toothache that gets worse with heat but is relieved by cold water or ice. It can be given in doses of 30-200c.

FERRUM PHOSPHORICUM

Given in doses of 12-30c, this medicine is used for throbbing pain or gums that bleed after brushing.

HEPAR SULPHURIS

Cases of ulcerated infection benefit from this remedy.

HYPERICUM

This is another good remedy for trauma, particularly for easing sharp pain associated with tender gum tissue. Not only does hypericum decrease pain and swelling, it fosters the regeneration of disjoined nerves. It is given at 30c potency.

MERCURIUS SOLUBILIS

This is used for festering gum tissue, indicated by a coated tongue and bad taste in the mouth.

STAPHYSAGRIA

This is good after surgery or incision wounds.

SILICA

This is used to drain out an acute abscess.

Other Approaches

Also, an herbal preparation that works to minimize inflammation is a paste consisting of a bit of myrrh and peppermint oil combined with goldenseal root powder. Place directly on the infected area.

Acupuncture can be used in dental treatment; research shows that this ancient technique is effective in relieving pain after dental surgery.

What to Avoid

It's most important that sugar and sugary foods be eliminated from the diet (particularly soft drinks which can remove calcium from the teeth). The consumption of processed foods should be restricted, and it is also important to refrain from alcohol, caffeine, and diuretics.

Treatment Summary

To prevent dental problems, eat a good diet consisting of whole, fresh foods and products rich in calcium; consider taking a variety of vitamin and mineral supplements and using the herbal extract aloe vera as a mouthwash; practice proper dental hygiene, including brushing with baking soda and hydrogen peroxide, flossing, and getting regular cleanings by the dentist.

Biological dentistry warns about the use of silver amalgam fillings and supports checking the biocompatibility of metals in the mouth in order to determine the right filling substance for a particular person. For infection and inflammation, conventional dentistry normally chooses to remove the bacteria and possibly remove the tooth.

A paste of myrrh, peppermint oil, and goldenseal root can be placed directly on an infected area to minimize inflammation.

Acupuncture is effective in relieving pain after dental surgery.

Homeopathic remedies can be used in dental treatment.

See also: Periodontal Disease

Depression

There is virtually no person who is immune to depression. Becoming depressed is a normal response to certain situations that arise as part of our daily lives. However, when low or blue feelings hinder our normal functioning in society, for an extended amount of time, they can be classified as a clinical depression requiring some type of treatment.

The incidence of depression has risen dramatically over the past several years; the condition affects over 30 million Americans. Its impact can range from mild—suggesting that the affected individual has the ability to defeat the illness through a variety of self-care techniques—to severe, a state that requires attention from a trained medical professional.

Depression can actually be classified as one of three types. Reactive depression is a consequence of a painful or anxiety-producing incident, such as the death of a loved one, the loss of a job, or an illness or family or relationship crisis. This is the most common type of depressive disorder, one that can affect anyone at any time of their life. A person suffering from a reactive depression generally displays a loss of interest in those things that used to provide pleasure, but is usually still able to function at a basic level.

A physically-based depression originates from an imbalance of chemicals in the brain. This type of depression tends to affect people after mid-life, although this is by no means always the case. There may be a genetic predisposition to this type of illness. It is characterized by a severe loss of interest or pleasure in almost everything, and the condition has the capacity to negatively impact normal everyday functioning in a significant way.

The last major type of depression, also physically based, is manic depression. This is manifested as severe mood swings. A person with manic depression will fluctuate between periods of extreme energy and vivacity and those of complete hopelessness.

Regardless of how the disease originates, the way it manifests itself, or the degree of severity, depression should generally be considered both a mind and a body disorder. Both realms should certainly be addressed when planning treatment.

Causes

When depression is externally caused, any type of extremely distressing situation may trigger it. Simply being exposed to depressed people can even be an influence, since children learn by imitation. While these are normal reactions, the condition can perpetuate itself when it affects the internal workings of the body, preventing the person from overcoming their pain. When it persists, the condition becomes clinical depression.

There are a number of nutritional factors that can affect a person's mood, contributing to depression. Vitamin deficiencies can play a part. The B vitamins are clearly related to the healthy maintenance of the brain. The level of folic acid, in particular, bears an inverse correlation to the severity of depression: the lower the level of folic acid in the blood, the higher the degree of depression. The mineral magnesium is also a substance found to be deficient in depressed people. Large amounts of fluoride, on the other hand, may lead to the onset of depression. These types of nutritional factors should not be surprising, even in the case of reactive depression. Once depressed, the person might lose interest in exercising and eating healthfully—or eating at all. Further, the person may be under a great deal of stress, which not only perpetuates poor eating habits but causes the more rapid loss of important nutrients.

Chemical imbalances in the brain can also be either the cause or effect of depression. Dopamine is the chemical that produces anxiety, stress, nervousness, and aggression. When the level of dopamine is elevated, a person may develop feelings of insecurity, paranoia, and fear. Serotonin is another important chemical in the brain that can affect a person's mental well-being. Individuals with low serotonin levels are usually controlled personalities who display mood swings and some sort of compulsion, such as alcoholism, overeating, or being a workaholic, perfectionist, or procrastinator. A serotonin imbalance can produce not only depression but internal anger.

Depression can also be linked to other physical factors, such as hypothyroidism and food or environmental allergies.

Symptoms

Depression is manifested both physically and emotionally. The classic physical signs of depression are headaches, fatigue, digestive problems, hyperactivity, sleeping disorders (these can be difficulty in falling or staying asleep or the need for an inordinate amount of sleep), loss of concentration, and distorted eating patterns—either the urge to consistently overeat or loss of appetite. A significant change in weight is often evident.

The emotional side of depression can include excessive crying, pessimism, a sense of worthlessness, guilt, or self-pity, loss of self-esteem, loss of enjoyment from normally pleasurable activities, decrease in sex drive, and suicidal tendencies. It is important to note that anyone who talks of suicide should be taken seriously, and professional help should be provided.

While many of the physical and emotional symptoms of depression are things that can be a normal part of everyday life, when several of these symptoms are experienced for any prolonged length of time (a few weeks or more), they may be an indication of depression, and, again, professional help should be sought.

Treatment

The conventional medical approach to depression is either drug therapy, psychotherapy, or a combination of the two. Drug therapy—antidepressants such as Prozac—can help people feel better, but there are negative side effects to these drugs, and we do not know the ramifications of long-term use. And while psychotherapy is a good outlet for depressive emotions, and may help some patients, it is also important to treat the body as well as the mind.

Natural approaches that treat both the mind and body gently are another avenue to try. Powerful, long-term results have been shown with these. Further, it's always a good idea not just to treat symptoms, but rather to focus on overcoming fundamental causes of a condition and to shore up long-term physical and mental health. Most important, a depressed person should speak with his or her doctor, as every individual's situation and needs are unique.

Exercise

Activity is not only an important factor in preventing depression, it can help people overcome it. Exercise can increase a person's energy level with lasting effect. As a result, the individual is left with a feeling of revitalization and accomplishment. The biggest problem in introducing any type of exercise regimen into a depressed person's routine is overcoming the difficulty of getting started. When one is depressed, it is very hard to begin any type of activity; the tendency is rather to withdraw. One suggestion, then, in getting started in an exercise routine is to begin with simple movements. First, just getting out of bed and going for a walk can start to afford the person a sense of well-being. Mild stretching exercises and active hobbies are also a way to introduce exercise into a person's life. As the activity begins to positively affect the mind and body, it can then be increased to a level and type appropriate for that individual.

Diet

Getting the proper amounts of amino acids in the system is very important. Therefore, the type of foods one should concentrate on are raw, fresh vegetables and a balance of protein foods. Complex carbohydrates are particularly important for the individual who has a low level of serotonin. A problem in getting the depressed person to eat healthfully is to overcome the feeling of not wanting to be bothered thinking about diet or not having the energy to prepare a nutritious meal. One suggestion is to make easy meals in quantity once a week. A large amount of salad, for instance, can be stored in the refrigerator. This will help an individual to eat wholesome food for several days without too much fuss.

Supplements

Nutritional status plays a key role in how we feel emotionally, and there are many recommended supplements one can take to optimize that. It is essential to get all the B-complex vitamins, since they work together to balance proper brain functioning. The essential fatty acids, such as omega-6 and omega-3, as well as magnesium and niacin, are of particular importance. Note, though, that niacin dosages and the length of time it should be taken will need to be carefully monitored as this nutrient can impact liver functioning. Vitamin C is important as an immune-enhancing antioxidant; it is also significant to the production of serotonin.

Social and Lifestyle Factors

Trying to persuade a despondent person out of his mood may be futile. However, distracting the depressed mind has proven beneficial. Interaction with other people is extremely important for a depressed person because it can get his or her mind off negative thoughts. In particular, doing things for other people, such as volunteer work, is a great way to get a depressed person out of his own dark thoughts and into something that will feel rewarding.

Herbs

There are herbal extracts that have properties similar to conventional antidepressant drugs, but that are gentler and without the drugs' side effects. Prime among these is St. John's Wort, which is very popular in Europe. Clinical double-blind, placebo-controlled studies exist to support the efficacy of St. John's Wort. Also consider valerian, skullcap, hops, kava kava root, passionflower, Chinese schizandra berry, wild oats, and calamus root.

Light Therapy

According to Dr. Michael Norden, author of *Beyond Prozac*, light therapy has shown positive results in overcoming mild depression associated with the winter season (called seasonal affective disorder, or SAD). The body chemistry of many individuals is thrown off by the decrease in the amount of daylight during this time. But treatments have been designed that utilize bright light to overcome this kind of depression. One of the newest treatments is called dawn simulation. A special lighting system in the bedroom is manipulated to mimic the sunrise. This technique has been proven to increase energy and help overcome difficulty in getting out of bed during this time of year.

Homeopathic Remedies

The following are the most common homeopathic treatments for acute, more temporary cases of depression. In cases of chronic depression, homeopathic remedies, while still beneficial, will need to be utilized in conjunction with other therapies. Always work with a qualified health professional.

AURUM METALLICUM

This remedy is prescribed by homeopaths to alleviate feelings of worthlessness, low self-esteem, and despair. It can help provide hope for a person with reactive depression, and is said to be particularly beneficial to those generally hard-working individuals who have had life-altering events that they feel suggest failure on their part. This type of person is usually idealistic and goal-oriented.

IGNATIA

In instances of depression caused by an event that produces profound sadness or grief, such as the loss of a loved one, and in which those feelings of deep sorrow are obvious, ignatia is prescribed.

NATRUM MURIATICUM

This treatment, like ignatia, is also used when depression is caused by an event that generates profound bereavement and distress. However, the difference is that this one is used for those individuals who cannot show their feelings. This is for people who appear strong and controlled and suffer in silence.

SEPIA

This remedy is used mainly for women going through menopause. While depression associated with menopause often appears and disappears at random, or for no apparent reason, the depression the woman feels is quite real and intense. She may feel disconnected from everything that once gave her pleasure, including family and friends. This type of depression can be characterized by irritability and indifference to others.

PULSATILLA
This is generally used for people who show signs of manic-depression.

What to Avoid

Our diet not only plays an important role in good health, it can also negatively impact emotions and result in depression. The following foods should be avoided so as to prevent a nutritional or chemical imbalance that could cause or contribute to depression: fast foods, simple carbohydrates (this is particularly important for people with low blood sugar), alcohol, artificial sweeteners, white flour products, and caffeine.

Treatment Summary

Psychotherapy may be helpful, but it should be used in conjunction with other approaches in order to address both the mind and the body.

Traditional drug therapy, while common, can produce negative side effects and tends to treat symptoms rather than causes of depression, something that is important for the long term.

Exercise can increase a person's energy level and produce feelings of revitalization and accomplishment. A person who is having difficulty getting started, can begin with simple movements. Once the effect of the activity is felt, it can be increased to a level and type appropriate for that individual.

A diet centered on raw, fresh vegetables and fruits, and a balance of proteins is recommended to ensure that the proper amounts of amino acids necessary for proper brain functioning are being ingested. Complex rather than simple carbohydrates (like sugar), should be the focus.

B-complex vitamins, niacin, and magnesium are important in preventing and overcoming depression.

Interaction with others may help in overcoming depression. Volunteer work, in particular, can help distract the person, as well as get him or her into something rewarding.

Some herbs have effects similar to those of antidepressant drugs, without drug side effects. St. John's Wort is widely used in Europe for this purpose, and double-blind studies have supported this herb's antidepressant effect. People have also had success with valerian, skullcap, hops, passionflower, Chinese schizandra berry, wild oats, and calamus root.

Light therapy can aid in the mild depression associated with the winter season.

The homeopathic remedies aurum metallicum, ignatia, natrum muriaticum, sepia, and pulsatilla are used for cases of acute, temporary depression.

Diabetes

Diabetes mellitus affects 14 million Americans and claims over a quarter of a million lives a year. The problem has grown increasingly worse, with a threefold increase in the past 35 years. The escalation in diabetes corresponds to a rise in heart disease, and both conditions have been associated with a greater concentration of refined carbohydrates in Western diets.

Diabetes is traditionally viewed as a failure of the pancreas to release enough insulin for sugar metabolism (insulin is the hormone needed to move sugar out of the blood and into tissues). Newer thinking in the field sees insulin deficiency as but one of three possible causes, the other two being insulin resistance and insulin insensitivity.

Juvenile diabetes, also known as type I, is generally characterized by a true insulin deficiency. This most serious form of the disease is believed to affect children and teenagers after their pancreas has been damaged from viral infections or extreme toxicity. It may also be genetically acquired. Juvenile diabetics must receive insulin regularly, and generally for life.

In most adult-onset, or type II, diabetes, the body produces sufficient insulin, but the cells do not respond to it. Normally, insulin enters the cells at points known as receptor sites. When receptor sites become plugged up by fat and cholesterol they become insensitive to insulin, and insulin cannot enter cells. Glucose remains in the blood, creating a condition of hyperglycemia or high blood sugar. This excess sugar is diagnosed as diabetes. In this scenario, there is a need to increase insulin sensitivity; taking more insulin will not accomplish this.

Insulin resistance is a closely related concept in which there is also sufficient insulin. Here, allergic responses to specific foods keep insulin from doing its job by disturbing carbohydrate metabolism. The foods creating the problem vary from person to person. Wheat may create high blood sugar in one individual while corn may adversely affect someone else. Allergy-provoking foods can be determined on an individual basis with food allergy tests.

Adult-onset diabetes is much more common than the juvenile type. It tends

177

to be an acquired disease, precipitated by overweight, poor diet, and lack of exercise. It may also be caused by frequently eaten foods in the diet that result in insulin resistance. Most of these cases can be controlled by addressing biochemical and nutritional needs.

The beginning stages of type II diabetes are often symptomless, although the prediabetic state can be accompanied by obesity, especially around the waistline. Classic diabetes symptoms are more often experienced by type I sufferers and include frequent urination, especially at night, great thirst and hunger, fatigue, weight loss, irritability, and restlessness. As diabetes progresses, the eyes, kidneys, nervous system, and skin become affected, and infections and hardening of the arteries can develop. In type I diabetes, a coma can result from a lack of insulin.

Treatment

Conventional Medical Approaches

After its development in the 1920's, man-made insulin was deemed a miracle cure. Indeed, it has prevented suffering and saved countless lives. Before the development of synthetic insulin, diabetes patients were given a bleak prognosis and suffered terribly from disease complications such as blindness, gout, and gangrene. Insulin has extended the lifespans of childhood diabetics from months to decades. Today, many diabetic children live normal, productive lives.

The problem with insulin is that it is prescribed universally, not just to those with true insulin deficiencies. Giving this hormone to a person with already sufficient levels does nothing to correct the underlying problem. Furthermore, its use can be counterproductive. This is because insulin stimulates the development of antagonists in the body that counteract its blood-sugar-lowering effects. When a diabetic receives insulin, and his or her blood sugar begins to fall, the body immediately responds with an output of growth hormones and epinephrine. These hormones keep blood sugar levels elevated. The result of aggressive insulin therapy, then, is a rebound effect.

Constant fluctuations in blood sugar can lead to a wide range of disorders. Clinical studies shows that diabetics treated aggressively with insulin have a 40-percent greater incidence of eye problems than those treated moderately. Nevertheless, aggressive insulin treatment is the modality of choice in mainstream medicine for diabetics with eye problems.

Another problem with insulin treatment is that it may contribute to inner arterial wall damage and lead to cardiovascular problems. In fact, the incidence of heart attacks and strokes is five to eight times greater among diabetics than in the general population. Seventy-five percent of all diabetic mortality is due to heart disease brought on by hardening of the major arteries.

Other complications from insulin are the result of damage to microvascular vessels, particularly those leading to the eyes, kidneys, and peripheral nerves. As these arteries become thick and brittle, it is more difficult for blood to pass through them, and they become less functional. In the eyes, sudden surges of blood sugar put extra stress on the retinal blood vessels. The repeated stresses that diabetics often experience cause these vessels to hemorrhage and break down. After several hemorrhages, blindness is a likely outcome. This is the second most common cause of blindness in older people, following glaucoma. In the kidneys, similar events can cause renal insufficiency, so that nitrogen wastes can no longer be eliminated from the body efficiently. Interference with blood circulation in both large and small vessels is responsible for the high incidence of neuritis and gangrene, which begins with peripheral sensations of tingling and ends with loss of feeling. A frequent outcome of this problem is amputation.

Insulin is not the only diabetic treatment of choice in orthodox medicine; there is also a group of oral medications that stimulate insulin secretion. Some of these drugs increase the sensitivity of receptor sites so that there are more locations for glucose to enter the cell.

In spite of their seeming benefits, oral agents, with names such as Orinase, Diabinase, and Tolinase, are a cause for concern because of their potential for adverse side effects. Most worrisome is an increased susceptibility to heart attacks. Diabetes itself makes a person more prone to heart disease, and diabetic drugs add to the likelihood of this event.

Orthodox medicine does also pay some attention to dietary modification, but again it may be missing the mark. Diabetic individuals are advised to avoid all carbohydrates, since these foods eventually break down into glucose. But no distinction is made between simple and complex carbohydrates. In addition, allergic responses to foods are not taken into account.

Unlike simple sugars, complex carbohydrates may be beneficial to diabetics. Although both are broken down into glucose, the latter do not go directly into the bloodstream. Complex carbohydrates go through a long digestive process, and release sugar into the blood gradually. Rather than contribute to high blood sugar levels, complex carbohydrates stabilize blood sugar levels, and improve health.

Diabetics are advised to eat high-protein diets, which can cause several additional problems, especially when protein is derived from animal sources. Animal proteins are high in fat, making the person more prone to cardiovascular disease. Receptor sites become clogged from fat and cholesterol, leading to greater insulin resistance. The inevitable rise in blood sugar results in the prescription of more medicine. Too much protein is also related to kidney damage. Since protein cannot be stored by the body, it needs to be immediately processed. A high-protein diet stresses nephron cells, causing diabetics to suffer from kidney deterioration. Many patients must receive dialysis or a kidney transplant as a result.

Natural Approaches

Diabetes is often reversible with the aid of a healthy lifestyle, diet, supplements, and exercise. When making these types of changes, it is important not to immediately go off any medication. Instead, a complementary physician should assist in the transition, which should be a gradual one. With a doctor's guidance, an insulin dependency may be reduced or completely eliminated. While type II diabetes responds most dramatically to such an approach, juvenile diabetes may improve as well, with patients needing less insulin and experiencing fewer complications.

DIET

Since diabetes and heart disease are so closely related, many complementary physicians recommend that diabetics follow the same type of low-fat diet used by heart patients. This diet consists of organic vegetarian foods, with lots of high-fiber vegetables eaten raw, sprouted, steamed, baked, or stir fried with little or no oil. The addition of bran and other forms of fiber will pull the extra sugar out of the system. Diabetics, as well as people prone to the disease, produce too much insulin in response to carbohydrates, so that many of the following foods should be completely omitted until insulin reactions normalize: bread, pasta, potatoes, rice, corn, parsnips, bananas, raisins, and other sweet fruits and vegetables. Good protein sources include organic turkey, chicken, egg whites, and tofu. The ratio of carbohydrates to proteins and fats should be in the range of 40:30:30.

EXERCISE

An exercise regimen is crucial for burning calories and normalizing metabolism, and is especially important for overweight adults who tend to be inactive. Exercise also heightens the body's sensitivity to insulin. By lowering cholesterol, exercise lowers triglyceride levels in the blood, making cells more available for glucose assimilation. This is why the insulin requirements of diabetic athletes always drop while they are engaged in swimming, soccer, and other sports. Conversely, athletes notice an increase in their insulin requirements when they cease their physical activities for any extended period.

Athletes are not the only ones to benefit from exercise. Ten to 20 minutes of light exercise after each meal helps to reduce the amount of insulin necessary to keep blood sugar levels under control. A brisk walk gets the body's metabolism working a little bit faster so that the absorption of food becomes more efficient. That prevents blood sugar from going up too high.

An exception to the exercise-after-meals rule is for diabetics with heart disease. In these patients, exercising after eating may precipitate an angina attack because of the transfer of blood from the intestines to the legs and other parts of the body.

ALLERGY TESTING

When allergies are the root of an insulin-resistance problem, testing for food allergies can be quite helpful. To determine whether a specific food is causing hyperglycemia, a doctor can monitor a patient's blood sugar before and after that food is eaten, looking for abnormal blood-sugar rises. Once allergy-provoking substances are identified and omitted, the patient with insulin resistance can often reverse his or her condition.

Eliminating allergens may also lead to weight loss. People tend to crave allergy-producing foods, but when these foods are taken out of the diet, the desire for them stops.

MINERAL SUPPLEMENTS

The most important mineral for diabetes may be vanadyl sulfate. Discovered in France in the late 1800s, vanadyl sulfate was used to control diabetes before insulin was developed. It's generally taken three times a day. Other important minerals are chromium picolinate, magnesium, and potassium, which help normalize glucose levels in insulin-dependent diabetics. Also, zinc is essential for normal insulin production.

HERBS

Dandelion root and eyebright cleanse the liver and blood, which indirectly helps treat diabetes.

Blueberry (also known as huckleberry) leaves are known to promote insulin production. Unlike many other medicinal herbs, blueberry tea is actually pleasant tasting. If you gather the leaves yourself (they grow all over the state of Pennsylvania) it's best to pick them before the fruit appears, or after it's gone. Otherwise, the berries absorb the strength of the plant.

By increasing circulation, ginkgo biloba can alleviate symptoms associated with diabetes, such as intermittent claudication and problems with the eyes.

Other herbs that can help diabetes and other pancreatic problems include pau d'arco, cedar berries, aloe, ginger, burdock, evening primrose, false unicorn root, onion, juniper berries, cranberry, fenugreek, goldenseal, alfalfa, and kelp. These herbs are safe to take along with any preexisting medications, and are especially good to take before pharmaceuticals are prescribed.

HOMEOPATHY

The remedy Mucokehl, from Germany, may actually reverse diabetic neuropathy. People have reported getting feeling back in their extremities, as well as eyesight improvement, with this medicine.

CHELATION THERAPY

This is helpful for its ability to reduce diabetic retinopathy and foot ulcers.

What to Avoid

Diabetics need to reduce their sugar intake and increase dietary fiber. Among its many detrimental effects, sugar works to lower chromium levels. As levels of this mineral go down, pressure in the eye increases. This can cause vision problems in diabetics.

Treatment Summary

Diabetics often do well on the same type of high-fiber, low-fat diet as heart patients are given, with a ratio of carbohydrate:protein:fat of 40:30:30.

Exercise can help correct a sluggish metabolism, normalize weight, and keep blood sugar under control.

It is essential to identify and omit allergy-producing foods from the diet.

Minerals that can help correct blood sugar imbalance are vanadyl sulfate, chromium picolinate, magnesium, and potassium.

The homeopathic remedy Mucokehl may help those with diabetic neuropathy to get feeling back in the extremities and improve eyesight.

Chelation therapy increases blood circulation to the microcapillaries in the eyes and extremities.

Digestive Disorders

One could call digestive disorders a virtual epidemic in this country, because they affect over two-thirds of all Americans. Dr. Kenneth Bock, of Rhinebeck, New York, refers to many of his patients as the walking wounded. While these people are well enough to lead normal lives, they are not functioning at an optimal level. Their early symptoms, though minor, indicate that the digestive system is unable to fully do its job of converting food to energy and carrying nutrients to other systems.

Left untreated, the slight discomforts of chronic indigestion gradually worsen, and the early warning signs of abdominal pain, cramps, diarrhea, bloating, gas, and constipation can graduate to full-blown diseases. Crohn's disease, ulcerative colitis, and irritable bowel syndrome may develop within the lower gastrointestinal tract. But bowel disorders can also help precipitate seemingly unrelated diseases, such as cancer, heart disease, arthritis, or renal disorders. At this point, diseases are generally treated with expensive, toxic treatments, which ignore the root of the problem.

Correcting digestive disorders in their early stages is the best way to avoid the need for invasive, harmful therapies later on. But even when caught late, many diseases can often be stopped in their tracks when attention is paid to correcting digestive imbalances.

First, it's helpful to understand the various types of digestive disorders.

Common Digestive Problems

Acid Indigestion

The term acid indigestion refers to the failure of the body to digest food properly due to insufficient stomach acid. Burping, stomach distension, flatulence, and sometimes diarrhea are indications of this condition. Low stomach acid can prevent the gastric mucosa from releasing sufficient intrinsic factor, a substance essential for the intestinal absorption of vitamin B12. This may result in pernicious anemia or in subclinical symptoms such as weakness, forgetfulness, and confusion.

Acid indigestion is commonly experienced after indulging in a rich, fatty, or overabundant meal. There is just too much for the body to handle, especially if food is gulped down. As a result, large chunks of poorly masticated food must be almost entirely digested in the stomach, and there simply is not enough acid for all that work. Acid indigestion may also be the result of aging, stress, or food sensitivities.

Bad Breath

Many of us take mints or use mouthwash to freshen our breath. But this will not get rid of the problem for long, as most bad breath stems from bacterial toxins in the gut. It is important to avoid being constipated, as this causes bacterial toxins to back up through the gut and be released through the mouth.

Constipation

If you are not having at least two easy bowel movements a day, you are probably constipated. Many people think it's normal to depend on laxatives to combat this problem, and, indeed, Americans spend a lot of money on these products. What this indicates is that, as a nation, we are not getting enough exercise, water, and fiber in our diet. Our high intake of processed foods is the biggest reason for constipation. Other causes of constipation are poor food choices, overeating, eating at night, drinking with meals, and high-protein diets. These habits tend to hinder the digestive process, and can create mucus in the colon.

Taking laxatives creates a dependency, and only worsens the problem, as the body forgets how to have a bowel movement on its own. Laxatives can also cause bowel inflammation and bleeding. Stress contributes to the problem by constricting colon muscles. Many people refuse to have a bowel movement away from home and need to pay more attention to their body's urges.

Long-term constipation can lead to more serious problems. Indeed, holistic doctors believe that nearly half of all diseases start in the colon. Sluggish bowels cause poisons to be absorbed into the blood, where they circulate and result in extra work for the other organs of elimination: the liver, kidneys, lungs, and skin. Any manner of disease, from colds and flu to arthritis, can eventually result.

Crohn's Disease

This is an inflammatory disease that usually affects the colon, but which can be found anywhere along the digestive tract, even as far up as the esophagus.

The inflammation goes deep into the tissues, and can cause structural changes. Symptoms of the disease include diarrhea, pain in the stomach, nausea, fever, chills, and loss of appetite.

Diarrhea

Loose, frequent, watery stools are usually a sign of another disorder, such as food poisoning, flu, malabsorption syndrome, or a more serious illness. The stool may contain mucus, pus, blood, or fat. Left untreated, diarrhea may lead to dehydration and the loss of trace minerals.

Diverticulitis

Small pockets commonly form in the colon, where food particles, bacteria, and viruses get stuck. Most people have these pockets and never know it, but sometimes they become inflamed and infected, a condition known as diverticulitis. This condition is accompanied by diarrhea and gas, and can be excruciatingly painful. Many doctors recommend avoiding seeded foods, such as raspberries and strawberries, which tend to clog the pockets, but once the infection is under control, a person can once again eat these high-fiber foods.

Flatulence

Flatulence is caused by the fermentation of carbohydrates in the small intestines. This may be a sign of inadequate intestinal flora, and a signal to take good quality probiotic supplements. Flatulence is also the result of poor digestion. Chewing food properly, building the liver, pancreas, and gallbladder, and rebalancing the enzymatic activity of the stomach, can all help to eliminate this problem.

Food Allergies

Classical allergies produce immediate symptoms. But masked, or cyclic allergies, which are more common, cause problems too, although the link may be harder to trace. This type of food allergy may be the result of eating the same foods too often, or of a system imbalanced by candida, parasites, or nonsteroidal medications. These factors can irritate the digestive lining and cause holes to develop in the mucosal lining of the small intestines, a phenomenon known as leaky gut syndrome. Oversized food particles can then enter the bloodstream. The immune system creates antibody reactions against the unusable food particles, and various problems can result, including asthma, arthritis, headaches, and chronic fatigue. Food allergies can cause a variety of symptoms, from fatigue and bloating to skin conditions, depression, and headaches. The food or foods causing the condition can be discovered through IgE antibody tests.

Gastric Reflux

A small sphincter at the base of the esophagus keeps stomach acid from splashing up as food goes down. When this does not work properly, acid from the stomach backs up into the esophagus and burns tissue to produce heartburn. Hiatal hernia may be the result of gastric reflux. Sometimes chiropractic manipulation and herbs, such as licorice and slippery elm, can help.

Irritable Bowel Syndrome

Ten to 20 percent of people suffer from irritable bowel syndrome, which is characterized by alternating constipation and diarrhea, and sometimes by abdominal pain, spasms, bloating, and flatulence. When the condition is severe, there may be blood or mucus in the stools, and fever. It may also result in poor appetite, even anorexia (which means absence of appetite), and varying degrees of anxiety and depression.

As with many digestive problems, the underlying cause of irritable bowel syndrome is often food sensitivities. Often the foods responsible have a delayed effect, causing a reaction 24 to 48 hours after being eaten. The most common offenders are wheat and dairy products, which are hidden in ingredients in many foods. Other common offenders include corn, coffee, tea, and citrus fruits. Irritable bowel syndrome may also be the result of candida, parasites, leaky gut syndrome, and chemical sensitivities.

Malabsorption Syndrome

Malabsorption syndrome is the failure of the body to absorb nutrients due to a digestive lapse. With this problem, after a food is eaten, the vitamins and minerals do not enter the cells, but are eliminated as waste products. The resulting lack of nutrition can be manifested in multiple symptoms, including weakness, anemia, loss of appetite, weight loss, swollen abdomen, muscle cramps, and bone pain. Malabsorption syndrome can be a side affect of other diseases, such as celiac disease, cystic fibrosis, and Whipple's disease. It can also be brought on by nervousness, anxiety, and fear, as well as by stomach or small bowel surgery, and by alcohol consumption.

Peptic Ulcers

Ulcers can be acute or chronic: acute ulcers are shallow and often symptomless, while chronic ulcers, known as true ulcers, are deep, painful, and damaging to muscles. Depending upon the part of the digestive tract affected, peptic ulcers are known either as gastric or duodenal. Both produce a gnawing pain in the upper abdomen, but the timing is often different. Distress from a gastric, or stomach, ulcer is usually experienced after a meal, while pain from a duodenal ulcer, which is located in the first part of the small intestine, is generally felt on an empty stomach. The person has pain between meals or is uncomfortably awakened in the middle of the night.

Orthodox Western medicine relates ulcers to excess stomach acid, and to the presence of certain bacteria, such as Campylobacter and Helicobacter pylori. In fact, some estimates attribute the bacteria to ulcers in 80 percent of cases. While stomach acid and bacteria can cause irritation leading to ulcers, the problem is mainly due to the susceptibility of the involved area. The epithelial lining of the stomach or duodenum is weak, and therefore vulnerable to attack.

Drugs designed to block stomach acid, such as Zantac, cimetidine, and Tagamet, are standard treatment. By masking symptoms, these appear to alleviate ulcers, at first. But since they do nothing to address the real cause of the problem, ultimately, they may cause more harm than good.

The Oriental medical approach has proven helpful to some ulcer patients. In Oriental medicine, not all ulcers are similarly treated. Practitioners carefully diagnose patients, looking for imbalanced systems (meridians), and base their recommendations on these findings. Some ulcer patients need to stay away from spicy foods, for example, while others do not. Some benefit from certain herbal combinations, and others need acupuncture.

Ulcerative Colitis

Ulcerative colitis is a chronic, episodic, inflammatory disease of the large intestine and rectum, often caused by food allergies. Symptoms are debilitating and can include excruciating pain; stools containing blood, pus, and mucus; explosive bowel movements; chronic gas; distension of the bowel; ulcers; excessive diarrhea and constipation; fever; chills; anemia; and weight loss. Complications can include peripheral arthritis, ankylosing spondylitis, kidney and liver disease, and inflammation of the eyes, skin, and mouth. The disease tends to come and go, and a person may be fine for months at a time. Parasites and bacteria are sometimes the cause.

Diagnosis

Minor digestive problems, with their small discomforts, tend to be ignored by orthodox medicine. As conditions become more severe, diagnoses are made through x-rays, scopes, and blood tests, and drug therapy is generally prescribed. But medications are only quick fixes, not permanent solutions, because they only mask the underlying cause of the problem.

Since a myriad of factors can cause digestive illnesses, all possible etiologies should be investigated. Complementary physicians employ multiple measures of diagnosis, including tests for food sensitivities, parasites, candida, thyroid functioning, and nutrient levels. Once the cause of the problem is identified, the individual can be appropriately treated.

Treatments

Digestive disturbances respond well to nutritional protocols that include changes in diet, supplements, herbs, and detoxification. In addition, stress reduction techniques can make a profound difference. Work with a holistically-oriented physician who can help you tailor a program to your individual needs. The following recommendations are basic to overall well-being.

High-Fiber Diet

Foods that work with the body are wholesome and natural, not processed and chemically altered. Basically, this means that the healthful diet contains many complex carbohydrates, which are fiber-rich foods. We ought to follow the example of primitive cultures, who do not suffer from gastrointestinal diseases seen in the modern world, and eat five to nine servings of fruits and vegetables daily. If constipation is a problem, include fresh fruits, especially apples, figs, peaches, berries, oranges, and prunes. Vegetables, raw juices, and sprouts are other good choices. Eat lightly, and go on a short vegetable or fruit juice fast, if possible. It is also helpful to drink a glass of warm water in the morning and take a tablespoon of olive oil before retiring at night. The rest of the diet should focus on whole grains and legumes, with small amounts of nuts and seeds. Note that, despite its name, whole wheat bread contains a lot of white flour. Consider, as better sources of fiber, brown rice, barley, millet, and buckwheat. In addition to fiber, green leafy vegetables are high in magnesium, a mineral that helps the muscles of the intestines contract in a rhythmic fashion (peristalsis) to help with bowel movements.

Note that a healthy diet need not be bland. Common spices and herbs are more than flavorful; they actually aid digestion. Allspice and rosemary can relieve indigestion, basil and dill can calm an upset stomach, while cayenne and horseradish stimulate circulation and quicken digestion. Spices move foods through the system more easily with little distress to the GI tract. They also promote elimination through the increase of perspiration through the skin.

Foods with Flora

We have more bacteria in our digestive system than we have cells in our body. We may not realize it, but these good bacteria do a lot for us by allowing us to benefit from the vitamins we take in, and by acting as our first line of defense against other microbial organisms. Unfortunately, modern living often destroys these friendly colonies through stress and drug use, particularly antibiotic use. It is therefore important to repopulate the digestive tract with natural flora by eating natural foods with high-quality bacteria, such as tempeh, sauerkraut, and yogurt.

Food Preparation

When preparing foods, it is important to maximize digestibility without altering the integrity of the food's cellular structure. This means the avoidance of irradiated foods, foods prepared in microwaves, and overcooked foods. Many foods should be juiced or eaten raw, as cooking destroys important enzymes. When cooking, steaming is generally preferable to boiling, although boiling in one inch of water is better than boiling in six inches of water, and boiling for five minutes is better than for 20. If prepared foods are chosen, it is best to eat those closest to their natural state. For example, frozen peas are preferable to peas that have been boiled and canned. The type of cookware is equally important; aluminum cookware should be avoided because it gets into the food and can lead to many serious health problems.

Herbs

As we've mentioned, nature supplies us with a great variety of herbs for strengthening digestion and overcoming everyday problems. Those with digestive problems should keep the following in mind:

ALOE VERA

The valuable phytochemicals contained in aloe vera can help correct many chronic conditions, including indigestion, malabsorption syndrome, leaky gut syndrome, spastic colon, and ulcerative colitis.

CHAMOMILE

This is a gentle yet highly effective remedy for irritable bowel syndrome and other digestive disturbances accompanied by anxiety. A cup of boiled water can be poured over a heaping tablespoon of dried chamomile flowers and strained after several minutes. Taken with honey, this is a delicious, soothing tea that can be consumed throughout the day, between meals, and before retiring at night.

FENNEL

Fennel helps alleviate flatulence, cramps, and indigestion. It can be taken as a tea, or the seeds can be chewed.

GINGER

A cup of ginger tea in the morning, with bee propolis and raw unheated organic honey, will invigorate the system and promote good digestion.

NETTLES

Nettles make a good tea to take for diarrhea. Usually, diarrhea causes a loss of trace elements, and nettles tea is a good source of these minerals, as well as of chlorophyll.

OATS

Oat tea will soothe a nervous stomach and strengthen a weak digestive system.

ORIGANUM

This is known to strengthen the stomach and stop flatulence.

LICORICE

Licorice is an herbal aid for alleviating heartburn and recovering from ulcers. In fact, this herb may be as helpful as standard medications for healing gastric and duodenal ulcers. Licorice stimulates the production of prostaglandins that promote healing to the whole gastrointestinal tract, but especially the stomach. The deglycyrrhizinated form of the extract (DGL) prevents blood pressure elevation. Taking licorice three to four times a day can provide tremendous relief.

Herbs that stimulate liver activity improve digestion as well, and include agrimony, dandelion, barberry, wild yam, and milk thistle. Herbs that soothe and coat the digestive tract include mallow, chickweed, mullein, and plantain. Other herbs to investigate include balmony, barberry, cayenne, gentian root, ginseng, goldenseal (on a temporary basis), coltsfoot, lobelia, wild cherry bark, skullcap, slippery elm, wormwood, and angelica.

When constipation is the problem, these herbs can be taken on a temporary basis: cascara sagrada bark, senna, flaxseed, bayberry root bark, goldenseal root, and red raspberry leaves. Herbs and olive oil can also be added to warm-water enemas.

Supplements

Supplements give the body extra concentrated support. It's a good idea to start slowly and build up to an optimum level, and to use supplements under the guidance of a knowledgeable health professional.

ANTIFUNGALS

These natural alternatives to antibiotics can help get rid of parasites and yeast overgrowth. Grapefruit seed extract, pau d'arco tea, garlic, artemesia, and various homeopathic remedies all have an antifungal effect. Sometimes antifungal medications, such as Nystatin or Diflucan, are prescribed by a physician. Antifungals work best when accompanied by a yeast-free diet.

ANTIOXIDANTS

To support the digestive system, a person may need up 800 IU of vitamin E, 1 to 6 grams of vitamin C, and between 25,000 and 50,000 IU of beta carotene. Patients with severe cases of inflammatory bowel disease may benefit from higher doses of nutrients given intravenously. Using this route, a person may be given 20,000 mg of vitamin C to start and graduated to 50,000 mg. In addition, nutrients such as magnesium, B vitamins, glutathione, and glycyrrhizin may be used.

BIOFLAVONOIDS

Vitamin C works even better in conjunction with bioflavonoids. Quercetin and pycnogenol are especially important because of their anti-inflammatory and immune-enhancing properties. Usually 300 mg of quercetin and 25 mg of pycnogenol, three times a day, are recommended.

COENZYME Q10

Inflammations respond well to this nutrient when 50 to 100 mg are taken two to three times daily.

DIGESTIVE ENZYMES

Stomach or pancreatic enzymes can be useful aids to digestion.

L-GLUTAMINE

L-glutamine nourishes and heals the entire lining of the upper and lower intestines, and is especially helpful for patients who are losing weight. Anywhere from 3 to 10 grams are needed. Since this is a large amount, glutamine should be taken under the guidance of a health practitioner.

MAGNESIUM

People who tend to get constipated are often deficient in this vital mineral. Using 200 to 300 mg of magnesium twice a day will not only help with the peristaltic activity of the GI tract, but will address a deficiency in a large number of individuals.

OMEGA-3 FATTY ACIDS

A number of studies prove that fish oils have anti-inflammatory effects. Between 1000 and 2000 mg can be taken 2 to 3 times daily with meals; take less if belching or nausea result.

PEPPERMINT OIL

Clinical tests have long shown peppermint oil to reduce colonic spasms. One capsule of enterically coated peppermint oil can be taken two to three times a day, on a temporary basis, to remove this discomfort. A handful of patients will get a burning sensation in the rectum after using peppermint oil, in which case the therapy should be discontinued. Chamomile tea can be taken instead.

PROBIOTICS

Literally translated, probiotics means for life, and the word refers to products that replenish the healthy bacteria in our digestive systems. Hundreds of studies show Lactobacillus acidophilus, Bifidobacterium bifidum, and fructo-oligosaccharides to promote overall good health. They are especially important to use after antibiotic therapy, vaginal yeast infections, and urinary tract infections.

PSYLLIUM SEED AND WHEAT BRAN

These products are helpful for overcoming constipation when a high-fiber diet alone does not seem to make a difference. Wheat bran should be used only by people who do not have wheat allergies.

BOWEL DETOXIFICATION

Getting rid of toxins is an important first step for many people with bowel disorders. Until this is done, none of the nutrients for rebuilding the system will make much difference. Detoxification can be approached in many ways. Bentonite is a clay-like substance, used in a drink, that draws out toxins from the colon. Colon therapy also eliminates stored wastes and restores proper tissue and organ function. Some physicians place their patients on elimination diets, consisting of hypoallergenic foods, until a time when the body can handle certain foods again on a rotational basis. Total parenteral nutrition, or intravenous feeding, is used in extreme cases to quiet down the colon before other dietary approaches are tried. These are all excellent methods for healing an overburdened digestive tract.

Stress Reduction

The expression butterflies in my stomach reflects an example of how our thoughts and feelings affect us physically. A large bundle of nerves, known as the solar plexus, is located in the stomach area. When our nerves are stressed in any way, this is often the first place to be affected. This is why we have gut reactions.

The best way to deal with mental and emotional problems is to address the issue at hand. When anxiety interferes with clear thinking, there are many techniques for helping us to overcome those stresses, including meditation, biofeedback, yoga, tai chi, hypnosis, and breathing techniques. Remembering to take time each day for the things we enjoy, such as gardening, playing a musical instrument, and spending quality time with friends and family is also important for our digestive wellness, and for our total well-being as well.

What To Avoid

Poor Food Choices

Digestive disorders often result from food sensitivities; therefore, problem foods must be eliminated from the diet. People suffering from inflammatory bowel diseases usually need to stop eating wheat and certain other grains, dairy products, sugar, and specific carbohydrates. Doctors who take people off foods they are sensitive to often see dramatic improvement in just weeks.

In addition to allergy-producing foods, there are some common rules of what not to eat for good health. In general, the substances to stay away from are processed foods; saturated fats; artificial colorings, flavorings, and preservatives; irradiated produce and herbs; canned foods; foods grown in chemical fertilizers and those treated with pesticides or wax; and overcooked foods. When one is constipated, foods to stay away from include starchy grains, meat, and dairy products.

Drugs

Antibiotic overuse is the underlying cause of many health problems that begin in the digestive system. Antibiotics do not discriminate between good and bad bacteria; rather they destroy bacteria indiscriminately, and alter the flora in the gut, leading to an overgrowth of yeast. Yeast infections are believed to be contributing factors to many illnesses, including inflammatory bowel diseases. Antibiotics can also have the effect of altering bacterial structure. When this happens, good bacteria may begin to produce toxins that harm the gut. Many problems may result, including illnesses that seem to be unrelated to the digestive tract, such as chronic fatigue syndrome and fibromyalgia. Non-steroidal anti-inflammatory medications, caffeine, nicotine, and alcohol, are other drugs that can wreak havoc on digestive health.

Parasites

Parasitic infections can cause chronic gastrointestinal problems and are quite common throughout the world. It is important to take as many precautions as possible against contracting these microbes, such as washing hands after using the toilet, and not ordering salad foods in restaurants. Anyone who suspects that they have this condition should see a doctor who specializes in the treatment of parasites. A testing procedure known as an endoscopy is the best method for identifying parasites that attach themselves to the intestinal wall, because these parasites are often missed in routine stool analysis.

Improper Chewing

Chewing constitutes the first stage of digestion, and sets the stage for how much nutritional benefit we receive. Unless chewing is slow and thorough, saliva will not mix sufficiently with food. Improper chewing leaves food chunks too large to pass easily through the esophagus and into the stomach for the next stage of digestion. When improperly chewed food reaches the stomach, excess stomach acid is secreted to break down oversized food particles. This subjects the inner linings of the stomach and intestinal tract to high levels of acid, which is extremely corrosive and, over time, damaging. This can aggravate digestive problems, causing everything from indigestion and heartburn to ulcers.

Drinking with Meals

Drinking with meals should be minimized or avoided, as fluid dilutes digestive juices, making the breakdown of food more difficult. Incompletely digested food causes irritation of the bowel lining and can lead to ulcerative colitis. Toxins from incompletely digested food can enter the bloodstream and activate an immune reaction. Drinking while eating also encourages gulping down food chunks that would otherwise be chewed more thoroughly. This is dangerous in that it can result in choking.

Eating Under Stress

People tend to not chew thoroughly when nervous, anxious or hurried. In addition, digestive enzymes are not properly secreted because stress adversely affects normal enzyme production. Up to 50 percent of the nutrients in a meal can be lost when one is eating under stress.

Eating Hard-to-Digest Foods

When foods are difficult to digest, the body oversecretes gastric juices. This highly acidic state can be internally damaging. Proteins are difficult to digest because they are made up of bonding peptide linkages, long beaded chains that must be broken down by gastric juices before they can be digested and utilized. Some peptides are more difficult to reduce than others. Those with lots of fat surrounding them, such as the peptides in meat, are difficult enough, but not nearly as bad as those in deep-fried or charcoal-broiled foods, which are held together by strong bonds of molecules that are very hard to separate.

Treatment Summary

Digestive disorders can be due to a myriad of factors. Therefore, a complete checkup is needed to uncover the cause of the problem.

Cultures that eat high-fiber foods have few digestive disorders. Spices further enhance digestion, and the addition of foods containing flora equips the gut with the microorganisms needed to ward off microbial invaders.

Foods should be eaten as close to their natural state as possible to avoid loss of vitamins and enzymes and prevent damage to the food's cellular structure.

Herbs and nutritional supplements are often used to strengthen digestion; a health professional can help tailor a program to your unique situation.

Ways of getting rid of stored-up toxins that interfere with digestion and elimination include the use of bentonite clay, colon therapy, elimination diets, and intravenous feeding.

Since our emotions and our digestive functions are intimately related, we must address emotional issues as they arise, and engage in activities that promote relaxation.

See also: Allergies

Dysmenorrhea

Commonly known as menstrual cramps, dysmenorrhea is part of the experience of millions of women worldwide. However, painful periods do not have to be accepted as an inescapable product of the female menstrual cycle, and can actually be prevented by adhering to several basic guidelines. First, it helps to understand the underlying causes of this common condition.

Causes

Dysmenorrhea usually begins when contractions within the uterus become distorted. These contractions are governed by receptors within the uterine lining, which receive stimulation from hormonal and psychological factors. Women who have an excess of prostaglandins, which are the chemical messengers that affect the uterine receptors, are left susceptible to overstimulation, and consequently, are more likely to experience dysmenorrhea. One way in which prostaglandin production can become exaggerated is by eating foods that the body is allergic to. For instance, some women are prone to yeast reactions; hence, indulging in baked foods, breads, pastries, and processed fruit juices can facilitate the onset of dysmenorrhea.

Another factor implicated in dysmenorrhea is poor nutrition. Unfortunately, most people tend to indulge in diets that lack nutritional value, and consequently, hazardous toxins in the form of synthetic preservatives, additives, and caffeine are able to undermine their systems' functioning. Proteins that are obtained via red meat and diary products contain dangerous hormones that can have an adverse effect upon our bodies, as can oily and fried foods.

Symptoms

Dysmenorrhea is usually characterized by spasmodic cramps, but achiness, sensations of heaviness in the lower abdomen, and pain in the lower back or thighs can manifest as well. Additional symptoms include vomiting, nausea, loss of appetite, headaches, dizziness, anxiety, lethargy, depression, and diarrhea. In most cases dysmenorrhea occurs at the start of menstruation and persists for only a few hours, but sometimes, acute cases can manifest premenstrually and persevere for days. Stress can sometimes exacerbate dysmenorrhea. Something that many women report lessens the problem is the birth of a child; periods experienced afterwards are not as problematic.

Treatments

In most cases conventional doctors will treat dysmenorrhea by prescribing ibuprofen, a drug that can hinder the production of prostaglandins, and eliminate the painful symptoms that accompany menstruation. Although this approach may alleviate cramps and other symptoms, continual dependence upon the drug on a monthly basis can precipitate several adverse side effects, including gastrointestinal bleeding and diminished blood flow to the kidneys. Another possible side effect of prolonged ibuprofen use is leaky gut syndrome, which is characterized by the assimilation of undigested food particles into the bloodstream.

Fortunately, there are a variety of natural approaches that can be effectively employed, beginning with improved nutrition.

Nutrition

Since poor eating habits can contribute to excessive production of prostaglandins, reforming the diet can have a profound effect in terms of curbing menstrual cramps. Cool, green foods are effective in abating inflammation and hot stabbing pains, while legumes, flaxseed oil, organic grains, oatmeal, and steamed green vegetables can provide further relief. Deep-sea fish, such as tuna, salmon, and mackerel, are also recommended.

Some nutritionists assert that menstrual cramps with emotional origins can be combated via tofu consumption. Cooking warm tofu with sweet spices, such as pumpkin pie spice or nutmeg, can be especially helpful in soothing the nerves and promoting overall relaxation.

Supplements

A deficiency of magnesium can encourage the release of prostaglandins and the occurrence of spasms; hence, daily consumption of magnesium citrate supplements can act as an effective preventative agent. Start at 300 to 500 mg daily, and gradually augment the dosage until bowel tolerance is attained.

For the headaches and blemishes that manifest prior to menstruation, evening primrose oil is a supplement that can be consumed on a daily basis.

Herbs

There are a variety of herbs that can be used to mitigate menstrual conditions:

Popularized by the Chinese, *gardenia and philodendron* can be obtained with a prescription from an herbalist.

The herb corn silk can be used to eliminate bloating that is induced by excessive hormones in the blood supply.

In addition, herbal formulas, such as "women's rhythm," can be used to ameliorate bloating. Another formula, Xiao Yao Wan, which can be obtained at herbal pharmacies in Chinese ethnic neighborhoods, aids the digestive process, reduces menstrual pain, and soothes angry emotions. Yunnan Pai Yao is a blend of herbs that can be employed to stabilize profuse bleeding, mitigate stabbing pains, and reduce swelling.

Green tea is a way of enhancing energy by stimulating the digestive system, without excessive quantities of caffeine. It is creates a cooling sensation, and can help alleviate sharp, stabbing menstrual pains. A pinch of green tea should be added to a pot of boiling water and allowed to sit for five minutes. Then the tea can be sipped throughout the day.

Aloe vera can be used to treat several symptoms that commonly accompany menstrual cramps, including headaches, irritability, stabbing pains, fever, blemishes, and bad breath Furthermore, aloe vera is effective in decreasing acidic levels in the stomach and liver, and it can be slightly laxative. Aloe can be consumed in a juice, tea, or water mixture.

Consumption of the herb dandelion can help the body eliminate impurities. Capsules or tea are available forms of this herb.

Sarsaparilla is useful in quelling hot, stabbing pains; this herb is also diuretic.

Homeopathic Remedies

Homeopathy is an effective way of treating dysmenorrhea with no side effects, as the dilution process used in creating the remedies renders substances completely harmless. Homeopathic medicines are always keyed to very particular symptoms:

The remedy colcynthis can be used to treat acute cramps that occur suddenly during the first day of menstruation. Severe irritability and extreme anger are also part of the picture for this remedy. In addition, if the pain is substantially reduced when your knees are held firmly near your stomach, then you may wish to try colcynthis.

When the body feels more comfortable near warmth and you are suffering from spasmodic cramps and bloating, magnesia phosphorica should be administered. This potent remedy has proven effective in approximately 85 percent of the cases in which it is used.

The remedy pulsatilla should be used when cramps and the blood flow are inconsistent. Pulsatilla can be used to alleviate cutting and tearing pains in the lower back or kidney regions. Emotional signs include gentleness and weepiness. Also, the patient will have a desire to be with other people during menstruation and will prefer to be in environments with fresh air, rather than in warm stuffy rooms.

Viburnum should be employed when the menses are exceedingly late and very light. Cramps affect the sacrum and thigh regions and are accompanied by a cessation in bleeding. In addition, the patient may feel faint.

Cimifuga is for women suffering from spasmodic cramps that radiate across the thighs and pelvis, and from premenstrual headaches. As the flow of blood intensifies, pain increases as well. Emotionally, the patient may seem exceedingly nervous or depressed.

Chamomilla should be consumed when the woman is either hypersensitive or insensitive to pain. Also, she may be extremely irritable and argumentative. When menstrual bleeding increases, reliance upon coffee, stimulants, and sedatives is also heightened. Furthermore, symptoms become intensified when they are accompanied by anger.

Aromatherapy

Marjoram, lavender, and clary sage all possess analgesic qualities that can be used to assuage dysmenorrhea. Eighteen to 20 drops of any of these essential oils can be assimilated into a lotion or oil and massaged into the abdomen and lower back. Inhaling the cooling fragrances of rose, lavender, or sandalwood can be helpful in subduing sharp, stabbing menstrual pains.

Exercise

Exercise, particularly of the type that stretches the body, can do a lot to minimize cramps. Relaxed swimming may be helpful. Also, a yoga class can be an invaluable aid in teaching dysmenorrhea sufferers helpful moves.

Stress Reduction

Stress can have a whole range of adverse effects upon the body, one of which is the exacerbation of dysmenorrhea. Consequently, engaging in a stress reduction program can help in both the long run and the short run. Engaging in deep abdominal breathing, meditation, and tai chi, are some suggestions for eliminating stress and stress-induced pain.

What to Avoid

Several foods encourage excessive production of prostaglandins, which interact with the uterine lining and ultimately, can induce the exaggerated uterine contractions associated with menstrual cramping. Foods that should be avoided include hot spices, sugar, fried, greasy foods, alcohol, and stimulating foods, such as garlic and onions. In addition, white potatoes have been implicated in the onset of dysmenorrhea.

Treatment Summary

A healthy diet can minimize the occurrence of menstrual cramps; recommended selections are cool green foods, legumes, flaxseed oil, organic grains, oatmeal, steamed vegetables, deep-sea fish, and tofu.

Evening primrose oil and magnesium citrate supplements can counter the effects of dysmenorrhea.

Herbs and homeopathic remedies can alleviate uncomfortable menstrual symptoms.

Fragrant essential oils, massaged into the abdomen or lower back, can help reduce cramps.

Exercise, with the accent on stretching, may provide relief.

Deep abdominal breathing, meditation, and tai chi are stress reducers that may help in overcoming painful periods.

Ear Infections

Ear infection is the number one reason for visits to pediatricians; by the age of three, two thirds of all youngsters have seen a doctor for this reason. This amounts to 30 million visits a year, at a cost of $2.2 billion.

Several groups are at high risk for ear infections: children with allergies, children who were exposed to alcohol or tobacco smoke in the womb, children who were not breast-fed, those exposed to cow's milk within the first six months of life, and those placed in day care.

The problem stems from a hypertrophy, or increase in cell size, of lymphoid tissue surrounding the eustachian tube. The eustachian tube becomes blocked, and, as a result, there is a backup of fluid. When the middle ear is affected, the condition is known as otitis media. When the external canal is involved, it is known as otitis externa. Here, boils and discharges may be present.

Treatment

Standard medical therapies for ear infections are antibiotics and decongestants. If these aren't effective after several trials, the next step is tubes in the ears. But according to research, these methods do not make a positive difference long-term. Studies show that children receiving antibiotics are just as likely to get recurrent infections as those who do not. Some even report a greater likelihood of recurrent infections when antibiotics are given. Similarly, tubes provide relief initially, but the ear infections do not stop. All the tubes do is provide a drainage system for the pus. This is because the cause of the problem is not addressed.

Natural treatments, by contrast, go to the root of the problem, and begin with pre- and postnatal care. Simple precautions before and just after giving birth can prevent ear infections from developing. Expectant mothers should completely avoid smoking and alcohol, eat nutritious foods, and take care of their mental and emotional health. After birth, breast-feeding is preferable to bottle-feeding, as many studies show that children who are breast-fed for six months or more have far fewer ear infections then their bottle-fed counterparts.

Treating Allergies

When ear infections first develop after a child is introduced to solid foods, parents should suspect allergies as the cause, according to Florida homeopathic physician Dr. Mark Frank. The first step, he says, is to discover what substance causes the allergy, and then to eliminate it. Most commonly, this is cow's milk; the earlier it is given to the child, the sooner infections start. Problems may also stem from wheat, corn, soy, and other foods.

To test for allergies, remove the suspected food for four days. On the fifth day, return it to the diet. If symptoms are exacerbated soon afterwards, the cause of the allergy has been discovered.

Supplements

An important step in recovery is building up the child's immune system with nutrition. If the mother is still breast-feeding, these nutrients can be taken by the mom:

OMEGA-3 ESSENTIAL FATTY ACIDS

These play a major role in breaking up inflammatory processes. One of the best foods for this purpose is flaxseed oil. Flaxseed oil must be stored in the refrigerator, and never cooked.

ANTIOXIDANTS

Zinc boosts the immune system, as do beta carotene, ascorbic acid, and the B-complex vitamins.

Homeopathy

Homeopathic remedies, which are chosen according to the patient's presenting symptoms, can be highly successful in the treatment of ear pain and infections, and in the prevention of reinfection. A physician looks for the severity of pain, and whether or not there is fever, nausea, vomiting, and diarrhea. In addition, the color of the ear and the presence of fluid are taken into account. These are some common remedies a homeopath might choose:

BELLADONNA

Keynote symptoms include tearing, burning, and throbbing pain in the ears, causing a child to cry out in sleep. The ear is clogged and the person hears humming noises. The ear may also be red, hot, and overly sensitive to sound. The eardrum appears to bulge and the parotid glands and cervical lymph nodes may be swollen. The patient feels worse when touched, with noise, in drafts, and when lying down, and better when sitting up.

FERRUM PHOSPHORICUM

This is a remedy to think of if belladonna fails. Here patients are pale with flushed cheeks. They tend to be anemic and to have repeated infections in both ears. Symptoms worsen at night, when the patient is jarred, and with motion. Cold applications provide relief.

MERCURIUS

Symptoms are like those for belladonna, but are more intense in regard to redness and pulsating pain. Glands are enlarged and the throat is deep red. The pharynx is red and pus-filled and the eustachian tube is inflamed. Breath is foul, a state that worsens at night and with warmth. Sweat accompanies fever.

CHAMOMILLA

This remedy helps earaches due to teething. The child is frantic, whiny, restless, and inconsolable, wanting to be held and nursed constantly. One cheek is hot, while the other is pale and cool. The youngster wants, but then refuses, everything. Symptoms worsen with heat, anger, open air, and at night, and get better when the child is carried and kept warm.

PULSATILLA

Symptoms resemble those for chamomilla. The remedy comes from the windflower and, likewise, symptoms are changeable. Infections may fluctuate between the right and left ear; discharges may alternate from yellow and green to clear. The child feels worse with heat, in the evening, and after eating rich, creamy foods, and better in the open air, with motion, and with cold application. Repeated ear infections make hearing difficult.

HEPAR SULPHURS CALCAREUM

This helps earaches accompanied by chills, splinter-like pains in the ear, hypersensitivity to touch and noise, and a tendency to have boils in the external canal.

KALI MURIATICUM

This remedy can be used to help the healing of the eardrums.

Adjunctive Therapies

Washcloths soaked in warm water, or a warm hot water bottle placed around or on the ear, often alleviate earaches. As long as no puncture wounds to the eardrums exist, drops of mullein oil with hypericum can relieve pain. Or olive oil, warmed slightly with a bit of crushed garlic (which is taken out before using the oil) can be dropped into each ear instead. This is a soothing antiviral and antibacterial remedy.

Treatment Summary

Expectant mothers who engage in healthful lifestyles are less prone to have children who suffer from ear infections. Breast-feeding after birth further reduces risk of infection and enhances the child's overall well-being.

Ear infections may be the result of allergies to cow's milk or other foods, such as wheat, corn, and soy. These substances should be identified and eliminated from the diet.

Supplements that build the child's immune system are essential fatty acids, zinc, beta carotene, ascorbic acid, and B vitamins. A mother can take these nutrients and pass them on to her child during breast-feeding.

Several homeopathic remedies can alleviate ear infections.

Eating Disorders (Anorexia Nervosa and Bulimia)

Anorexia nervosa is a long-term refusal to eat, stemming from physical, mental, and emotional factors. It's a problem seen mostly in women, particularly teenagers, who typically start out on a weight-loss program but then don't know when to stop. Bulimia, which involves periods of intense overeating, or binging, followed by vomiting or purging, is also more common in women than in men.

Unfortunately, the media have glorified an unnatural ideal of feminine thinness, adding greatly to the prevalence of these eating disorders. Couple these two conditions with a third, obesity, and distorted eating patterns become a virtual epidemic in our culture.

Causes

Research has shown that anorexia nervosa, bulimia, and obesity can often be attributed to a deficiency of the mineral zinc. Evidence of the impact of zinc deficiency upon the body was discovered during the 1930's, when animals fed zinc-deficient diets developed anorexia. Further indication of the significance of zinc is provided by people who suffer from morbid obesity, a condition in which the victim's lifespan is considerably shortened and susceptibility to disease is heightened. Studies reveal an inverse relationship between the level of obesity and the level of zinc in these people's bodies. Although the zinc factor has not been identified as being either causal or an effect of obesity, it's interesting that patients on the opposite side of the spectrum—those with anorexia—have also demonstrated zinc deficiencies. Further studies of people who suffer from eating disorders have revealed that patients who do not overcome their mineral deficiencies have less of a chance of recovering from an eating disorder.

The richest supply of zinc within the female body is located within muscle tissue. Not surprisingly, a common symptom of anorexia involves the deterioration of muscle mass. Anorexics who do not receive a sufficient amount of zinc in their diets actually consume their own muscle tissue to compensate for the lack. When the body begins to "scrounge" for zinc from the heart, irreversible damage can occur. When the supply of zinc within cardiac tissue is consumed, the heart, which is comprised of one percent zinc, is at risk of several disorders, including bradycardia, tachycardia, and arrhythmia. Eventually, heart failure can occur, which is why anorexia nervosa should always be treated with utmost seriousness. Even the recuperation process for an anorexic person can be hazardous, since any weight gain can overburden the recovering heart.

Yet another adverse effect of zinc deficiency is loss of taste. Studies have shown that zinc-deficient individuals have difficulty synthesizing the proteins that would enable them to experience various flavors. Interestingly, eating disorder patients who are given an initial dosage of zinc supplement are often unable to taste the zinc when it is in their mouths. If you have ever consumed zinc supplements, you are probably well aware of their pungent metallic taste. An inability to experience zinc's potent flavor is a lucid indication of a zinc deficiency.

Another common contributory cause of eating disorders is stress, and stress can facilitate the onset of mineral deficiencies as well. Since women are more susceptible to stress-induced mineral deficiencies than men, they comprise a greater percentage of eating disorder cases. A possible explanation for the difference is that the male prostate contains a rich supply of zinc; indeed, zinc located within the prostate is vital to the production, mobility, viability, and quantity of male sperm. When a man encounters stress, zinc depletion is improbable due to the man's inordinate auxiliary supply. Women, though, are forced to withdraw quantities of zinc from surrounding tissue; hence, a deficiency is more likely to develop.

Unfortunately, most victims do not realize that the cessation of eating will inevitably culminate in malnutrition. While the manifestation of a zinc deficiency remains a common occurrence among eating disorder patients, other minerals vital to the body's functioning can become depleted as well. Two of these, potassium and iodine, are essential to proper thyroid maintenance. Since the thyroid is responsible for metabolism rates, any interference in its operation can actually inhibit our ability to remain thin. When a thyroid malfunction occurs, the rate at which calories are burned is dramatically decreased. So, women who think that they can prevent weight gain by throwing up their meals or going on extreme diets can end up actually compounding their problem.

Symptoms

Besides obvious weight loss and muscle deterioration, symptoms of anorexia nervosa include loss of menstruation, an extreme fear of becoming overweight, and a distorted self-image; in other words, a very thin person will see herself as being overweight. The bulimic's compulsive eating binges are followed by self-induced vomiting, or the person may take laxatives or diuretics on a consistent basis. The continual cycle of bulimia will result in malnutrition and dehydration. As with the anorexic, heart functioning may become adversely affected.

The final form of eating disorder, obesity, is characterized by excessive storage of fat inside of the adipose tissue and organs of the body. Usually, the effects of obesity become quite evident on the exterior aspect of the body as well. Obesity makes exercise more difficult, which, in turn, increases the problem. The heart becomes affected here too; it has to work harder and harder to move all that weight.

Treatment

Minerals

Since zinc plays such a pivotal role in the mechanism of appetite, zinc supplementation is a significant part of the treatment of eating disorders. Liquid zinc is the recommended form. Supplements in the form of powders, tablets, or capsules first have to be broken down by stomach acids, and since many eating disorder patients are unable to properly digest nutrients, these are not as effective as the liquid form of the mineral.

The importance of liquid zinc is hard to overstate. Prior to the discovery of this versatile supplement, the expected recovery rate for eating disorder patients was only between 20 and 30 percent, while the current recovery rate is approximately 65 percent for bulimics and 85 percent for anorexics. Patients who have had a long history of eating disorders often report that they no longer have any desire to binge or purge after adherence to a zinc supplementation program.

A valuable benefit that liquid zinc provides is its ability to combat depression. This is important because many people with eating disorders are clinically depressed. Often, eating disorders develop as part of a response to a traumatic event, with depression being another facet of that response. For this reason—and because anorexia, in particular, can be life-threatening—eating disorder patients should be under the care of a competent medical professional. Zinc supplementation, although highly beneficial, is only part of the picture of the anorexic's or bulimic's recovery plan. Attention to the person's emotional outlook is another vital aspect.

Other important minerals for those with eating disorders can be obtained via sea vegetables, such as dulse, kelp, sea palm, and nori. In addition to their valuable mineral content, sea vegetables also contain an ample quantity of other vital nutrients, including beta carotene and vitamin B12. Since sea vegetables provide such a concentrated source of minerals, only a minimal quantity is necessary to eliminate a deficiency. In fact, mineral supplementation can be effectively achieved by adding a meager two tablespoons of a dried sea vegetable to a soup.

During the early phases of a supplementation program, many eating disorder patients have an intense phobia of gaining weight and are thus reluctant to eat large quantities of food. Consequently, small concentrated sources are often initially prescribed to quell their fears. While sea vegetables remain an ideal selection, other rich mineral sources are available in the form of green foods, such as chlorella, spirulina, and blue-green algae, or of grasses, such as barley greens, barley grass, and alfalfa. Since many eating disorder patients tend to suffer from dehydration, taking these remedies in a drink can be especially beneficial. The malnutrition state of anorexia and bulimia can often inhibit a patient's ability to perceive the body's need for liquid; hence, ensuring proper saturation should be an integral part of the treatment process.

Prevention

Prevention of eating disorders starts with the education of youth. Young people should be taught the importance of exercise as a way of strengthening and beautifying their bodies. Food, then, can be seen as a fuel to keep us moving, feeling good, and functioning at our best. Also, children should be taught exactly what constitutes a healthful diet, and how to prepare simple dishes. And they should understand how junk food can contribute to obesity and other problems.

Finally, we have to keep stressing to young people that most of the advertising and show business images they see of the female body, both on screen and in print, are thinner than most girls can hope to be while still eating healthfully. Only a small percentage of women have body types that can fit into the current idea of glamour without compromising their nutrition.

Treatment Summary

Liquid zinc greatly improves the chances of recovery from anorexia and bulimia.

Other important minerals are available in sea vegetables and green foods, such as chlorella and alfalfa.

Eating disorders must always be treated in the context of the patient's emotional state.

Good exercise and nutrition habits, as well as an understanding of our culture's distorted images, should be part of children's education.

See also: Obesity

Endometriosis

Endometriosis is a condition in which the cells that line the interior of the uterus dislodge and grow outside the uterine cavity. The cells in their normal state build up in the uterus every month when estrogen levels are high. In this way, they assist in making the lining of the uterus suitable for pregnancy, serving as a nest in which the fertilized egg will be implanted. If pregnancy does not take place, the lining breaks off when the estrogen level becomes low, and it emerges as menstrual flow. In the case of endometriosis, though, these cells can attach to a variety of areas. They may grow anywhere in the pelvis, on the fallopian tubes, ovaries, bladder, intestinal surfaces, rectum, colon, ligaments, or appendix. Endometrial tissue has even been found in more distant places within the body, such as the lung or armpit.

The cells that grow outside the uterus act as if they were in the uterus; in other words, they grow during periods in which the estrogen level is high and create blood when estrogen levels are low. However, when endometrial tissue grows in areas other than the uterus, there is no exit for the blood when estrogen levels drop. Therefore, the blood will then collect in these areas, causing cystic structures, scarring, and other types of damage to these organs. Over 5 million women in the U.S., mainly in the 20- to 40-year-old age group, are afflicted with this problem.

Causes

The causes of endometriosis are unknown at this time. However, there are theories as to why the condition develops.

One possible cause may be that, during menstruation, the blood flows backward as opposed to outward. If that is the case, menstrual blood is able to go through the fallopian tube and gain access to the pelvic and abdominal cavity. The cells from this blood can then embed themselves outside the uterus in other tissues and organs. Another theory is that the cells in the uterine lining migrate through lymphatic channels for implantation outside the uterine cavity. Genetic predisposition to the condition may play a part. So may a deficiency in the immune system. The theory here is that through some hormonal and chemical influence, endometrial tissue becomes activated at different times in the cycle, causing tissue to proliferate in abnormal areas. There are also studies showing that exposure to dioxin, a chemical found in pesticides and certain types of waste incineration, may be an additional cause of endometriosis. Lastly, childbearing in conjunction with various methods of birth control may also be responsible.

Symptoms

There are generally two symptoms of endometriosis: pain and bleeding. Pain is the main symptom and may be either minimal or severe. It occurs because of inflammation and scarring of affected tissues. The area where the pain is felt and the degree to which it is experienced will depend on the site of the endometrial tissue and the degree to which it is implanted. The pain might occur just prior to menstruation and be attributed to menstrual cramps. However, some women experience pain during intercourse at any time during the month. It is also possible for pain to be felt during urination, due to implantation of the cells in the bladder; during bowel movements as a result of colon and rectal implants; and in the ovaries and extending to the back and buttocks, or down the legs. There may also be pelvic pain during a gynecological examination.

Bleeding problems might persist as well. There may be internal bleeding as well as bleeding from various orifices in the body (such as nosebleeds). It is important to note that recurrent bleeding at specific times of the month should lead one to suspect endometriosis.

Other symptoms may include bladder infections and fatigue.

Diagnosis

The only way to truly confirm endometriosis is through a surgical process known as laparoscopy. This procedure allows the doctor to biopsy the tissue. Sonograms and MRIs can also be helpful in diagnosing the problem, but are not completely accurate.

Treatment

The ultimate treatment for the most severe cases of endometriosis is a hysterectomy in which reproductive organs that are scarred and damaged are removed. However, this is a serious surgical procedure that should only be explored as a last result when the condition has become very serious and other approaches have failed.

One of these approaches is traditional drug therapy, which generally consists of medical prescriptions for pain, and suppression of estrogen, to reduce endometrial growth. Medications given may include indomethacin, ibuprofen, Naprosyn, and danazol. However, there may be adverse side effects, such as arteriosclerosis, bone loss, weight gain, edema, changes in breast size, acne, excess hair growth, hot flashes, and deepening of the voice.

Hormones are another aspect of conventional therapy. They are given to simulate pregnancy in order to slow down and prohibit the progress of endometriosis. This method, too, may produce unpleasant side effects, such as depression, painful breasts, nausea, weight gain, bloating, swelling, and migraine headaches.

Some newer compounds, which diminish pain and reduce the mass of endometrial tissue, may produce fewer sides effects. They are called gonadotropin releasing hormone compounds and are sometimes given by injection.

Diet

Since conventional treatments for endometriosis have their drawbacks, it may be beneficial to explore natural solutions, starting with a dietary approach, to alleviate symptoms and reverse the problem. There are foods that may reduce estrogen levels, and thus diminish or slow the growth of endometriosis. A mostly vegetarian diet is recommended, with an emphasis on soy products, alfalfa spouts, flaxseeds, and legumes. Another dietary strategy is to consume foods that aid in excreting estrogen from the body through the intestinal tract. A high-fiber diet works to this end; think in terms of whole grains and fresh fruits and vegetables. Also, you want the diet to be low in fat; avoid, particularly, products high in saturated fat, e.g., dairy products and red meat. Lastly, the liver may aid in lowering estrogen levels. Therefore, it is a good idea to eat foods high in B-complex vitamins, such as whole grains and legumes, and avoid alcohol, fat, and sugar, in order to promote a healthy liver.

Supplements

Vitamin and mineral supplements can also be helpful in reducing inflammation. Recommended supplements include:

Vitamin C. The dosage can be based on a woman's bowel tolerance; stop short of a level causing diarrhea.
Beta carotene. 150,000-200,000 IU.

Selenium. 400 mcg.
Vitamin E. 800-1200 IU.

Herbs

Herbal supplements work similarly to vitamins in that they can assist in decreasing inflammation. Recommended herbs include white willow bark and a formula suggested by a Portland, Oregon gynecologist, Dr. Tori Hudson, which contains equal amounts of chaste tree berry, dandelion root, motherwort, and prickly ash. The recommended dosage is one teaspoon taken three times daily.

Hellerwork

Hellerwork is a body technique that helps to refine body structure through deep tissue work. It has been shown that patients with endometriosis have muscle spasms, which is one of the causes of pain. Thus, Hellerwork instructs women to relax their muscles to ease the symptoms. This therapy strives to create a healthy balance of mind and body by freeing misalignments in body structure, working to improve everyday habits that contribute to the problem, and working through emotional issues that may affect a woman physically.

Oriental Medicine

Women with endometriosis may want to consider some natural therapies used in Oriental medicine. One approach is to decrease the size of the endometrial mass through the use of laser acupuncture. Other Oriental techniques are retention enemas or injection into the endometrial nodes with common sage root. Oriental practitioners advise abstaining from sexual intercourse at the time of menstruation as it can cause the migration of endometrial tissue into the pelvic cavity and result in an imbalance of energy. They also advocate using acupuncture to release obstructions from the liver, spleen, heart, lung, and kidney in order for energy to move freely within the system.

Treatment Summary

Switch to a mostly vegetarian, high-fiber, low-fat diet, and be sure to consume foods high in the B-complex vitamins.

The following nutrients and herbs can help reduce inflammation: vitamin C, beta carotene, selenium, vitamin E, white willow bark, and a formula containing chaste tree berry, dandelion root, motherwort, and prickly ash.

Hellerwork is a body technique that teaches women to relax their muscles to ease the pain caused by muscle spasms associated with endometriosis.

Oriental medicine recommends increasing pelvic flow, avoiding sexual intercourse during menstruation, and using acupuncture to release obstructions.

Environmental Illness

The environment in which we live affects the way both our mind and body function. This is not a new concept. In fact, even thousands of years ago people knew that they could become ill from certain foods and products. Today, as our society continues to produce more toxic chemical substances that can result in immune deficiencies and mutations, researchers and some practitioners within the medical community are beginning to give more credence to this area of study. As *Environmental Magazine* writer, Alyssa Burger, points out, naturalists have recently seen how chemical contamination of animals' habitats have caused mutations in certain species. That chemicals can affect humans in physically subtle as well as overt ways, is beyond question.

Females are most likely to develop ailments related to toxic chemicals in the environment because exposure to certain toxins can create an imbalance of estrogen in a woman's body. Once in the body, many chemicals mimic estrogen, and are therefore known as xeno-estrogenic compounds (xeno meaning foreign). But males too can be adversely affected by xeno-estrogenic compounds. Animal studies show that a variety of male reproductive disorders, ranging from sterility to undescended testicles to odd sexual behaviors, may result from environmental factors.

Causes

From silicone breast implants to the nerve gas encountered by our Gulf War troops to the hormones used in the dairy industry, today's society exposes us to a wide variety of chemicals that can affect our systems. Dioxins, to name one infamous group, are byproducts of the manufacture of herbicides; they increase the likelihood of cancer as well as negatively impact the endocrine system. Organochlorine pesticides, of which DDT is the most notorious example, affect fertility. Other widely used chemicals found in toiletries, spermicides, household detergents, plastics, and food can linings can affect the health of susceptible individuals as well.

Foods and beverages are also potential causes of environmental illness. Tap water, foods containing additives, inorganically grown vegetables, certain meat products, and hydrogenated oil all bear toxic chemicals. Even the products with which we furnish our homes, such as carpeting, paint, and mattresses, can release chemicals at a low level. We commonly have all of those in our bedrooms, and if they are giving off toxic fumes this is not a good situation because the bedroom is one room in the house that really needs to be safe. Our bodies tend to detoxify at night while we are sleeping. However, if the bedroom is a toxic environment, not only can't we detoxify, but we also increase the amount of chemicals to which we are exposed, which continually weakens our systems.

In addition to chemicals, there are other environmental factors that need to be addressed. Exposure to radiation, radon, car exhaust, tobacco smoke, and heavy metals are other factors that can create immune system deficiencies.

The more poisons a person ingests or inhales, the more inclined he or she is to become sick. The poisons collect in body fat until capacity there is at a maximum. They then move all around the body through the circulatory system, manifesting themselves in a variety of symptoms. While anyone may become ill from environmental factors, those most at risk are people who reside or work in a sealed building that lacks windows or a good ventilation system; those who work with chemicals, computer chips, gasoline, or formaldehyde; those who are allergic or sensitive to certain foods, molds, or chemicals; those who take a variety of antibiotics; those who live near commercial properties involved in chemical manufacturing or toxic incineration; and those who are under a great deal of stress, which leads to poor eating habits.

Considering all the risk factors and the products to which we're exposed, it may seem as it everybody is fated to suffer environmental illness. That's not the case, though, because we can educate ourselves to lessen risks and build our immune systems.

Symptoms

Different people react to environmental conditions in different ways. Symptoms can include the following: exhaustion, muscle aches, heart irregularities, asthma, flu-like symptoms, ringing in the ears, burning in the eyes, mild or severe headaches, colon problems, sleep disorders, loss of balance, skin disorders, inability to concentrate, memory loss, anxiety or panic attacks, depression, and sensitivities to changes in the weather.

Since there are so many possible symptoms, environmental illness can be difficult to diagnose. Routine blood tests frequently yield normal results and lead doctors to believe that no problem exists. It is always a good idea for a person who suspects environmental illness to examine the following: where they feel ill (e.g., at work, at home or in a new residence or office); whether their surroundings or lifestyle expose them to toxic substances; and whether they have recently had any new products introduced into their home or office, such as new carpeting or paint. Fortunately, there are some medical practitioners who do recognize environmental illness as a possibility when unexplained symptoms arise. Occupational or environmental physicians can order tests that examine, for example, pesticide and mineral concentrations in the blood, to help determine whether a person suffers from chemical exposures.

Treatment

While no conventional medical treatment exists for environmental illness, there are some things that people can do to minimize or reverse the damage and better protect themselves from continued exposure.

Detoxification

Two forms of detoxification have had encouraging results in the reversal of environmental illness. One is heat stress detoxification, which involves wood saunas, hot sand packing, steam baths, and sweat lodges. This method requires the guidance of trained practitioners, since it necessitates understanding of toxins and their effects on the body. Another approach is biotoxic reduction. This is a two-week medically managed program that incorporates aerobics, sauna therapy, and increasing niacin levels. Professional supervision is, of course, needed here too. There are additional treatments that can be included, depending upon the individual.

Diet

The foods we eat have a great impact on our system. Many of the meat products in this country contain toxins, concentrated in the tissues since animal feed is often treated with chemicals. Also, crops are treated with pesticides, which can then get into our systems, through the fruits, vegetables, and grains we eat. That's why buying organically grown food, whenever possible, is recommended. Poultry that is organically fed can also be considered. Further, before you drink or cook with your tap water, it should be purified.

Supplements

There are many nutrients that can help reverse the effects of chemical exposure. Since exposure to chemicals affects people in different ways, the recommendation will vary depending upon the individual. However, some of the supplements that have proven helpful are vitamins C and E, L-glutamine, carnitine, glucosamine sulfate, magnesium, and chelated manganese.

What to Avoid

There's a lot that people can do to minimize the toxicity of their environment. If you suspect that you are suffering from environmental toxins, test the effect of removing suspect products containing harmful chemicals from your surroundings. Plastic-lined tin cans, as well as foods microwaved in plastic wrap, should be avoided. If you must microwave, be sure to use microwave-safe containers. Stay away from fatty animal products, as these contain toxic chemicals, including dioxin. Synthetic fragrances in personal care products, such as perfumes and after-shave lotions, can also cause harm. It's better to buy unscented products and add pure, natural fragrances. Hot showers produce steam that may emit chlorine compounds, which we inhale. A simple way to reduce these compounds is to use a carbon shower filter. In addition, ensure that at least the bedroom is one room in your house that is free of toxins.

Don't overlook your travel habits. Did you know that car exhaust affects people inside the vehicle more than those on the outside? Always keep a window rolled down. Carbon and hepa car filters, found in newer, upscale models, may help. Finally, if you're a jogger, try to follow a route that's away from heavy traffic. You don't want to undermine your health while engaged in an essentially health-enhancing activity.

Treatment Summary

Heat stress detoxification and biotoxic reduction have provided relief for people with environmental illness. Both programs require the guidance of trained practitioners.

Given that many foods contain chemicals that weaken the immune system, the following are recommended: fruits, vegetables, and grains that are organically grown, organically fed poultry, purified water, and avoidance of foods containing food additives or other chemical substances.

Supplemental nutrients that can help reverse the effects of chemical exposure include vitamins C and E, L-glutamine, and carnitine.

Measures to remove toxic substances from your environment include avoiding foods microwaved in plastic wrap, buying unscented personal care products, using a carbon shower filter, and keeping car windows open when you're on the road.

Eye Disorders

The eyes are a part of the body that can easily be taken for granted until a problem emerges. Most of the problems people have with their eyes occur gradually and generally do not produce many symptoms at first. Therefore, without regular visits to the doctor, immediate attention and early prevention are essentially sacrificed. To further complicate the issue, conventional treatments tend to achieve only short-term solutions that can sometimes make the eyes worse. Therefore, given the discomfort eye conditions can create, in addition to the potentially serious, long-term ramifications, it is important to understand the most common disorders and their impact.

What Can Go Wrong with the Eyes

Cataracts

This is when the lens of the eye becomes fogged, due either to a decrease in the fluid surrounding the lens, to poor circulation, or to nutritional deficiencies. Cataracts can impair the detail of a person's vision by causing a haze and preventing light from penetrating the lens. This condition tends to get worse over time—even to the point of blindness in the most extreme cases. Cataracts can affect either one or both eyes.

Glaucoma

Similar to cataracts, this disorder also causes a gradual loss of sight, initially affecting a person's peripheral vision. The optic nerve is quite sensitive and can be affected by fluid, sunlight, infection, circulatory problems, exposure to toxins, and nutritional deficiencies. When this nerve is damaged, pressure on the eye will tend to progressively increase. This causes gradual vision loss and, without proper care, can eventually lead to blindness. In fact, glaucoma is one of the principal causes of blindness in the U.S.

Macular Degeneration

Another primary cause of blindness is the condition that occurs when the tiny area in the center of the retina, the macula, deteriorates. This is a condition primarily of the older population, and it occurs for a variety of reasons, including nutritional deficiencies, circulatory trouble, and atherosclerosis. Exposure to electromagnetic fields, particularly through heavy computer use, has also been implicated.

Myopia

This is the condition generally referred to as nearsightedness. It occurs when the lens of the eye becomes motionless and locks into one spot. Thus, the light entering the eye achieves clarity in front of the retina as opposed to on the retina, where it would normally come into focus. This results in difficulty seeing objects that are far away.

Hyperopia

When the lens of the eye freezes with the opposite effect, the result is hyperopia or farsightedness. Here, the carrier wave of light adjusts to achieve images behind the retina. Thus, a person with hyperopia has trouble seeing objects in very close range.

Symptoms

One symptom common to all of the aforementioned disorders is vision impairment, whether it's the inability to see objects up close or far away or the gradual loss of vision. In the case of glaucoma, there are additional symptoms, including headaches, eye pain, redness in the eyes, nausea and vomiting, and an abnormally wide pupil.

Treatment

Conventional treatment for eye disorders includes surgery, drug therapy, and corrective eyewear. Surgery is generally used in the case of cataracts and glaucoma. However, there is always some risk with surgery, and the conditions may not be reversed. Drug therapy, used for glaucoma, can produce serious side effects, such as asthma, depression, loss of libido, and high cholesterol. It too does not guarantee a cure. In the case of corrective eyewear for both near- and farsighted individuals, the muscles in and around the eyes tend to worsen, since they begin to rely on prescriptive lenses to improve vision. As for macular degeneration, traditional medicine does not even have a way of dealing with it, viewing it as an untreatable condition.

Some natural solutions have been found not only to prevent and improve all these disorders, but, sometimes, to correct them as well. Plus they can provide results in a manner that is much easier on the system than conventional medical treatments. Some of these therapies are cited below:

Nutrition

Nutrition is key in dealing with eye problems not only because it can help correct a disorder, but because it will prevent problems from occurring. Keep in mind that the eyes are dependent upon the rest of the body for nourishment. In particular, the eyes rely on the liver and kidneys, as well as on the circulatory system, to eliminate toxins from the bloodstream and to metabolize and deliver the appropriate nutrients.

The vitamins and minerals associated with eye care are vitamins E and D for the general maintenance of healthy eyes, vitamin A for proper liver metabolism and digestion, vitamin C to help rid the bloodstream of toxins, glutathione to help rid the eye of excess fluid, selenium, the carotenoids, niacin to increase circulation, all the B vitamins, omega-3 and 6 fatty acids (found in fish oils) to decrease inflammation, and a balance of magnesium and calcium for proper muscle control. While these nutrients can all be taken in the form of supplements, it is important to get them from one's diet as well. Overall, a low-fat, dairy-free, vegetarian diet is a great way to get the nutrients essential for proper eye care. In particular, carrots, green leafy vegetables (such as beet greens, spinach, and broccoli), and yellow, green, and orange fruits (particularly in the form of fresh organic fruit juices) are excellent sources of vitamin A. Further, sulfur-rich foods, such as eggs, garlic, and asparagus, increase the amount of vitamins C and E in the body.

Herbs

Herbs complement the nutrients a person receives from his or her diet. Specifically, herbs that allow for better circulation so that more nutrients can reach the eye are gingko biloba, gotu kola, and hawthorn berry. The same effect can be found in the common spices marjoram, cayenne pepper, ginger, and garlic.

Bilberry, pine bark extract, and grape seed extract can be used to fortify the capillaries that furnish the eye with fluid and aid in the prevention of lens impairment. Recommended dosage is 120 to 160 mg daily.

Diagaku eye drops and shi hu are Chinese herbs useful for healing dry or inflamed eyes. For the correction of early cataracts, the Chinese herbs zhang yan, baineiting eye drops, and ming mu may be beneficial.

Lycium rehmannia is an herb that helps to maintain the health of the retina.

Vision Therapy

Dr. Robert Michael Kaplan, author of *The Power Behind Your Eyes,* is a behavioral optometrist who practices vision therapy. One of the best methods, Kaplan says, for correcting vision problems on an emotional and physical level is breath work. One technique he recommends is called the integrated breath. The method involves breathing in, breathing out, and then pausing. This is performed three to five times consecutively, in a slow manner to prevent hyperventilation.

Kaplan follows this foundation exercise with a procedure that he calls eye crossing. While classical vision care warns people not to cross their eyes for fear of getting stuck in this position, Kaplan believes that eye crossing, when done in a relaxed manner without straining, can increase vision fitness. The easiest way to cross the eyes is to position one of the thumbs about 8 inches in front of the eyes. Focusing attention on the thumb, notice how everything behind it doubles. This is a good sign because it shows that the left and right eyes are participating equally.

Kaplan believes that the cross-eye exercise will increase one's ability to stay centered in life because when you pull the left eye and the right eyes in, you are looking closer at the self. This is also a valuable exercise for children who are developing vision, for people who experience motion sickness when reading in a vehicle, and for individuals who experience concentration difficulties and stress from working on computers or reading books for sustained periods.

Kaplan recommends visual hygiene practices that can easily be incorporated during the day. First, he advocates taking vision breaks while working. A person should periodically look up from the book or computer, and focus on the distance. Another tip for improved vision includes writing on an angled surface rather than a flat desk. This avoids leaning over, which strains the shoulders and back, and limits blood flow to the eyes. Additionally, good lighting is important. People should surround themselves with natural light by working near windows, skylights, or full-spectrum lighting. Lastly, it is important to take frequent body-stretching breaks every 20 minutes to an hour—to increase nerve flow from the spine, shoulders, and neck. Kaplan explains that after people practice vision therapy, eyeglasses may become too strong. A vision therapy oriented practitioner can lower the prescription. In that way, eyesight can improve.

More Eye Exercises

Exercises can be helpful in preventing or correcting particular conditions. Overall, daily activity is recommended to help lower interocular pressure and increase circulation. This could even take the form of a brisk walk. Specific exercises that may be included in an individualized program include the following:

To enhance peripheral vision, imagine a clock. In visualizing the clock, rotate the eyes counterclockwise from 12 to 9 and then back again. Then move the eyes in the opposite direction, from 12 to 3 and back. This should be done without the help of corrective eyewear, using the thumb as a guide. During the exercise, the person should be attentive to objects on the perimeter of the scope of vision. This drill can be done three times daily.

For strengthening the muscles in and around the eye, focus clearly on an object, and bring it in closer until that object becomes blurred. At this point, stop and take deep breaths until sight turns clearer. Then the object can be brought in closer again and the procedure repeated.

Another muscle-strengthening exercise involves sitting in the middle of a room and, without moving anything but the eyes, gazing up to the ceiling and then following the visual path in a straight line down to the floor. This can be repeated several times. Then the same process should be done looking from one side of the room to the other. Deep breathing should be performed during this exercise.

To release tension in the eyes, while in a comfortable position, cover the eyes with the palms of the hands. Visualize a peaceful place while performing deep breathing. One can also visualize a time in the past when one's vision was better, in order to picture the eye in its proper shape.

Massage can increase circulation to the neck, and subsequently to the eyes.

Additional Therapies

Acupuncture and acupressure are sometimes used to lessen tension and improve vision. Practitioners apply pressure to specific points surrounding the eye and clear the energy paths connected to the eye, including the stomach, urinary bladder and gallbladder meridians. Reflexology is also used for eye problems. Practitioners of this technique explain that there are reflex points in the foot—specifically located between the second and third toes—that, when massaged, can clear nerve blockages to the eyes. Biofeedback techniques can assist in regulating eye focus and muscle movement to result in improved vision. These are performed with special instruments that use sound to help teach muscle control.

What to Avoid

Particular foods and environmental factors can be harmful to the eyes, resulting in vision impairment. These include artificial sweeteners, as they contain toxic substances which can negatively affect the optic nerve; caffeine, which affects circulation; alcohol, as it can damage liver function; sugar, which may hinder enzyme function; lactose, a form of sugar found in dairy products; tobacco; steroids; the toxin mercury, found in dental amalgam fillings; and exposure to direct sunlight, which can increase oxidative damage to the eyes.

Treatment Summary

Nutrients important to eye health include vitamins A, C, E, and D; glutathione; selenium; the carotenoids; niacin; all the B vitamins; omega-3 and 6 fatty acids; and the proper balance of magnesium and calcium.

Some herbs that help the eyes by allowing for better circulation are gingko biloba, gotu kola, and hawthorn berry.

The field of vision therapy offers exercises and lifestyle advice that can help strengthen the eyes. Daily activity is important to help lower interocular pressure and increase circulation. Also, specific vision exercises can help with particular problems.

Acupuncture, acupressure, reflexology, and biofeedback are other techniques used to improve vision.

Fever

Contrary to what most of us think, a fever is really a friend in that it tells us that our body is handling an internal crisis. The hot feeling we experience is an indication that the body is working hard to burn up pathogenic microbes. High, prolonged fevers can be dangerous, however, and can result in convulsions or even death.

The definition of a fever is an abnormal rise in temperature. Some consider a fever to be a body temperature of 100 degrees Fahrenheit or higher. Others define it simply as an increase above normal daily variations.

Fevers are caused by infectious agents, such as bacteria, viruses, and other microbes, and by noninfectious agents, such as inflammation and immune response. They may also be brought on by exercise, anxiety, dehydration, cancer, anemia, nerve disease, and drugs.

Treatment

Since fever is a part of the body's natural healing process, eradicating it should not necessarily be your goal. If a mild to moderate fever is part of your case of the flu, or a cold, you can work with it to cleanse the body by consuming foods—particularly in juice form—high in chlorophyll, vitamin C, and other antioxidants. Save the aspirin or Tylenol for those times when fever lasts for more than a day, or is high.

Note: Aspirin has been associated with the serious condition known as Reye's syndrome in children and teenagers who have taken it while they had the flu or chicken pox. Consult a physician before giving aspirin to children.

Homeopathy

Homeopathic physicians key their remedies to very specific symptoms and sensations experienced by their patients. Here are some of the remedies they use when fever is a problem.

224

ACONITUM

The fever appears suddenly after exposure to cold, dry winds, and rises rapidly within the first few hours, going up to 104 or 105 degrees Fahrenheit. The patient feels restless, anxious, and frightened of never recovering.

BELLADONNA

If aconitum does not take effect within 12 hours, homeopathists give "the deadly nightshade," belladonna. Indications for this remedy are being flushed and congested, with dry, hot skin. Covered areas perspire, while the feet remain icy cold. There is no thirst and the tongue is bright red. Extreme sensitivity to light, noise, and motion may result in a throbbing headache. This is a remedy used for fever with convulsions or hallucinations.

BRYONIA

Think of "bry" rhyming with "dry," and you know when this remedy is recommended. Bryonia is for dry, hacking coughs, and for dry, parched lips accompanied by thirst. Symptoms worsen in cold, dry, wind. Unlike the restless belladonna patient, the bryonia individual remains motionless to avoid achiness.

GELSEMIUM

This is a remedy often used for patients with the flu or summer colds. The yellow jasmine plant from which it is derived resembles this person's appearance: dull, droopy, drowsy, and yellow. Low energy causes lethargy and a heavy sensation in the limbs. Fever is slow to start, but is long-lasting, and is accompanied by a chill and great thirst.

BAPTISIA

Onset of fever is sudden and high, and often accompanies intestinal flu. There is sudden vomiting, diarrhea, foul breath, and a dull, reddish, unhappy appearance. Symptoms worsen at 11 a.m. Emotionally, the patient is fearful and frustrated.

See also: Colds and Flu

Fibroids and Uterine Bleeding

One in five women over the age of 35 is afflicted with fibroids, with women of African American descent being especially prone to the problem. Fibromyoma uteri and leiomyoma uteri, the medical terminology for fibroids, are benign tumors that originate from muscle tissue and adhere to either the inner or outer uterine wall. Fibroids usually develop as a result of varying estrogen levels in the body, and provide a natural way for the body to cope with hazardous toxins. Most fibroid patients have indulged in unhealthy diets and exercise habits. The Asian medical perspective is that fibroid development can be a product of angry emotions, prolonged or dilatory menstruation, or abortion. After an abortion cells from the terminated fetus may remain in the endometrial wall and eventually serve as the foundation for fibroid production.

Symptoms

While the presence of minute fibroids cannot be ascertained by symptomatic evidence, larger fibroids, which take time to develop, are frequently accompanied by agonizing menstruation, urinary tract infections, chronic infertility, and uterine bleeding. Fibroids positioned on the inside of the uterine wall are often responsible for uterine bleeding, which commonly results in the performance of a hysterectomy. Fibroids located on the muscle wall of the uterus are not associated with uterine bleeding, and are therefore seldom removed from the body.

Treatments

The medical establishment usually follows one of two approaches. The first, myomectomy, is used to eliminate small, harmless fibroids and does not alter a woman's ability to bear children. Hysterectomies are prescribed for women who have fully developed fibroids and suffer from chronic symptoms, such as heavy bleeding. A significant percentage of the hysterectomies performed are totally unnecessary, and actually, quite hazardous. In addition to an abundance of physical complications, a hysterectomy can have severe psychological ramifications. What's more, out of the 750,000 hysterectomies performed each year, 2500 result in the death of the woman.

Recent estimates are that fibroid development will eventually become a reality for up to 40 percent of all women. Another prediction is that if the medical establishment's reliance upon hysterectomies continues, it is quite possible that within a few years one third of all women will have had the operation by the time they reach 60. Clearly, alternative treatment modalities need to be explored.

Myoma Coagulation and Reconstruction

Too often, women who receive hysterectomies are not offered safer alternatives by their physicians. Unfortunately, the public is unaware of benefits of a recently developed laser procedure, known as myoma coagulation, or myelosis. Myoma coagulation originated in Europe, where fibroids are eliminated with the use of special lasers that puncture the tumor and deflate it. The operation is effective because it restricts the flow of blood to the fibroid, after which the tumor can be lanced. After the fluid drains, harmless tissue is left behind and there is no need for extraction.

This technique is currently being taught to doctors across the nation, and the number of successful operations continues to rise. Since the uterine wall is debilitated by the procedure and unable to sustain pregnancy, likely candidates for myoma coagulation are women who are uninterested in post-operative pregnancies. In addition, the procedure can only be performed if the tumor is less than six inches in diameter. Fibroids that surpass the size limit can be treated with Lupron, a medication that decreases the production of estrogen in the body and causes a 30- to 50-percent reduction in size of the tumor. The fibroid reduction lasts only for a limited amount of time, but during this period, myoma coagulation can be performed, further reducing the fibroid by up to 75 percent. When this occurs, the threat of uterine bleeding is virtually eliminated.

Nutrition, Supplements, and Exercise

The development of fibroids can be lessened by dietary modification. Women who wish to reduce the size of their fibroids, or prevent their further growth, should incorporate large quantities of protein into their diets. But the protein should come from healthy sources—i.e., vegetables and whole grains, such as quinoa, amaranth, millet, buckwheat, oats, and brown rice. Legumes can also be beneficial in hindering the formation of fibroids. Soy products, including soy beans, tofu, soy milk, miso, and tempeh, contain a good supply of isoflavones, which have been found to combat tumor growth. The numerous types of beans, including black beans, pinto beans, lentils, lima beans, and chick peas, are useful in preparing a variety of meals and constitute a good protein source.

In addition to consuming adequate quantities of protein, it is important to drink a minimum of two quarts of purified water daily to promote proper functioning of the kidneys and bowels. Organs involved in the excretion process can facilitate the discharge of excess estrogen, and consequently, lower the potential for fibroid development. A high dietary intake of fiber can act as a deterrent to fibroid growth due to fiber's estrogen-reducing capabilities. Citrus fruits and berries, which contain ample quantities of vitamin C, can further stabilize the body's estrogen levels.

Sometimes excessive uterine bleeding is brought on by liver poisoning and can be effectively treated by abstaining from food consumption for limited periods of time throughout the month. Be sure to seek medical guidance, though. When paired with an extensive hygiene regimen, temporary fasting can alleviate symptomatic bleeding in cases that do not necessitate hospitalization. Although the medical explanation is still unclear, supplements of oil-soluble liquid chlorophyll have also demonstrated their ability to treat abnormal cases of bleeding. For maximum results, two or three capsules should be taken two to three times per day. In addition, a balanced mixture of natural organic oils, including flax and borage, can fortify the uterus and protect it from chronic bleeding.

Women with abnormal uterine bleeding accompanied by anemia should supplement their diets with iron, but remember to seek medical supervision and adhere to recommended dosages, as excessive quantities of iron have been linked with cancer and coronary disease. Vitamin E should be taken in quantities of 400 IU daily, while 1000 mg vitamin C with bioflavonoids can be taken five times per day. A recent medical investigation correlated symptoms of uterine bleeding with deficiencies of vitamin A; hence, daily consumption of vitamin A supplements is recommended. Additional supplements include 100 mg of evening primrose oil three times daily, plus silica.

The incorporation of an exercise routine into your daily routine can enhance the discharge of excess estrogen from the body, thus reducing the possibility of fibroid development.

Herbal Remedies

There are several herbal remedies that can alleviate fibroid symptoms. Fifteen drops of shepherd's purse taken three times daily can aid in controlling uterine bleeding, while the herb white ash can facilitate the reduction of fibroids. False unicorn root can be useful in treating severe bleeding when 15 drops are mixed with water and consumed on an hourly basis. The Chinese herb dong quai, which contains useful phytoestrogens and acts as a muscle relaxant, has demonstrated its ability to alleviate cramps attributed to fibroids. This herb should be consumed in quantities of 500 to 1000 mg per day. Han man chow, another Chinese herb that is also known as warrior's grass, enhances functioning of the spleen and uterus, and can control severe bleeding. Some additional herbs commonly prescribed by holistic practitioners to treat fibroids and uterine bleeding include red raspberry, ladies' mantle, yarrow, white dead nettle, partridge berry, goldenseal, motherwort, stone root, and ginger.

Homeopathic Remedies

The homeopathic remedy aurum muriatium can aid in the reduction of fibroid size when the patient does not suffer from any adverse symptoms, such as bleeding. Hydrastinum muriaticum has demonstrated its ability to decrease the size of larger fibroids that form on the anterior uterine wall. Fibroids in this location often burden the bladder and promote frequent urination and pain.

Acupuncture

Acupuncture points that correspond to the uterus are located on the ankle. Electrical acupuncture is used to promote the elimination of fibroids; it is believed that the electrical currents create stimulation that contributes to the removal of the fibroids from their position on the uterine wall.

What to Avoid

As discussed earlier, the most nutritious sources of protein are whole grains and beans. Meat should be avoided. If you do eat meat, limit intake to three ounces per day, a quantity that can fit in the palm of your hand. Furthermore, meat products should originate from healthy sources. Avoid consuming meat from animals that were not free-range or grass-fed. Animals injected with synthetic hormones and antibiotics are quite unhealthy for the human body.

It is also important to avoid an excessively fatty diet because fatty foods are estrogen stimulators. Furthermore, studies have correlated obesity with heightened estrogen production within the body. The liver, which aids in the elimination of excess estrogen, can be protected by avoiding fried foods, illegal drugs, coffee, alcohol, and processed or refined foods. Additional foods to be avoided include diet sodas, pizza, donuts and other pastries, and potato chips.

Treatment Summary

Standard medical practices for fibroids include myomectomy, to eliminate small, harmless fibroids, and hysterectomy, to remove fully developed fibroids accompanied by severe, chronic symptoms. The latter approach is not always necessary, though, and since it can have serious repercussions, alternatives should be sought first.

Myoma coagulation and reconstruction is a surgical technique in which lasers deflate tumor growth. When performed by a well-trained medical doctor, it is far safer than the standard hysterectomy.

Eating wholesome proteins, and drinking four quarts of purified water daily, as well as concentrating on citrus fruits and other vitamin C-rich foods, can create an internal environment less conducive to the growth of fibroids.

Short-term fasting and liquid chlorophyll can diminish uterine bleeding.

Vitamins E, C, and A, as well as evening primrose oil and silica, offer extra protection.

Exercise lowers estrogen levels, thus lessening the chance of developing fibroids.

Herbs for strengthening the uterus include shepherd's purse, white ash, false unicorn root, dong quai, and warrior's grass, another Chinese herb.

Stimulating points connected to the uterus, via acupuncture, can aid in the elimination of fibroids.

Foot and Leg Problems

People take their feet and legs for granted—until something goes wrong and suddenly their personal transport system isn't working so well. The fact is, foot and leg problems slow down large numbers of individuals each year. In general, most foot and leg problems are preventable or can be treated effectively with simple home remedies. At other times a condition may require professional guidance. Fortunately, there are a number of holistic podiatrists who can help.

Because we're so dependent on our feet and legs, it's worth becoming familiar with common conditions affecting them, and with how best to prevent and treat these.

Types of Problems

Peripheral Neuropathy

Peripheral neuropathy is characterized by a burning, pins-and-needles, tingling, or itching sensation in the feet. This condition commonly begins as a result of either sensory dysfunction or malfunction in the motor nerves. Improper functioning of these nerves can be induced by metabolic disorders, such as diabetes, and by other diseases. Patients with diabetes tend to suffer from extreme cases of neuropathy and often experience complete numbness in the lower extremities. When proper nerve enervation is hindered, tissues tend to break down, leaving the external aspects of the foot susceptible to abrasions, wounds, and sores. In light of the fact that approximately 20,000 diabetics undergo leg amputation each year, getting treatment for these problems is essential.

Other metabolic disorders that are frequently responsible for peripheral neuropathy are thyroid hyperactivity and hypoactivity. Also, patients with kidney disease, liver disease, or hepatitis A, B, or C have a tendency to suffer from mild cases of numbness or pins and needles. Injury to the nerves can be induced as well by even the most moderate forms of trauma, including

231

pounding the feet. In addition, toxic chemicals and medications, such as pesticides, antidepressants, and especially chemotherapy, have been found to induce peripheral neuropathy.

Recent advances in modern technology have enabled doctors to establish the origin of a neuropathy problem by analyzing both motor and sensory nerves. Painful nerve conduction studies that utilize needles have become virtually antiquated, as new holistic and noninvasive techniques provide doctors with computerized analysis of the foot that can trace peripheral nerves to their roots in the spinal cord. Today's instrumentation is capable of determining whether a patient's neuropathy is a result of heavy metal toxicity from mercury amalgam dental fillings or excessive exposure to lead, cadmium, or arsenic. People can be exposed to these harmful elements simply by drinking unfiltered tap water. As metal accumulates within the body, the nerves in the lower extremities begin to degenerate, and peripheral neuropathy is compounded. Prolonged exposure to these types of hazards necessitates immediate attention before the damage becomes irreversible. Mercury fillings can be removed and replaced with less hazardous substances, while heavy metal accumulations can be eliminated via chelation therapy.

There are two holistic remedies that have proven to be especially effective in ameliorating neuropathies: ozone therapy and vitamin C therapy. Ozone therapy enhances the detoxification of tissue by heightening the elasticity of red blood cells, which are then able to infiltrate small arteries and nourish the nerve cells. Vitamin C therapy can have a profound effect upon every tissue within the body. This versatile vitamin can act as a direct healing agent or as a coenzyme—a facilitator of essential chemical processes within the body.

External Problems

People who engage in rigorous athletic activity, such as long-distance running, sports, or even race-walking, are often prone to exterior foot and leg injuries. Participating in an athletic activity for a lengthy period of time can be especially detrimental, while engaging in an activity after a period of abstinence can also facilitate injury.

BLISTERS

Sometimes, a new pair of shoes can adversely affect the foot by causing blisters. Areas of the foot that are susceptible to abrasion or the formation of blisters should be treated with Superskin, a relatively new innovation that has proven effective in preventing external foot irritations. Superskin is a liquid that is applied by rubbing directly into the skin. Before using this product on your entire foot, it is advisable to test a small hidden area on the skin to determine if an allergy exists.

WOUNDS

Seek medical care for serious wounds where infection could be a problem. During the initial treatment of a wound it is advisable to apply an evaporating wet dressing that will allow the cut to reach a desirable level of dryness. Once this is achieved the wound should be covered with an emollient dressing that can further aid the injury. A simple dressing that allows proper wound drainage is important. Vitamin E, aloe vera, and vitamins A and D are some natural substances that can be used in such a dressing. The potent healing ability of vitamin E was demonstrated in a study of patients suffering from gangrene. Scientists concluded that even advanced forms of the condition could be treated with large dosages of vitamin E.

An internal approach to wound healing involves large intravenous supplements of vitamin C. Furthermore, intravenous ozone therapy can eliminate viruses, fungi, and bacteria that may be hindering the healing process. Finally, a topical solution of ozone gas, which is comprised of an ozone/oxygen mixture encased in a balloon-like plastic container, can be applied to further cleanse the skin. Ozone has met widespread popularity in Europe, where it has proven to be quite useful in treating burn victims.

WARTS

Warts stem from a viral infection that infiltrates the body's immune system and debilitates its supply of T cells. These are the cells designed to combat this type of invader, but when the immune system is weak, they are unable to successfully perform their duties, and consequently, the viral intruders are able to form a small tumor on the skin's surface. Warts that develop on the underside of the foot are given a special designation: plantar's warts. Treatment of warts encompasses two main aspects. First, immune system functioning needs to be rejuvenated via vitamin and mineral supplementation and stress reduction. External treatment is the second approach. The external use of salicylic acid is an old treatment that is still administered. However, newer remedies, including ozone therapy and the use of liquid nitrogen, have proven more effective.

DRY SKIN ON THE FEET AND LEGS

This condition can be caused by poor nutrition or hindered circulation. A simple homemade moisturizer can serve as an inexpensive and effective substitute for costly products. Most commercial moisturizers contain hydrogenated vegetable oil, an ingredient that can be effectively replaced with several home products. Safflower, sunflower, and canola oil are all excellent moisturizers, while a mixture of vegetable oil and the oil from vitamins E, A, and D capsules is another effective solution for dry skin. The latter concoction can be refrigerated to ensure its potency.

When using a homemade ointment, spread a small amount directly onto the skin and rub away any excess. For maximum results, apply the ointment right after your shower or bath while the skin is still wet. This way the moisture is locked into your skin under the coat of oil.

CALLUSES AND CORNS

Calluses tend to develop on the bottom of the foot, and corns form on the top, on the side, or under the foot. Calluses are caused by thick accumulations of dead skin, while corns originate from calcified protrusions on the bone that either press against the skin from inside the foot or receive external pressure from a shoe, the ground, or another toe. Since corns and calluses consist primarily of dead skin, they are not terribly dangerous and can be eliminated via the use of a pumice stone or other abrading apparatus. Since metal can cut through skin, resulting in infection, it is advisable to avoid any type of metal tool. In addition, before using a pumice stone or other tool, you should clean it with peroxide or alcohol in order to eliminate the possibility of bacterial or viral infection.

In most cases, the development of a corn can be averted by selecting a pair of shoes that do not squeeze or put pressure on the toes. The formation of calluses and corns underneath the foot can be prevented with shock-absorbent insoles. If this method is not successful, you may require an orthotic device that can correct any bone misalignments. Sometimes the formation of calluses or corns under the foot can be induced by a malfunction in a completely different region of the body. For example, if the spine, neck, head, or pelvis are even slightly out of alignment, your gait will be adversely affected, and consequently, excess pressure will be placed upon certain areas of the foot, which may lead to the formation of a corn or callus. A meager 2 percent of corns or calluses necessitate professional attention. Surgery should be avoided whenever possible, as there is no guarantee that it can provide worthwhile relief. Unfortunately, many times the performance of foot surgery will leave the bottom of the foot permanently susceptible to pain.

RASHES

Sometimes people acquire a blistering skin rash when they come into contact with a certain kind of soap or detergent. A mixture of liquid aloe and purified water added to a bandage or gauze pad can be effective in combating this type of condition. A key element of the treatment process is allowing the solution to evaporate directly from the skin. After it dries, the concoction should be repeatedly reapplied, and eventually the irritation will disappear. It is important to continually rewet the bandage once it has dried, in order to prevent it from adhering to the wound. In certain cases of rash that necessitate it, when the acute blistering has completely vanished, intravenous vitamin

C therapy can provide long-term relief, while more severe cases may necessitate ozone therapy.

Ozone therapy can also be administered for psoriasis, a serious rash in which the body exudes toxic waste products from the surface of the skin.

ATHLETE'S FOOT

Athlete's foot is a common, fungal skin infection that is usually a product of a weak immune system, excess acidity, and warm, moist conditions. Poor T-cell function, which can be contributory, may be corrected through stress reduction and nutritional supplements, and ozone therapy can aid the immune system further. Keeping the feet cool and dry is essential. It is important to remove sweaty socks and to avoid the use of talcum powder. The substance often contains asbestos, which can be absorbed by the lungs, leading to illness later in life.

There are several new sock materials that have proven useful in preventing the accumulation of sweat. During the winter, Thermostat and Thermax can keep the foot dry and warm, while during the summer, Coolmax can be used to keep it dry and cool.

Since athlete's foot is an acid condition, acid-forming foods, such as red meats, should be eliminated. Other foods to avoid include foods high in phosphates, such as sodas, sugary foods, and fried foods. It may be beneficial to include cultured foods, such as yogurt, tofu, or kefir, and to drink plenty of water to help flush out toxins.

Herbs with antifungal activity are recommended for athlete's foot. Pure aloe vera skin gel, or ointments containing cat's claw, echinacea, or tea tree oil, can be applied topically. Myrrh and goldenseal powder, dusted on the foot and covered with a sock, may also help.

Another way to treat the condition is with magnets. Advocates of this method explain that magnets can be effective because they increase oxygen to the area, creating an environment that is not conducive to pathogenic microorganisms.

Fungal peeling may be due to dehydrated skin, and is a sign that essential fatty acids are low. Evening primrose oil can help here.

It is also helpful to wash the fungus under the toes with negatively charged water, to wear cotton socks, and to go barefoot in a clean home whenever possible. And to prevent susceptibility to reinfection, boosting the immune system with healthful nutrients is the best idea.

Joint Pain

Many adults develop arthritis in their lower extremities. Osteoarthritis, which develops after a long history of wear and tear on the joints, can be prevented by maintaining alignment in all parts of the body. A proper alignment regimen incorporates treatment of the upper body by a trained chiropractor or osteopath. A foot examination can also be beneficial, and in some cases, the use of orthotics may be necessitated. Appropriately fitted orthotics can help certain people eliminate unnecessary wear and tear on their feet. Stretching exercises are important for eliminating muscle strains, while strengthening exercises can aid in balancing muscle groups and preventing joint strains. When joint aches have already manifested, consumption of several nutritional supplements, such as boron, glucosamine sulfate, boswellia, vitamin C, and vitamin E, can help combat the pain. In addition, vitamin C and ozone therapy can be employed to quell the symptoms of osteoarthritis.

Rheumatoid arthritis is a condition in which one's own immune system turns against the body, leaving the bones and joints of the lower extremities susceptible to degeneration. When this form of arthritis manifests, high dosages of vitamin C can be used to restrain the immune system from causing any further damage. After the immune system has become pacified by the vitamin C, it can reinitiate functioning at a more tranquil level.

Many people develop bunions during the course of their lives. While there's a common belief that bunions are a product of ill-fitting shoes, in reality they are inherited from one generation to the next. Although improper footwear can facilitate the development of a bunion problem, a genetic predisposition for bunion formation must exist regardless of your shoe selection. Young children with the genetic tendency for bunion formation can be fitted with corrective shoe inserts that are capable of eliminating the potential problem. Shoe inserts used during the early stages of development can prevent further degeneration of the bone structure and allow the bones to become realigned. Once a child has reached the age of 12, his or her foot is almost fully developed; hence, the potential for future bunion development becomes more difficult to eliminate. Although bunions usually do not appear until later in life, the use of a properly fitted orthotic during the early stage of development and throughout life can act as an effective preventive agent. In addition to being unattractive, advanced forms of bunions frequently result in the development of arthritic joints, which cannot be corrected without surgery.

Another common joint disorder that affects the foot is gout. This disease frequently manifests in the big toe joint, the ankle joint, and the heel. When the kidneys are unable to assimilate the purines found in certain foods, an excessive accumulation of uric acid infiltrates the blood supply, leaving the body prone to the disease. Both carnivores and vegetarians should be wary of gout, as certain foods in both of their diets contain inordinate quantities of gout-inducing purines. Some examples include meat, poultry, red wine, beer, fish, cauliflower, and kidney beans.

Ingrown toenails

Almost everyone incurs an ingrown toenail at some point in life, and this problem can be quite frustrating and painful. The best way to deal with a persistent ingrown toenail condition is to cut toenails straight across. Unfortunately, people have a tendency to cut out only a small section of the nail in the corner of the foot, allowing the nail to grow directly into surrounding flesh.

To eliminate an ingrown toenail, take a small piece of cotton and roll it between your fingers. Using a toothpick, lift the ingrown nail and slip the cotton under the nail. Instead of irritating nearby skin, the nail will grow over the cotton buffer. The piece of cotton should be replaced every few days. It is important to remember that an ingrown toenail can become an expensive and agonizing problem if it does not receive adequate attention when it first develops.

Athletic Injuries

In general, if an injury does not improve significantly within 24 hours, you should seek professional help. In the meantime, here are several suggestions that can help extinguish the pain of minor internal injuries. (Broken bones, of course, always require professional care.) The first step in treating an internal injury is the application of ice. Apply ice for 10 minutes straight, and then keep the ice off for another 10 minutes to prevent the skin from becoming frozen. Ice therapy should be continued for at least the first two days after the injury occurs, or until the pain desists. Sometimes people resume activity prior to initiation of the healing process, and consequently, the injury becomes aggravated and swelling can once again occur. If you experience pain, it is important to apply ice, but once the pain has stopped and healing has begun, warm, wet compresses should be used for 10- to 15-minute periods on the injured region. This second form of therapy can aid circulation and enhance the healing process. So, in summary, during the initial stages of an injury use cold therapy, while sensations of sensitivity during the actual healing process should be treated with heat.

Another important element of the healing process is the performance of non-weight-bearing exercises immediately after the occurrence of the injury. It is important to engage the joints and muscles of the foot, ankle, and leg in full-range-of-motion exercises. Since any initial movements may hurt at first, you should rub ice over the injured area to numb it. Once you have applied ice for several minutes, move the muscles and joints in a full range of motion. These motions will enable the body to naturally eliminate scar tissue and prevent adhesions from developing. Massage therapy can be especially beneficial for muscle, tendon, or ligament injuries in the lower extremities, while additional treatment can be obtained via ozone and vitamin C therapy.

Forty-eight hours after the occurrence of an athletic injury, moderate stretching exercises should be incorporated into the daily treatment regimen. Stretches should be executed slowly in a long, continuous, pulling manner. Each stretch should be performed for approximately 20 seconds, but never use a bouncing motion. Proper stretching can enhance circulation in the injured area, can mitigate spasms by extending the tendons and ligaments to their correct length, and can prevent future spasms. After several days, you should move on to strengthening exercises. Before you initiate exercise, you should identify any weak muscles that may have actually contributed to the occurrence of the injury. Once you have done this, you can work on restoring equilibrium to all of the body's muscle groups so that future injury can be averted. Professional guidance is always helpful when beginning exercises, especially when the injury is acute.

Internal Foot and Leg Problems

A heel imbalance can be induced by a variety of factors, including arthritic ankles and joints, plantar fasciitis, which is an inflammation of the muscle under the foot's arch, and heel and bone spurs. People who are plagued by heel imbalances can benefit from another new product, known as the *Heel Hugger,* a small elastic ankle brace that can stabilize both the ankle and the knee. People who incur multiple ankle sprains usually have a tendency to suffer from chronic knee ailments as well. The Heel Hugger can provide an effective means of preventing these types of injuries.

Many people mistakenly believe that heel and bone spurs are the result of too much calcium, but the opposite is true. When there is too little calcium, the body leaches this mineral from the bones, and then deposits it into the heel and foot. Calcium works best when it is taken together with magnesium, in a ratio of 1500 mg:750 mg. Unless heartburn is a problem, the addition of hydrochloric acid can further enhance the effect of these nutrients. Several other nutrients and herbs have analgesic and anti-inflammatory properties; these can be used singly or in combination for the treatment of bone spurs. Vitamin C relieves swelling, and works best in combination with bioflavonoids. Between 2000 and 4000 mg of C and 100 mg of bioflavonoids are needed on a daily basis. Additionally, one gram of shark cartilage daily may help alleviate inflammation and pain. Sage, rosemary, and alfalfa can be made into a tea. Alfalfa is particularly good for this type of problem because it contains calcium. Bee pollen, yucca root, and devil's claw may also produce excellent effects. Externally, a hot linseed or castor oil pack can be comforting. Just place the oil on a heated cloth and wrap it around the affected foot.

Foot injuries can often be traced to improper walking. The F-scan is a recently developed diagnostic device that can discover the presence of a foot imbalance with the use of a pressure-sensitive mat. First, a patient is instructed to walk across the mat, which registers the amount of pressure being applied by each foot. Then, the data are converted by a computer into color printouts. Analysis of these by a doctor can offer an explanation as to why a patient is experiencing pain when he or she is walking.

Circulatory Problems

Varicose veins are one of the most common circulatory problems, yet most people remain unaware of the variety of alternative treatments that are available. In general, the health of our veins can be enhanced by maintaining proper weight, exercising to improve circulation, and eating foods and nutritional supplements that support the liver. Much blood circulates through the liver, and if the liver becomes congested, the whole venous system can back up. This, in turn, adds pressure on the veins, damages valves, and results in varicose veins. Foods that support the liver include beets, artichokes, and dark-skinned fruits and berries, such as blueberries, cherries, and dark-skinned grapes. Also, milk thistle and dandelion are helpful herbs for the liver. In addition, gotu kola, horse chestnut, and butcher's broom help strengthen veins. Supplemental phosphorous, and vitamins E and C can be beneficial for the veins in the legs and feet. People with deep varicose veins should also invest in supportive stockings.

Deep varicose veins are usually characterized by red and brownish markings, light dots, and especially dark, concentrated areas above the ankle and lower leg. Severe cases are characterized by a permanent discoloration of skin. When skin discoloration is exhibited, the body is providing us with a warning that elements deep within the body, such as the valves, are not functioning properly. As the veins swell, the legs and feet can become plagued by itching and, eventually, sores and open wounds known as varicose ulcers will develop.

Another common product of varicose veins, phlebitis, is characterized by inflammations within the veins and clotting of the blood. If a blood clot breaks away from the vein, a sudden stroke or heart attack may ensue. Obviously, discovering a varicose vein problem during its early stages and immediately instituting an appropriate treatment plan is essential in eliminating serious health risks.

Another widespread circulatory problem that frequently affects the legs and feet is intermittent claudication brought on by arteriosclerosis, or hardening of the arteries. The most effective preventive measure for this condition is regular aerobic exercise. Supplements of vitamins C and E can also be beneficial because of their ability to promote blood flow, while chelation or ozone therapy can be used once the condition has already developed. Ozone therapy helps because it increases the flexibility of red blood cells, enabling them to slip through clogged arteries, while chelation therapy removes toxic byproducts from the arteries, rendering them more pliable. Both methods can provide an effective alternative to coronary bypass and leg surgery.

Proper Foot Attire

When selecting a shoe, choose a size that allows you at least half an inch from your big toe to the end of the shoe. One way of determining whether or not a shoe fits properly involves taking the insole out and placing your foot upon it. By using this method, you can see if the shoe is appropriate in both the length and width. After you have made your selection, break the shoes in gradually by wearing them for short periods every day. This way you can avoid injury or irritations. As your tolerance grows, you will be able to comfortably wear the shoes for the entire day.

As for sneakers, there are a multitude of sneaker manufacturers, and each manufacturer offers an extensive selection of products; hence, consumers are under the impression that finding proper foot attire to suit a specific need takes some time. In reality, the best type of sneaker for walking, shopping, or doing housework is the running shoe. This type of shoe offers a significant degree of protection from the elements. It is comprised of highly advanced shock-absorbent materials that can shelter the entire foot, from heel to toe. Furthermore, these shoes are extremely flexible in the ball of the foot and offer stability in the rear.

Treatment Summary

Peripheral neuropathy can often be successfully countered with ozone and vitamin C. These increase the blood's elasticity and help detoxify and nourish cells.

External wounds of the legs and feet should be properly dressed to prevent infection and speed up the healing process. An effective dressing allows the wound to drain properly. Initially, an evaporating wet dressing should be used. Next, the wound should be covered with an emollient dressing incorporating vitamin E, aloe vera, vitamin A, or vitamin D.

Corns can usually be arrested by wearing well-fitting shoes. Corns and calluses can also be prevented by wearing a shock-absorbent insole or an orthotic device.

For athlete's foot, ozone therapy is an effective remedy, especially when used in conjunction with stress reduction, nutritional supplements, and keeping the feet dry and cool.

Maintaining proper body alignment with the help of a chiropractor or osteopath can prevent joint pain. In some instances, orthotics and strengthening exercises may be necessary, as well as supplementation.

To prevent ingrown toenails, cut the nails straight across. Cotton over a toothpick can be used to lift the ingrown toenail out of the skin.

Sports injuries that do not resolve within 24 hours should be handled by a medical professional. First aid involves the application of ice. Once pain subsides, this is followed by the application of warm, wet compresses. Non-weight-bearing exercises, stretching, and massage therapy may be indicated later to restore full range of motion.

Heel imbalances may be corrected with a product known as the Heel Hugger. Heel and bone spurs may be healed with extra calcium, magnesium, and other nutrients.

Varicose veins can be treated with nutrients and supportive stockings.

A regular exercise routine, vitamins E and C, and chelation or ozone therapy can help eliminate intermittent claudication.

Gallstones

Approximately 20 million Americans, most of them over 65, suffer from gallstones. These are a concentration of bile components, like cholesterol, biopigments, and salt, that form into little stones and block the common or cystic bile duct. As these pieces accumulate and enlarge, the gallbladder becomes inflamed, resulting in severe pain. If left untreated, the stones can cause digestive incapacity and become life threatening.

Causes

According to new research, it appears that the problem underlying gallstones is related to a deficiency in hydrochloric acid or to a food intolerance. Gallstones are also occasionally due to cysts, tumors, Crohn's disease, pancreatitis, or roundworm infection. Obesity, diabetes, and hypothyroidism can lead to increased cholesterol in the blood and the formation of gallstones.

Symptoms

Most people with gallstones never know they have them and are able to lead normal, comfortable lives without medical intervention. When symptoms do appear, however, they can include bloating, belching, and a sharp pain or spasm under the ribs or under the right shoulder blade after eating fatty foods.

Treatment

Diet

Basically, a person needs to be on a low-fat, no-sugar diet, and abstain from coffee and other forms of caffeine. A vegetarian diet is generally the best one to follow, and the following foods should be included: dandelion root, beet greens, and black radish greens. These foods help to increase the flow of bile, needed to break down fat.

Gallbladder Flush

Gallstones are easier to prevent than treat, but once they are there, a gallbladder flush is sometimes effective in getting rid of the problem. According to Linda Rector Page, author of *Healthy Healing: An Alternative Healing Reference*, the flush consists of a three-day fast on olive oil and lemon juice, and six days of olive oil, lemon, carrot, beet, and cucumber juice, as well as a potassium broth containing carrots, spinach, celery, and parsley. The liquids should be taken four to five times a day. Page adds that enemas using coffee, garlic, catnip, or wheatgrass can further enhance the cleansing process.

Following the flush, it's best to follow an alkaline diet with lots of sea vegetables and concentrated green juices, such as chlorella, barley grass, spirulina, and wheatgrass, to boost the liver and gallbladder.

Supplements

People with gallstones should check to see whether they are deficient in hydrochloric acid, which would indicate a need to add this substance as a supplement. Lipotropic supplements, like choline, omega-3, and flaxseed oil, are good to take three times a day. Other useful supplements include inositol, methionine, vitamin C, and phosphatidylcholine, which is a refined form of lecithin. The amino acid taurine can help increase bile formation. Also, the plant enzymes bromelain and papain help digest protein and are anti-inflammatory.

Herbs

Bitter herbs that normalize liver function and help to produce bile should be taken. The herb milk thistle, also known as silymarin, is one such herb. Other good herbs to take are goldenseal, cardamom, and Oregon grape, which are high in the active ingredient berberine. Dandelion is also excellent for the liver and can be taken in large quantities. Additionally, tumeric is excellent for its anti-inflammatory properties. Gravel root or chamomile tea will help to dissolve gallstones.

What to Avoid

Certain foods aggravate gallbladder disease, the most common offenders being eggs, onions, and pork. Dairy products and any other foods high in fat also tend to intensify the problem. Sugar may aggravate the gallbladder and should therefore be avoided. Note that being overweight places a person at high risk. Certain prescription drugs do as well; check with your physician if this is a concern.

Treatment Summary

A low-fat, no-sugar, no red meat, no dairy, caffeine-free diet should be followed.

A nine-day liquid fast, called a gallbladder flush, may help dissolve gallstones.

A variety of supplements and herbs help dissolve gallstones and support the return of health.

Headaches

Each year a seemingly infinite number of Americans are plagued by headaches. While sometimes the degree of severity is trivial, at other times headaches can lead to excruciating agony. There are two basic categories of headaches: tension headaches and migraines. Tension headaches are common to everyday life and are usually associated with a sensation of pressure or band-like tightness on either side of the head. Migraines, on the other hand, do not occur on a daily basis and are characterized by intense discomfort. Starting with a slight throbbing sensation, migraines can rapidly crescendo into an oppressive pounding in the head.

The number of Americans affected by migraines has been estimated at 23 million. Since hormones play a decisive role in the onset of migraines, an overwhelming majority (about 18 million) of migraine sufferers are women. Clinical evidence shows that migraines are brought on by an abrupt dilation of the blood vessels that burdens the brain with excessive amounts of pressure. This can be caused by a variety of conditions.

Causes

First of all, migraines are commonly exacerbated by allergic reactions to elements in the diet or the environment. Dietary reactions include allergies to foods, artificial food additives, and food combinations. Reactions to alcoholic beverages, especially red wine and beer, are quite common, as are reactions to tyramine and MSG. Tyramine is an amino acid found in cheese, yogurt, yeast extracts, and smoked fish, while MSG is a flavor enhancer sometimes used in Chinese food and other products. People who are allergic to wheat, dairy products, eggs, and corn may experience migraines if they indulge in these foods. Sodium nitrate, which is common in most cold cuts and frankfurters, and aspartame, an artificial sweetener that reduces the level of serotonin in the body, have also been implicated in migraines. Furthermore, reactions to caffeinated products, such as coffee, soda, and chocolate can trigger a migraine. Environmental reactions include reactions to hazardous fumes emitted from home furnishings, cleaning products, carpeting, and other sources.

Sometimes migraines can result from cranial faults or deformities in the cranial bone structure. The position of cranial bones can be adversely altered by intense traumas to the head, such as whiplash, being hit on the head, or birth trauma. According to the beliefs of Chinese medicine, a meridian imbalance, which can be diagnosed by an acupuncturist or practicing kinesiologist, can also influence the occurrence of migraines. The meridians are a system of 12 bilateral electromagnetic channels of energy within the body. When energy is entrapped within one of these channels, a meridian dysfunction occurs, and consequently, a painful migraine results.

Hormones, too, can play a role in causing migraine headaches. Sixty percent of all female migraine sufferers relate the occurrence of migraines to their menstrual cycle. Although the medical community is still uncertain as to the exact relationship between the development of migraines and the level of the hormone estrogen in the body, it is evident that this hormone somehow plays a key role in their occurrence. One hypothesis is that estrogen affects the functioning of the nervous system and the level of serotonin in the body, a substance that may facilitate in the onset of migraines. Women who use birth control pills are more likely to experience acute migraines, while women who have recently experienced menopause are less susceptible to them due to the reduced quantities of estrogen in their bodies. Reliance upon hormonal replacement therapy in post-menopausal women can contribute to reoccurrence of migraines.

A deficiency of magnesium in the blood is another predisposing factor. An insufficient intake of this vital nutrient has also been correlated with the onset of a myofacial disorder known as fibromyalgia that is characterized by migraine-like symptoms.

It is not generally acknowledged, but prescription drugs administered by medical doctors and even over-the-counter drugs can promote migraines. Simple painkillers, including mixed analgesics, acetaminophen, and aspirin, which are supposed to treat headaches, can actually contribute to their onset. In fact, overuse of these products has been cited as a cause of migraines. When painkillers are used in excess, the body becomes accustomed to their presence in the bloodstream and will experience withdrawal symptoms when the supply is depleted.

Another factor contributory to migraines is a cervical subluxation in the upper portion of the neck, a condition common among people who frequently talk on the telephone. Often, people have a tendency to cradle the telephone receiver between their shoulder and neck, causing the vertebrae to assume a distorted position. People who like to read in bed are also likely candidates for cervical subluxation because the propped position of the head shifts the vertebrae and places excessive pressure upon the nerves, resulting, possibly, in a migraine.

Although stress cannot be considered a direct cause of migraines, prolonged exposure to stressful situations and anxiety can compound the symptoms.

Symptoms

Some cases of migraines are preceded by the presence of certain warning signs on one side of the head, including sensations of flashing lights or zigzag lines. The appearance of these ominous warning signs, called an aura, foreshadows the occurrence of a migraine. The actual headache usually occurs within 20 minutes of the warning signs on the opposite side of the head. Although the aura is usually characterized by visual stimuli, sometimes it can take the form of other sensations, such as the detection of odor, lingual difficulties, disorientation, tingling, or numbness. Early detection of these warning signs can allow the victim some time to prepare for the onset of a migraine.

Unlike regular headaches, migraines are characterized by pain on only one side of the head. In addition, nausea, vomiting, fatigue, irritability, vision problems, and sensitivity to light and sound commonly occur.

Treatment

Since many over-the-counter painkillers can create a rebound effect, migraine sufferers are usually given nonsteroidal anti-inflammatory medication, such as ibuprofen, or special migraine medicines that can be used during acute attacks. Muscle tension headaches are commonly treated with minor analgesics, and a combination of massages, hot showers, and other muscle relaxation techniques.

Pressure Point Therapy

Pressure point therapy can be used to alleviate even the most intense tension headaches. There are several pressure points that promote muscle relaxation. One is the hand. By placing the thumb in the webbed area between the first and second fingers, and applying pressure in the direction of the first finger, headache pain can often be lessened.

Since most tension headaches begin in the back of the neck and the shoulders, there is a special procedure designed to manipulate the head. While sitting down and bending the head forward, position the thumbs just above the neck and below the occipital bone, approximately one and a half inches away from the midpoint of the neck. When you locate a bump, apply pressure for 10 to 15 seconds. A useful technique for treating headaches on the side of the head involves placing the finger one and a half inches above the ear on the temple. When you locate a tender area, press for several seconds until the tender area disappears. Also, pressing a half inch above the eyebrows for several seconds can further reduce headaches. There are a few reflex points below the eyebrow as well. Each point is located approximately a half inch apart and should be pressed in an upward motion for five or ten seconds. Squeezing the bridge of the nose for five or ten seconds can also be useful. The reflex points under the cheekbones should be manipulated starting near the nose and slowly moving the index fingers a half inch at a time toward the ears. After these points are treated, proceed to the neck and shoulder region.

Massage Therapy

Sinus headaches can be alleviated by massaging under the neck and proceeding upward through the hairline to the top of the head. Remember to squeeze the muscles located at the back of the neck and shoulders, and carefully manipulate the various acupressure points, including the bridge of the nose, below the cheekbones, under the eyebrows, and under the forehead. When you are treating a migraine, you should lie down and place a cold compress over the eyes and head for a few minutes. Gently massage the temples for a few seconds, and then stretch the head back in order to release any energy blockages. This procedure alleviates migraines because it relieves tension in the muscles, increases circulation, and facilitates the transport of oxygen to the brain.

Reflexology

The practice of reflexology is founded upon the principle that manipulation of the foot can aid the rest of the body. Therapy for migraines is usually initiated by creating a relaxed environment, which can include using a shallow basin of water to soften and warm the feet. There are several points on the foot that are involved in the treatment process. The big toe, reflexologists explain, corresponds to the head, while the other toes also pertain to the head and to the sinus region. The ridge located under the toes relates to the neck and shoulders, and the ball of the foot corresponds to the chest and lungs.

A key factor in quelling the onset of a migraine is relaxing and comforting the body. The little notch just under the ball of the foot relates to the solar plexus, which is vital to emotional processes. Reflexologists explain that by placing the thumb on this point during inhalation and removing it during exhalation, the solar plexus is relaxed, allowing emotions to flow freely. Another activity that can aid in relaxation involves wringing the foot as if it were a washcloth. And a technique called the lung press constitutes pressing the ball of the foot with the right fist while supporting the foot with the left hand. The pressing motion of the fist should gradually be brought down to the heel. This technique also promotes relaxation and should be performed three times consecutively.

During a session with a reflexologist, a wide variety of techniques are used, and both feet are treated. Sessions end with both feet being massaged, followed by a few minutes of quiet rest and a glass of water to flush out harmful deposits.

Aromatherapy

Aromatherapy, or a combination of aromatherapy and other treatment modalities, can be quite effective in subduing headaches. Lavender oil can aid in combating migraines by relaxing the neck muscles and releasing tension. This oil should be massaged into the back of the neck and the temples prior to pressure point therapy. One or two drops of peppermint oil can be applied as a massage oil like lavender oil, added to drinking water, or inhaled from your palm or a tissue.

Herbal Remedies

Aloe vera is especially beneficial in alleviating headaches induced by pollution or acidic foods. The herb feverfew can be used to combat migraines. Lungtanxieganwan is used in Oriental medicine to ameliorate headaches brought on by anger or constipation, and the herb Xiao Yao Wan treats headaches prompted by allergies, premenstrual syndrome, and hypoglycemia. Valerian is of use for headaches characterized by nervousness and insomnia, and can also treat migraines and dizziness associated with air travel.

Allergy Control

Since migraines induced by allergic food reactions may take hours to fully develop, patients often need to keep a journal listing all of the foods they have consumed in order to effectively expose the culprit. In ascertaining the presence of a possible food allergy, patients can place a sample of the suspect food under their tongue. If there is truly an allergic reaction, muscles that were once strong will be weakened by the food, and there will be variations in the intensity and frequency of the pulse. Future migraines can be prevented by eliminating the allergy-inducing food from the diet.

The frequency of migraines caused by environmental allergic reactions can be reduced by keeping household plants. Plants have the ability to assimilate various toxins that are found in our homes. For instance, spider plants demonstrate the capacity to absorb formaldehyde, which is commonly discharged by plywood, synthetic carpet, particle board, and new upholstery, while chrysanthemums can aid in absorbing fumes released by glue, varnish, and lacquer.

Alternatively, one can attain a similar effect by drinking an herbal tea that contains chrysanthemums.

Craniosacral Therapy

Although an examination of the skull for cranial faults is considerably more difficult than detecting a food allergy, proper diagnosis, followed by corrective measures, can help prevent future migraines. Cranial faults often escape detection due to the subtle motions of the cranial bones. Many people who suffer from migraines with cranial origins have internally rotated frontal bones. This condition frequently results in the occurrence of a migraine accompanied by eye pain. What craniosacral therapists do is manipulate bones to relieve pain. Treatment with this modality consists of pressure, applied at varying levels, to different parts of the head.

Other Modes of Treatment

Migraines induced by hormonal imbalances can be combated with supplements that stabilize hormonal levels, such as vitamin B6, and evening primrose oil. Migraines characterized by a meridian imbalance can be treated by either an acupuncturist, who will rely upon the use of needles, or a kinesiologist, who will manipulate the meridians using a finger. Either type of practitioner can be effective in restoring the balance of energy. The treatment of migraines caused by upper cervical subluxation should be performed by a competent chiropractor, who can adjust the region and eliminate the subluxation. As we've mentioned, some cases of migraines are induced by excessive reliance upon medication. People who suffer from this category of migraine should, while under the supervision of a holistically-oriented physician, halt consumption of these products. Gradually, the body will lose its dependence upon the medication and can readjust to normalized conditions. Migraines induced by a magnesium deficiency can be remedied with a combination treatment of magnesium supplements and malic acid. Since the necessary dosages vary from one individual to the next, a physician should be consulted before beginning supplementation. Stress-related migraines can be treated with the herb feverfew, which acts as a sedative, and can be consumed in either a tea or in capsules. Recommended dosage is one cup of tea per day, or one or two capsules of the freeze-dried extract version. Meditation, progressive muscle relaxation, yoga, and moderate exercise, such as swimming and walking, can be employed to further reduce stress and improve the emotional state.

Additional Supplements

When the herb feverfew is accompanied by 250 to 500 mg of magnesium and 125 mg of ginkgo biloba on a daily basis, the symptoms of migraines can be drastically reduced. This combination of supplements has met remarkable success in the treatment of people who regularly suffer from migraines, and can serve as an effective substitute for conventional treatments. Supplements of niacin have a tendency to create a flushing sensation in the head, which in turn eliminates excess blood and quells the onset of migraines. Finally, recent studies have shown that daily supplementation of 1000-2000 mg of omega-3 fatty acids, found in fish oil, and riboflavin can decrease the frequency and severity of migraines.

What to Avoid

Although some causes of migraines are beyond our control, others, such as food allergies, can be effectively combated by avoiding certain products. Clinical research has correlated the consumption of red wine and other alcoholic beverages with the occurrence of migraines in certain people, while other research has implicated chocolate as a contributing factor. Monosodium glutamate is another frequent cause of migraines. While Chinese food is infamous for its use of MSG, surprisingly, a variety of other foods, including salad dressing, sauces, frozen and prepared foods, and soups, incorporate the ingredient. Caffeine and artificial sweeteners, such as aspartame, have also been found to promote migraines. Studies have revealed that foods that contain quantities of the mineral copper, such as wheat germ, shellfish, and nuts, can act as migraine-inducing agents. Citrus fruits should also be avoided, due to their tendency to increase intestinal absorption of copper. Many people who suffer from allergy-induced migraines have cited reactions to dairy products, particularly various types of cheese, as the root of their problems. Cheese, smoked fish, yogurt, and yeast extracts contain an ingredient known as tyramine, which has been known to increase susceptibility to migraines. Sodium nitrate, common in cold cuts and frankfurters, is yet another cause.

In addition to abstaining from foods that provoke allergies, it is important to avoid missing meals and to avoid excessive exposure to stress, as these are both factors that contribute to the onset of headaches.

Treatment Summary

Pressure point therapy is useful in treating tension headaches.

A qualified massage therapist can promote recovery from sinus headaches, migraines, and tension headaches.

Pressure applied to specific areas on the feet can be effective in the alleviation of headaches, even migraines.

Several essential oils work to release tension, thereby alleviating headaches.

Migraines are often reactions to allergy-producing foods. Tests for food allergies will let you know which foods to eliminate.

Cranial faults in frontal head bones can cause migraines accompanied by eye pain. A craniosacral therapist can manipulate these bones to promote wellness.

Supplements that can provide support to the system for overcoming headaches include vitamin B6 and evening primrose oil.

The herb feverfew, magnesium, and ginkgo biloba work to reduce migraine symptoms.

Niacin, as well as omega-3 fatty acids and riboflavin, are other anti-migraine nutrients.

Acupuncture can be an effective migraine treatment.

Chiropractors eliminate subluxations in the upper cervical region, which may result in the elimination of migraines.

To reduce the chance of headaches, don't miss meals, and try to reduce your stress level.

Heart Disease

Heart disease kills more Americans than any other ailment, and each year approximately $47 billion is consumed attempting to combat it. There are a wide variety of factors that contribute to heart damage. Anything that serves to damage the inner lining of the blood vessels and impedes the transportation of oxygen and nutrients to the heart can be defined as a risk factor. During the initial phases of heart disease, destructive agents ranging from tobacco, artificial food additives, and gasoline fumes to sustained high blood pressure contribute to hardening of the arteries, commonly known as arteriosclerosis. As time progresses, the accumulation of calcium deposits, scar tissue, fat, and cholesterol in the arteries leads to the formation of atherosclerotic lesions and eventual arterial blockage. The blockage of arteries going to the brain often results in a stroke, while blockage pertaining to the heart can cause heart attacks.

Types of Heart Conditions

Arteriosclerosis is the most common type of heart disease in the U.S. It is characterized by a slow, progressive thickening and hardening of the arterial walls, and loss of elasticity due to excessive calcium buildup along the vessel linings. Diet is a big factor in this process, as it is the buildup of cholesterol and fats on the inner walls of coronary arteries that narrows these arteries, impedes the circulation, and can eventually cause heart attacks.

Angina pectoris is a spasm of the heart muscle that occurs when clogged arteries do not permit adequate oxygen flow to the area. This creates a situation analogous to that of a person exercising beyond their oxygen capacity. The angina pectoris patient will experience pains in the chest or deferred pains to the shoulder, wrist, or jaw. Most of the time, the problem stems from a blockage of blood flow caused by atherosclerosis (a kind of arteriosclerosis).

Congestive heart failure is another condition that can result from the progressive hardening and thickening of the arteries. It occurs when inefficient functioning of the tissues creates an imbalance in the amount of blood being pumped in and out of the heart. In this situation, the narrowing of the vessels causes the blood inflow to exceed the outflow, which can eventually overwhelm the heart and result in hazardous fluid backup in the lungs, legs, and other organs.

Congenital heart disease is caused by a persistence in the fetal connections between the arterial and venous circulations. Under normal circumstances these connections are terminated at birth, but in babies who suffer from congenital heart disease, these connections continue to exist. A prime example of this is the presence of the ductus arteriosus, which attaches the pulmonary artery and the aorta. In addition, congenital defects involve the partitions between the cardiac cavities and the vessels surrounding them. In newborn "blue babies," who suffer from a condition known as cyanosis, the pulmonary artery is excessively narrowed, and the ventricles are connected by abnormal openings, resulting in insufficient oxygen intake and a bluish skin tone. Modern technology has helped improve the outlook for infants suffering from this problem.

Rheumatic heart disease, associated with rheumatic fever, is characterized by damage to the entire cardiac region. It was once the leading form of heart disease among children and adolescents, but is now quite uncommon due to the widespread use of antibiotics.

Myocarditis, which is common in older adults, can be described as a degeneration or inflammation of the heart. It often results in dilation, which is enlargement of the heart muscle due to weakness, or hypertrophy, which is overgrowth of the muscle tissue.

Cardiac arrhythmia refers to abnormal beating of the upper (atrial) or lower (ventricular) chambers of the heart. These palpitations, which may be experienced as pounding or thumping in the chest and the sensation of having missed a beat, generally indicate that the heart needs nutrients, and that it is overworked and tired. The condition is related to poor intestinal function, associated with gas and fermentation in the stomach, and allergy. Caffeine may be a precipitating factor.

A major factor associated with various forms of heart disease is high blood pressure, or hypertension. Hypertension is commonly caused by poor dietary habits, including excessive intake of sugar, caffeine, alcohol, or salt; lack of exercise; high stress; or being overweight. Over time, subclinical hypothyroidism can also make a patient prone to hypertension, a fact that often gets missed by the medical profession.

Heart disease is sometimes associated more with men than with women. But women at menopause and beyond should be aware that as estrogen levels go down so does estrogen's protective effect on the cardiac system. Medical data shows that twice as many women die from heart disease than from all forms of cancer combined. In short, risk factors associated with the onset of heart disease should be of concern to everyone.

Symptoms

During the initial phases of heart disease, there are no clear indications that the disease is present, since the illness develops quite gradually and can take years before it assumes its deadly status. Symptoms of heart disease usually become evident only after the arteries become severely blocked, as is the case with arteriosclerosis. This disease is sometimes called "the silent killer" because its victims are often unaware of its presence until the first heart attack.

Some early warning signs that may indicate arteriosclerosis include leg cramps during walking, changes in skin tone and temperature, chest pain, shortness of breath, headaches, fatigue, dizziness, and memory defects. People who suffer from congestive heart failure may also experience shortness of breath, accumulation of water in the lungs, and swelling of the ankles, while angina pectoris patients will encounter pains in the chest and other body parts. The deferment of pain to other parts of the body associated with angina pectoris may bewilder people, but it is important to acknowledge the cardiac origin of these sensations.

Treatment

Finding a qualified professional advisor is crucial to preventing and treating heart disease. Your doctor should be personally interested in your situation, and should possess extensive knowledge of your family history of heart disease, blood pressure, cholesterol level, stress level, and weight. Only after taking these factors into consideration can a proper cardiovascular health program be administered.

Traditional Approach: High-Blood-Pressure Medication

People who suffer from high blood pressure have traditionally been treated with medication. But pharmaceutical propaganda notwithstanding, there's one problem with this approach. Studies indicate that prolonged dependence on prescription high-blood-pressure medication can cause adverse side effects and can actually compound heart disease. Should people, then, discontinue medication use? Not without a physician's guidance. It is recommended that patients do not discontinue use on their own without first consulting their doctor, because this can lead to a dangerous elevation of blood pressure and eventual stroke. Before discontinuing your consumption of prescription drugs you should work with your physician on discovering a method that will allow your body to cope naturally with high blood pressure. Changes in lifestyle and diet will be key in this process and understand that the process may take some time, and that your dependence on the pharmaceuticals may continue for several more years, or even the rest of your life.

The First Linchpin of a Natural Approach: Nutrition

Dean Ornish's classic study, in which heart disease patients were placed on strict vegetarian diets and were instructed to follow aerobic exercise and relaxation programs, have provided clear evidence that heart disease can be effectively treated and even reversed. Many nutritionists feel that the reduction of dietary fat intake is vital to preventing heart disease, especially angina. The intake of fatty foods, which on average comprises 40 percent of an American's diet, should be reduced to, at most, 20 percent. In fact, some health practitioners feel that fat intake should be as low as 10 percent.

While saturated fats are the worst culprits, too many unsaturated fats have also proven to have potentially harmful effects on the body. People who consume a large amount of unsaturated vegetable oils will experience a fall in blood sugar level when the body becomes tired. When this occurs, the adrenaline level rises and the unsaturated fats that the body has stored are drawn out, causing the lining of the blood vessels to become polluted.

People should try to consume a diet of vegetarian whole foods. Complex carbohydrates—fruits, vegetables, beans, and whole grains—are the basis of such a diet. Plant pigments known as flavonoids, which can be found in vegetables, fruits, and some beans and grains, provide healthy protection against heart disease that cannot be provided in other forms. However, since studies show that up to 75 percent of the population release too much insulin in response to carbohydrates in the diet, the type and amount of carbohydrate foods may need individual monitoring.

Many Americans were brought up with the notion that only animal products could supply the necessary amounts of protein. But this assumption is false, as research has demonstrated that grains and legumes, such as rice and beans, can provide a healthy source of protein without harmful fats. Clinical studies have shown that increased intake of fish can be useful in combating heart disease and some forms of cancer. Fish oils from sardines, mackerel, salmon, and cod contain the valuable omega-3 and omega-6 fatty acids. Consumption of tofu, which is low in fat and high in fiber and protein, is yet another way to promote the development of a healthy heart and prevent cancer.

Plenty of pure water will help to normalize blood pressure and end angina pain, according to Dr. Batmanghelidj, author of *Your Body's Many Cries for Water*. As we grow older, we tend to lose our perception of thirst and drink too little water. As a result, our cells become dehydrated, and a process of reverse osmosis occurs. This means that, to maintain vital cell function, the body filters water into the cells from outside them. The result of this transfer of water is increased blood pressure.

Angina can be set off by too little water, Dr. Batmanghelidj warns. So to regulate blood pressure and put an end to angina pain, he recommends drinking half of one's body weight in ounces. In other words, a person weighing 150 pounds needs to consume 75 ounces of water daily, which is over nine glasses' worth.

Supplements

The consumption of certain dietary supplements can assist in the maintenance of a healthy heart and reduce dependence on prescription medication. Antioxidants, in particular, such as vitamins C and E, can shelter the arteries and heart from free radical damage by protecting the tissues that line the artery walls.

VITAMIN C

Vitamin C supplementation should be an integral part of everyone's life, as it works to prevent cancer, heart disease, and other serious disorders. This vitamin should be consumed in quantities of 500 to 1000 mg three to five times per day because of its tendency to be excreted from the body.

VITAMIN E

Vitamin E can be especially useful in preventing blood clots because it reduces the adhesive qualities of clot-inducing platelets. Thus E helps prevent strokes and heart attacks. It has been estimated that if everybody supplemented their diet with 200 to 800 IU of vitamin E per day, the incidence of stroke in our country could be reduced by up to 20 percent. By having E reduce the occurrence of blood clotting and oxidation in the arteries, these vessels are able to heal and recover briskly, guaranteeing the clear passage of oxygen through the arteries and into the tissue. Vitamins C and E work even better with the addition of beta carotene and selenium.

BIOFLAVONOIDS

Studies show that bioflavonoids protect against cardiovascular disease and heart attacks. The bioflavonoid quercetin is particularly important in this regard. Good food sources of these substances include the white membrane in oranges and grapefruits, as well as grapes, plums, apricots, cherries, currants, and blackberries. Between 100 and 300 mg should be taken daily.

COENZYME Q10

Coenzyme Q10 is a heart-helping nutrient in that it assists the cell mitochondria—the main source of cell energy—in the burning of fats and reduces high blood pressure and arrhythmias. This substance serves as an antioxidant by preventing oxidation damage and hardening of the arteries. Coenzyme Q10 is especially important for angina and congestive heart failure patients. Recommended dosage for people with less severe heart ailments is 50 to 200 mg per day, while people with more serious conditions may require 400 mg.

ESSENTIAL FATTY ACIDS

We need to include the essential fatty acids (omega-3 and omega-6) in our diet to minimize heart disease and other ailments. Good sources of omega-3 fatty acids are fish, fish oil supplements, and flaxseed oil. Omega-6 fatty acids are found in evening primrose, borage seed, or black currant seed oils. The two complement each other and both should be taken daily. Generally, 3000 mg of omega-3 and 2000 mg of omega-6 should be divided into three doses.

FOLIC ACID AND VITAMIN B12

These nutrients assist in the reduction of blood levels of homocystine, a substance linked to heart disorders.

L-ARGININE

The amino acid L-arginine facilitates the body's production of nitric oxide, which has an antiangina and antistress effect upon the arteries in that it enables the muscles in the arterial walls to relax. Supplements of L-arginine can also prevent platelet-induced arterial spasm by hampering the buildup of plaque on the arterial walls. Supplementation is generally at a level of 2 or 3 grams of L-arginine per day.

L-CARNITINE

The burning of fat within the cell's energy-makers, the mitochondria, is enhanced by the amino acid L-carnitine, whose presence is required to lure the fat into the cell. Once inside the mitochondria, the fat is burned for energy that our bodies use. L-carnitine enables the body to recover quickly from fatigue, and when combined with supplementation of vitamin E, this nutrient is a capable combatant of heart disease. Taking 500 mg twice a day on an empty stomach is recommended.

LECITHIN

Derived from soy, lecithin supplies the body with inositol, choline, and phosphatidyl choline, three nutrients that aid in the maintenance of healthy arteries and the emulsification of fat. Lecithin can reduce plaque in the arteries, lower blood pressure, and ameliorate angina pectoris. Lecithin granules are like finely chopped nuts, and can be sprinkled on cereals; liquid lecithin can be blended into healthful beverages.

MAGNESIUM

Approximately 80 percent of the American population is magnesium-deficient. Magnesium, which should be consumed in quantities of 600-1000 mg daily, is an advantageous nutrient because it enhances circulation by permitting the muscles in the arterial walls to rest. It's useful in ameliorating many forms of heart disease, including hypertension and arrhythmias. About 100-200 mg should be taken in the morning on an empty stomach; the remainder is best absorbed before bedtime.

NIACIN

Clinical studies have indicated that niacin, also known as vitamin B3, can help prevent heart attack and heart disease fatality. In addition, evidence suggests that it can be an effective combatant of cancer. Note, though, that niacin should only be taken under medical supervision because of its tendency to hamper liver function.

SELENIUM

A lack of this important trace mineral has been associated with hypertension. Generally, 200 mcg daily is recommended.

TAURINE

Supplementation of taurine, an amino acid that acts as an antioxidant, can help fortify cardiac contractions and consequently enhance the outflow of blood from the heart. The consumption of 500 mg of taurine twice a day can be a key factor in avoiding congestive heart failure and arteriosclerosis.

ACIDOPHILUS AND FRUCTO-OLIGOSACCHARIDES

Both products increase helpful intestinal bacteria and thus eliminate the harmful germs. As a result, heart palpitations due to intestinal problems diminish and heart strength increases.

CALCIUM AND POTASSIUM

These are important since low levels of calcium and potassium may also result in heart palpitations.

MAXEPA/EFA

People who do not consume adequate quantities of fish should be pleased to learn that the heart-disease-deterrent essential fatty acids found in fish oil can be provided with the supplement Maxepa.

Some additional supplements to consider are vitamin B complex, B6, choline, inositol, niacinamide, phosphorous, GLA, cod liver oil, brewer's yeast, and wheat germ. Also, for people who are deficient in thyroid hormone, supplements of thyroid extract are important because—among other reasons—they reduce the risk of heart attack. The natural form is better than the synthetic.

Herbal Treatments

Herbs are a source of nutrition that can assist in treating and preventing heart disease. Among the many choices available, garlic shines as a cardiovascular disease preventive: It contributes to the lowering of cholesterol levels and elevated blood pressure, and helps prevent blood clots in the arterial walls when taken along with vitamin E. It also helps stimulate and revitalize the heart muscle and strengthen the peripheral circulation, as well as circulation within the heart. Eating a crushed garlic clove, once in the morning and once at night, has a revitalizing effect on the heart. For those sensitive to the social implications of eating raw garlic, 500 mg of deodorized garlic can be taken twice a day. Two other cooking spices that help to counteract atherosclerosis are ginger and turmeric (the yellow spice used in curry powder).

Cayenne, which contains the active ingredient capsaicin, has multiple functions, including the abilities to lower blood pressure and cholesterol levels and prevent heart attacks and strokes. Studies find that using the entire herb is more effective than using capsaicin alone.

Hawthorn berry is versatile, with the ability to improve arrhythmias, angina, blood pressure, and arterial hardening. In addition, the daily consumption of hawthorn berry can enhance circulation and treat valvular insufficiency, irregular pulse, and abnormal acid levels in the blood. The herb is used widely in Europe for early-stage congestive heart failure, as it has been found superior to medications for slowing down the condition. The recommended dosage is generally 160 mg, divided into two doses a day, although people with more challenging conditions may need up to 160 mg three times daily.

Bugleweed can help alleviate heart palpitations and high blood pressure, and lily of the valley is also effective against palpitations.

Gingko biloba aids small blood vessel circulation.

Mistletoe can relieve heart strain, stimulate circulation, and lower blood pressure. Fifteen drops of the extract or three cups of the tea can be taken three times a day. Remember not to misuse this particular herb by exceeding the recommended dosage, and do not eat the mistletoe berries.

Motherwort can be used to secure cardiac electrical rhythm, but be sure to seek medical supervision when taking this herb. It can be added to warm water (10 to 20 drops) and consumed as a tea.

Tansy is another herb used for heart palpitations and can also be ingested as a tea. It can be taken three to four times a day, an hour before meals and just before sleep.

Wild yam enhances the body's production of DHEA, a hormone needed to prevent the onset of heart disease.

Alfalfa, which is especially useful in preventing arteriosclerosis and calcium deposits, should be consumed in the seed form, either mixed in salads or by taking six teaspoons per day.

Arjuna is an Ayurvedic herb for improving circulation to the heart and normalizing high blood pressure. It also helps to reverse soft tissue damage to internal organs and muscles.

Indian snakeroot, also known as Rauwolfia, possesses hypotensive properties, according to clinical studies from the U.S., Britain, and India. The plant grows wild in India and Africa, and has been used for centuries to treat various conditions affecting the nervous system, including anxiety, fear, snakebite, and abdominal pain. Rauwolfia is used in hypotensive medications and is found most effective for mild conditions when the whole herb is taken, and when it is used over an extended period of time.

Black cohosh is an American herb that has the ability to help lower blood pressure and act as a sedative by inhibiting vasomotor centers in the central nervous system.

Some additional herbs that can be used to alleviate and prevent heart disease are bilberry, valerian root, kelp, and butcher's broom.

Chelation Therapy

Many health practitioners agree that chelation therapy is the most effective way of treating heart disease because of its ability to fully reverse all the disorders associated with the arteries and cardiac region. This form of therapy provides an attractive alternative to bypass surgery, which treats only a limited portion of the body's arteries and blood vessels. One of the major advantages of chelation therapy is its ability to improve the functioning of the brain by ameliorating the symptomatic dizziness and mental degradation associated with artery blockage in the upper body. The average patient will experience significant results after 30 exposures to the therapy. After the initial treatments, maintenance treatments are usually needed once a month or every other month to preserve the benefits the patient receives.

Chelation therapy consists of the usage of an IV apparatus and a chemical known as EDTA. During the procedure, the patient is seated in a comfortable chair and a bottle containing the EDTA is situated several feet above the head of the patient. The EDTA solution slowly flows from the bottle, through the IV, and finally into the patient's veins, where it filtrates into the blood and circulates around the fluid spaces that surround the cells. The entire procedure usually lasts for approximately three hours.

What chelation therapy does is cleanse the body by removing potentially harmful substances, such as lead, uranium, and nickel. The EDTA is also able to combine with calcium deposits in the arterial walls, which are then discharged by the kidneys out of the body. Furthermore, the EDTA promotes softening of the arteries by eliminating the buildup of scar tissue within them.

People in their 40's are prime candidates for chelation therapy, since most people in this age group will experience some amount of arteriosclerosis as a result of excessive cholesterol intake and the buildup of calcium, scar tissue, and fat within the arteries. The performance of chelation can successively eliminate these risk factors and can turn back the clock for many potential heart disease victims. It is an excellent idea to initiate therapy during the early stages of heart disease, as evidence has indicated that the reduction of arterial calcium accumulation between the ages of 40 and 60 can be vital to curbing the development of arteriosclerosis.

Chelation therapy has also achieved widespread success in the treatment of people who already suffer from advanced forms of heart disease, such as angina or intermittent claudication. Treatment of these people frequently results in the complete disappearance of the symptoms that have plagued them. In numerous cases, people with angina who were unable to participate in relatively simple activities experienced remarkable improvement in their abilities. People in their 70's and 80's sometimes require a number of treatment sessions beyond the average 30 because of the accumulation of pollutants that have attached to their arterial walls over the years, but their systems can eventually be cleaned out as well.

Overall, when chelation is combined with an extensive regimen of aerobic exercise, correct dietary intake, proper supplementation, and stress reduction, this therapy can provide an extremely effective means of averting heart disease or dealing with a condition that already exists.

Exercise

Any exercise program should be initially supervised and okayed by a medical doctor to ensure that medical problems do not worsen with activity. Many people benefit from an exercise routine that burns 2000 calories a week. Three kinds of exercises therapeutic for the heart are lifting of light weights, yoga, and aerobics:

LIGHT WEIGHT EXERCISES

Lifting light weights benefits the heart when exercises are directed at expanding the chest area. This allows the heart more room to breathe. These three exercises are particularly helpful.

1. Lie down on a bench with two- to three-pound dumbbells and perform lateral flies. As you inhale, stretch both arms to the side. Hold the breath in as you bring the dumbbells back overhead. This exercise opens the rib cage and gets more oxygen and energy into the chest area.
2. Lie down on a bench and bring the dumbbells straight back overhead while breathing in deeply. Bring them back down to the front while breathing out.
3. Squat down to perform a deep knee bend while holding a light (20-pound) barbell or broomstick across the shoulders. Breathe in deeply as you bend. Hold the breath and then blow it out audibly as you rise.

YOGA

The best yoga exercise for opening up the chest area is the cobra posture. In this exercise you lie on the floor with your stomach to the ground and your feet together. Slowly arch the body up towards the ceiling, beginning with the eyes, head, and neck. Take care not to overarch the neck. The palms of the hands can touch the floor in a push-up position, or the hands can rest alongside the body with the palms facing up. This second option will give less of a stretch but necessitate more work for the head, neck, and chest.

Breathe in deeply as you lift. Once in position, breathe lightly in and out. After holding the posture for several seconds, gradually come back down, chest first and head last. Generally, the cobra is performed three times. During the first round, the arms are stretched out alongside the body. During the second two rounds, the palms are down on the floor. The body is raised higher with each successive round.

AEROBIC EXERCISE

Walking is an aerobic exercise that is beneficial to the heart and highly recommended by physicians, as it is something almost anyone can do. Other types of aerobic exercise are jogging, running, water-walking, swimming, and bicycling. Choose an exercise or exercises that you enjoy doing, so that you will be more likely to continue with your routine. Remember, though, to get medical clearance before you begin any new activity.

The Power of the Mind

Although physical factors such as diet and exercise play a big part in preventing or combating coronary disease, it is crucial not to overlook the spiritual health of the mind in relation to the body's ability to heal itself. People should try to let their minds, as well as their bodies, relax by engaging in cardiovascular exercise, deep breathing, biofeedback, yoga, and massage therapy. A mixture of aromatic oils, such as ylang ylang, lavender, peppermint, or marjoram, combined with massage oil, can enhance a massage by calming the body and lowering the blood pressure.

A positive relationship and understanding with one's soul can enable the body to combat disease more effectively, as a healthy soul is able to influence an effective bodily response. People who have undergone traumatic experiences, such as divorce or death of a loved one, will often suffer from symptoms of heart disease because they have lost touch with the desire to remain healthy. These people need to reconnect with their souls, regain confidence in themselves, and work on effectively expressing their emotions.

Many times people inappropriately internalize the stress in their lives, converting it into self-destructive habits, such as overeating, alcoholism, or recreational drug use. Prolonged exposure to stress can actually induce red blood cell clotting by increasing the adhesive qualities of the platelets. Increased clotting contributes to the accumulation of atherosclerotic plaque, arterial blockage, and eventually, heart attack. When people are able to relax, their blood pressure decreases, halting the buildup of waste along the walls of the arteries.

Improvement of a patient's mental health can have a profound effect upon the functioning of the immune system as well. When we feel loved, favorable hormones are produced by the endocrine system, enabling the muscles to relax and oxygen to flow more freely. In short, paying kind attention to one's own emotional state, making positive changes in attitude when necessary, can be a rewarding complement to the physical treatment of coronary disease.

What to Avoid

An overly sedentary lifestyle and obesity are to be avoided, as these factors can contribute to high blood pressure. In addition, it is important to eliminate your dietary intake of animal protein, saturated fats and saturated oils, salt, fried foods, caffeine, tobacco, alcohol, and heavy starches, because these foods contribute to the deposit of pollutants within the walls of the arteries. The presence of hydrogenated vegetable oil or vegetable shortening on a product's ingredients list should serve as a reminder to stay away from that product. Avoid margarine at all costs. At one time, people believed that polyunsaturated oil assisted in the reduction of cholesterol levels, but we now realize that the high trans fatty acid content in margarine only promotes heart disease. Unfiltered tap water can be a problem; it can eventually lead to coronary damage due to pollutants in the water supply. While sufficient amounts of pure water protect the heart, other beverages are not good substitutes, particularly caffeine and alcohol, which are dehydrating.

Finally, let go of stress in any way that you can. Stress reduction is not a frill. As discussed earlier, the reduction of stress in one's life decreases the risk of heart disease and heart attack by eliminating unnecessary free radical damage to the tissues and by relaxing the walls of the arteries.

Treatment Summary

There is clear evidence that heart disease can be effectively treated and reversed through a low-fat diet program.

Drink sufficient amounts of pure water.

Supplements and herbs can be taken to combat many forms of heart disease. Antioxidants, in particular, are vital.

Chelation therapy can reverse disorders of the arteries and cardiac region.

Light weight exercises, yoga, and aerobics are excellent forms of exercise that can benefit people at risk or suffering from heart disease.

Spiritual, emotional, and mental health play a role in the body's ability to heal itself.

Heat Exhaustion and Heatstroke

Heat exhaustion and heatstroke (also known as sunstroke or heat hyperpyrexia), come from an overexposure to the sun or high temperature. While most people are careful not to overdo it, there are times when they may not be mindful of the power of the sun, such as when they are vacationing in a tropical country where they are not used to the weather.

Symptoms

Heat exhaustion is characterized by weakness, dizziness, nausea, and muscle cramping from a loss of fluid and salt, while heatstroke is more severe, with the possibility of permanent brain damage or even death. Symptoms of heatstroke include a lack of sweat, high temperature, quick pulse, headaches, confusion, shivering, and blackouts.

Treatment

First Aid

A common-sense first-aid approach would be to get the person out of the sun, and to provide rest, fluid replacement, and cooling. Cooling can be accomplished by applying ice packs and wrapping the person in a cool, wet sheet. When the condition is severe, the individual should be rushed to a medical facility as soon as possible. This applies especially to the person who is in shock, as evidenced by shivering, incoherence, and confusion. Fluids containing electrolytes are also important. These drinks supply the person with calcium, potassium, and magnesium, minerals that must be replaced as they drain out of the body quickly during heat exhaustion or heatstroke. Many companies sell these drinks, but their effect can also be obtained from a solution that incorporates lemon juice, lime juice, green drinks, mineral water, or salt water.

Herbs

Second- or third-degree burns that can occur from either condition are minimized with the help of pure aloe vera. The gel, placed directly on the skin, will hydrate the skin immediately. Taken internally as a juice or gel, aloe vera further promotes healing by providing the body with a multitude of electrolytes.

Homeopathy

The main homeopathic remedy for sunstroke is belladonna. Homeopathic practitioners use it when symptoms include a throbbing and pulsating headache. The face is flushed and hot, and the extremities are cold. The pupils may be dilated, and the person feels worse being touched or laying down flat.

What to Avoid

The worst thing to give a person felled by heat is alcohol. Some people are under the impression that alcohol will revive the person, when in actuality it only dehydrates the tissues further.

Treatment Summary

A person suffering from heatstroke or exhaustion should be given immediate aid in the form of rest, fluid replacement, and cooling. The condition may be a medical emergency that requires hospitalization.

Aloe vera can be applied topically or taken internally.

Belladonna is a homeopathic remedy for sunstroke.

Hemorrhoids

Hemorrhoids, also known as piles, are swollen blood vessels that cause the mucous membranes of the lower rectum or anus to protrude. When the projection is above the inside opening of the anus, it is referred to as an internal hemorrhoid. This tends to be painful, and causes bleeding with bowel movements. Hemorrhoids that appear outside the anal opening are called external hemorrhoids; these do not usually cause bleeding or discomfort.

Generally, hemorrhoids affect people with sedentary lifestyles, as well as people who eat too many dairy products and constipating protein and starch. The problem may also be due to the overuse of laxatives, poor circulation, putrefaction of old wastes, and straining to defecate. Pregnant women are especially susceptible, and are advised to avoid constipating foods for this reason.

Treatment

Diet and Lifestyle

Although we tend to think of hemorrhoids as a local problem, the condition is generally due to a systemic imbalance. As mentioned above, straining to have a bowel movement places pressure on the blood vessels and is a primary cause of the problem. This can be avoided by eating a high-fiber diet, getting sufficient exercise, and drinking eight to ten glasses of water daily. Magnesium aids peristalsis and can be very helpful. And vitamin C loosens stools, making bowel movements easier. The addition of bioflavonoids reduces swelling.

Herbs

Some simple herbs may have a healing effect. Aloe vera juice is, for one, a gentle laxative that increases circulation and soothes the alimentary canal. A person can begin with one teaspoonful of the gel and work up one tablespoonful or more, if needed. A Chinese herbal formula called Fargelin may remedy the condition quickly by improving circulation to the area. Slippery elm and marshmallow also soothe an irritated digestive tract. Either one can be used to relieve constipation. They should not be used, however, if there is diarrhea or mucus in the stool. Additionally, butcher's broom and horse chestnut are useful for this problem, especially when there is pain and numbness in the feet and legs.

External treatments, combined with internal ones, speed up the recovery process. Herbs and oils added to bath water can provide further relief to an irritated system and improve circulation. Botanicals can also be made into a poultice by grinding up herbs, placing them inside a cloth, and applying to the skin. This helps to break up congestion, lessen inflammation, and remove toxins. Suggested botanicals for such a compress include lemon juice, vitamin E, and witch hazel.

Also, cyprus oil is a venous tonic that is used in the treatment of hemorrhoids. Five drops of the essential oil can be added to bath water. Alternatively, a therapeutic bath can be made by covering three handfuls of chamomile and one handful of witch hazel, nettle, echinacea, or calendula with boiled water. The herbs should be covered and allowed to steep for about an hour. The herbs should then be strained and the liquid poured into a tubful of water.

Finally, adding a quarter of a cup of Epsom salts to four inches of bath water will reduce all swelling.

Treatment Summary

A high-fiber diet, exercise, and 8 10-ounce glasses of water daily allow for elimination without straining. Magnesium, vitamin C, and bioflavonoids are additionally helpful.

Numerous herbs can be taken internally or applied externally to soothe and heal hemorrhoids.

Hepatitis

Hepatitis is a viral infection that damages the liver. There are three types of hepatitis, called A, B, and C. Hepatitis A is usually spread by food or water contaminated with feces, while hepatitis B comes from tainted blood products used in transfusions or unsterile needles, and C is spread sexually through infected blood. Hepatitis A has a slow onset and most people fully recover, while Hepatitis B begins and progresses rapidly. It can lead to prolonged illness, including cirrhosis of the liver, or death.

Having a weakened liver makes one more susceptible to hepatitis. Factors that may contribute to weakening of the liver are other viruses, such as cytomegalovirus and Epstein-Barr virus. Degenerative substances that harm the liver include toxic chemicals in the environment, as well as alcohol, and drugs that cause liver cells to die. Liver-harming medications can include tranquilizers, chemotherapeutic agents, antibiotics, and anesthetics.

Symptoms of hepatitis include mild or severe fatigue, upper respiratory problems, nausea, vomiting, multiple joint aches or tenderness, muscle aches, headaches, loss of appetite, fever, jaundice, low blood sugar, anxiety, depression, nervousness, and visual changes.

Treatment

Nutrition

Recovery from hepatitis depends largely on restoring the integrity of the liver. Many holistic approaches therefore focus on liver detoxification and strengthening. A whole-foods vegetarian diet prevents the liver from being overworked. Such a diet also contains phytochemicals, plant chemicals that help prevent acute damage or even protect a person from developing problems in the first place.

A good daily drink for liver cleansing consists of lemon juice or cider vinegar in water with a teaspoon of honey and royal jelly. A mid-morning snack of apple, carrot, or cranberry juice, or a vegetable juice with green powder, will further purify the liver. Roasted dandelion, peppermint, pau d'arco, and Japanese green teas are also good for this purpose. Ten 8-ounce glasses of fresh, organic dark green and yellow vegetable juices with only 1 ounce of aloe in 5 of the glasses.

Supplements

Important supplements to consider include quercetin, vitamin C (taken intravenously and orally), vitamin E, essential fatty acids, B-complex vitamins (especially B12), and selenium. New information shows that glutathione can detoxify the liver and stop cirrhosis.

Herbs

The best herbal support is derived from silymarin, a milk thistle extract. This herbal aid protects and renews cells, and is widely used in India, where hepatitis is seen in epidemic proportions.

Curcumin, an ingredient in turmeric, has anti-inflammatory properties.

Astragalus stops free radical damage and aids detoxification processes.

The Japanese frequently eat burdock root, a bitter herb known for its ability to cleanse the liver.

The Chinese herb phyllanthus and the ganoderma mushroom have been shown to act against hepatitis B.

Dandelion root is used for hepatitis and jaundice because it stimulates the liver and gallbladder. When large quantities are taken, patients are sometimes cured in a short period of time.

Red clover fights free radicals attacking liver cells and helps the system to detoxify.

Evening primrose oil will also benefit the liver and spleen and is especially good together with echinacea. The oil contains prostaglandins, which help reduce inflammation.

Another valuable herb for the treatment of hepatitis is Oregon grape root. This herb contains berberine, a substance that aids liver metabolism. Interestingly, similar species of the herb grow throughout the world and are used by separate cultures for blood and liver cleansing; while Native Americans have long valued Oregon grape root, Chinese and Indian cultures have their own species of the plant.

Barberry is yet another herb useful for this condition, especially when combined with goldenseal and lobelia. However, as barberry is quite bitter, only small quantities can be tolerated.

Alfalfa is important because it relieves liver inflammation. Additionally, alfalfa is a good source of vitamin K, which helps prevent bleeding.

Jamaicans have long used Jamaica weed, a form of phyllanthus, in the treatment of hepatitis. This plant contains ingredients that can kill the hepatitis B virus in vivo, something that is difficult to accomplish using allopathic medicine.

Many liver disorders accompany candida problems. In these instances, pau d'arco or garlic should be taken for its antifungal effects and for immune support.

Other herbs that improve liver function include aloe vera, buckthorn, wild yam, wood betony, and yellow dock.

Ozone therapy

All forms of hepatitis have been known to be reversed with intravenous ozone, and hepatitis can sometimes be fully eliminated after several sessions. The modality appears to step up immune system activity, enabling the body's own defenses to wipe out aggressive viral organisms.

What to Avoid

All foods that stress the liver must be avoided. This includes food additives, preservatives, and artificial sweeteners. Sugar can promote liver inflammation and free radical damage. Alcohol kills liver cells and leads to cirrhosis. Many drugs can aggravate the problem as well.

Treatment Summary

Foods that replenish the liver are detoxifying and strengthening, and include many plant foods, as well as vitamins C, B, and E, selenium, and glutathione.

Numerous herbs strengthen the liver. The most noteworthy is the milk thistle extract, silymarin, which can actually reverse liver damage.

Ozone therapy can sometimes reverse hepatitis in a matter of a few sessions.

Herpes

One aspect of the aftermath of the sexual revolution was an epidemic of herpes outbreaks. While much feared in the 1970s, this contagious condition was overshadowed by the advent of AIDS in the early 1980s. Today, though less publicized than AIDS, herpes is far more prevalent, affecting, in one form or another, 80 percent of the American population. Over half the population gets cold sores from time to time, the result of herpes simplex virus 1 (HSV1). Others become afflicted with shingles, a herpes zoster infection, years after they get chicken pox. Additionally, people get Epstein-Barr, the form of herpes that causes mononucleosis. Still others break out in genital herpes, an infection caused by herpes simplex virus 2 (HSV2).

Causes

Herpes is a contagious virus that lives at the base of the spine in the nerve cells. Periodic attacks occur whenever the immune system is below par. Any kind of emotional, mental, or physical stress can lower the body's defense system and create the perfect climate for an outbreak. Common physical stressors include illness, menstrual periods, vaginal yeast infections, too much sunlight or friction (which breaks down skin cells), allergies, and certain foods. Prescription drugs that lower immunity can set off an attack. Examples of such medications include antibiotics, steroids, and antidepressants. Also, genital herpes can be sexually transmitted, and pregnant women can transmit the virus to their unborn children via blood or through direct contact with infected tissue during delivery.

Symptoms

Genital herpes causes surface sores on the skin and lining of the genital area. In men, penile blisters may appear on the tip of the foreskin and turn into surface sores for several days before healing. In women, sores can appear on the cervix, vagina, or perineum. These sores may be accompanied by a discharge or vaginal blisters. There is often a burning sensation, especially at the onset of an outbreak. Other symptoms may include urinary problems, fever, and lymphatic swelling. Intercourse is painful and should be avoided during an outbreak to prevent sexual transmission. HSV2 occurs intermittently and usually lasts from five to seven days.

Oral herpes attacks the skin and mucous membranes on the face, particularly around the mouth and nose. These cold sores tend to appear as pearl-like blisters. Although they are short-term, they can be irritating and painful.

Herpes zoster, the result of the varicella zoster virus (VZV), causes agonizing blisters on one side of the body, usually on the chest or abdomen. Pain is usually felt before effects are seen. Symptoms may last from a few days to several weeks.

Treatment

While there are no cures for herpes, drugs are commonly given to lessen symptoms. The most famous of these is Cyclovir, also known as Zovirax, which supposedly reduces the rate of growth of the herpes virus. Herpes medications have many potential side effects, including dizziness, headaches, diarrhea, nausca, vomiting, general weakness, fatigue, ill health, sore throat, fever, insomnia, swelling, tenderness, and bleeding of the gums. In addition, Cyclovir ointment can cause allergic skin reactions.

Natural remedies, which are kinder to the system, are effective in shortening the length of outbreaks and in diminishing their frequency. These are some to know about:

Nutrition and Lifestyle

When herpes strikes, it's always a good idea to rest and eat lightly. Short fruit fasts, with plenty of pure water and cleansing herbal teas, can be helpful. Good herbs to include are sage, rosemary, cayenne, echinacea, goldenseal, chaparral, red clover, astragalus, and burdock root. Beneficial bacteria, such as those found in yogurt, or supplements of lactobacillicus and acidophilus, support the digestive processes necessary for the maintenance of the immune system. Other nutrients that directly enhance the immune system include garlic, quercetin, zinc gluconate, buffered vitamin C, and beta carotene or vitamin A. In addition, 500 mg of the amino acid L-lysine, taken two to four times a day, can produce excellent results. Bee propolis is anti-inflammatory, and high in B vitamins, which combat stress. Also good are bee pollen, blue-green algae, and pycnogenol.

Homeopathy

Homeopathy will build the immune system, not merely suppress symptoms. The following remedies are used to treat herpes homeopathically. Note that you shouldn't touch the formulas directly; that may disturb their vibration. Rather, they should be placed under the tongue until dissolved. Also, coffee, mint, camphor, and chamomile must be avoided, as they act to cancel the effects of the remedies. It is also important to note symptoms; as they change so must the homeopathic remedy.

FOR COLD SORES

Natrum muriaticum —When sores are on the lips, especially in the middle of the lips, the 30c potency should be taken twice a day.

Phosphorus —Cold sores that manifest above the lips, accompanied by itching, cutting, and sharp pain, need the 30c potency twice a day.

Petroleum —For cold sores that erupt in patches, and become crusty and loose around the lips and mouth, petroleum is indicated. A 9c potency is needed three times a day.

Apis —Apis helps cold sores around the mouth and lips that are accompanied by stinging, and painful blisters that itch and burn. A 6c potency is needed three to four times daily.

FOR FEMALE GENITAL HERPES

Natrum muriaticum —This remedy is indicated when the herpetic lesions are pearl-like blisters and the genital area feels puffy, hot, and very dry. A 6c potency may be beneficial when taken four times a day.

Dulcamara —Women who tend to get a herpes outbreak in clusters on the vulva, or on the hair follicles around the labia and vulva, every time they catch a cold or get their period, are given dulcamara in a 12c potency, two to three times a day.

Petroleum —This may help if herpes eruptions form in patches and the sores become deep red and feel tender and moist. Outbreaks usually occur during menstrual periods, and most often affect the perineum, anus, labia, or vulva. A 9c potency should be taken three times a day.

FOR SHINGLES

Arsenicum album —This remedy benefits most cases of shingles, especially when the individual feels worse in the cold, worse after midnight, and better with warmth. If taken at the onset of an attack, it is best taken in a 30c potency twice a day for two to three days. After the first three days, arsenicum album is indicated if there is a burning sensation in the areas that were affected by the zoster eruptions (typically the chest and abdomen). At this point 12c, taken two to three times a day, is best. This remedy is excellent for getting rid of the burning sensation that is often present.

Hypericum perforatum —Hypericum is a remedy for any kind of nerve pain. It is indicated whenever there is intense neuritis and neuralgia, with burning, tingling, and numbness along the course of the affected nerves. Hypericum perforatum should be taken in a 30c potency, two to three times a day.

Essential Oils

In France, essential oils are well respected for their medicinal properties, and used in place of antibiotics to combat various inflammatory ailments, including cold and canker sores. Aromatherapist Valerie Cooksley, author of *Aromatherapy: A Lifetime Guide to Healing with Essential Oils,* suggests this mouthwash recipe: Mix 5 drops of peppermint, bergamot, or tea tree oil with raw honey. Then add this to a strong sage or rosemary tea. Rinsing with the formula, several times a day, balances the pH of the mouth and helps to heal infections. Daily use may even prevent outbursts from arising.

Cooksley recommends dabbing a Q-tip with myrrh oil and applying directly onto cold and canker sores to relieve pain. Another aromatherapist, Sharon Olson, dabs a cotton swab with diluted tea tree oil and places that on the cold sore to kill the virus. She follows this up later with soothing lavender oil and aloe vera gel. A side benefit of the therapy, she explains, is its ability to lift the spirits and clear the mind.

Ozone

Intravenous infusion for 4 weeks plus IV vitamin C and water-soluble vitamin A plus glutathione.

What to Avoid

Stay away from anything that upsets the nervous system, such as caffeine, alcohol, and hard-to-digest meats. Foods high in the amino acid arginine, such as chocolate, peanut butter, nuts, and onions, are also associated with higher incidences of outbreaks.

Toothbrushes should be changed frequently, and completely dried before reuse to prevent reinfection. Soaking them in baking soda also fights germs. Since stress promotes more outbreaks, it is important to make time for activities that alleviate tension. Possibilities include biofeedback, yoga, meditation, deep breathing, and exercise.

Treatment Summary

Antiviral drugs are routinely given to herpes sufferers to alleviate symptoms, but these have many potential side effects.

During a herpes outbreak, one should rest, avoid stress, and eat light, cleansing foods. There are many beneficial herbs that can be taken as teas, and a variety of nutrients support the immune system directly.

Homeopathy offers several remedies for combating herpes.

Essential oils can be used internally or externally in place of antibiotics to stimulate the immune system and relieve inflammation and pain.

See also: Cold and Canker Sores

High Cholesterol Level

Most Americans, including doctors, are victims of a mass campaign against a substance produced by our own bodies. Cholesterol is not necessarily the monster we've been led to believe that it is. In fact, cholesterol is vital to the health of every cell in our systems. It helps the liver digest fats, and works with protein and lecithin to transport fats through our blood. Not only that, but sex hormones are made from the stuff. In addition, cholesterol helps keep skin moist. Cholesterol is so important that if not enough comes from food, the liver manufactures it.

Most of us think of cholesterol as a type of fat, but it is really a special kind of alcohol, called a steroid alcohol or sterol. Normally, most cholesterol is found in cells, and a small amount is found in the blood. Doctors do not worry about cholesterol in the cells, but when levels in the blood get high, the substance can clog arteries and put a strain on the heart.

A serum cholesterol level that is between 125 and 200 milligrams per 100 milliliters of blood is generally a safe one, in my opinion. Opinions on this differ widely, though; some experts say a 175-mg cholesterol level is high; others place the acceptability cutoff as high as 275. You should discuss this issue with your own practitioner.

Actually, the cholesterol number alone is not enough to say that a potentially dangerous situation exists. It is also important to test triglyceride and lipoprotein levels (as part of a regular SMA-24 blood test). An elevated triglyceride level indicates a poorly functioning liver or pancreas. This is dangerous because triglycerides are blood fats and may play a part in clogging the arteries with harmful plaque. Lipoproteins are compounds composed of fat and protein, and of particular interest to the health-conscious are high-density lipoproteins (HDL's) and low-density lipoproteins (LDL's). HDL's are low in cholesterol and high in phospholipids, and are considered the "good guys" by heart specialists because they actually lower blood pressure and lessen the chance of heart disease. Too many LDL's, on the other hand, are what doctors worry about. LDL's contain high levels of cholesterol and have a tendency to stick to the walls of arteries and build up as plaque. Too many LDL's, therefore, increase the risk of atherosclerosis, a condition in which the arterial walls are damaged by cholesterol and normal blood flow is blocked. An important factor to consider when testing cholesterol is the ratio of HDL versus the total serum cholesterol level. Ratios of 4:1 or better (i.e., the first number is lower than 4) are desirable.

Treatment

Dependence on cholesterol-lowering medications is unnecessary and unsafe. Unless a person suffers from a rare genetic disorder called hypercholesterolemia, where high blood cholesterol levels begin at birth, there are safer, more natural ways to keep cholesterol levels down.

Eating less cholesterol-containing food would seem to be a good approach, and indeed the goal of lowering high dietary cholesterol intake has received much publicity in recent years. The problem is that cutting out eggs, steak, and dairy products does not necessarily correct high blood cholesterol. While cutting down on fatty foods is an excellent suggestion for most Americans, who eat far more fat than they need, this approach alone may not be sufficient for lowering cholesterol because the substance is produced by the body. The body may respond to a sharp reduction in cholesterol by manufacturing more on its own. It can make as much as 1500 mg of cholesterol a day, more than six times the amount normally eaten!

It is interesting to note that certain ethnic groups, such as the Masai tribes of Africa and the Eskimos, have high-cholesterol diets, and yet have low levels of serum cholesterol and few incidences of heart disease. So factors other than cholesterol intake must obviously come into play. Some of these factors are genetics, nutritional status, stress, exercise, age, and blood triglyceride levels.

Diet

Instead of cutting out cholesterol-rich foods completely, a better approach might be to add more fiber. Roughage increases the speed at which the body eliminates cholesterol. It does this, basically, by mopping it up and getting it out of the blood. Pectin, found in apples, is especially good for this. Also, eating old-fashioned hot grain cereal, such as rolled oats, barley, or buckwheat, is helpful in this regard. Adding pectin-rich apples to the cereal doubles the benefit.

Another interesting finding is that a small amount of polyunsaturated fat may lower serum cholesterol levels by 5 or 10 percent. Like roughage, polyunsaturated fat forces cholesterol concentrations out of the blood. Linoleic acid, found in cold-pressed oils, fish (not shellfish), nuts, seeds, and nut butters, is especially good.

Foods high in vitamin B6 (pyridoxine) are helpful. As this is a water-soluble vitamin, and thus gets lost in cooking, it is best to include plenty of raw fruits and vegetables in the diet. Leafy green vegetables are especially high in B6. Lecithin-rich soy products, such as tofu and tempeh, are important as well.

Supplements

Many people are deficient in vitamins and minerals that keep cholesterol levels under control. Niacin (vitamin B3) is important for cholesterol control and can be found in a variety of foods, including leafy greens, wheat germ, beans, peas, salmon, and tuna; it can also be taken as a supplement (50 mg daily). This helps to lower triglycerides as well as cholesterol, and to raise beneficial HDL levels. Note that niacin should be used cautiously by those with a history of gout, liver dysfunction, or diabetes, and that its effects are enhanced by vitamin C.

One of vitamin C's many wonders is that it helps to lower cholesterol; anywhere from 1000 to 10,000 mg are needed each day (requirements increase in colder months and during periods of illness and stress). Vitamin C is best in combination with bioflavonoids, especially rutin and quercetin. When combined with lecithin, this helps to dissolve arterial plaque. (Encapsulated liquid lecithin should have a phospholipid choline content of at least 35 percent, and should deliver a minimum potency of 51.5 percent phosphatides. Granulated lecithin should be labeled 25 percent phosphatidyl choline, and should not have soy flour added to it.)

Vitamin E (400-600 IU daily) will help improve circulation to the heart. Vitamins B6 and methionine balance triglyceride levels, and ultimately help to normalize cholesterol.

Studies reveal the best cholesterol-lowering minerals to be chromium, calcium, magnesium, and zinc.

Herbs

Ginger and cayenne decrease liver production of cholesterol and triglycerides, according to studies. In addition, plenty of garlic should be eaten, as it lowers cholesterol and thins the blood, lessening the chances of dangerous blood clots. Raw garlic is most effective, but even cooked, this herb has a therapeutic effect. Deodorized capsules and pills are least effective, though, because it's the allicin, the smelly part of garlic, that makes it useful. The ganoderma mushroom helps reduce cholesterol, triglycerides, and total number of fats in the bloodstream.

Exercise

Exercise seems to help raise HDL and lower LDL levels, although it may take several months before you see a noticeable change.

What to Avoid

Many people replace cholesterol-rich foods with artificial ones—fake eggs, margarine, imitation bacon, nondairy cream, etc. But there is no evidence proving that these fake foods prevent heart trouble, and they are associated with a higher incidence of cancer.

Foods containing refined sugars lead to an unhealthy buildup of fats in the liver and tissues. They also lower the level of healthy HDL's and increase the unwanted LDL's. Refined foods should be replaced with complex carbohydrates—fruits, vegetables, and whole grains. Note that alcohol is high in refined sugar and should also be avoided.

Many medications, including steroids and contraceptives, can increase cholesterol and triglyceride levels and destroy nutrients needed for maintaining normal levels. In fact, studies reveal that people on steroid medications have a 50-percent increase in blood cholesterol level. Excessive amounts of protein and cooked foods can also destroy cholesterol-controlling nutrients. Finally, another factor that tends to raise cholesterol levels is stress, which is one of the reasons that stress avoidance—or management—is so important.

Treatment Summary

Cholesterol-lowering medications are unsafe and unnecessary except for people suffering from the rare disorder hypercholesterolemia.

Fiber, especially pectin, helps to eliminate excess cholesterol from the body. Small amounts of polyunsaturated fats may lower cholesterol levels as well.

Exercise raises good cholesterol (HDL), and lowers bad cholesterol (LDL), over time.

Supplements that keep cholesterol under control include niacin, vitamin C, bioflavonoids, liquid lecithin, vitamin E, and the B vitamins, as well as chromium, calcium, magnesium, and zinc.

Ginger, garlic, and the ganoderma mushroom lower cholesterol and triglycerides.

See also: Heart Disease

Hypoglycemia

Hypoglycemia is a defect in the carbohydrate metabolism whereby blood glucose reaches lower than normal levels. As glucose is a particularly important metabolic fuel for the brain, lowered glucose can result in a host of central nervous system disorders. The main cause of low blood sugar is a diet high in refined carbohydrates. Unfortunately, the average American diet, which is rich in processed foods, sugar, soda, and coffee, is practically a prescription for hypoglycemia. These foods require little digestion and get absorbed too rapidly into the bloodstream. As a result, the blood sugar level becomes unstable. With sugary food consumption, the level shoots up. As a result, too much insulin is secreted by the pancreas, and so the blood sugar level drops. At this point, people tend to reach for more refined carbohydrates, and the cycle continues.

Symptoms

Hypoglycemia causes sustained stress, which can result in a variety of symptoms, including weakness, headaches, visual disturbances, food and chemical allergies, chronic fatigue, emotional problems such as anxiety and mood swings, confusion, chronic yeast infections, and even asthma. Often, people don't realize that low blood sugar underlies their symptomatology. Nor do medical professionals realize that hypoglycemia is the problem in many cases. For a lot of people, this ignorance has sad consequences. Hypoglycemic individuals have been institutionalized because they were thought to be emotionally imbalanced and incapable of making rational decisions. Complicating the issue is the fact that tests rarely detect hypoglycemia. If a diabetic undergoes a five hour glucose tolerance test, the condition shows up. Otherwise, it usually goes undetected.

Treatment

Naturopathic Viewpoint

Naturopaths view hypoglycemia as a disease of civilization. The overburdening of the system that culminates in hypoglycemia stems from the kinds of diets most people eat and the high stresses they endure. According to Dr. Paul Epstein, a naturopathic physician practicing in Norwalk, Connecticut, alleviating the problem usually involves attention to diet, supplementation, and emotional support. He advocates making the following changes in order to banish this problem.

ANALYZE YOUR CURRENT DIET

To find out what foods may be causing the problem, a naturopath often takes a complete patient history, and uses the information to make the patient aware of what is being eaten that is causing distress. Troublesome foods are then eliminated and replaced by those that provide the body with optimal support.

Avoid Simple Sugars. Simple sugars must be avoided at all costs since they cause the pancreas to overproduce insulin. They also lack B vitamins and other essential nutrients found in complex carbohydrates that are needed to metabolize sugar into energy.

Simple sugars come in a variety of forms: sugar, fructose, glucose, corn sweeteners, corn syrup, fruit sugar, table sugar, and brown sugar. They are found in alcoholic beverages and are hidden in many canned, packaged, and frozen foods as well.

Eat a Diet High in Complex Carbohydrates. For years, hypoglycemics have been told to eat high-protein diets when abundant complex carbohydrates are what they really need. If a person with low blood sugar eats a piece of fruit to overcome fatigue, 30 minutes later the fruit is digested. As a result, glucose enters the blood, raises the blood sugar level, and restores energy. If that same person eats a lean steak instead, he or she has to wait six to seven hours for the meat to leave the stomach. It takes even longer for the amino acids derived from the meat to be translated into usable energy. Carbohydrates deliver required energy rapidly and efficiently while protein not only takes longer to get energy to the cells but even depletes the body in the process because it takes a lot of energy to create energy from protein.

Eat Vegetable Protein. As protein sources, vegetable foods are generally preferable to animal-derived foods. Foods such as nuts, seeds, grains, and Jerusalem artichokes provide time-released energy.

Add Fiber-Rich Foods. People with sluggish digestion or constipation may benefit from additional dietary fiber. This can help slow down the absorption of glucose into the intestinal capillaries. Slower absorption allows a more gradual release of insulin and a faster normalization of blood sugar levels after meals.

Avoid Caffeine and Nicotine. Caffeine and nicotine overstimulate the adrenal glands. When these substances, other stressors, and a generally poor diet are combined, the adrenals can enter into a state of emergency. They become depleted of important vitamins, such as B-complex vitamins and vitamin C.

Use Herbs Known to Rebalance the Blood Sugar. Herbs associated with balanced blood sugar include black cohosh, panax and Siberian ginseng, dandelion, gentian, ginger, and cinnamon, uva ursi, licorice root, and huckleberry leaves. Goldenseal is helpful but should only be used for short periods to prevent the depletion of B vitamins. Astragalus, by contrast, is a tonic herb that can be safely used on a daily basis. It boosts energy by providing adrenal and immune support, and can be taken as an extract or made into a soup by boiling the root.

Pay Attention to When You Eat. When you eat is just as important as what you eat. The hypoglycemic person generally needs to eat frequent, small meals to provide the body with a steady supply of food that is easily and slowly converted to glucose.

SUPPLEMENT THE DIET

Supplementation further restores homeostasis by providing overall support to the entire system, and by providing specific help to digestive organs associated with sugar regulation: the liver, the adrenal glands, and the pancreas.

Overall Support. Dietary changes alone may be sufficient to overcome hypoglycemia. Still, you may want to reinforce an improved diet with supplementation. First, consider supplements that support the regulation of blood sugar. These include adrenal extracts, glucose tolerance factor, zinc, and chromium, nutrients that allow insulin to do its job more effectively. In addition, B vitamins supply crucial enzyme cofactors essential for carbohydrate metabolism. L-carnitine, L-glutamine and vitamin B6 help lessen cravings for sugar. Vitamin E increases energy naturally, so a person doesn't feel the need for an artificial jolt from caffeine or sugar.

Also, consider supplements which nourish specific digestive organs associated with hypoglycemia:

Liver Support. The liver stores glucose as glycogen and breaks it down in the process called gluconeogenesis. Certain botanicals, such as dandelion root, Siberian ginseng and beet leaf, aid in this process. Celandine, methionine, and choline are substances that work to maximize liver efficiency. Lipotropic factors also help control blood sugar by boosting liver function. These are especially helpful for people who have flatulence, hemorrhoids, difficulty digesting fats, light-colored stools, or elevated fat levels.

Adrenal Support. A person who is highly stressed or suffering from allergies, chronic inflammations, fatigue, or nervous and emotional disorders should consider supplements that support the adrenal glands. The number-one adrenal strengthener is pantothenic acid. Other beneficial supplements include freeze-dried adrenal gland extract, Siberian ginseng root, vitamin C, and zinc. Royal jelly also provides excellent nourishment for the adrenals.

Pancreatic Support. Digestive aids that support the pancreas might be indicated when there is impaired digestion.

GET EMOTIONAL SUPPORT

Knowing what to eat and what not to eat is one thing; following is another. Naturopaths often offer their patients support as they alter lifelong habits and struggle with issues at the core of their resistance to change.

The American Academy of Family Physicians has stated that 80 percent of all visits to family physicians are due to stress-related complaints. Stresses are critically important factors to address when hypoglycemia is the problem. According to Dr. Epstein, one doesn't treat hypoglycemia, one treats a person who has hypoglycemia.

What to Avoid

People with hypoglycemia need to avoid simple sugars, processed foods, concentrated foods, alcohol, nicotine, high-protein diets, caffeine, and stress. Aspartame, the chemical used in artificial sweeteners, should be omitted as well.

Treatment Summary

While dietary needs may differ from person to person, a general rule of thumb is to avoid all simple sugars and to eat complex carbohydrates, vegetable proteins, and fiber-rich foods.

Eating frequent, small meals is a good idea, as it slowly converts food to glucose.

Avoid caffeine and nicotine.

Herbs that help to normalize blood sugar levels include black cohosh, ginseng, and dandelion, among others.

Supplements that provide overall support may be beneficial, as well as those that benefit specific organs, including the liver, adrenal glands, and pancreas.

Hypoglycemia patients often need emotional support to encourage the development of new habits.

Hypothyroidism

The thyroid gland makes hormones that control metabolism. Hypothyroidism occurs when too few hormones are produced due to decreased thyroid gland activity. The condition often goes undetected; estimates, though, put the number of people affected as high as 20 percent of the U.S. population.

Symptoms are numerous and can include chronic fatigue, feeling cold all the time, inability to lose weight, and skin conditions such as acne and eczema. In addition, there can be psychological components of the condition, particularly chronic depression, anxiety, and panic, as well as poor concentration and poor short-term memory. Sexual complications may include a low sex drive, impotence, and infertility (especially low sperm count). Chronic constipation, hair loss, heart palpitations, brittle nails, muscle weakness, and muscle and joint pain are additional symptoms. Women often experience menstrual problems, such as excessive bleeding, painful or irregular periods, scanty flow, cessation of menstruation, premenstrual syndrome, and very late or very early onset of menses.

Also, an increase in age-related and immunodeficiency diseases, such as arthritis, cancer, and heart disease, is associated with populations that are low in thyroid hormone.

When thyroid hormone levels are low the body doesn't produce enough heat, so the extremities tend to be cold. Cold fingers, cold toes, and cold tip of the nose are common indicators that not enough heat is being produced. In general, being colder than other people can be an indicator that one's thyroid output is insufficient.

Treatment

Conventional treatment for hypothyroidism is often clouded by misdiagnosis and by incomplete testing. Because there is such a great variety of symptoms, other diseases are often blamed, and the condition goes undiagnosed. For example, hypercholesterolemia, or too much cholesterol in the blood, is often diagnosed in place of hypothyroidism. Treatment with restrictive diet or choles-terol-lowering medication often causes liver irritability and does nothing to address underlying thyroid malfunctions.

Another problem is that T4 or thyroxin hormone levels are commonly used as the sole diagnosis for hypothyroidism. But levels of two other hormones should also be tested: T3 and thyroid stimulating hormone, or TSH. Additionally, thyroid antibody levels should be tested in order to rule out autoimmune thyroid conditions.

Hypothyroidism may be caused by poor general nutrition, especially too little high-quality protein. Water fluoridation is also thought to be a potential thyroid suppressant. Huge quantities of foods in the cabbage family can suppress thyroid function as well, but this is extremely rare.

Standard treatment for hypothyroidism consists of prescription synthetic thyroid hormone. Natural thyroid hormone is much more efficacious, but this has become increasingly difficult to obtain. Patients may be started on the lowest possible dosage of thyroid hormone and gradually built up. Improvements should be noticeable after 30 days, with full effects occurring after 90.

Some naturopathic physicians find a formula called Energetics to be helpful in normalizing thyroid function. The formula consists of tyrosine (a precursor of thyroxin), organic iodine (in the form of thyroxin-3), vitamin B2, niacinamide, zinc, chromium, and liver concentrate. Depending on the patient's requirements, this formula is given from one to three times daily in one or two tablets each time. Thyroid supplements need not be taken indefinitely. Once the body gets a little help, it begins functioning properly on its own.

Aerobic exercise may provide additional support. A regular routine is recommended, one that burns up 2000 calories a week and centers on long walks or intense activity like jogging or bike riding.

Treatment Summary

The conventional approach to hypothyroidism usually consists of giving a synthetic thyroid hormone.

Natural thyroid hormone is more effective than the synthetic type, but more difficult to obtain. The formula Energetics may be helpful. Thyroid support is only necessary temporarily, until the gland picks up and functions optimally by itself again.

Aerobic exercise may help to correct a low-thyroid condition.

Infertility

Infertility is a widespread problem today. In the U.S., it affects approximately 17 percent of all couples who are of childbearing age, which translates to about five million Americans. There are many factors—physical, emotional, and environmental—that contribute to infertility.

To understand infertility, it helps to understand the conditions necessary for a couple to be able to have a baby. First, eggs need to be produced from the woman's ovaries. Second, the man has to be able to produce healthy sperm. Third, the woman's fallopian tubes have to be clear and open in order to allow for the sperm to reach the egg while it is in the fallopian tubes, and to allow for easy passage of the egg to the uterus. Fourth, the lining of the uterus needs to be suitable for the fertilized egg to be implanted. And finally, once the egg is implanted, the necessary hormones must be created by the woman in order to sustain the fertilized egg. Obviously, there are many things that can go wrong along the way.

Causes

The most common causes of infertility prevent the first condition necessary for conception: ovulation. The failure to ovulate is most commonly due to some kind of hormone imbalance. Birth control pills and other sources of estrogen are sometimes the cause of hormonal imbalances. Fertility specialists report that women who have taken birth control pills for an extended period of time have difficulty reestablishing their monthly cycles. This may be due to oral contraceptives causing pituitary hormone deficiency, as well as their precipitating a deficiency of B vitamins, both of which contribute to hormone imbalance. Excessive exercise may also be an impediment to proper hormonal balance. Further, an inordinate amount of weight loss or gain, excessive stress, poor diet, sleep deficiency, and thyroid problems may disturb normal endocrine function. (According to Dr. Dahlia Abraham, a complementary physician from New York City, a woman can determine whether she has a problem with hypothyroidism by taking her temperature. On the third, fourth, and fifth day of a woman's cycle, she should place a thermometer under her armpit first thing in the morning. If the mean average on those days is below 97.5 degrees Fahrenheit, then she is most likely hypothyroid.)

In addition to hormone imbalances, there are other potential causes of ovarian failure. Zinc deficiency, abnormal body fat distribution, obesity, or being underweight may also result in abnormal ovarian dysfunction.

If it is found that a woman is able to ovulate regularly and successfully, then another potential cause of infertility problems that can be explored is blockage of the fallopian tubes. A sloppy abortion may lead to blocked fallopian tubes. Further, chlamydia (which may be promoted through the use of birth control pills), use of IUD's, and use of certain drugs may cause this problem, as these factors can result in pelvic inflammatory disease and subsequent scarring, which may hinder the ability of the ovum to get through the tube and into the uterus.

Another possible problem is male infertility, which occurs in 40 percent of all infertility cases. Male infertility may be due to low sperm count, decreased sperm motility, or aberrant sperm morphology. There are several reasons this happens. Saunas and ultra-vigorous exercise can contribute to impaired sperm production. Further, a topic of some debate in Europe is the effect of birth control pills and estrogen-like chemicals on male infertility. These chemicals are not biodegradable by stomach acids and get into the environment, i.e., the soil, water, and through urine. Thus, they get into the food chain and in that way can affect both males and females alike.

As mentioned, the lining the uterus must be able to nurture the fertilized egg. Endometriosis may deter this from happening as cells that normally build up in the uterus each month in preparation for pregnancy can actually grow outside the uterus, resulting in fertility problems. Nutritional insufficiency may also affect the ability of the uterus to sustain the embryo. In these cases, conception may actually transpire but the ovum may not have appropriate nutrients to develop. What results is unrecognized spontaneous abortions, which may lead to a label of infertility.

Other possible causes of infertility are low plasma copper concentrations, abnormalities of the reproductive system, heavy metal toxicity, genetic damage from electromagnetic radiation, and antibodies that the woman may produce against the man's sperm.

Symptoms

The obvious symptom of infertility is the inability to conceive after an appropriate amount of trying, often considered to be a year's worth. However, what is not always acknowledged by society is the emotional aspect of the problem. Couples can experience anguish, mourning, loss of self-esteem, and marred self-image. Infertility can also result in difficulty between partners, as it is so related to sexual issues. If there is a communication problem between the partners, this can be exacerbated as they grapple with infertility.

Treatment

Treatment for in fertility ranges from drugs to surgery to in vitro fertilization, the method in which the man's sperm is used to fertilize his female partner's egg outside of her uterus. The embryo is then implanted inside the womb for her to carry to term. This may cost approximately $10,000 per cycle. Modern assisted reproductive technology (ART) also offers the ability to fertilize donor eggs and then implant those in the infertile woman. Thus, a woman is able to bear a child that is not genetically related to her. This method is generally even more costly, as it could run up to $15,000. However, it is important to know that there may be alternative natural solutions that can be tested prior to using ART or other conventional methods of treatment, or in conjunction with these. Some natural approaches are outlined below, although couples should of course work with a holistically-oriented health practitioner to get individualized guidance.

Learn How to Identify When Ovulation Begins

A woman is most fertile at certain times of the month, and it is important that she know how to pinpoint these. In order for a woman to determine when she is ovulating, she should take her temperature just before she gets out of bed in the morning. She should observe that her temperature will increase slightly in the second half of the cycle, two weeks prior to menstruation. This will indicate ovulation. Further, vaginal discharge during this period is usually clear in color and slippery in texture, permitting the sperm to penetrate the cervix.

Select Healthy Lifestyle Choices

First, it is important to provide the body with proper nutrients by eating a well-balanced, healthy diet. Therefore, it is suggested that fat and food additives, such as nitrates, nitrites, and MSG, be avoided. Fasting for a few days may even provide assistance in the case of fallopian tube blockage. It is further recommended that the following substances be avoided completely, as they inhibit fertility in both men and women: tobacco or nicotine products; caffeine; alcohol; heavy metals; environmental hazards (e.g., pesticides and herbicides); and drugs such as marijuana and cocaine. Additionally, relaxation techniques have been proven to enhance fertility by increasing vigor and reducing stress, anxiety, depression, and fatigue. Lastly, one or both partners may be anxious about becoming pregnant, and a lot of tension can build up around this issue. It's important to address this through some type of emotional or spiritual work. Support, whether it comes from an individual counselor or a group, can make a big difference in one's outlook.

Supplements

While a good diet will benefit the system and positively impact chances for becoming pregnant, the addition of specific nutrients can further enhance the male and female reproductive systems. Talk to a nutritionally-oriented health practitioner. In general, these are some of the more important nutrients to consider:

ESPECIALLY IMPORTANT FOR MEN

Zinc. Studies show that consuming 25-50 mg of zinc a day has positive consequences for overcoming male impotence. In addition to supplementation, foods containing zinc should be eaten; these include nuts, seeds, whole grains, and brewer's yeast.

Vitamin E. This nutrient may improve the sperm's impregnating ability. Food sources rich in vitamin E are wheat germ, whole grains, and uncooked nuts.

L-Carnitine. Infertility due to low sperm motility may be due to insufficient carnitine levels. Carnitine is generally recognized as being important for the heart muscle, and indeed it is, but studies have also shown that 3,000 mg of oral L-carnitine, taken daily for four months, will increase spermatozoa motility as well.

Reishi (Ganoderma) Extract. Recent studies of infertile men with chronic genital inflammation secondary to infection by the human papilloma virus (HPV) find reishi extract effective for overcoming the condition. Taking the extract significantly reduces inflammation of the skin in these patients and improves sperm parameters.

Other nutrients helpful to men are selenium and vitamin D.

ESPECIALLY IMPORTANT FOR WOMEN

Vitamin B6. This vitamin is particularly important for women as it can help adjust progesterone and estrogen levels. The recommended dosage of B6 is generally from 100 to 300 mg per day. Good food sources of B6 include eggs, rice, soybeans, oats, and whole wheat products.

Other vitamins that have been proven to help increase fertility in women are: iron (35 mg); folic acid (1 mg 3 times daily) to help normalize blood chemistry; vitamin B12, to help normalize reproductive function; colloidal silver, to help cleanse the system when chlamydia is causing infertility; and bioflavonoids (found in broccoli, green peppers, parsley, and citrus fruits), to help develop a healthy uterine lining.

IMPORTANT FOR BOTH MEN AND WOMEN

Vitamin C. This nutrient is beneficial to both men and women as it has the capability to dispose of toxic metals from the body that can interfere with pregnancy. Generally, recommended dosage is 100 to 200 mg daily. Food sources of C include broccoli, cantaloupe, and any type of berry.

Oriental Naturopathic Medicine

This type of Eastern approach to infertility strives to create an overall healthy environment within the woman that allows for proper digestion, menstruation, and hormonal balance. It also focuses on raising the man's sperm count and sperm motility. One aspect of Oriental treatment involves increasing pelvic blood flow to correct fallopian tube obstruction and/or problems with ovulation. This method encompasses the use of laser acupuncture, retention enemas, and injection of common sage root into the endometrial nodes.

Oriental naturopathic medicine advocates practicing good sexual hygiene to reverse endometriosis and enhance fertility. Practitioners suggest that couples avoid intercourse at the time of menstruation, saying that it can result in an imbalance of energy and cause the migration of endometrial tissue into the pelvic cavity.

The use of acupuncture is another Eastern approach to infertility. The idea is to release obstructions from the liver, spleen, heart, lung, and kidney, in order for energy to move freely within the system. This can potentially impact fertility by overcoming possible hormonal, psychological, and emotional factors that are connected to those organs.

Herbs to tone renal/adrenal function are part of the Oriental approach, since reproduction is considered related to the kidney. Recommended herbs include wormwood, which is actually a European herb that can be consumed along with the Chinese herbs daughter seed and fructose litchi (a red berry); dong quai, which can be taken as a tea or in capsule form; kelp, which is rich in iodine and thus beneficial for hypothyroidism; and ginseng, an herb that may help strengthen the male reproductive system, as it contains a lot of zinc.

Western Naturopathic Medicine

According to Dr. John Pizzorno, naturopath and midwife, one type of treatment that may counter infertility is a hydrotherapy procedure used to ease pelvic inflammatory infection. Essentially, this procedure uses sitz baths and has a woman submerge herself in a tub of hot water for five minutes with her extremities outside the tub. The water level should extend to her umbilicus. She should then alternate to a bucket of cold water for one minute (here the water level should be just underneath the umbilicus, so there is less cold water than hot water). This procedure should be done three to four times daily. After a period of participating in this regimen, she should start getting a discharge which may indicate that the body is emitting scar tissue and toxic material from the ovaries and fallopian tubes. However, it is recommended that women avoid unprotected sex for several months during this treatment. The reason is that prior to completion of the treatment, there may be partial blockages, which could result in problem pregnancies should conception occur during this time.

Herbs

Lastly, there are some herbal supplements that have been known to increase fertility and so should be kept in mind. Fennel and anise have both been known to promote menstruation and facilitate birth. Red raspberry leaf tea contains a lot of iron, as well as other nutrients, making it beneficial to the reproductive system overall. Gingko biloba improves circulation, and therefore may help to overcome impotence.

Treatment Summary

Learn to identify when ovulation begins. This can be done by observing: (1) an increase in temperature approximately two weeks prior to menstruation, in addition to (2) a change in the color and texture of vaginal discharge to more of a clear, slippery substance.

Because proper nutrients and optimal chemical balance offer the best chance of becoming pregnant, it is important to make healthy lifestyle choices. A well-balanced diet, relaxation techniques, and avoidance of bad habits or substances known to inhibit fertility should be considered.

Vitamin and mineral intake can make a difference. Specific recommendations for men are zinc, selenium, and vitamins E, D, and C. Particular suggestions for women include vitamins C, B6, and B12, in addition to iron, folic acid, colloidal silver, and bioflavonoids. It's worth talking to a nutritionally-oriented health practitioner, because each individual's system and situation are unique.

Oriental naturopathic medicine uses acupuncture and herbs in treating infertility.

A hydrotherapy procedure can be used to ease pelvic inflammatory infection. It prescribes that a woman alternate between a tub of hot and cold water to help the body emit scar tissue and toxic material from the ovaries and fallopian tubes.

Learning Disorders

Teachers from past decades may recall an occasional hyperactive student. This is in dramatic contrast to today's world, where more and more children are being classified as having some type of behavioral or learning disorder. In the United States, over 6 million youngsters are currently diagnosed with one of the most common of these, attention deficit disorder. By the year 2000, it is estimated that the number labeled as having ADD will rise to 8 million. Many adults too are being told that their learning suffers because of this condition.

One might ask, why the sudden epidemic? Is our modern world, with its exposure to too many chemical pollutants, causing brain disturbances that make learning difficult? Or are medical advances enabling us to detect a condition that was there all along? Since the diagnosis is subjectively based, perhaps the condition is not real at all, but only a fabrication.

Medical practitioners differ widely in their beliefs. At one extreme, ADD is said to be a bona fide medical condition that needs pharmaceutical control. At the other end of the spectrum, doctors believe ADD to be nonexistent. Many of these physicians express alarm at the growing population of medicated children, especially since a diagnosis is based on observations of behavior, and not measured through neurological tests. Thus, any child who exhibits noncompliant behavior may be diagnosed with a learning disorder. According to Nina Anderson, author of *ADD: The Natural Approach*, in many cases, children are being labeled with a disorder such as hyperactivity when, in fact, they may simply be normal kids who are particularly bright and require a more active social and educational experience as an outlet for their intelligence. Others in the medical field take a middle ground. They believe that learning disorders do exist, but that they should be viewed in a broader context. They see these disorders not just as psychological or behavioral disturbances, but as nutritional, biochemical, and medical issues as well.

Causes

Learning disorders may be a consequence of several factors, toxicity and nutritional deficiencies being two of these. With increasing amounts of pesticides, processed foods, and environmental toxins to contend with, our bodies—and more specifically, our brains—are being deprived of important nutrients. When this happens, normal brain chemistry is impaired such that this organ will send irregular signals to the rest of the body, which subsequently results in abnormal mental, emotional, and behavioral patterns.

Another possible reason for the increase in learning disorders is the introduction of certain vaccines and immunizations. Dr. Alan Cohen explains that some of these vaccines may produce a minor swelling in the brain, called encephalitis. When children show symptoms of encephalitis, such as a high fever, within 72 hours of being inoculated, they can be treated. However, many do not present immediate symptoms. Instead, the problem persists, and later in life this may hinder their ability to learn, focus, and behave normally in society. It might also negatively impact their immune system and cause a variety of allergies and continual infections. As a result, these children are given a lot of antibiotics, which can produce an imbalance of normal bacteria and create digestive problems, making it easier for toxins to enter the bloodstream and penetrate the brain, which will also alter normal brain chemistry.

Food allergies may be responsible for some leaning problems, as they allow inflammatory compounds to permeate the bloodstream and affect normal brain function. Additionally, hypothyroidism may be an underlying factor in that an underactive thyroid gland may cause the brain to operate incorrectly.

Treatment

Conventional treatment relies on drugs, such as Ritalin, to control behavior. Children often take drugs every day, for years and years. But there are side effects to long-term drug use. Also, drugs only mask symptoms and do not get at the underlying pathology, if there is one. Therefore, it's preferable to get at the source of learning disabilities and try to correct the fundamental problem.

Supplements

It is important to nourish the brain with the types of nutrients it needs to function properly. Dr. Cohen has found that many people have responded to the correct diet and supplement program. Magnesium and selenium are two vital minerals that everyone needs, but that we don't all get enough of. In fact, low magnesium levels are related to cases of hyperexcitability and inattention. The recommended daily dosage is 200 to 500 milligrams of magnesium and 100 to 200 micrograms of selenium. Zinc is another key nutrient, since an insufficient amount of this mineral in the body may impede enzyme function and subsequently hinder normal brain function. As a supplement, 20-40 mg a day are suggested. Sulfur amino acids are also significant, as they help in eliminating toxins from the body. Children will also respond to vitamin B6 and calcium supplementation. Do remember, though, that while these nutrients can all be taken as supplements, diet is of prime importance. An organic diet, free from all additives and preservatives, is recommended so that exposure to toxins is limited and the amount of nutrients the body receives will be maximized.

Clean Schools, Clean Diet

Dr. Doris Rapp is a board-certified environmental medicine specialist, pediatric allergist, and author of many books, including *Is This Your Child's World?* Dr. Rapp emphasizes the connections between chemical sensitivities, poor nutrition, food allergies, and alterations in behavior: "The tendency is to place children with learning and developmental problems into special classrooms with special education teachers. But maybe stopping the dyed sugary cereal for breakfast would eliminate the problem. I had one child whose IQ was verified at 57. After discovering her sensitivities and making the appropriate changes, her IQ zoomed to 125. This switch is from retarded to superior. How many other children are getting D's and F's, when they can be getting A's and B's?"

Dr. Rapp adds that medical science has now documented the fact that children's brains can actually be altered by exposure to certain chemical odors. These odors can interfere with the blood flow into the brain, which, in turn, can alter functioning in particular parts of the brain. She explains that if the speech area is affected, the child may stutter, speak too fast, or not be able to remember words. If the frontal lobe is affected, the child may suddenly bite or hit, or become irritable, withdrawn, moody, or depressed. Dr. Rapp mentions that in the past, psychologists often blamed parents for problems that actually stemmed from an environmental illness.

Rapp cites the experience of the Ontario school system, after psychologists there noted that standard treatments for learning problems were not taking effect. The schools called in environmental physicians, such as herself and Drs. Lyndon Smith, Alex Schauss, and Marshall Mandell. All basically gave the same advice: Improve the children's nutrition and keep classrooms free of chemicals.

These suggestions worked. Better nutrition and clean classrooms not only increased academic performance and attendance, but some children who were being taught at home were able to return to school. As Dr. Rapp points out, there's no good reason that we in the U.S. can't follow Ontario's lead.

What to Avoid

Dr. Cohen suggests that heavy metals, such as antimony, aluminum, arsenic, lead, and cadmium, should be avoided, since a percentage of autistic children have been found to have high concentrations of these substances in their bodies. Also, many children with learning disorders seem to have a gluten and casein sensitivity. Casein is a protein found in milk, so that dairy products may have to be removed from the diet. Gluten is found in grains, and therefore wheat, spelt, oats, barley, and rye may also be problematic. Further, since many children with learning disabilities have compromised immune systems, indicating an overgrowth of candida yeast which allows for increased production of toxins, they should be placed on a yeast- and mold-free diet. Lastly, while food allergies are individual in nature, there are certain common food allergens that parents may want to keep in mind. These are corn, soy, eggs, tomatoes, yeast, and peanuts.

Treatment Summary

Nutrients that can enhance brain function include magnesium, selenium, zinc, sulfur amino acids, vitamin B6, and calcium.

An additive-free organic diet maximizes learning potential.

Evaluating the diet for possible allergens, and then eliminating them, can be helpful.

Keeping school and home environments free of harmful chemicals can enhance learning.

Lupus

Lupus erythematosus is an autoimmune disorder in which the body attacks its own connective tissue or collagen. For most sufferers (overwhelmingly women between the ages of 20 and 40), lupus is a mild disease affecting only a few organs. But for others it can be serious and life-threatening. People of African, Native American, and Asian ancestry develop the disease more frequently than those of European background.

Symptoms can include achy joints, fever, nausea, dizziness, vertigo, prolonged or extreme fatigue, arthritis, a rash that goes across the bridge of the nose and cheeks, kidney problems (including renal failure), pleurisy (chest pain), sun and light sensitivity, hair loss, Reynaud's phenomenon (fingers turning white or blue in the cold), seizures, anger and depression, mouth or nose ulcers, nail fungus, headaches, and anemia. These indications can be aggravated by infections, antibiotics, extreme stress, hormones, especially estrogen, and certain drugs.

Treatment

Lupus is often treated with steroids, such as Prednisone and corticosteroid compounds. Taken long-term, these can cause great damage to the liver, eyes, and other organs, as well as weakening of the bones. This is one of the reasons that alternative approaches to the condition are worth looking into.

Herbs

Herbs that promote detoxification may be of benefit to lupus sufferers. Pau d'arco, a blood cleanser, and aloe vera juice or gel, which neutralizes and flushes toxins from the body, can both help in this regard. Cat's claw, flaxseed oil, and omega-3 fatty acids can reduce inflammation. Other helpful nutrients include black walnut, which is anti-inflammatory and antiparasitic, and gotu kola, which nourishes the nervous system.

DHEA

DHEA is a hormone produced by the adrenal glands. Many diseases are associated with low levels of this hormone, including lupus. In studies, women with lupus were given high levels of DHEA replacement, in studies, and some dramatic improvements were seen.

Acupuncture

An acupuncturist will take into account the whole range of symptoms each individual manifests, and tailor treatment accordingly. In general, acupuncture increases circulation of blood and what the Chinese refer to as qi, or vital energy, which in turn decreases pain.

Exercise

A regular exercise program helps to keep mobility in the joints and detoxify the body.

Flushes

Enemas and colonics are of great importance in cleansing the body, which is necessary for the alleviation of lupus symptoms. Massage further stimulates detoxification. Colloids, metals (such as silver) suspended in solution, are designed to bypass the intestines and enter directly into the cells. These have detoxifying, antifungal, and antibacterial effects, and help to clear arthritic symptoms.

Aromatherapy

Aromatic oils have a positive effect on the emotions as well as the body. Joint pain can be alleviated with pine, cedar, and other tree oils. A technique aromatherapists recommend for relaxation is placing a drop of chamomile, lavender, lilac, or neroli on the palms, rubbing them together, cupping the hands around the nose, and breathing in. It is important to use natural oils of a pure quality, and to dilute these before applying directly to the skin.

What to Avoid

Lupus symptoms vary widely and can be adversely affected by stress and lifestyle. Working at a job one dislikes, for instance, can exacerbate symptoms. Foods that stress the system include the obvious villains: processed foods, sugar, caffeine, and carbonated beverages. There are also less obvious triggers, healthy foods that set off an allergic inflammatory response. People commonly have problems with peanuts, soy, wheat, corn, milk, and acid-producing foods such as meat, dairy, and oranges. Problem-causing foods can be individually identified through allergy testing.

Treatment Summary

Lupus is conventionally treated with steroid drugs, which can damage organs and bones.

Herbs are a natural treatment that can benefit lupus sufferers as they cleanse the blood, flush toxins from the body, and reduce inflammation.

Studies reveal that DHEA supplementation yields improvement in the condition.

Acupuncture can decrease the pain associated with lupus.

A regular exercise program, massage therapy, enemas, and colonics flush the system of toxins, and help to remove arthritic symptoms.

The essential oils used in aromatherapy can alleviate joint pain and create a feeling of relaxation.

See also: Allergies, Arthritis

Lyme Disease

Lyme disease is an acute inflammatory condition that can cause joint pain and heart and nervous system symptoms. Its name comes from the place it was discovered, Lyme, Connecticut. Although Lyme disease occurs in other parts of the U.S., as well as in other countries, the highest concentration of Lyme disease is in the northeastern United States.

Causes

This disease is caused by the borrelia spirochete, which is a type of bacterium in the same family as the one that causes syphilis. This spirochete is transmitted through the bite of a deer tick. Not all deer ticks are infected, but a good percentage are. Note that deer ticks do not reside just on deer; various animals can pick them up. In fact, it is not at all uncommon for people to get deer ticks from their pets after the pets have been running around in the woods or even on a lawn that has trees and bushes.

Symptoms

Some people manifest the classical identifying sign of an inflamed, slightly raised bull's-eye rash. The rash is usually painless, but can be stinging, and often occurs from several days to weeks after the tick bite. It may manifest in an area other than where the original bite happened.

Many other symptoms can be present. Some of these are unexplained fevers, sweats, chills, flushing, weight loss or gain, fatigue, and tiredness. Neurological signs include muscle cramps, twitching, headaches, neck creaks and cracks, neck stiffness, tingling, numbness, and facial paralysis, such as in Bell's palsy. Mood swings, irritability, and depression, as well as memory problems, can occur too.

Signs are not necessarily persistent; they tend to come and go, so that a person with Lyme disease may feel severe symptoms for a week and only mild effects for several months.

The Importance of Tick Removal

Once a person is bitten by a tick, the longer it remains, the more chance there is of infection. Usually, a tick must feed for 24 hours before it will transmit infection. Most people will therefore reduce their major problems if the tick is spotted fairly soon and removed.

The way to dislodge a tick is with tweezers, never with fingers. (If tweezers are unavailable, protect the fingers with a paper towel.) Grab the insect close to the head, and pull it straight out. The tick should then be cellophane-taped to a card for identification purposes, so that a doctor or health department can see whether or not this was a deer tick.

If some tea tree oil is available, before attempting to remove the tick place the oil on a piece of cotton and then onto the head of the tick. This will help kill the tick within minutes, making it even easier to yank out and further minimizing the amount of harmful bacteria absorbed into the system.

Diagnosis

According to Dr. Michael Schachter, of Suffern, New York, Lyme disease cannot be diagnosed by one single antibody test alone, since tests give false negatives 30 percent of the time. There are also about 10 percent false positive readings, where the patient doesn't have the disease even though the blood test says he does. For this reason it is best to make a diagnosis based on a combination of laboratory tests and manifesting symptoms.

New York City's Dr. Martin Feldman says that although the antibody test is the most common diagnostic tool used today, there is also a PCR enzyme test, which is superior for identifying spirochetes. Even better is electrical acupuncture, which can tap into the spirochete's energy fields right away. The device used can also test a person's reaction to different therapies, and, ultimately, help test the individual's return to wellness.

Dr. Feldman adds that people can be infected by Lyme to different degrees, depending on the state of their immune systems. In order to see whether or not the body has the ability to effectively fight off the spirochete, Feldman begins his diagnosis by taking a complete profile of the person's immune system status. Some signs of lowered immunity include frequent or lingering colds; recurrent infections; sinus problems; digestive disorders; skin problems; PMS; candida overgrowth; parasitic, viral, or fungal infections; allergies; and chemical sensitivities.

Treatment

Antibiotic therapy is the primary treatment given for Lyme disease. Basically, four groups of antibiotics are used. These include those in the penicillin family, the tetracycline family, the cephalosporin family, and the macrolide family.

There is a controversy within the medical establishment regarding the best way to utilize antibiotic therapy in treating Lyme disease. Many doctors treat the condition with short courses of antibiotics. These physicians argue that you can get rid of the disease after a one- or two-week course. Others say that the Lyme disease organisms can hide in the tissues for long periods of time, and that short courses of antibiotics frequently do not get to them. They feel that large doses of medicine over long periods of time, generally from four to six weeks, may be needed.

The way antibiotics are administered depends on various factors. In milder cases, in the newly infected, and as a prophylaxis (for people who have just gotten a tick bite and think they might be getting Lyme disease), it is sometimes recommended that people take oral antibiotics for a period of time. In more severe circumstances, or in cases that do not respond to oral treatment, antibiotics may be given intravenously.

Some holistic practitioners do agree that antibiotics can be an important therapy when taken at the early stages of the disease. However, that treatment alone is not enough. At a minimum, anyone on antibiotics, particularly on long courses, should be taking yogurt or an acidophilus supplement to prevent the overgrowth of yeast. Additionally, many other measures for destroying the spirochete and enhancing the immune system should be taken.

Diet

Organically grown foods should be eaten in their natural form whenever possible, with an emphasis on fruits and vegetables. Nuts and seeds, as well as whole grains, should be used. When a person eats meat, organically raised animals should be the source, to avoid weakening from chemical contamination.

Supplements

Dr. Schachter feels that large amounts of the amino acid glutamine feed the immune system so that it can quickly overcome any infection, including Lyme disease. Although glutamine is naturally made by the body, insufficient amounts are produced during times of stress. When an infection is present, the body will resort to breaking down muscles to get more of this vital substance, resulting in a wasting away of the body. Glutamine is even more important when antibiotics are taken because large doses of antibiotics can cause yeast overgrowth, damage to the intestinal lining, leaky gut syndrome, and poor absorption of nutrients, all conditions that glutamine can help repair. Additionally, glutamine is an essential part of the glutathione molecule, a major antioxidant produced by the body. The best way to take glutamine is as a teaspoon of powder, somewhere in the range of 5 grams, three times a day, or a teaspoonful three times a day. Higher doses may be needed for some Lyme disease patients.

Sometimes, vitamins and minerals need to be injected into the patient. This is because the Lyme spirochete, and other bacteria, viruses, and fungi in the person's system, weaken the intestinal tract so that oral supplements are not fully absorbed. Injectable nutrients bypass the gastrointestinal system, and, at the same time, help to heal the digestive tract, so that oral nutrients can have a greater effect. Some nutrients a doctor may administer in this fashion are vitamin C, B vitamins, particularly B6 and B12, and the minerals chromium, magnesium, calcium, zinc, manganese, copper, molybdenum, selenium, and glutathione.

The joints can be nourished with calcium, magnesium, manganese, copper, and vitamins A and D, as well as glucosamine sulfate, and chondroitin. Other basic nutrients for immune repair are bioflavonoids, gamma linoleic acid, essential fatty acids, zinc, and selenium.

Bio-oxidative Therapies

Bio-oxidative therapies can restore health, even after other methods have failed. Some patients benefit from a very low concentration of intravenous hydrogen peroxide. Others do well on ozone therapy, where a portion of the patient's blood is mixed with ozone and then injected back into the body. Studies show that ozone therapy stimulates cytokines, chemicals in the white blood cells that help the immune system kill off offending organisms.

What to Avoid

It's important for Lyme disease patients to avoid products that weaken immunity, whenever possible. The list of these is long, and includes sugar, alcohol, caffeine, tobacco smoke, white flour products, hydrogenated fats, chemicals added to foods, fluoridated and chlorinated water, aluminum cookware, and certain medications. Some people have impaired immune systems because of their mercury amalgam dental fillings, and may benefit from their removal, with the addition of a chelating agent that helps to remove mercury from the body. It may seem troublesome to avoid all these substances, but optimizing the condition of the immune system is vital in fighting an illness like Lyme disease.

Preventing tick bites is obviously a good idea for everyone. High-risk activities include walking in the woods or on the beach near tall grassy areas, and gardening. Woodpiles tend to attract mice, and therefore Lyme problems. Bird feeders attract animals too when the seeds spill over. Dogs and horses may carry ticks, and get Lyme disease themselves. When entering high-risk areas, cover the body completely, wearing long pants, a long-sleeved shirt, and a hat, and check for ticks afterwards. Ticks show up better on light colored clothing. Be sure to shower thoroughly, while inspecting the body for ticks. Ticks usually crawl around for at least a few hours before biting, so you have some time before the tick might attack.

Treatment Summary

Cover up to avoid ticks in high-risk areas; if you find a tick on your body or your pet's, remove it promptly to avoid infection.

Antibiotics are the primary method of treatment, although there is controversy regarding how long a course is needed.

Foods selected should be chemical-free to support immune health.

A variety of supplements are helpful in combating Lyme disease, with glutamine being particularly noteworthy.

Bio-oxidative therapies can aid in treating this condition.

Lymphedema

Lymphedema is the ongoing, abnormal swelling of an arm or leg (sometimes both legs), and very occasionally other parts of the body, such as the head or intestines. Besides swelling, symptoms can include skin thickening, the leaking of lymphatic fluid when the skin is cut or broken, and bursting pain, where the skin feels like it is about to explode.

An estimated 1 percent of the U.S. population has lymphedema, which results from not having enough vessels to carry the lymph. Most cases in the U.S. are the direct result of trauma associated with surgical and radiation treatments for breast cancer. Other causes include parasites, automobile accidents, and other physical injury. Also, some 2 million people worldwide are born with inadequate lymph circulation.

The most frequent complication associated with lymphedema is cellulitis, or streptococcal infection of the skin and subcutaneous tissue. Patients will run a high fever; the arm or leg will turn red. Other complications include leaking of lymph fluid, known medically as lymphorrhea; some people leak fluid all the time. Rarely, patients develop malignant tumors in the swollen arm or leg, so-called lymph angiosarcoma.

Lymphedema should be treated immediately, as it can be life-threatening. Early indications include tight jewelry, and skin that does not lose its indentation after being squeezed for several seconds.

Treatments

Manual Lymphatic Drainage

This simple method employs light, slow, rhythmic movements to stimulate lymphatic flow. It can be used as a preventive measure following a mastectomy, before lymphedema occurs. When used after breast removal surgery, studies show that it can reduce scarring, increase arm mobility, and alleviate pain and uncomfortable sensitivity.

Diet

An abundance of fresh, organic, live foods, such as sprouts, salads, and fresh juices, aid detoxification and promote good health. The best foods to eat are complex carbohydrates; animal protein and sodium should be avoided. Green juices, such as wheatgrass, celery, and parsley, contain chlorophyll, which purifies the blood and lymph. Green juices are too strong to be taken alone, however, and should be diluted with other juices and pure water.

Herbs

The following herbs are known for their anti-edema qualities: hyssop, rosemary, black licorice root, astragalus, and dandelion root. Alfalfa, corn silk, juniper berries, lobelia, and pau d'arco are also helpful. Garlic is valuable for its antimicrobial and antibiotic properties.

Supplements

Certain nutrients help to cleanse the lymphatic system and move materials through. These include vitamins B1, C, and E as well as L-taurine, potassium, and raw kidney extract.

Magnets

When properly applied to the affected region, magnets stimulate lymphatic flow. The negative pole is the one used.

Respiration

Breathing deeply is the most cost-effective way to activate stagnant lymph fluid. One technique, recommended by California lymph specialist Dr. William Martin, is the following: Breathe deeply in through the nose and out through the mouth, in cycles of three. With each exhalation, push the air out strongly. The third time, before exhaling, hold the breath as long as possible. While the breath is being held, imagine where the healing breath should go, and mentally direct it to that part of the body.

This exercise opens up the lymphatic ducts and speeds lymphatic flow. It also releases pain, because pain can come from a lack of oxygen at the cellular level. A word of caution: Never hold in air to the point of stress. And stop to rest if this causes dizziness.

Other ways to improve respiration include light bouncing on a small trampoline, while breathing deeply, as well as bio-oxidative therapies, which employ ozone or oxygen. Aerobic exercises prompt lymphatic drainage, and sweating removes toxins from tissues.

Minimizing Symptoms

Patients already affected can take many steps to minimize their problems. Here are some important ones to follow:

Heat should be avoided, as it causes the body to produce more lymphatic fluid. This means no hot showers, hot tubs, or saunas, and wearing long sleeves and hats to avoid sun exposure.

To minimize the chance of skin cuts, gloves should be worn when gardening. Electric razors, rather than manual ones, provide less of a chance of cutting the skin.

Patients are urged to avoid strenuous exercise and the lifting of heavy objects.

Women who wear a breast prosthesis should find the lightest one possible, and bra straps should be padded. Whenever possible, bras should not be worn as they restrict lymphatic flow.

Skin and nail care should be meticulous to avoid infections, and patients should avoid going to manicurists who use their instruments on other patrons.

Patients must avoid injections to affected areas or to the arm nearest where the breast cancer was. They must avoid having a doctor take blood or blood pressure readings from that arm. Nor should they receive chemotherapy in that arm.

Mosquito bites can lead to serious infections and must be avoided.

Maintaining a normal weight minimizes symptomatology.

If airplane travel is necessary, the arm or leg should be wrapped and elevated before take off. Preparation for travel includes taking extra garlic and other natural antibacterials.

What to Avoid

The most detrimental foods contain salt, sugar, and caffeine. It is also important to stay away from processed foods and artificial chemicals.

Treatment Summary

Stimulating lymph flow through manual lymphatic drainage, especially after a mastectomy, can prevent the occurrence of lymphedema.

Healing foods promote cleansing and include live green foods and complex carbohydrates. Caffeine, sugar, and salt must be avoided.

Beneficial herbs have anti-inflammatory, antimicrobial, and antibiotic properties.

Nutrients that promote further detoxification include vitamins B1, C, and E, L-taurine, potassium, and raw kidney extract.

The negative pole of a magnet placed over the affected region will speed up healing.

Deep breathing accompanied by visualization is a powerful way to promote healing.

Menopause

Menopause can be defined as the conclusion of the female reproductive phase of life. In most women the onset of menopause occurs between the ages of 45 and 50, but it has been known to occur anywhere from age 40 to 60. In addition, menopause can be provoked at an earlier time due to uterine or ovarian surgery or certain types of illness. Menopause is characterized by the decreased functioning of the ovaries, which results in reduced quantities of the hormone estrogen in the body. Not just a discrete event, menopause is actually a process, one that lasts several years, or even a decade.

Although menopause is an experience common to women all around the world, those in Asian cultures tend to adapt more easily to the hormonal changes involved, due to their willingness to accept the aging process as a natural transition. In Asian countries, age is associated with wisdom and respect; hence, women in these countries do not dread this stage of life. In the United States and other Western nations, advanced age is feared profoundly by women, due to cultural conditioning. This negative outlook is often correlated with the acquisition of acute menopausal symptoms. Women who are about to experience menopause, or have already, should reexamine their attitudes and try to eliminate any preconceived ideas regarding aging. It should also be noted that acute symptoms are frequently avoided by Asian women because their diets contain ample quantities of soy products, which are high in phytoestrogens and phytoesterols. In addition, Asians benefit from the widespread use of medicinal herbs.

What Women Experience

The menopausal process usually begins with variations in the menstrual cycle. The time between cycles often becomes irregular, and sometimes periods are skipped. Although menopause is usually accompanied by reduced menstrual flow, some women report heavy, irregular bleeding. Hot flashes are another common experience, while some women may experience dry skin, irritability, vaginal dryness, night sweats, urinary tract infections, mood swings, fatigue, and sleep disturbances. It should be kept in mind that some women have no troublesome symptomatology at all. It's also important to mention that menopause is characterized by diminished estrogen production by the ovaries, and when this occurs, the manufacturing process is transferred to the adrenal glands. Consequently, women with healthy adrenal glands are less susceptible to experiencing acute symptoms.

A common misconception is that women will lose their sex drive once they have experienced menopause. In fact, only a small percentage lose their ability to become aroused, and these cases can be effectively treated. Actually, many women report heightened sexuality because the risk of pregnancy is absent. Another assumption whose time has gone is the belief that, after the change of life, life will no longer be enjoyable. Many women fear that their later years will be characterized by intense psychological problems. This is untrue, as women who have reached 50 years of age are not at any increased risk of clinical depression. Although some women may experience mood swings due to decreased levels of estrogen, serotonin, and endorphins, these levels can effectively be corrected by natural means, and thus symptomatic mood swings can be eliminated.

Treatment

The medical establishment has traditionally approached menopause as a disease, and, in that paradigm, offered hormone replacement as a "cure." In reality, menopause is not a disease; it is a natural transitional period that can be coped with using natural techniques. Unfortunately, hormone replacement therapy has become commonplace in our nation in the past few years. Although most doctors insist that replacement therapy involves the use of natural hormones, the fact is that the hormones being used are not manufactured by our own bodies, nor are they derived from natural plant sources, such as soy products or yams. Premarin, a popular hormone replacement product, is obtained from the urine of pregnant horses. Currently, 10 million women are being administered this product in capsules or in patches. Clinical studies have confirmed that the administration of synthetic hormones to patients can increase the risk of breast cancer by up to 33 percent. Furthermore, hormone replacement has been linked to upper body obesity and insulin resistance, a condition commonly associated with low blood sugar levels, elevated blood pressure, and excessive insulin levels.

Nutrition and Supplements

Fortunately, synthetic hormone replacement can be averted in favor of natural treatments that have no harmful side effects. Studies have shown that plant estrogens, such as those found in soy products, are quite helpful in combating symptoms. And soy products (e.g., tofu, tempeh, soybeans) hamper the proliferation of cancerous cells. Oats, cashews, almonds, alfalfa, apples, and flaxseeds also contain natural sources of estrogen enhancement, although in more modest amounts. Women who incorporate these foods natural estrogen-containing foods into their diets can experience remarkable relief of hot flashes. In addition, sufficient intake of magnesium, found in soy products, whole grains, and beans, is important in curbing hot flashes. Increased dietary intake of fiber and reduced quantities of animal products can limit irritability, while sunflower seeds, walnuts, hazelnuts, cabbage, asparagus, broccoli, oats, and barley can serve as additional combatants of menopausal symptoms.

A multivitamin/mineral supplement that has more magnesium than calcium and adequate quantities of B vitamins and vitamin C can enhance adrenal functioning and alleviate emotional disturbances. Supplements of vitamin E are recommended too. This useful vitamin promotes the production of the brain hormones FSH and LH, which act as vital agents in the prevention of hot flashes. In addition, vitamin E reduces vaginal dryness and thinning. Natural sources of vitamin E, including the various mixed tocopherols, are more efficient than artificial versions. The mineral zinc is useful as well.

Supplements of the vitamin B complex are especially important during the menopausal years and can be extracted naturally from whole grains and green vegetables. Three to four hundred mg of vitamin B5 and 150 mg of B6 should be consumed on a daily basis, while prescriptions of folic acid can serve as natural hormone replacements. Adequate quantities of essential fatty acids should also be consumed because they act as natural hormone supplements, prevent cancer, and can alleviate the symptoms of aging. Essential fatty acids are also crucial in preventing dryness of the vaginal region. People on low-fat diets often suffer from deficiencies of essential fatty acids and, consequently, need to incorporate certain foods into their diets to correct the problem. Omega-6 fatty acids can be obtained from pumpkin, sesame, safflower, and flaxseed oils, while omega-3 fatty acids are sufficiently supplied in diets that contain fish, fish oil capsules, and flaxseed oil.

Vitamin D, which can be supplemented in quantities of 400 to 600 IU per day, is also absorbed directly from sunlight, or extracted from salmon oil. This is an important vitamin for menopausal women, especially those who live in polluted regions. Calcium supplements can prevent or curb osteoporosis and can be particularly beneficial when supplementation is initiated considerably before menopause. While many women have difficulty assimilating dairy products, calcium citrate, amino acid chelate, and calcium carbonate offer alternative sources of calcium that can be easily digested. Regardless of which source you select, remember that the body requires 1300 mg of calcium on a daily basis, and even more if you have difficulty assimilating it. An analysis of an individual's calcium absorption can be performed prior to supplementation. Gamma linolenic acid, which is available as evening primrose oil, borage oil, and black currant seed oil, should be supplemented by menopausal women in quantities of 200 mg per day. Boron is yet another valuable source of both female and male hormones and can be effectively supplemented.

There are several other natural products that can stimulate the production of hormones during the menopausal years. Natural DHEA, commonly obtained from yam extract, can invigorate the body. Progesterone cream or serum guards against fibrocystic conditions and breast cancer, improves the effectiveness of thyroid hormones, and prevents osteoporosis by replacing depleted calcium. Progesterone should be administered three to four weeks out of every month. Wild yam cream, which is an over-the-counter product, and oral progesterone supplements can provide effective natural hormone replacement. Estriol is a beneficial hormone that has demonstrated its ability to hinder the development of breast tumors in animals and is currently being prescribed as an alternative to synthetic hormones by some gynecologists. Finally, Triple Estrogen, a formula comprised of 80 percent estriol and 20 percent estrone and estradiol, can prevent the onset of breast cancer, osteoporosis, and cardiovascular disorders without any harmful side effects.

Herbal Treatments

In addition to dietary modifications and natural supplements, there are numerous herbs that can enhance a woman's ability to cope with menopause if she is having problems. First of all, the herb chaste berry, commonly marketed under the name Vitex, can augment the progesterone level in the body and consequently eliminate many of the symptoms associated with menopause, including vaginal dryness, hot flashes, and mood swings. Chaste berry can be obtained in capsules, teas, and in dry or liquid extracts. Note that the medicinal capabilities of this herb, which affect the pituitary gland and hypothalamus, can take a considerable amount of time to show up. Usually at least one or two complete cycles are required before the effects become apparent, and six months of use may be needed for sustained improvement.

Herbs that serve as natural sources of phytoestrogens and progesterone include dong quai, wild yam, alfalfa, black cohosh, sarsaparilla, and blessed thistle. To assist with proper functioning of the nervous system, consider skullcap, motherwort, valerian root, passionflower, ginseng, fresh oat, and blue vervain.

Homeopathic Remedies

There are several homeopathic remedies that can be effective in treating flooding in younger women. (Flooding is the condition in which menstrual bleeding stops for a period of time and then resumes profusely.) The remedy China is used by homeopaths in remedying heavy bleeding with dark, clotted blood. To treat the painful discharge of heavy, bright red, clotted blood, sabina can be used. Sabina can also be used to alleviate feelings of irritability. Secale is helpful in reducing heavy and persistent bleeding of almost black colored blood, while the remedy phosphorous can control frequent bleeding of bright red blood without any clots. Additional symptoms that can be treated with phosphorous include multiple fears, non-severe depression, chilliness, and memory loss.

Homeopathic remedies can be useful in lessening the vaginal dryness and thinning that frequently accompany menopause. Sepia should be used when the vagina is itchy and dry. When vaginal dryness interferes with sexual inter-course, natmur is the remedy administered. In addition, natmur can be used to control burning vaginal secretions, loss of pubic hair, depression, and irritability that intensifies with consolation. These symptoms often become compounded in the later part of the morning. When dryness and headaches occur simultaneously, the herb bryonia can act as a healing agent. The homeo-pathic remedy nitric acid is used to treat cases of severe vaginal dryness in which extreme desiccation of the mucosa results in splinter-like sensations in the vaginal region.

Aromatherapy

Aromatherapy is an approach to menopausal symptoms that incorporates both the mind and the body. Menopausal women may want to try the applica-tion of fennel, clary sage, and cyprus in a lotion or body oil two or three times a day. Inhaling peppermint or basil oil on a tissue numerous times a day is recommended by aromatherapists for hot flashes. Remember, though, not to use excessive quantities of essential oils and to avoid direct skin contact. In addition, essential oils should constitute only 3 percent of lotions or body oils. People interested in aromatherapy should seek professional supervision when they begin treatment in order to prevent harmful side effects and ensure that high-quality oils are being used. Also, professional aromatherapists can create specific oils tailored to the individual needs of their clients.

Exercise

Research demonstrates that exercise can diminish the occurrence of hot flashes in menopausal women. In order to completely reap the benefits of physical fitness, regular exercise should be initiated significantly before the onset of menopause, although any time is a good time to begin—with medical guidance.

Exercise can also be a good counter to menopausal depression and mood swings because it enhances the production of endorphins and serotonin in the brain. And considering the disease-preventive benefits of exercise, everyone should partake, at some level. Beneficial forms of exercise include biking, running, swimming, walking, and dancing. Discover what you enjoy, and then keep at it. Cross-training can also be advantageous, but be sure to perform different exercises on different days of the week in order to avoid overexerting any one part of the body.

Ayurvedic Medicine

Ayurveda, which translated means "the science of life," has had a widespread following in India for 4000 years. The key to Ayurveda lies in the belief that balance can have a profound influence upon a person's health. Practitioners of Ayurveda examine the patient's psychological and physical health, and then custom-design a proper diet and exercise program based upon their evaluation. To alleviate menopausal symptoms, this form of therapy uses herbal phytoprogesterones and phytoestrogens.

What to Avoid

Although all women will experience menopause, some will be victimized by adverse symptoms more than others. Remember that the severity of symptoms may be dependent upon one's willingness to accept the aging process and the person's ability to adapt to the tremendous hormonal changes that occur. Adaptation includes taking some preventive measures, specifically, avoiding several foods that have a tendency to compound symptoms. Clinical research has revealed that excessive intake of sugar, caffeine, and alcohol can modify the blood sugar levels of the body, leading to or compounding psychological disturbances. Furthermore, it should be noted that studies have correlated alcohol, meat, and cigarettes with premature menopause.

Treatment Summary

Beneficial plant estrogens are found in soy products, and, to a lesser extent, in other foods, such as oats, cashews, almonds, alfalfa, apples, and flaxseeds.

Some important nutrients for the menopausal years are the B-complex vitamins, vitamins C, D, and E, magnesium, calcium, and zinc.

Herbs that may be helpful are chaste berry, dong quai, and wild yam, among others.

Homeopathic remedies can help balance menstrual flow if flooding is a problem. Other homeopathic remedies are used to alleviate vaginal dryness.

Aromatherapy can be a helpful modality for menopausal women.

Exercise alleviates hot flashes and depression.

Ayurvedic medicine uses plants with progesterone and estrogen to alleviate menopausal symptoms.

Motion Sickness

Motion sickness is usually attributed to an inner ear problem, but the condition may also stem from a poor diet or allergies.

Treatment

Chewing ginger may help prevent nausea, including motion sickness and sea sickness. According to scientific studies, ginger is more effective than Dramamine, a common over-the-counter motion sickness drug, and, unlike pharmaceuticals, it does not create drowsiness. To help prevent jet lag and motion sickness during air travel, 1-3 mg of melatonin, taken during the trip, may be effective.

Homeopathy

Tobaccum is a remedy recommended by homeopathic practitioners for helping dispel motion sickness, especially sea sickness, characterized by a sinking feeling in the stomach and nausea. As its name implies, tobaccum is made from tobacco. Cocculus can help motion sickness when there is nausea at the smell of food. The person for whom this is prescribed feels worse when looking at something moving and better when focusing on a still horizon. Arnica can be taken to overcome the achiness and jet lag that follows a long flight.

Multiple Sclerosis

Multiple sclerosis is an autoimmune disease in which the myelin sheath, a fatty protective coating around nerve cells, is destroyed by the body's own defense system. The disease presents a wide variety of symptoms, which range in severity and can come and go. MS symptoms include weakness of an arm or leg, unexplained tingling or funny sensations in various places in the body, double vision, loss of vision, problems with speech or walking, increased urinary frequency, incontinence, and memory impairment.

Allopathic medicine is uncertain as to the exact cause(s) of MS, but environmental, dietary, and even viral factors are implicated. For some reason, people who live further from the equator have a higher incidence of the disease. Some theories attribute this difference to degrees of sunlight. Others connect it to diet, as people in northern regions tend to eat greater amounts of saturated fat.

Treatment

Because MS is an autoimmune disease, most neurologists believe that shutting down immune function is the best treatment approach. In the process, though, harmful steroids, such as Prednisone and Solu-Medrol, and even chemotherapeutic agents, may be used. Recent studies show that beta interferon injections decrease the frequency of flair-ups (which are called exacerbations), but these injections can also produce flu-like symptoms, including severe body aches, high fever, and debilitating weakness.

What conventional medicine tends to neglect are low-tech approaches, which can be highly successful. Changes in diet, the use of nutritional supplements, and reduction of environmental toxins can all have a positive impact on MS patients.

Diet

A neurologist by the name of Dr. Swank has been studying dietary factors related to MS and publishing his results in peer-reviewed medical journals since the 1950s. His long-range studies show that strict adherence to a low-fat diet, consisting of no more than 20 grams of fat per day, produce the best results. Saturated fats, including those found in red meat, dark meat, and palm and coconut oils, should be eliminated or eaten rarely. This approach can improve disease management and greatly increase life expectancy, even in severe cases. More specific dietary recommendations are found in Dr. Swank's book, *The Multiple Sclerosis Diet Book*.

Supplements

Taken daily, these important nutrients have a variety of benefits. They can enhance neuron functioning, prevent free radical damage, improve circulation, and increase oxygen:

> Garlic—1,000-2,000 mg
> L-cysteine—500 mg
> Inositol—1,000 mg
> Choline—1,000 mg
> Vitamin C—1000 mg six times daily
> Vitamin E—600 IU
> Sodium selenite—200 mcg
> Coenzyme Q10—up to 200 mg
> Niacin—200-500 mgs three times daily
> Vitamin B12—1000 mcg
> Vitamin B6—100–500 mg
> DMG—100-400 mg
> Evening oil of primrose—1500 mg

In some instances, DMG contributes to a remyelinization of the sheath protecting the spinal column. Garlic is beneficial for its high sulfur content. And borage, black currant seed, and evening primrose oil are valuable for their gamma linolenic acid. Studies indicate use of this substance is related to decreased severity of symptoms.

Since people in the north get less sunlight, and therefore less vitamin D, it may help to take more of this vitamin. In fact, one study showed that up to 5,000 units of vitamin D, taken in combination with 16 mg per kilogram of body weight of calcium, and 10 mg per kilogram of body weight of magnesium cut MS exacerbations in half. Since vitamin D can be toxic in such high doses, this plan should be followed under a physician's guidance.

Magnets

Magnets can help to heal damaged muscle and nerve tissue. Wearing magnets or sleeping on a magnetic bed can thus play a role in the management of MS symptoms.

Biological Dentistry

Toxic vapors from mercury amalgam fillings, or bacteria lodged in the gums and teeth, can cause any number of debilitating symptoms seemingly unrelated to the mouth—even central nervous system damage. Anyone with MS should work with a biological dentist to remove toxic fillings and make other dental and periodontal corrections for improved overall health.

Treatment Summary

Studies show that adherence to a low-fat diet can improve management of MS and greatly increase life expectancy.

Nutrients taken supplementally can enhance neuron functioning, prevent free radical damage, improve circulation, and increase oxygen.

Use of magnets can help to heal damaged muscle and nerve tissue.

Since toxic vapors from mercury amalgam fillings can aggravate a host of problems in the body related to MS, it is suggested that a biological dentist be consulted for removal of these fillings.

Obesity

Obesity refers to an abnormal increase in body fat, and is usually, but not necessarily, synonymous with being overweight. The distinction is most clearly seen in athletes, when muscular 300-pound football players are not obese until they stop working out; then muscle turns to fat. Conversely, a person whose weight falls within an acceptable range on a chart can actually have too much body fat. An impedance test is useful in determining whether one is overfat.

In the U.S., people often are. This is largely due to the massive consumption of high-fat and sugary foods in the typical American diet. Children become addicted to this fare, and grow into overweight adults who are prone to a variety of diseases, including gastrointestinal and cardiovascular disorders. But even health-conscious individuals, who restrict their fat and sugar intake, are becoming heavier, according to government statistics. Dr. Alan Cohen, medical director of the Health and Rehabilitation Center in Danbury, Connecticut, explains that people are eating less fat and replacing it with more carbohydrates. Yet, 75 percent of the population are carbohydrate intolerant. This means that these individuals convert carbohydrates very quickly into high doses of sugar, which, in turn, stimulates the pancreas to produce insulin. When there is a high level of insulin, or hyperinsulinemia, sugar is converted into body fat, making weight loss difficult. Whether one is carbohydrate sensitive can be determined by a health care practitioner who performs a complete physical in conjunction with a complete health and family history. A family background of heart disease, diabetes, and obesity, as well as high levels of cholesterol and triglycerides, are signs of hyperinsulinism and carbohydrate sensitivity.

Additionally, many overfat people have subclinical hypothyroidism, that is, the kind that does not necessarily show up on blood tests. The thyroid gland sets the rate at which we burn calories. When the thyroid slows down, our metabolism becomes sluggish, meaning that we burn calories less efficiently. To learn whether or not subclinical hypothyroidism exists, people can take their temperature by placing a thermometer under the arm for 10 minutes before getting out of bed in the morning. Five readings yielding an average of at least 97.8 degrees indicates normalcy; an average below that may indicate hypothyroidism. Besides a low body temperature and weight gain, other signs of subclinical hypothyroidism are cold hands and feet, memory and concentration problems, dry skin, constipation, PMS and other menstrual problems, and hair thinning or loss.

Treatment

Obtaining and maintaining a normal level of body fat depends on lifelong habits that encompass a healthy way of eating and exercising. The traditional weight loss tactic of dieting, by contrast, implies a temporary restriction of food intake or calories, not permanent change, and is thus doomed to failure from the beginning. Diets create a rebound effect whereby the person not only gains back lost weight, but adds additional pounds. Repeated attempts result in a yo-yo syndrome, with the person continually losing and gaining poundage. This is not only bad for self-esteem; it slows down metabolism, making it more difficult to lose weight with each subsequent try.

Most people blame failure on their lack of willpower, but they need not be so hard on themselves. The reason diets do not work can be explained by considering the way our ancestors lived in prehistoric times. For much of the time that humans have been around, there was no steady source of food. Sometimes there was plenty to eat, and at other times there was nothing. In order to survive, people's bodies had to adjust to these conditions of feast or famine. When food was scarce, metabolism would slow down to preserve energy, and when there was plenty, it would speed up.

Dieting places the body in the famine or starvation mode, which is why metabolism slows down when people go on strict diets. When they begin to give into cravings, metabolism speeds up—when one is young. Up until the age of 30, the body can adapt to metabolic changes brought on by dieting and then quitting, but after that it becomes less flexible. With added age, metabolism slows down and stays down. To make matters worse, the weight lost is often muscle, but the weight gained tends to be more fat than lean body mass. Fat burns fewer calories than lean tissue, with the result that the next time around in the yo-yo diet cycle, the pounds will be more difficult to shed.

Many people mistakenly believe that a high-protein diet is a good way to lose weight. While such a diet may have dramatic effects at first, it can produce unwanted consequences over time, such as irritability, agitation, sluggishness, and even damage to the kidneys and liver. Additionally, animal protein foods are usually marbled with saturated fat that clog the arteries.

Proper Eating

The best diet to follow is one that teaches proper eating as a way of life. It is generally higher in complex carbohydrates, and lower in protein and fat. The ratios of calories from carbohydrates, protein, and fat should be approximately 60:20:20. But for people with a carbohydrate intolerance, the proportion should be more like 40:30:30. As mentioned earlier, this will keep insulin levels down and burn more body fat. People with carbohydrate sensitivities should avoid bread, pasta, potatoes, rice, corn, bananas, and raisins, getting their carbohydrates instead from other sources.

Good fruits to include are apples and blueberries, because of their gel-forming fibers. As these foods travel through the intestines, they provide a sense of fullness, which signals the brain to turn off its hunger appestat. Additionally, sea vegetables, such as kelp, nourish the thyroid, which in turn keeps the metabolism running smoothly. Drinking plenty of pure water is important as well.

Dieters should be wary of the no-fat craze, as avoiding fats completely can be dangerous. Each cell in our body is lined with cholesterol or fat. Plus the fat-soluble vitamins A and E can only be absorbed when fat is present. These antioxidants work to prevent a variety of diseases, including cancer, heart disease, and immune disorders. A distinction needs to be made between good and bad fats. Good sources are found in fish, avocados, nuts and nut butters, and olive oil.

Supplements

Nutrients have many important functions for the individual working to lose weight healthfully. Some help to eliminate cravings by balancing blood sugar, while others burn calories quickly by speeding up the metabolism. Here are some important ones to consider:

CHROMIUM PICOLINATE

Chromium helps stabilize blood sugar levels, so that there is less of a craving for sweets. It also helps to increase lean body mass and boost energy. Furthermore, chromium reduces insulin resistance, which in turn decreases the storage of adipose (fatty) tissue and increases its metabolism. Between 200 and 400 mcg of the chelated form is preferred, as it is more easily absorbed into the intestinal tract.

ESSENTIAL FATTY ACIDS AND GAMMA LINOLEIC ACID

The body needs two types of essential fatty acids: omega-3 and omega-6. Omega-3s are found in flaxseed oil, which should be cold-pressed, organic, and stored in a cold place in a dark container, as essential fatty acids are light-sensitive. This oil can be used on salads and should never be cooked. If a product tastes bad, it may be rancid and should be discarded. Omega-3s contribute to weight loss by helping the kidneys get rid of excess water.

The body needs to balance omega-3 fatty acids with omega-6's. Gamma linoleic acid contains omega-6 and can be found in evening primrose, borage, or black currant seed oil. Five hundred mg of evening primrose oil taken in the morning may help reduce appetite.

L-CARNITINE

L-carnitine 500–1000 mg helps take fatty acids inside cells, where energy-producing mitochondria burn them up.

LECITHIN

Lecithin helps emulsify fat, and one tablespoon is best taken in the morning with breakfast.

POTASSIUM

About 300 mg daily, taken in divided doses, will increase energy and muscle strength.

PSYLLIUM HUSK

A tablespoon, once or twice daily, along with 8 to 16 ounces of water, provides extra fiber for better digestion.

ADDITIONAL SUPPLEMENTS

Research has shown that daily supplementation of ascorbic acid (vitamin C) can have a positive effect for obese people who are attempting to lose weight. Other supplements to know about are hydroxy citric acid (HCA), spirulina, yerba mate, and kola nut, which have been found to speed up metabolism. Supplementing a normal diet with gel-forming fibers such as quar gum produces a feeling of fullness that can make adhering to a diet easier. In addition, fiber can improve metabolism.

Exercise

Eating right without exercise offers little hope for success in fighting fat. Exercise has to be part of any body-reshaping effort, and for best results, a combination of aerobic and anaerobic exercises should be performed. Aerobics burn body fat and lower the body's setpoint, or weight-regulating mechanism, making weight loss easier. Anaerobics help to build lean body mass.

A person's setpoint will work against a weight-loss effort, which is why exercise has to be brought to bear in that effort. If you are used to being 150 pounds, for example, and then drop to 145, the brain creates signals in the form of hunger until your original weight is restored. But if you exercise and make intelligent food choices when you're hungry, this will help the body get comfortable with a lower setpoint.

The type of exercise you do is not as important as consistency. The idea is to enjoy the exercise enough to make it part of a routine. A half hour of walking each day is a beneficial exercise that most anyone can engage in. The pace should be comfortable, not too hard. But dancing, swimming, and even gardening are other good choices.

One word of caution: Before beginning an exercise program, it is important to get a complete physical from a doctor to rule out any underlying cardiac or pulmonary problems that may preclude exertion.

Breathing exercises

When Pam Grout, author of *Jump Start Your Metabolism with the Power of Breath,* began doing breathing exercises for energy, she found, to her surprise, that she was able to lose 10 pounds without trying. Grout subsequently learned that shallow breathing accompanies being overweight, and that deep diaphragmatic breathing improves metabolism, and, secondarily, appearance. Proper breathing contributes to weight loss because it sends more oxygen to the cells, which then allows cells to rapidly burn up and eliminate wastes. When we clean out the cells with each breath, fats do not get the chance to deposit themselves there. We have a lot more energy, and far better health.

These are some of the breathing exercises Grout recommends:

Lie on the floor, relaxed, with hands down at the sides and palms up. Place a slightly heavy book on your stomach. With each inhalation, allow the book to raise up as high as possible, without straining. Bring the book back down with each exhalation. This is a good exercise for learning to pay attention to breathing.

Inhale though your nose to a comfortable count. Hold the breath for four times as long as the inhalation. This allows the body's cells to get lots of oxygen. Then exhale for twice as long as you breathed in. The ratio, then, is 1:4:2. So, if you count to 5 to inhale, you hold the air in to a count of 20, and then you exhale through your mouth to a count of 10. As you exhale, your tummy flattens and you get all the carbon dioxide out. For optimal benefit, this exercise should be performed for 10 rounds, three times a day.

Colon Cleansing

Sometimes people overeat because they are not absorbing nutrients. The brain does not perceive nutrients in the blood and therefore does not signal the body to stop craving food. By restoring intestinal health through colon cleansing, more nutrients are absorbed and a person tends to eat less.

What to Avoid

As mentioned earlier, dieting is ineffective and sometimes dangerous. Healthful eating should be a way of life, which means the elimination of processed foods, bad fats, and certain carbohydrates, if an intolerance to them exists. Additionally, a lack of exercise, a clogged colon, and shallow breathing are counterproductive.

Substitutes for fattening foods are particularly harmful. First, they are based on the assumption that a person is not willing to change his or her eating habits, thereby reinforcing unhealthy food selections. Second, they introduce harmful chemicals into the system. Be particularly wary of artificial sweeteners. Aspartame, for one, is used in a popular sugar substitute and in many diet foods. While no detrimental effects have been proven in controlled studies, there have been reports of neurological reactions, such as hallucinations, dizziness, and even epilepsy. And studies on rats have linked the product to brain tumors.

A new artificial food posing a potential challenge to consumer health is the fake fat Olestra. This product has a vacuum effect on the fat-soluble vitamins A, D, E, and K, and on the carotinoids. These vital nutrients are dissolved into the Olestra and passed out of the system before they can be utilized. As a result, the body is deprived of important protection against cancer and other illnesses.

Treatment Summary

Dieting has been the traditional approach to obesity. However, done in conventional fashion, this implies a temporary restriction of food intake or calories—not permanent change. The best approaches are ones that strive to reverse the condition long-term.

Learning proper nutrition and eating habits is essential. A healthy diet is high in carbohydrates and lower on protein and fat.

Nutritional supplements that help eliminate cravings and burn calories include chromium picolinate, essential fatty acids, gamma linoleic acid, and others.

Exercise is an essential complement to a healthy diet. More important than the type of exercise is consistency of routine.

Breathing exercises will teach proper breathing, which will improve metabolism and contribute to weight loss.

Colon cleansing restores colon health so that more nutrients can be absorbed, lessening the tendency to overeat.

Osteoporosis

Osteoporosis is a serious condition in which the bones become porous, leading to the weakening of the skeletal system and increased occurrences of fracture. Women become afflicted with the disease more often than men, with postmenopausal women being at the highest risk. Women who have recently experienced menopause often endure heightened bone loss and the cessation of bone growth as a result of the hormonal changes that have taken place. The onset of osteoporosis is characterized by a sustained loss in calcium, a process that occurs at a rate of 1 to 2 percent per year in women in their mid-30's and increases to 4 to 5 percent during the postmenopausal years. Some people with osteoporosis suffer from defective calcium assimilation due to a deficiency of silica or phosphorous, while others may have a malfunctioning of the thyroid and parathyroid glands, which are responsible for calcium metabolism. The parathyroid glands control the level of calcium in the blood by secreting hormones that can balance the level when a shortage arises. During a calcium shortage, excess calcium, which is stored in the bones, joints, and soft tissue, is discharged into the bloodstream, resulting in the reduction of bone mass. Acid blood, a condition induced by the consumption of acidic foods, excessive quantities of animal protein, stress, and the accumulation of hazardous waste products within the body, fosters osteoporosis because the parathyroid glands are forced to balance the pH level of the blood by releasing excess calcium from the bones.

There are several risk factors for the condition, including a family history of the disease and excessive dietary intake of meat, caffeine, sugar, refined carbohydrates, or phosphates contained in soda and processed foods. Frequent consumption of alcoholic beverages, cigarette smoking, and a sedentary lifestyle are additional contributory causes. Furthermore, evidence has shown that women of Northern European ethnic origin and women with small frames are at an increased risk of osteoporosis.

Contrary to what we've been told, large quantities of calcium-rich dairy products in the diet can actually contribute to the condition's onset. Researchers who travel to China often anticipate a high incidence of osteoporosis because of the country's lack of dairy intake, but to their surprise, there are actually few cases of skeletal disorders. Interestingly, in the U.S. and other Western nations, where abundant dairy intake is common, there is a higher rate of osteoporosis.

Symptoms

People who suffer from osteoporosis often experience pain in the lower back and the occurrence of sudden fractures due to fragile bone mass. Loss in height and skeletal deformity are other symptoms. Some early indications of calcium deficiency are gum disease and loose teeth, insomnia, back pain, height loss, and cramps in the legs at night.

Treatment

The conventional medical approach to osteoporosis involves the introduction of synthetic estrogen into the body. Unfortunately, estrogen replacement therapy has been linked to an increased risk of uterine and breast cancer. Obviously, alternative approaches to the condition are worth examining.

Nutrition

A low dietary intake of animal products and a high intake of plant foods facilitate the growth and repair of the bones. Green leafy vegetables provide abundant sources of vitamin K, beta carotene, vitamin C, fiber, calcium, and magnesium, all of which promote the development of a healthy skeletal structure. Vitamin K is responsible for the formation of osteocalcin, the essential calcium building matrix protein involved in bone mineralization. Calcium sources include broccoli, milk, nuts, and seeds. The Chinese, who have a low incidence of osteoporosis, frequently consume calcium-rich sesame seeds and cook with sesame oil.

Supplements

Women over the age of 25 require 500 to 1000 mg of calcium per day in addition to their dietary intake, a quantity that can be obtained in supplements of calcium citrate with magnesium. Women over the age of 40 should take 1500 to 2000 mg per day, while estrogen replacement patients require between 1200 and 1500 mg. Other important supplements include magnesium citrate, vitamin D, vitamin C, vitamin K, beta carotene, selenium, boron, strontium, folic acid, silica, copper, zinc, and manganese. A balanced vitamin/mineral supplement can supply most of these nutrients, but it is advisable to supplement the zinc separately in order to avoid decreased nutrient absorption.

A hormonal supplement that can be of value is DHEA, a substance that is depleted during the later years of life and that is useful in the treatment of chronic aging symptoms.

Herbs

The herb horsetail can be a valuable source of calcium, while nettles and dandelion can supply vitamin D.

An alternative to the use of synthetic hormones is the consumption of natural ones. Natural progesterone, which can be obtained from the herb wild yam, is preferable to synthetic estrogen because it promotes the development of healthy bones without harmful side effects. And while estrogen can only eliminate calcium loss, progesterone can actually replace depleted calcium in the bones. This useful substitute can be purchased in pill form or in a cream. For maximum benefit, half a teaspoon of the cream should be massaged into the skin twice a day over soft tissue and the spinal region for a period of two weeks out of every month.

Homeopathy

Homeopathy can serve as a valuable complement to diet and exercise in the prevention and treatment of osteoporosis. Calcarea phosphorica can be relied upon for extended periods of time for the treatment of soft, weak, curved, or brittle bones. Corticoid helps alleviate the symptoms of post-traumatic osteoporosis and can be especially useful for older people who have recently fractured a hip. Parathyroids can aid in the treatment of pains in the long bones, ankles, knees, and hips, and can be beneficial to people who experience pain while walking.

Homeopathic remedies should be administered at a potency of 200c for acute pain, while people with chronic symptoms should begin treatment with 12c or 30c. Recommended dosages should be administered in groups of three to four pellets placed under the tongue and should be consumed on an empty stomach. It is advisable not to eat 15 minutes before or after taking homeopathic medication.

Exercise

The performance of weight-bearing aerobic exercise and weight-lifting can be a crucial factor in avoiding osteoporosis. And even after a patient has been diagnosed with the disorder, these forms of exercise can be beneficial. Of course it is important to obtain medical supervision at this time in order to design a program that will not result in injury.

Ideally, women should initiate an exercise program long before menopause to prevent osteoporosis. Aerobic exercise can be advantageous because it allows the muscles to engage in a continuous, rhythmic workout. Weight-bearing aerobic exercise, such as jogging, dancing, stair climbing, and brisk walking, promotes mechanical stress in the skeletal system, contributing to the placement of calcium within the bones.

Although non-weight-bearing aerobic exercise, such as biking, rowing, and swimming, does not contribute to the strengthening of the bones as much as its counterpart, it does enhance flexibility and can be especially beneficial to women susceptible to arthritis. People involved in aerobic programs should exercise for 15 to 30 minutes, two or three times per week. A full day of rest between workouts is required to allow adequate time for the muscles to recuperate.

A warm-up and cool-down routine should become an integral part of the workout. Warm-ups, which are frequently confused with stretches, are relatively simple movements that enable the body to produce heat by enhancing the circulation of blood through the muscles. The performance of a warm-up routine prevents unnecessary injury to the muscles. The legs can be properly warmed up by lying on the floor and rotating them in a bicycle fashion or by walking in place, while the arms and upper body muscles can be engaged in full range of motion exercises. After the conclusion of your exercise routine your body should be quite flexible and you can proceed to the stretching segment of your workout. Remember that stretches should resemble long, continuous pulls, and that bouncing will only tighten the muscles and can cause injury.

According to Ann Berwick, a practicing aromatherapist, the incorporation of warming and stimulating massage oils, such as rosemary, ginger, sage, blackberry, and eucalyptus, into the warm-up routine can help improve its effectiveness. During the cool-down portion of your workout, a mixture of juniper, rosemary, and lemon can help eliminate waste products and treat stiffness.

Yoga is an effective method of evading osteoporosis because it contributes to the development of healthy bones, corrects posture, and allows the muscles to remain firm and limber. In addition, participants will benefit from improved coordination and balance. By strengthening the arms, yoga helps prevent fractures of the wrist, upper arm, and forearm, which are common to women who fall with outstretched arms. Furthermore, improved strength and flexibility of the muscles can aid in the aversion of fractures by absorbing the shock of a fall, and a correct posture lessens the possibility of spinal fractures. Older women often become involved in yoga in the hopes of avoiding getting dowager's hump. This condition, characterized by the slumping of the shoulders and caving in of the chest, significantly limits the movement of the body and puts extraordinary pressure on the spine, which can result in compression fractures of the spinal column. Improvement in balance and coordination can prevent fractures by reducing the chance of falling and improving response time.

There are several fundamental yoga poses that are effective in combating osteoporosis. In Downward Facing Dog, an exercise that aids in the fortification of bones in the arms and wrists, the body is positioned in a standing position with the hands on the ground, forming a triangular shape under the torso. There are actually three parts of this triangle. The first part consists of the area from the hands to the hips and the second is formed from the hips to the heels, while the final part is comprised of the space on the floor between the hands and feet. When this yoga position is properly performed the burden of body weight is placed upon the arms, and consequently, bone mass in the upper extremities is strengthened.

The Warrior Pose, which helps increase muscle strength, balance, and flexibility, involves standing with the legs three to four feet apart (depending on one's height) and rotating one leg slightly inward and the other outward. Meanwhile, the arms can be positioned either out to the side or above the head. This exercise strengthens the hip muscles, which is crucial to preventing osteoporotic hip fractures.

The Cobra improves posture and increases flexibility and strength of the paraspinals, which are the muscles in the rear portion of the spinal chord. This yoga position is performed by laying face down on the floor and using the back muscles to lift the head and chest away from the floor.

Women who already suffer from osteoporosis should beware of forward-bending exercises, since they have a tendency to overexert the back and cause compression fractures. In addition, it is advisable to seek professional assistance (i.e., at a certified instructional facility) while participating in yoga to ensure that proper technique is practiced and potential injury averted. Ideally, again, women interested in yoga should begin participating considerably before the onset of menopause in order to prevent unnecessary pain and suffering later in life. When performed correctly, yoga can indeed effectively enhance the skeletal system and serve as an early deterrent to osteoporosis.

Women susceptible to slouching can improve their posture by practicing a relatively simple exercise. Fold a blanket to the size of a box of roses and then lay down with your head and spine centered on it. Your arms can either be placed at your sides with palms facing upward or can be held in the air creating a V-shape, while your shoulders should remain on the ground on either side of the supportive blanket. When the body is slouched, the intercostals, which are the muscles between the ribs, are constricted, causing a reduction in lung capacity and compression of nearby organs. By breathing deeply in the position described above, the intercostals are able to expand and potential organ compression can be averted.

Acupuncture

Chinese women have an exceptionally low incidence of osteoporosis, and when someone does acquire the disease in China, it is effectively treated with acupuncture. This method of treatment utilizes an electrical impulse along the spinal chord, which causes the reproductive cells, known as bone stem cells, to multiply and fortify the bone structure. When combined with the supplementation of calcium and weight-bearing exercise, this type of acupuncture can be an effective means of combating osteoporosis. In addition, studies have indicated that the performance of peripheral electrical stimulation in the legs can also aid in the strengthening of bone mass.

What to Avoid

People can prevent osteoporosis by avoiding excessive intake of sugar, white flour, caffeine, alcohol, carbonated sodas, meat, and salt. Prolonged consumption of these substances promotes the depletion of calcium from the bones and diminishes calcium production. Clinical studies have demonstrated a positive corrclation between caffeine and alcohol intake and the occurrence of fractures in women. However, consumers of tea have less to worry about than coffee drinkers because tea contains a moderate level of caffeine in comparison to coffee.

Medical evidence has also established a direct link between the smoking of tobacco products and the decrease of bone mass. Note that heavy reliance upon cow's milk and other dairy products will not ameliorate the symptoms of osteoporosis, as evidence has demonstrated that cultures that do not eat these products have lower incidences of the disease. Furthermore, dietary intake of protein-rich fish, eggs, and chicken should be limited, because these foods contain inordinate amounts of the amino acid methionine. Methionine is transformed by the body into homocysteine, a chemical known to encourage the development of osteoporosis and arteriosclerosis. Finally, people who are involved in homeopathic treatment should avoid coffee and aromatic substances, such as perfumes and breath mints, as these can hinder the effectiveness of treatment. In addition, avoid excessive handling of the pills because residue from perfumes or other aromatic substances can debilitate the potency of the medication.

Treatment Summary

A low dietary intake of animal products and a high intake of plant foods, especially green leafy vegetables, facilitate growth and repair of bones.

Vitamins and minerals important to bone health include calcium, magnesium, vitamins D, K, and C, beta carotene, zinc, and others.

The hormonal supplement DHEA may be helpful.

Some herbs that can help supply the body with substances necessary to keep the bones strong are horsetail, nettles, dandelion, and wild yam, from which natural progesterone is obtained.

Homeopathy can serve as a complement to a bone-building diet and exercise program.

Weight-bearing aerobic exercise and weight-lifting can be crucial in avoiding or alleviating osteoporosis.

Yoga is beneficial in combating skeletal problems.

Acupuncture offers a method that can treat osteoporosis by sending an electrical impulse along the spinal cord that fortifies bones.

Parasites

Many people have parasites and don't know it. Neither do their doctors. Often, when doctors are prescribing treatments for urinary tract infection, chronic fatigue, pelvic inflammatory disease, vaginitis, candida, and other diseases, they are oblivious to the actual cause of their patients' ailments—parasites. If you have a condition that has not benefited from medical care, you should consider the possibility that your condition is a product of parasites. Recent estimates have indicated that 7 million people suffer from parasites in our country alone.

Invasive parasites can be broken down into two categories: worms and protozoa. Worms, such as hookworms, pinworms, roundworms, tapeworms, and ringworms, are able to infiltrate the body and subsist on undigested food which accumulates on the intestinal walls. These intruders especially enjoy refined carbohydrates and sugar, which become lodged in the lower intestinal region as a result of decreased nutrient absorption. Insufficient pancreatic production of digestive enzymes or enzyme malfunction are often responsible for this maldigestion and the accrual of leftovers within the intestines.

While the presence of worms in the system can have many adverse effects, most people with parasites are affected by the second group, protozoa. The simple single-cell structure of protozoa facilitates infinite reproduction and enables the organism to defeat the body's complex defense system. Protozoa can thrive for prolonged periods inside the cells of the body, creating a potentially difficult situation for our immune systems, which are unable to formulate a suitable response.

Causes

Although we in the U.S. are widely known for our general adherence to sanitation and health laws, parasites continue to pester many Americans, for several reasons. First, parasite infestation is commonly caused by eating in restaurants where employees do not properly cleanse their hands before preparing food. In addition, if you or a sexual partner has traveled to a foreign country that does not adhere to strict sanitation laws, the risk of contracting a parasitic infection is increased. Another risk factor for parasite infection is drinking from an infested water supply, which is commonplace in many cities and suburbs abroad, and even domestically. The consumption of raw fruits and vegetables and undercooked meat and fish can promote parasite infection, as can working in a hospital, day care center, garden, or sanitation facility. Evidence has linked the use of antibiotics and immunosuppressive medications to infection because of their tendency to alter the intestinal system and create a climate conducive to parasite development. Parasites do not usually survive in a healthy host; therefore, the presence of parasites within a human implies that he or she may suffer from a defect in the elimination process, an unhealthy diet, or poor health habits. Public tap water is also a source of parasites. Finally, the escalating frequency of parasitic infection within our nation can be partially attributed to the increasing importation of foreign delicacies, such as sushi.

The detection of parasites in the body cannot always be effectively achieved by examining stool samples, since parasites fasten themselves to the mucosal surfaces of the intestines, and are thus able to avoid the stream of waste exiting the body. Intestinal biopsy can also produce misleading results because, often, an uninfected area is extracted and studied.

A more accurate method of ascertaining whether parasites are present is a rectal swab examination. This test, which was designed by Dr. Herman Bueno, utilizes fluorescent stains in the identification of protozoan parasites.

Symptoms

The invasion of the human body by parasites can cause a wide variety of chronic symptoms, which, if left untreated, may expedite the onset of other serious disorders. The presence of parasites can have an adverse effect upon the intestinal system, causing flatulence, abdominal bloating and pain, foul-smelling stool, heartburn, constipation, anal itching, vomiting, bloody or mucousy stool, and diarrhea. Psychologically, parasites can promote mood swings, varying degrees of depression, nightmares, irritability, spaciness, and hyperactivity. Parasites can also drain the body's energy, resulting in chronic fatigue. Additional symptoms include fever, night sweats, weight loss, loss of appetite, rashes, hives, abnormal itching, arthritis, allergy, Crohn's disease, colitis, food allergies, anemia, and insomnia. In women, parasites can promote the development of cervicitis, pelvic inflammatory disease, and vaginitis, and can contribute to a decreased libido.

The eclectic assortment of symptoms associated with parasitic disease is attributable to the ability of the parasite to interfere with a variety of essential bodily functions. For example, research has demonstrated that parasites are capable of manufacturing enzymes that can corrode the intestinal walls and allow toxins to infiltrate other parts of the body. Also, parasites can effectively disorient the immune system, creating a situation in which our own immunosupressive agents attack healthy tissue and thus induce autoimmune disorders.

Treatment

Herbs

The use of herbs in treating patients with parasitic infections is often more effective than prescription medications, such as Flagyl, because herbs can be safely consumed for extended periods of time, while prolonged dependence on drugs can lead to harmful side effects. Although most medical textbooks state that the treatment of chronic protozoal infection should last only 5 to 14 days, this is proven untrue by recent research, which has demonstrated that successful therapy usually takes several weeks, or even months.

The daily consumption of raw garlic or odorless supplements can eliminate most strains of parasites, and can be an effective combatant of fungi, bacteria, and viruses as well. Garlic can also be administered in jucies and in colonics. Goldenseal, which contains an active ingredient known as berberine, is another herb with antiparasitic potential, and can be especially useful in defeating the Giardia lamblia amoeba. Unfortunately, goldenseal, unlike garlic, cannot be relied upon for more than a month at a time.

Several drops of green black walnut tincture, Western wormweed, cloves, capsicum, quassi chips, mullein leaf, cascara sagrada aged bark, thyme sweet Annie, cinchana, and elecampane root added to purified water can effectively cause parasites to be exuded from various parts of the body. This concoction should be consumed when you first awaken and again at the end of the day. Chaparral is yet another herb with antibiotic, parasiticidal properties. A small quantity of citrus seed extract can also be an effective means of expelling parasites from the body.

In addition, there are several traditional Chinese herbs that have proven their ability to combat parasitic infection. The herb baibu can eliminate pinworms from the body when it is added to a cloth containing alcohol and worn while sleeping. When ku shen is assimilated into a tea, it can aid in the purification of the lower intestinal and urogenital regions. Lei wan is yet another versatile Chinese herb that can be helpful in defeating a wide variety of parasites. A knowledgeable herbologist can guide you further.

Nutrition and Supplements

The consumption of raw garlic, onions, horseradish, and raw pumpkin seeds can help prevent the contraction of parasitic infections. In addition, supplements of magnesium, vitamin B12, capsicum, and calcium can aid the body in its battle with parasites. Certain foods can actually heighten the possibility of parasitic infection, so avoid excessive dietary intake of these products; See the What to Avoid section, below.

Other Treatment Modalities

The weekly performance of colonics can aid in the prevention and treatment of parasitic infections because the cleansing of the bowels eliminates a potential breeding ground for microorganisms. Furthermore, colon therapy contributes to the fortification of the digestive system.

Some additional forms of therapy include hydrogen peroxide therapy, ozone therapy, and the application of tea tree oil, acidophilus, probiotic homeopathic 59, and colloidal silver.

What to Avoid

Being careful about what you eat is always a good idea. To minimize risk of parasitic infection, beware of crustaceans, such as crabs, lobster, and shrimp, and avoid consumption of pork, pork products, raw beef, and sushi. If you do eat meat, when preparing the raw meat, be sure to separate your meat cutting board from your vegetable cutting board, because during the handling of raw foods millions of parasites can easily be transferred from surface to surface. In addition, avoid intake of coffee, sugar, alcohol, milk, and dairy products, as evidence has shown that they can contribute to the debilitation of the immune system, and consequently facilitate the influx of parasites. Although fruit, honey, and tofu have significant nutritional value, people with parasitic infections should abstain from these products in order to allow time for the body to effectively combat the parasites.

Unfortunately, restaurants usually lack ideal sanitary conditions, or even the conditions of your home kitchen, so you should try to limit your consumption of meals at outside establishments. Salads and other raw foods can be especially dangerous because they're not exposed to the parasite-killing heat of cooking and, often, food preparers do not properly wash their hands after they leave the bathroom.

When cleaning utensils, the use of a food-grade hydrogen peroxide can aid in the prevention of infection Many times people will only wipe fruits and vegetables with a cloth before they eat them, but this is an ineffective means of ridding them of parasites. So it is important to wash these foods in a solution of food-grade hydrogen peroxide.

Although urban and suburban water supplies are treated with chlorine, parasites frequently survive nevertheless, so beware of consumption of unfiltered tap water. And even though pets may be fun to sleep with, they can carry parasites and transfer them to their owners. Also, be sure to remove parasitic worms on a regular basis, try not to walk barefoot when around animals, and avoid letting pets lick your face or eat from your plate. Remember not to leave the bathroom without properly washing your hands. Finally, if you are experiencing any type of elimination difficulties, be sure to correct the problem before the onset of putrefaction, a condition that is ideal for the breeding of parasites.

Treatment Summary

Herbs can be more effective than prescription medication in treating parasitic infections because they may be safely consumed for extended periods of time. Garlic is particularly recommended.

Supplements useful against parasitic infections include magnesium, vitamin B12, capsicum, and calcium.

Colonics can aid in the prevention and treatment of parasitic infection.

To minimize risk, beware of shellfish, pork, raw beef, and sushi.

Beware of raw food, such as salad, when eating out.

Unfiltered tap water can present a hazard.

Parkinson's Disease

Parkinson's disease is a degenerative central nervous system disorder, the result of damage to brain cells. Although the disease is usually associated with aging, young people may become affected due to encephalitis, carbon monoxide, heavy metal poisoning, or drug use.

Symptoms

The first sign of Parkinson's is a small tremor in the hands or a slight dragging of one foot. Symptoms grow more pronounced when the person is stressed or fatigued. Over time, voluntary movements become increasingly difficult. Walking becomes stiffer and slower. This is followed by speech difficulties and visual problems. Then the face becomes expressionless due to increased muscular rigidity. Since the person cannot control his or her facial muscles, there is often drooling. There may also be numbing of the hands and feet. Thinking processes remain normal, but they are stuck inside a debilitated body. For this reason, as symptoms worsen, a great depression may set in, and lead to a shortened life span.

Treatment

Drugs are usually given in an attempt to correct imbalances of brain chemicals, such as dopamine and acetylcholine, but these often have unpleasant side effects. In order to relive tremors, treatments have also been given to destroy parts of the brain. For example, the nerve to the area may be cut, or alcohol may be injected into certain areas.

In the natural arena, major lifestyle changes must be addressed. Parkinson's patients do require a great deal of therapy, but major improvements are possible through natural means.

Nutrition

A fresh, live-foods diet helps to start the healing process. The diet should incorporate mostly alkaline foods, with green drinks, such as chlorella, spirulina, barley grass, or wheatgrass, once or twice a day. Only bottled or filtered water should be used, to minimize the ingestion of toxins.

Antioxidants are critical for overcoming oxidative damage to the brain and for slowing down progression of the disease. Some of the best antioxidants for this purpose contain compounds known as PCO's, found in extracts of grape seed and white pine bark. About 100 mg three times daily are generally recommended. Vitamin C is another important antioxidant for this condition that helps to flush toxins from the system. In addition, the brain nutrient phosphatidylserine should not be overlooked. Also, when a person is depressed, the amino acid DLPA has been found to work well.

Herbs that work with Parkinson's patients include hawthorn extract and ginkgo biloba. Over time, these can improve circulation, minimize leg cramps and tremors, and increase a feeling of well-being. Nervines, such as skullcap, valerian, hops, and lady's slipper, can help to rebuild the nervous system.

Aromatherapy

Massage with fragrant essential oils will not cure Parkinson's disease, but can have beneficial effects. Clary sage, marjoram, and lavender are recommended. Anxiety, lack of energy, muscular pain, stiffness of gait, and sleeping problems are all aspects of Parkinson's that may be alleviated by aromatherapy.

What To Avoid

Older adults commonly develop drug-induced Parkinson's disease after having been prescribed antipsychotic drugs, such as Haldol, Thorazine, Mellaril, and Stelazine. These antipsychotics are used to sedate nursing home patients with dementia and chronic anxiety, two nonpsychotic disorders. When these drugs are discontinued, most newly diagnosed Parkinson's patients return to normal.

Studies show that toxic pesticides routinely used in agriculture and lawn care are linked to Parkinson's disease. People tend to discount low levels of exposure, but in children, the elderly, and people already ill, even small amounts can be damaging, leading to any number of problems, including nervous disorders and cancers.

Heavy metals harm the central nervous system. Therefore, avoid aluminum cookware, remove amalgam dental fillings, and stay away from cigarette smoking, as cigarette papers contain cadmium. Hair analysis can be performed to see if high levels of these and other metals need to be chelated out of the body.

Treatment Summary

Drugs are conventionally given to correct chemical imbalances, but they often have unpleasant side effects.

Destruction of parts of the brain is sometimes attempted to stop tremors. A nerve may be cut or alcohol may be injected into a motor area.

Maximizing nutrition, emphasizing a live-foods diet, with alkaline foods and green juices, is beneficial.

Antioxidant nutrients are extremely important for Parkinson's patients. In particular, they may benefit from L-carnitine 500 mg x 2 per day, phosphatidyl choline 500 mg x 2 per day, L-glutathione 1000 mg, L-cysteine 500 mg, ginko 125 mg, DHEA 25 mg, Melatonin 5 mg, CoQ10 200 mg, L-phenylalanine 500 mg, L-taurine 500 mg, Chelation therapy, IV vitamin C and Glutathione Therapy, Choline 1000 mg, Inositol 1000 mg, B-Complex 50 mg 3 x per day, PCO's, vitamin C, and phosphatidylserine.

The amino acid DLPA works to counter depression.

Herbs can improve circulation, minimizing cramps and tremors. Hawthorn extract and ginkgo biloba are noteworthy in this regard. Soothing, nervine herbs include skullcap, valerian, and hops.

Aromatherapy may alleviate Parkinson's symptoms. Additionally, antioxidants also help; L-glutathione 1000 mg, vitamin C 5,000–10,000 mg, N.A.C. 1500 mg, Alpha lipoic Acid 500 mg, Quercetin 700 mg, Pycnogenol 200 mg.

Periodontal Disease

Normal healthy gums are pink and do not bleed, but this is rarely seen. In fact, 90 per cent of Americans suffer from gum conditions, the most common ones being gingivitis and periodontitis. Unfortunately, most periodontal disease goes largely unnoticed, as it progresses slowly and silently over a period of years. That's why it's vital to understand what gum disease is, how it develops, and how to prevent and treat it.

Types of Periodontal Disease

Gingivitis

Gingivitis is an infection of the gums usually associated with poor dental hygiene and the accumulation of bacterial plaque on the teeth. Food debris, bacteria, and the normal turnover of skin cells create sticky deposits that accumulate along the gum line and around the necks of the teeth, leaving a thin, white coating. If not removed, this bacterial plaque will harden to form calculus or tartar, material that can't be brushed off. This makes it difficult to remove bacteria, which is the cause of swollen, infected, and bleeding gums. As the gum continues to swell, pockets form near the teeth. Eventually, calculus lodges within these pockets, setting up an environment that contributes to the development of gingivitis.

Gingivitis may be triggered by a variety of factors. These can include ill-fitting fillings, constant breathing through the mouth, certain illnesses, such as diabetes mellitus and leukemia, and vitamin deficiencies. In addition, bacterial formations in the mouth are often the result of too many of the soft, sticky foods that are common to American diets.

Periodontitis

While gingivitis is reversible, the patient who ignores the problem may advance to periodontitis, a more severe, degenerative condition causing irreversible bone loss. According to the American Academy of Periodontology, 32 million Americans are currently suffering from this silent, progressive condition. In people over the age of 35 periodontitis is the leading cause of tooth loss.

If a patient with gingivitis does not regularly disturb bacterial formations, the bacterial colonies will get more dense, resulting in less oxygen available to support typical healthy and gingivitis-related bacteria. Now anaerobic bacteria begin to accumulate. These are highly pathogenic, and the result is degeneration of the underlying tissues and bone resorption.

There are several reasons people develop periodontitis. First, smoking can be implicated, as well as chewing tobacco. In addition, ill-fitting bridges, fillings, crowns (caps), harbor and encourage the proliferation of harmful bacteria. Poor dental hygiene obviously promotes periodontitis. And a significant contributing factor to the onset of periodontitis is diet. Research has shown that periodontitis was not nearly as prevalent in primitive civilizations as it is today. Without a doubt, this is due in large part to the dominance of refined foods, such as white flour and white sugar, in modern diets. Also, today, people live longer and teeth are subject to longer exposure to a wider variety of organisms. It is therefore especially important to develop good gum care habits early and to carry them throughout life.

Symptoms

Since gum disease progresses silently, some people will notice no symptoms at all. Others will be aware of subtle changes that occur in stages. As mentioned earlier, when a person is healthy, the gums are light pink, very firm, and do not bleed. As plaque accumulates, the teeth will appear to have a white coating at the gum line, and within five days gingivitis will manifest. During this preliminary stage of gum disease the gums will bleed more often, especially in the morning when a person is brushing, flossing, or eating something hard. In addition, the gums will exhibit moderate inflammation. This inflammation can be characterized by swelling, redness, heat, loss of function, and sensitivity. Sometimes a peculiar taste and odor will develop in the mouth.

As periodontal disease becomes more chronic, a bluish or purplish tint can appear. If the disease is not treated in its initial stages, the gums can start to recede. At this time, bleeding can worsen. Sometimes, however, bleeding stops. Pockets develop and deepen in size to about the 4-to 6-mm range, and slight bone loss is exhibited. As periodontitis progresses, pockets deepen further, measuring 6 to 8 mm, or more. Continual bone loss will cause spaces in between the teeth to develop, and eventually, permanent tooth loss.

Treatment

There are two basic treatments traditionally used for periodontal disease. One is surgery. During surgery, part of the gum is cut away, and some bone may be reshaped. The focus of surgery today is regeneration of tissue.

The second approach is antibacterial therapy. This involves long-term behavioral change with careful adherence to a rigorous self-cleaning program that can significantly improve gum health. Many patients using this approach report gratifying gradual success. First, they notice that the gums no longer bleed when they brush or floss. After some more time, the gums stop receding and become firmer. As this occurs, loose teeth become more secure, and the bacterial infection within the gum line subsides. Consequently, inflammation resolves, pain is alleviated, and the infection in the mouth is finally controlled.

Of course, prevention is the best approach to gum disease, and there is a lot that people can do in this vein, namely brushing, flossing, irrigating, and receiving dental cleanings on a regular basis. Many dentists believe that preventive dentistry can quell harmful bacteria during the preliminary stages of a gum problem, but that in serious cases, it becomes more difficult to eliminate the bacteria because toxins become lodged below the surface of the gums. Pockets in excess of 10 mm deep should be treated with a special applicator device designed to cleanse deep pockets. Now accessible to the general public, this type of applicator utilizes a safe, low-pressure stream, and can be used to bathe the pocket with an antiseptic solution containing hydrogen peroxide or table salt.

There are several natural rinses that are recommended for gum infections due to their ability to eliminate the bacteria responsible for periodontal infections. One such remedy is an herbal rinse containing calendula, which is a mixture of marigolds, goldenseal, and myrrh brewed into a tea. When preparing calendula, dilute the herbs with an amount of water that suits your personal tolerance. After the ingredients are brewed into a tea, the tea should be strained. Then use the liquid to irrigate the gum line, while the remaining granules can be applied during brushing. Other herbal rinses that have proven effective in treating gum disease are made from propolis, echinacea, garlic, and tea tree oil.

Baking soda may be the best combatant of shallow infections. It can also aid in neutralizing the acids emitted by infectious bacteria. Baking soda can be mixed with water, or if the infection is especially bad, hydrogen peroxide. This is also a great trick for stain removal. By adhering to a strict irrigation, brushing, and flossing routine, you can alleviate surface infections and quell some of the painful symptoms of periodontitis. However, you should not become overconfident, as infections hidden deep within pockets in the gum line can continue to proliferate and ravage the underlying gum structure. Most dentists will attest to the fact that surface precautions cannot reach beyond a 4-mm threshold. It is therefore advisable to work in conjunction with your holistic dentist and dental hygienist. Then, and only then, can periodontitis be controlled.

Nutrition

Proper dietary intake is crucial in preventing gingivitis and periodontitis. Fresh fruits and vegetables, whole grains, and fiber should be mainstays of the menu, according to biologic dental practitioners. Raw fruits and vegetable are especially beneficial because of their ability to enhance enzyme functioning. People who are able to assimilate dairy products should continue to do so, many practitioners advise, because dairy products can provide the body with an abundant quantity of calcium. Fermented dairy products, such as yogurt, are best, since they help maintain intestinal health. Cow's milk is also recommended; however, people who are intolerant of it should supplant cow's milk with goat's milk. If you are completely intolerant of dairy products you can obtain an ample amount of calcium via green leafy vegetables, especially kale or dandelion greens, collard greens, or turnip greens. Not only is the calcium in these last suggestions easier to assimilate than that in dairy products, but these vegetables also contain several other useful nutrients, including beta carotene, vitamin A, vitamin C, vitamin E, enzymes, and minerals.

Supplements

Sometimes proper nutrition cannot be completely obtained through our diets. If a person with periodontitis is not receiving a satisfactory quantity of calcium from his or her food intake, supplementing with calcium is a good idea. Periodontitis is frequently accompanied by blood sugar problems like hypoglycemia or diabetes, which make it more difficult for the person to effectively combat infections. Often these particular people, especially those who suffer from low blood sugar levels, will benefit by supplementing their diets with zinc, manganese, and magnesium. Magnesium and calcium are both crucial to the bones that provide the foundation for the teeth. Manganese, also serves to maintain the ligaments that surround the teeth, but is a nutrient often neglected by both conventional and holistic dentists. Chromium fortification should also be part of the treatment regimen, as almost 90 percent of Americans are deficient in this mineral. Chromium aids in transporting insulin into the cell mitochondria, where it is consumed and converted into energy. The micronutrients vanadium and boron are needed for proper bone structure, and silicon and zinc are important as well. Essential fatty acids are beneficial because they facilitate the transportation of calcium and magnesium through the cell membrane.

Coenzyme Q10 is a nutrient that has been used by the Japanese to treat mouth and gum diseases for quite some time. Q10, a valuable antioxidant, is naturally found in the body, but it gradually becomes depleted as time progresses; hence, it is essential to provide the body with additional sources. It can be obtained via salmon and mackerel, but for those who do not enjoy fish, Q10 is readily available in capsule form. Recommended dosage is 100 mg per day. (Although it is safe for most people, consumption of coenzyme Q10 during pregnancy is not recommended.)

Garlic 2000 mg can act as a natural antibiotic, and vitamin A can also be useful in combating periodontal conditions. Supplementation of A can be initiated at 100,000 IU, and then gradually decreased to 25,000 IU. (Again, pregnant women should not take supplements of this nutrient without consulting their doctors.) Additional nutrients that can be supplemented to improve gum health include vitamin D, vitamin E 400–600, selenium 200 mg, folic acid, riboflavin, and bioflavonoids, which are effective in mitigating capillary fragility. Cod liver oil is helpful, and 1000 mg of evening primrose oil is recommended for menopausal women because of its ability to fortify bones.

Perhaps the most important nutrient to add to your diet is vitamin C, an antioxidant that is especially effective when it's combined with bioflavonoids. Most Americans do not consume an adequate quantity of fruits and vegetables, and therefore are not receiving the needed amount of C. Holistic dentists and periodontists often advise their patients to begin taking between 5000 to 10,000 mg of vitamin C supplementation daily, and to increase dosage as needed.

> Alpha lipoic acid—300 mg
> L-cysteine—500 mg
> Lutein—50 mg
> Rutin—50 mg
> Zinc picolinate—30 mg

Homeopathy

There are several homeopathic remedies that have been shown to alleviate gum conditions. During the early stages of gingivitis, when the tongue appears to be coated, mercurius solubilis could be consumed at a 30c potency three times per day, while cases in which the tongue is not coated can be treated three times daily with nitricium acidum at a 30c potency. If the tissue in the mouth is in especially poor condition, consumption of cali chloricum at 30c, three times daily, may be necessary.

When gingivitis progresses into periodontitis, mercurius solubulis can still be used, but this time the dosage should be administered twice a day in the 6 to 12c potency range. This remedy can be used to ameliorate cases of gum disease in which the patient suffers from severe inflammation, strange tastes, abscesses, pus accumulations within the gum pockets, significant pain, and halitosis (bad breath). Cali corbonicum can be used to treat cases of periodontitis in which a person is plagued by purulent pockets without the abscesses, excessive saliva, halitosis, strange tastes, digestive pain, and a pale or coated tongue. Calcarea fluorica is prescribed by homeopaths for patients with loose teeth, digestive problems, dry tongue, and a painful burning sensation, while staphysagria can aid in combating cases characterized by black stained teeth, bleeding, bone loss, tooth decay, and pain.

Homeopathy also offers preventive treatment for gum disorders with the idea that by discouraging the initial accumulation of debris on the teeth, gingivitis and periodontitis may be averted. One remedy that can be used to prevent calculus accumulation is fragaria, which should be consumed at 6c potency twice daily. This treatment aids in dissolving existing accretions, so when the dentist scales your teeth, the process is easier.

What to Avoid

Although sometimes a genetic predisposition to gum disease exists, most cases can be averted by incorporating several simple precautions into our daily routines, and by avoiding certain activities.

Since nutrition can play such an important role in gum disease, it is obviously important to eat correctly. Try to avoid refined carbohydrates, alcohol, and caffeine whenever possible. Soda should also be avoided—especially dark soda—because it will encourage the loss of calcium. Also, smoking can facilitate the onset of periodontitis. Remember that refined sugars should be eliminated, as sugar hampers several vital immune system functions, including white blood cell migration and phagocytosis, which is the ability of white blood cells to eliminate bacteria, viruses, and other infectious intruders. Plus sugar can contribute to the gradual depletion of minerals needed for healthy bones and teeth. Most Americans could also benefit from avoiding excessive phosphorus consumption. Although most of us eat calcium-rich foods, only a limited quantity of this essential nutrient is actually absorbed by the body due to the fact that phosphorus, which is in red meat, soda, and fast foods, can force calcium out of the body. In an attempt to replace the nutrient, the body takes calcium from bones and deposits it as tartar on teeth and in arteries. The ideal diet has a phosphorus to calcium ratio of approximately 4:10.

Treatment Summary

Surgery may be needed in some cases of gum disease.

Proper dental hygiene is vital, both to prevent periodontal conditions and to treat them.

Noninvasive approaches to gum disease include massaging the gums to dislodge and eliminate infectious debris, natural rinses to help get rid of harmful bacteria, and baking soda to combat shallow infections.

A fruit- and vegetable-rich diet, with whole grains and fermented dairy products, promotes gum health.

Calcium, magnesium, zinc, manganese, chromium, and vitamin C are some of the nutritional supplements a person may need to combat periodontal disease.

When combined with a good diet and regular cleanings, homeopathic remedies can help reduce gum conditions.

Phobias

Phobias are overwhelming, irrational fears of specific objects or situations. People feel intense discomfort, sometimes to the point of panic, when faced with the feared object. The usual way of dealing with this problem is to avoid the stimuli entirely, which can create varying degrees of hardship.

Types of Phobias

There are three types of phobias, the first and most common being simple phobias, which affect about 10 percent of men and women, in equal proportion. Typical simple phobias are fear of animals, heights, medical procedures, needles, elevators, water, and air travel.

The second category is social phobias, which involve the fear of being embarrassed or humiliated in public. Number one on the list here is the fear of public speaking. In fact, surveys show this to be more frightening to many people than the thought of death. Other social phobias include fear of being in restaurants and other public places, using public toilets, blushing in public, dating, and meeting new people. With a social phobia, a person feels self-conscious about being judged to the point of not being able to function around others.

About one in 20 people are affected by the third and most severe type of phobia, agoraphobia (literally, "fear of the marketplace"). Individuals with this condition avoid public places for fear of having a panic attack. Usually, the condition begins after such an attack occurs spontaneously. Then, the person avoids going to places where he or she might be embarrassed should another attack occur. Or the person may fear being unable to escape if he must. The panic a person feels is tantamount to a severe stress reaction. Symptoms include heart palpitations, rapid heartbeat, chest pain, and shortness of breath, which can leave the person thinking that he or she is having a heart attack. There may also be dizziness, nausea, sweat, a choking sensation, and chills. Feelings of unreality and loss of control take over, and the individual feels detached, as if dying. In milder cases of agoraphobia, people tend to avoid closed places, like grocery stores, bridges, tunnels, and subways. They may go to places close to home with a person they consider safe. In the worst-case scenario, individuals remain homebound. Some will not even go from one room to another in their own home.

Causes

Phobias usually begin after the brain associates some object or situation with a frightening or traumatic event. Sometimes the connection is clear. A person who almost drowns as a child develops a water phobia, for example. But at other times the relationship is far less obvious. Elaine Magidson, of Creative Counseling in New York, tells of a client who had a phobia of butterflies. Although the woman lived in the city and was not likely to see any, she was obsessed with the possibility, and it was making her day-to-day life difficult. Special counseling techniques helped her to recall a traumatic incident in her life that took place when she was just three years old. At that time, her mother was having a nervous breakdown and being placed in a straitjacket by men about to take her away. As she watched, screaming and crying, a butterfly flew past. From that moment on, all the horror of the event became subconsciously associated with these insects.

Sometimes phobias are simply the result of people being afraid of something early in life and then spending their whole lives avoiding it. A fear of dogs may cause a child to stay away from them. This becomes a pattern and the person still avoids them years later. Because it occurs for so long, the person's fear of dogs turns into a phobia.

Of course, parental conditioning can contribute to this. Another way a phobia might form is through modeling. A child watches a phobic parent, and begins to copy his or her behavior. Some believe a genetic tendency is involved as well. Research with identical twins shows, in fact, that agoraphobia has a genetic component.

Another factor contributing to agoraphobia is upbringing, where a child has overprotective, perfectionistic, or hypercritical parents. Or their parents may continually give them the message that life is a dangerous place. As a result, the child becomes sensitive and frightened of the world.

Nutritional imbalances may play a role. Too much sugar, caffeine, or alcohol can cause physiological imbalances that increase stress and cause hypoglycemia, hypothyroidism, and mineral deficiencies, making agoraphobia more likely to be manifested in susceptible individuals. Certain foods and food additives can cause allergic reactions that increase susceptibility to the disorder as well. Unless these stresses are addressed, they can build up in the system until one day some incident triggers a full-fledged panic attack.

Treatment

The traditional psychological approach to phobias involves imagery and real-life desensitization. Imagery begins with placing the person in a state of deep relaxation. He or she may be asked to visualize a peaceful scene, like a beach or a mountaintop. Progression relaxation techniques may be used. Then, gradually, the person goes from imagining that safest space to ones that are more difficult, involving the feared object or experience. Someone with a phobia about elevators may go from the peaceful beach scene to a relatively unthreatening elevator scene, such as seeing himself with someone he trusts pressing the button outside the elevator door. A session or two later, he may feel comfortable enough to watch the door open. Then he sees himself going into the elevator with that person and so on until he finally envisions himself going up and down many floors alone. This is followed by real-life desensitization, wherein small steps to overcoming a phobia are actually taken. People become accustomed to each small success before moving ahead. But the road is not always direct. Generally people make progress and then fall back a few steps before moving forward again.

While this commonly accepted method works for many people, it has its problems. It involves a lot of time, which means a long-term commitment to the process. This is often difficult for phobic individuals, who may not have the time or not want to make it because of the discomfort involved.

Also, anxiety-reducing medicines are commonly prescribed. While these may be helpful at low dosages when a person is first beginning desensitization, the disadvantage is that the person may only feel better while on the medication. After it is stopped, the phobia may still exist.

Neurolinguistic Programming

Newer techniques take a quicker, more direct approach. Neurolinguistic programming, like the traditional approach, does use relaxation, but it uses several short-cut techniques that can be quite effective. Instead of involving the person in progressive relaxation techniques each time, where each muscle is tensed and then relaxed, the person gives himself a cue to get into that same calm state. The cue could be visual, auditory, or kinesthetic, and might involve gazing at a candle, squeezing the elbow, or saying something nice to oneself. This technique, called anchoring, saves a lot of time by creating a relaxed state immediately.

After anchoring, the next step in the "fast phobia cure" is called double-stepped association, and gets the person to step away from a scene while imagining it. It's as if the individual is watching an actor in a movie. This makes the phobia less personal and therefore less frightening.

Other interesting techniques are used to take power away from negative emotions. For example, when people are upset about something, they tend to remember it in vivid colors. Having people see the experience in black and white lessens the intensity of feeling.

The philosophy behind these methods is that a person becomes conditioned to a phobic response very quickly, and can become unconditioned just as fast.

Educational Kinesiology

This technique is used alongside neurolinguistic programming, and involves exercises that promote better mind/body balance. These exercises distribute energy throughout the brain in such a way as to promote greater relaxation and reduce stress. For example, the brainstem becomes active under duress. When that energy is transferred to the cerebral area, more rational thought processes take over, and a lot of discomfort disappears.

A simple way to do this is to place the fingers on the middle of the eyebrows, and move them about one-half inch up into a soft space in the forehead. Pressing into the area for several seconds when one is anxious immediately promotes relaxation by transferring energy from the brainstem to the cerebrum.

Acupressure

There is an acupressure technique used against anxiety or nervousness. Apply slight pressure to the indentation in the center of your breast bone, known as the sternum. Holding four fingers over the area opens up breathing and releases tension.

To relieve irritability or an agitated feeling, rub the top of your shoulder and notice where it feels tightest. This will probably be close to your neck. Hold this point and breathe slowly and deeply.

Acupressure can be done on oneself, or a friend or family member can help. The idea is that the application of pressure relieves tension, as well as alleviating pain and increasing circulation.

Affirmations

Affirmations are based on the principle that our thoughts and words create our experiences. Taking a situation that ordinarily frightens us and using thoughts and words to affirm the type of situation we want for ourselves can make a world of difference. An agoraphobic who has difficulty traveling can say, "I travel with ease and feel relaxed." Initially, we do not believe what we are telling ourselves. Otherwise, we wouldn't need to be making affirmations. But affirmations do make a difference over time. Positive thoughts and words impact our subconscious mind, enabling us to create new patterns of behavior.

Counseling

Building self-esteem and improving communication skills are essential elements in recovery. Phobias serve to protect the person in some way and once they are eliminated the person needs support.

Affirmations can be used in conjunction with counseling, as can journal writing. One journal-writing exercise has a person divide a page in two and write on one side, "I accept myself no matter what." On the other side all the objections to that thought can be recorded. Sometimes, by writing down negative thoughts, their power can be diminished. Then, positive thoughts can be explored.

Nutritional support

Research shows certain nutrients to have a positive effect on brain chemistry. Some nutrients that work to reduce anxiety are the B-complex vitamins, calcium, magnesium, and GABA. Also of value in this regard are the amino acid L-tryptophane, the omega-3 fatty acids, and inositol.

Herbs

Herbal agents that calm the nerves are known as nervines. A common one that's easy to find is valerian. Valerian is a tonic for the nerves that is best taken when an anxiety attack is imminent. It is especially recommended for nervous problems that are due to emotional stress or pain. While small amounts of valerian are helpful, large doses should be avoided as they can bring on depression. Lady's slipper is an eastern woodlands plant that has traditionally been used by Native Americans as a nervous system soother. People sometimes make a flower essence of it, leaving this rare species intact in the ground. Lady's slipper is often combined with other nervines, such as hops, scullcap, chamomile, passionflower, or celery. Hops will calm a nervous stomach and, when placed beneath a pillow, it is said, promote sleep in an insomniac. Skullcap is a remedy for overcoming sleep disorders and agitation. Chamomile and passionflower help nervous conditions in people of all ages. Celery is yet another tonic for nervousness.

In Ayurvedic medicine, the herb that specifically alleviates anxiety attacks is called Ashwagandha. Much scientific research from India confirms that Ashwagandha calms because it is actually a nutrient for the brain and nerves.

Recently, the South Pacific herb kava kava was approved in Germany for its antianxiety effects. The plant is a species of pepper that aboriginal peoples have taken for over a millennium for relaxation purposes. Kava kava has become popular recently, but some cautions should be taken. First, it works synergistically with alcohol, so the two should not be used together. Second, due to its potency, a person can become impaired to the point of not being alert enough to perform such tasks as driving or operating machinery. And third, a pigment in the plant can build up in the body, causing an itchy, scaly skin condition. Fortunately, the problem will go away once kava kava is discontinued. However, this is nature's warning to use the herb sparingly.

What to Avoid

Alcohol, caffeine, sugar, and nicotine cause chemical imbalances in the brain. Many people rely on these substances to avoid anxiety, not knowing that they actually cause it.

Treatment Summary

Imagery and desensitization are the traditional method of treatment for phobias. While this works for many people, it usually involves a long-term commitment and sometimes involves medications. However, there are some newer techniques that take a quicker, more direct approach.

Neurolinguistic programming is a newer method that involves short-cut psychological approaches to decondition the person from their phobic responses.

Educational kinesiology is used in addition to neurolinguistic programming and involves exercise that promotes better mind/body balance.

Acupressure can be used as a tool against phobic responses.

The use of affirmations is based on the principle that positive thoughts and words impact the subconscious mind, facilitating creation of a new pattern of behavior.

Antianxiety nutrients include the B-complex vitamins, calcium, magnesium, GABA, and L-tryptophane.

Valerian and several other herbs have an antianxiety effect.

Pregnancy-Related Problems

Pregnancy is a time of promise, joy, and vitality. But there can be physical problems associated with it too. Morning sickness, breast tenderness, fatigue, and constipation are some of the many complaints commonly associated with pregnancy. Further, after childbirth many women experience depression due, in part, to hormonal shifts in the body. Women should be aware that there are many natural, safe ways to alleviate pregnancy-related discomforts. Discuss these with your doctor or midwife, with the understanding that each pregnancy is different.

Common Pregnancy Discomforts and their Management

Morning Sickness

Hormonal shifts during the first trimester decrease the secretion of hydrochloric acid in the stomach. This can lead to poor functioning of muscles that move food along the digestive tract, which in turn can lead to the nausea and vomiting in early pregnancy known as morning sickness. The best way to alleviate morning sickness is to get plenty of rest and to eat several small, easily digested meals, since nausea typically starts on an empty stomach. Crackers should be kept by the bed and eaten before getting out of bed in the morning. Protein snacks eaten before going to bed or upon awakening at night also help.

Here are some additional ideas: Cucumber may relieve congestion quickly. A good preventive and treatment consists of a teaspoon of lemon juice or apple cider vinegar mixed with a teaspoon of honey in a cup of warm water. This can be taken before breakfast or ahead of each meal if nausea continues past morning. Vitamins that help with this problem include 50 mg of vitamin B6 and vitamin K. The latter is often low during pregnancy. Good sources of K include green leafy vegetables as well as cauliflower, broccoli, and cabbage. An injection of this vitamin can help stop intractable vomiting. Acidophilus may help by balancing the intestinal pH. Ginger is great for nausea. Wild yam is an herb that can help stop nausea. While it does not contain hormones itself, it works by helping the body to balance its own progesterone levels. Other herbs to consider include fennel, peppermint, and cardamon in warm milk. Catnip tea is another gentle remedy. A very dilute amount of peppermint oil can be rubbed onto the stomach or inhaled to relieve nausea and vomiting.

Constipation

This problem may also be the result of hormonal shifts and can be corrected by increased fluid consumption with at least eight to twelve glasses of water daily, as well as more fiber from whole grains, bran, and fresh fruits and vegetables. In severe cases, whole psyllium seeds often help. One teaspoon of seeds are placed in a cup of water, and after drinking this, it is important to drink an additional cup of water. Castor oil and other irritating laxatives should be avoided, including herbs such as cascara sagrada and senna. Anything causing peristalsis may bring unwanted contractions. Homeopathic remedies for constipation include nux vomica, sepia, bryonia, and lycopodium.

Diarrhea

Diarrhea can be helped by following the BRAT diet—bananas, rice, apples, and toast. Additionally, four capsules of charcoal, taken one to three hours apart, binds toxins in the bowels. However, charcoal should not be taken for more than three days, as it also binds up nutrients. Homeopathic remedies for diarrhea include podophyllum peltatum, sulfur, thuja occidentalis, veratrum album, and cinchona officinalis.

Flatulence

As with other bowel problems, this occurs because the gastrointestinal tract is not moving as well as it should. Also the baby's head sometimes presses on this area. It may help to avoid carbonated drinks and to chew food well.

Sugar Imbalances

Symptoms of sugar imbalance during pregnancy can include exhaustion accompanied by puffiness, especially in the hands or feet. Gestational diabetes can develop at this time. Although it ends when pregnancy does, if left untreated, this type of diabetes can cause problems for the baby and complicate delivery. Sugar should be minimized or avoided completely; chromium picolinate lessens cravings for it and keeps blood sugar balanced. Dandelion tea or tincture (30-60 drops, three times a day) can also help.

Breast Tenderness

Breast tenderness occurs in the first trimester as the body prepares for breast-feeding, and lasts only a few weeks. Hot compresses, hot showers, and well-fitting bras without underwires can alleviate sensitivity.

Exhaustion

Fatigue is a common problem, especially during the first trimester, due to hormonal changes and the needs of the fetus. Anemia may be a factor and is often prevented by eating lots of green, leafy vegetables. Herbs, such as yellow dock, nettles, and dandelion, can be taken as a tea or tincture to counter tiredness from anemia.

Heartburn

Frequent small meals are preferable to three big ones. And as is true for everyone, lying down after eating should be avoided, as this causes stomach acids to wash back up into the throat. A good herb for heartburn is slippery elm. One teaspoon of the powder can be added to water or juice, or lozenges can be taken throughout the day. Papaya enzymes are another handy item to have available. Also, two to three drops of diluted peppermint oil, placed on the back of the tongue, may relieve this problem.

Episiotomy Problems

Approximately 80 percent of women in the United States undergo this surgical procedure during childbirth to enlarge the vagina during delivery. The operation is often improperly performed, leading to problems later on when the cervix begins to push through the vagina and it appears as if the uterus is being forced out. Doctors often mistakenly diagnose this as a prolapsed uterus and recommend a hysterectomy. Tragically, 100,000 to 200,000 women are misdiagnosed with this condition each year. Corrective surgery, recently developed by gynecologist Dr. Vicki Hufnagel, easily ameliorates the problems. Repairing the vagina is a simple procedure that can be performed in 45 minutes in a doctor's office, allowing patients to go home the same day.

Treatment

Diet

Certain conditions during pregnancy—i.e., anemia, hypoglycemia, and diabetes—necessitate special diets and close supervision by a physician, but there are some general rules of thumb that benefit most women. These include eating a wide assortment of whole organic foods, such as grains, legumes, vegetables, fruits, nuts, and seeds; eating only when hungry; and eating small, frequent meals instead of a few larger ones. Pregnant women need lots of extra protein, which vegetarians can get through extra soy products, including soy milk, tofu, tempeh, beans, nuts, and seeds and fish. Plenty of pure water is needed but should be taken before and between meals. Drinking during meals dilutes stomach enzymes, making digestion more difficult. Cravings should be responded to with the most wholesome foods possible. Finally, calcium-depleting foods, such as coffee, chocolate, and sodium, should be avoided.

Supplements

Folic acid is especially important during pregnancy for preventing neural tube defects. Since heating food destroys this fragile nutrient, it is important to take it in supplement form. Other important nutrients during pregnancy include a multiple vitamin/mineral supplement, vitamin C, B12, zinc, vitamin E, and acidophilus. A doctor's guidance is needed when taking supplements during pregnancy.

Iron has traditionally been stressed for good health. But too much iron can be dangerous, and extra iron should not be taken unless tests indicate a need for it. Also, note that the best source of calcium is whole foods, especially green leafy vegetables. If a supplement is desired in addition, calcium citrate is easiest on the stomach; other forms sometimes cause digestive upsets or constipation.

For women with postpartum depression, research has shown that vitamin B6 can help reestablish hormonal balance by raising serotonin levels. Patients given B6 for 28 days after delivery did not have a recurrence of postpartum depression.

Herbs

There are many herbs that can aid in relieving the discomforts associated with pregnancy. Raspberry leaf is a tonic that helps relieve almost any complaint and can be taken as a tea freely throughout pregnancy. The tea can be combined with peppermint for morning sickness. To soothe cramps during pregnancy, women can try black haw or cramp bark. Ginger is one of the best natural remedies for preventing nausea, especially when accompanied by a diet of small, frequent, meals, as well as fresh air, and plenty of rest. Black cohosh is an old-time woman's remedy that grows in the deep, dark forests of eastern America. It was used by pregnant Native American women to ease childbirth and diminish labor pains. When taken in the last two or three weeks of pregnancy, black cohosh helps ripen the cervix and bring down the fetus. Sometimes the herb is taken together with blue cohosh.

In general, herbs to avoid are bitter (such as goldenseal and pennyroyal), those with antihistamine properties (such as ma huang and osha root), and diuretics (including buchu, horsetail, and juniper berries).

Exercise

Most pregnant women benefit from a mild to moderate exercise program. The best level of exercise depends on how active a woman was before pregnancy, but most women can increase their endurance and should be encouraged to start at a comfortable level and build up. The exceptions are women whose doctors advise against an exercise program due to specific health concerns, such as pregnancy-induced hypertension, premature rupture of membranes, incompetent cervix, persistent second- and third-trimester bleeding, and premature labor in a prior pregnancy or current one. Get your practitioner's go-ahead before embarking on a pregnancy exercise program.

In general, though, 60 minutes of aerobic exercise, approximately three times a week, is a good goal to work toward, although shorter workouts can be beneficial as well. Non-weight-bearing activities, such as cycling and swimming, are best, as they minimize the risk of injury and allow activity levels to remain closer to pre-pregnancy levels. Stretches that open up the pelvic area are also recommended.

Some precautions include not standing for prolonged periods and avoiding high-intensity exercises and any risks of falling. The woman should not push to the point of breathlessness, and try not to raise her body temperature. After the first trimester, exercising in the face-up position limits blood supply to the baby and should be avoided as well.

Alexander Technique

Teachers of the Alexander technique seek to restore the freedom of movement so necessary for women dealing with the added demands of pregnancy. Learning to bend, breathe, and even rest properly can decrease pain and tension, and ease delivery. Changes can extend beyond pregnancy and enhance stamina and overall functioning after birth.

During a session, the pregnant woman takes an active role in therapy, while the teacher acts mostly as a guide. A woman may learn to squat in preparation for delivery or learn how to pick something up without stressing her back. Many of these movements are ones we naturally make as children but lose as adults. In addition, the teacher has one important hands-on role. Touching the client stimulates the nervous system to respond in new, more beneficial, ways. After a lesson, people find that their movements are freer, and they report feeling lighter.

Massage

Maternity massage promotes relaxation, which is of significant value to an expectant mother and her unborn child. It also helps to stimulate lymphatic drainage of toxins and can alleviate muscle spasms, back pain, cramps, swelling in the legs, varicose veins, hemorrhoids, and fluid retention. In addition, massage can promote hormonal balance and a strong immune system, as well as decrease irritability, mood swings, and overheating. The therapist who understands pregnancy massage knows to adjust pressure and focus to each stage. During the first trimester, touch must be gentle. For example, mild pressure to the bridge of the nose and forehead, and under the eyebrows and cheekbones, can unblock sinuses. In the second trimester, massage can be more rigorous and used to stimulate circulation, increase flexibility, and reduce pain and spasm. Specific focus on the chest may alleviate breathing problems. In the third trimester, work is concentrated on the lower hips and sacrum to reduce back pain.

Just before delivery, a woman may be taught how to relax muscles in the perineum, the area between the vagina and rectum that needs to loosen up during childbirth. By enlarging this area, the need for an episiotomy may be eliminated. The technique involves self-massage: With clean hands and warm vitamin E or vegetable oil, the mother places thumbs or index fingers an inch to an inch and a half inside the vagina. Firm, gentle pressure is applied downward and outward until the stretch results in a burning sensation. This is held for a few minutes. The exercise is repeated once or twice a day.

During labor, applying pressure to certain acupressure points can reduce pain and anxiety, and even speed up labor. One technique involves walking the thumbs up from the sacrum to the top of the spine, holding each point for several seconds. Another is to press thumbs along the outline of the shoulder blades. A reflex point for quickening labor is located on the inside of the legs, approximately three inches above the ankle. Another is just below the ankle bone on the inside (uterus point) and outside (ovary point) of the foot. These areas are pressed for approximately ten seconds.

During the postpartum period, massage can stimulate milk flow, and help the uterus return to its normal size. Massaging the abdomen in a circular fashion helps to expel blood as the uterus contracts, and circling the breasts with light oil, followed by placing a flat hand on the nipple, and moving outwards and upwards, helps milk glands to flow.

While massage is useful for enhancing overall health during and after pregnancy and for treating a variety of conditions, there are times when it should not be used. Contraindications include vaginal bleeding, fever, abdominal pain, edema, severe headaches, blurry vision, excess protein, diabetes, high blood pressure, heart disease, and phlebitis.

Aromatherapy

Using essential oils, either alone or in conjunction with massage, works on both physical and emotional levels. Aromatherapists suggest for that common bane of pregnancy, hemorrhoids, five drops of cyprus oil added to a bath. For sinus problems, try eucalyptus added to a cold air humidifier or a pan of hot water. Varicose veins may improve with cyprus and lemon oil added to a body lotion and applied to the veins morning and evening. Postpartum depression blues may be lifted by jasmine and clary sage added to the bath.

Only pure oils should be used, and many good ones are available from health food stores. While most are safe to try, some women experience allergic reactions to certain oils and may benefit from the guidance of an aromatherapist.

Homeopathic Remedies for Postpartum Depression

Postpartum depression, generally blamed on hormonal shifts, may also be due, in part, to overwhelming major lifestyle changes that a woman is experiencing. All of a sudden, the woman may have gone from being the center of attention to the caretaker of a helpless new individual. She may have had no experience in this new role. And even if she already has a child, each new one brings a big change in family dynamics, and in the mother's responsibilities. Also, fatigue can be a factor in postpartum depression, which can range from "the blues" to a serious, life-threatening condition.

Women experiencing depression should be under medical care. And ideally, although this is far from always the case in our society, all new mothers should be the beneficiaries of a familial and neighborhood support system.

Part of a woman's medical support system may be a homeopathic physician. Classical homeopathy offers a wide range of remedies for postpartum depression, and a homeopathic physician can provide individualized guidance on which is appropriate for a particular woman's symptoms. The remedies include sepia, natmur, ignatia, arnica, pulsatilla, cimicifuga, kalicarbonicum, phosphoric acid, cocculus, and aurum metallicum.

Another (nonhomeopathic) treatment for postpartum depression is natural progesterone. It's generally started about a month after delivery. And nutrient supplementation, undertaken with the guidance of a physician knowledgeable in this area, can make a difference.

What to Avoid

When one is pregnant, special care should be taken to avoid exposure to toxic ingredients found in such items as chemical hair dyes, household cleaners, paint and paint fumes, thinners, solvents, benzene, dry cleaning fluid, wood preservatives, and pesticides. Radiation from x-rays and other sources is to be avoided, especially during the first trimester. It should go without saying that cigarettes, alcohol, and recreational drugs are to be avoided as well.

Toxic surroundings are also harmful. Negative people and aggravating situations cause stress. It's best to spend as much time as possible with loved ones and to fill surroundings with beauty.

Treatment Summary

Eating a wide assortment of organic foods, eating only when hungry, and eating small frequent meals, with extra protein, are some general rules of thumb for a pregnancy diet.

It's preferable to drink water between meals rather than during them.

Folic acid and other supplements, as prescribed by one's doctor, are important.

Raspberry leaf tea, and other herbal remedies, can help women feel better during pregnancy.

A pregnancy exercise program will generally be based on how active the individual was prior to pregnancy, as well as any specific conditions that may emerge during pregnancy. However, aerobics tend to be the best form of activity during this time.

The Alexander technique is a method designed to restore the freedom of movement necessary for women dealing with the added demands of pregnancy.

Certain massage therapies are beneficial during and after pregnancy.

Aromatherapy can alleviate specific conditions.

Homeopathic remedies and natural progesterone are two approaches to postpartum depression. Also, nutrient supplementation can relieve this problem.

Premenstrual Syndrome

For years, premenstrual syndrome was not recognized by the medical establishment as an actual clinical condition. Women suffering from PMS were told that their symptoms were imaginary, and were sometimes diagnosed with psychological disorders. Between the 1920's and the 1950's, women with this problem could even find themselves institutionalized and administered shock therapy, while more recent treatments have included Valium and Prozac. Fortunately the medical community has since acknowledged PMS as a true medical condition, and more effective remedies are currently available to alleviate its symptoms.

Symptoms

Premenstrual syndrome is characterized by a wide range of symptoms with different women experiencing the problem in different ways. Common symptoms are bloating, headaches, cramps, swelling, fluid retention, and lower back pain. Others are breast tenderness, sugar cravings, and acne, as well as depression, insomnia, anxiety, mood swings, irritability, withdrawal, and forgetfulness. While the diagnosis of most other diseases involves the recognition of specific symptoms, ascertaining the presence of PMS is most dependent upon the time frame within which symptoms manifest. Specifically, PMS symptoms appear a few days before the start of menstruation and usually subside within 48 hours after it begins.

Treatment

The usual medical approach to PMS involves administration of prescription drugs. As is always the case, though, prolonged dependence upon prescription drugs can have adverse side effects. Some doctors, with the idea that PMS is due to an imbalance of the hormone progesterone and estrogen, prescribe progesterone supplements. Although this treatment may adjust the hormonal levels of the body, it does not address the true origin of the problem.

Alternative practitioners provide another perspective on remedying the imbalance. They explain that excessive quantities of estrogen in the body may be a product of liver malfunction, a condition that can be effectively treated by limiting the intake of estrogen-rich foods in the diet and by improving the woman's exercise habits.

Diet and Supplements

A healthy diet is in fact key to both preventing and combating PMS. Women who suffer from PMS should consume foods high in fiber and complex carbohydrates, and should have snacks in between their meals in order to stabilize blood sugar levels and ameliorate symptoms. Cool green foods, such as salads, can be beneficial.

The diet should be as pure as possible. Contaminants found in pesticides, artificial food additives, drugs, and environmental chemicals can raise the body's estrogen level, creating a deficiency of progesterone and provoking PMS. Thus, food should be organically grown and unprocessed, whenever this is possible. Excessive estrogen within the body can also result from a surplus of animal fats in the diet or a deficiency of essential nutrients, such as the vitamin B complex, vitamin C, and vitamin E, which are essential for the proper disposal of unnecessary hormones.

During severe bouts of PMS a good diet may have to be supplemented with additional nutrients. Vitamin B6, also known as pyridoxine, serves as a natural muscle relaxant and can reduce cramps associated with PMS. This versatile vitamin also acts as a diuretic, relieving swelling, fluid retention, and breast tenderness. Vitamin B6 should be consumed on a daily basis in quantities of 200 to 400 mg and can be supplemented throughout the month. This may be part of a B-complex supplement. Remember not to exceed the suggested dosage of B6, as excessive intake of this vitamin can cause neuropathy, or inflammation of the nerves.

Magnesium, which soothes the nervous system, alleviating anxiety, irritability, nervousness, insomnia, and depression, can be quite advantageous when added to one's daily dietary intake in quantities of 500 to 1000 mg. The antispasmodic qualities of magnesium can reduce cramps and lower back pain associated with the menstrual cycle, and can also help eliminate sugar cravings. Supplements of vitamin E 200 to 600 IU can aid in the reduction of breast tenderness and are beneficial in treating cramps and fibrocystic breasts, which have a tendency to enlarge prior to menstruation. The mineral zinc 30 to 60 mg can be a useful tool in minimizing depression and irritability.

Another supplement to know about is gamma linoleic acid (GLA), a precursor of prostaglandin-E1, which is vital in coordinating neurological and hormonal functioning. This hormone-like substance can aid in the treatment of cramps, sugar cravings, muscle spasms, mood swings, depression, irritability, and breast tenderness. Common sources of GLA include evening primrose oil and black currant oil. Also, borage oil, which is actually 24 percent GLA, can provide a concentrated source of the substance in a single capsule and is an effective substitute for six evening primrose oil capsules. One 1000 mg pill of borage oil, which will supplement the body with 240 mg of GLA, should be consumed daily.

1000 mg of essential fatty acids, which can be obtained from fish and flaxseed oil, aid in the production of prostaglandin-E3, a hormone-like substance that can reduce breast tenderness. Although the essential fatty acid content of flaxseed oil is sacrificed during cooking, an ample supply can be obtained when the oil is used in salad dressings or on top of heated foods.

Natural sources of progesterone, such as Mexican yams, can prevent various forms of cancer and fibrocystic breast disease, and can also stabilize hormonal imbalances.

Isoflavones are substances useful in alleviating the mood swings of PMS. These are forms of phytoestrogen obtained from soybeans and other legumes that can help correct hormonal imbalances by joining in the competition for estrogen receptor sites. When the isoflavones occupy these receptor sites, inactive estrogen is displaced and eventually eliminated by the liver and colon. Organic sources of isoflavones, which include soybeans, peanuts, lentils, green peas, split peas, and beans, have demonstrated their equality to prescription hormonal supplements without the adverse side effects.

Exercise

As with so many conditions, exercise will make a positive difference with PMS. Research has shown that regular participation in aerobic exercise can prevent negative mood swings, alleviate cramps, reduce fluid retention, and limit sugar cravings. For maximum results, exercise should be performed three or four times per week.

Chinese Herbal Remedies

From the wide array of Chinese herbs, Lungtanxieganwan has demonstrated its capacity to reduce angry emotions associated with PMS. Another Chinese herb, Xiao Yao Wan, aids in the treatment of depression, indigestion, bloating, and poor circulation. The herbal formula called Women's Harmony can also be used to improve circulatory functioning.

Homeopathic Remedies

Several homeopathic remedies have proven their effectiveness in countering PMS, but it is important to remember that only one product should be used at a time. If the remedy you have chosen does not alleviate your symptoms, homeopaths advise discontinuing use and trying another.

The remedy lachasis can be used to combat a wide variety of symptoms, including ovarian pain, breast tenderness, and headaches. Laccaninum can be used to treat swollen breasts, while bovista eases gastrointestinal symptoms, such as diarrhea. Pulsatilla is prescribed to help alleviate the emotional state in which women become forlorn and seek consolation, and natmur is used to combat the kind of melancholy and depression that tend to intensify with consolation. Additional symptoms that can be treated with natmur include headaches and cravings for salty foods. Intense depression, severe discouragement and indifference, and a sensation that the uterus has become congested and will soon drop through the vagina are a few of the symptoms that homeopathic practitioners treat with sepia. Finally, folliculinum, a relatively recent French innovation, is reported to soothe symptoms of PMS when administered on the seventh day of the menstrual cycle in a 30 to 200c potency.

Reflexology

The ancient practice of reflexology is founded in the concept that the foot contains reflex areas that correspond to various other parts of the body. By manipulating specific parts of the foot, reflexologists seek to enhance the performance of the corresponding organs and glands. Women who have used reflexology to treat PMS often praise its benefits. The pampered treatment, soft music, and dimmed lights that often accompany reflexology treatments provide additional comforts and can promote the relief of stress.

According to reflexologist Laura Norman, the best way to understand the locations of reflex points is to visualize the human body superimposed on a foot. Accordingly, the toes correspond to the uppermost region of the body, including the eyes, nose, mouth, ears, and brain, while the ball of the toes coincides with the chest region—the heart, lungs, and bronchial tubes. The center of the foot represents the internal organs, while the heel and ankle area is associated with the pelvic area and reproductive organs. The uterus, which is symbolized on the foot by a diagonal line midway between the heel and ankle bone, can be treated by using the reflexology technique of thumb-walking around the inside area of the ankle. Rotating the thumb in a circular motion and finger-walking near the uterus point can aid in alleviating PMS.

A reflexologist can guide you on the manipulation of other reproductive reflex points. Beyond this, massaging the remaining parts of the foot can be beneficial in treating PMS because all of the systems of the body interact on a daily basis. Overall relaxation can be enhanced by running the thumbs across the bottom of the feet. While reflexology is most useful in alleviating PMS when it is practiced three or four days before menstruation starts, it can be used during and after menstruation as well.

Pressure Point Therapy

Another way of coping with PMS involves the manipulation of the body's natural pressure points. Positioning your hand three inches below the hip bone on the side of your leg, use your fingers to locate a tender spot. When you discover a suitable area you can initiate massage therapy. If the pressure point that you have selected is too sensitive for manipulation, work on the areas just above and below the spot. This procedure can also be performed on the outside of the ankle, midway between the heel and ankle bone. Once again, if this point is too delicate, try to use an area nearby.

What to Avoid

It's a good idea for everyone, but if you're concerned about PMS, be sure to avoid caffeine, alcohol, and sugar. Since many victims of PMS also suffer from hypoglycemia, sugar intake should be restricted in order to eliminate wide fluctuations in blood sugar levels. When people consume large quantities of sugar, their blood sugar level increases dramatically, and consequently, the body is forced to respond by rapidly diminishing the sugar level. Mood and energy levels plummet as a result.

Note that clinical evidence has correlated the consumption of caffeine with breast tenderness and sleep disorders. Also, the consumption of dairy products should be limited because of their tendency to increase estrogen levels within the body. As discussed, a heightened level of estrogen can lead to a deficiency of progesterone and thus bring on PMS. Foods that are hot, spicy, or acidic should be avoided by women who suffer from acute PMS. They should stay away from foods high in sodium and starch as well.

Treatment Summary

A healthful diet low in animal products and inclusive of snacks, green salad foods, and legumes, will work to minimize PMS.

Chinese herbs are available that will counter premenstrual symptoms.

Homeopathic remedies, keyed to specific complaints, have proven effective in dealing with PMS.

Research has shown that regular participation in aerobic exercise can prevent mood swings, alleviate cramps, reduce fluid retention, and limit sugar cravings.

Reflexology and pressure point therapy are manipulative techniques that can alleviate PMS.

Prostate Conditions

The prostate is a gland found between the bladder and penis. Though small, its functions are vital. Urine leaves the body through a tube in the prostate called the urethra. The prostate also provides seminal fluid, which nourishes sperm. There are two common conditions that affect the prostate, prostatic hypertrophy and prostate cancer.

Prostatic hypertrophy is an enlargement of the prostate. The condition is common in older men. Fifty to 75 percent of men over the age of 50 have prostatic hypertrophy, and 30 percent of these men have an operation for the condition. Prostatic hypertrophy is associated with the excessive intake of fat, especially saturated fat. It is also connected to the production of male hormones. Prostatic hypertrophy may develop into prostate cancer. Symptoms associated with prostatic hypertrophy can include any of the following: urination at night, decreased force of the urinary stream, hesitancy or difficulty in starting urination, dribbling, burning of the urine, discomfort when passing urine, and blood in the urine. Sometimes a mass is felt in the area of the prostate. Occasionally, there are problems with sexual potency. When prostatic hypertrophy blocks urinary flow, urine backup can result in kidney damage, bladder infections, or kidney stones.

Prostate cancer is almost as prevalent as lung cancer and is quickly becoming the number-one cancer killer of men. There are 165,000 new cases, and 35,000 deaths annually from this disease in the U.S. Prostate cancer occurs at higher rates among African Americans and older men, but is not unusual in men in their 30's and 40's. The disease is unusual in that it is generally very slow-growing; many men who have prostate cancer are unaware of it and die of other causes. Prostate cancer is linked to excess testosterone, which is believed to increase with a high-fat diet. An analogous condition in females is breast cancer, where too much fat increases estrogen levels.

There are few symptoms associated with prostate cancer. Nodules in the prostate may be felt on digital examination, although these are not necessarily malignancies. Bone pain can indicate an advanced stage of the disease after there have been metastases to the bones. Other symptoms may include inflammation and difficulty urinating. The presence of the disease is determined by the prostatic specific antigen (PSA) test. A raised PSA level almost always indicates prostate cancer. This test can even indicate the presence of microscopic cancers or the condition known as benign prostatic hyperplasia, an enlargement of the prostate. Unfortunately, the test is not always reliable, in that as many as 30 percent of patients with prostate cancer have normal PSA's. Additional diagnostic methods include transrectal ultrasounds and digital rectal examinations. Note that biopsies potentially spread cancer and are not recommended in the early stages of this disease where the cancer has not spread outside of the prostate.

Treatment

In the case of prostatic hypertrophy, the drug Proscar is the conventional therapy. The FDA warns, however, that the drug may inhibit PSA levels. Since excessive amounts of PSA are a strong indication of prostate cancer, Proscar may obscure this diagnostic sign.

If prostate cancer develops, mainstream medicine typically offers prostatectomy, or removal of the prostate, chemotherapy, and radiation. All are ineffective and often dangerous. Surgery, like biopsy, can actual spread cancer cells, and often decreases sexual potency and urinary control. PACT, a prostate support group, advocates hormonal blockers to induce cancer shrinkage, which may hold the disease at bay for several years, followed by a prostatectomy or cryosurgery (freezing of the prostate). The most common hormonal blockers are Lupron and Fludamide. As prostate cancer is generally slow growing, patients, especially those in the early stages, have time to try less harmful methods of treatment.

Nutrition

Low-fat diets are recommended, with special emphasis on complex carbohydrates, chiefly organic fruits and vegetables, raw juices, and some whole grains for their alkaline effect. A modest amount of nuts and seeds may be added. (See section on alkaline diet in Cancer article.) Foods specifically related to decreased prostate cancer risk include beans, especially soybeans, lentils, peas, tomatoes, raisins, dates, and other dried fruits. In some cases, small amounts of organic chicken and fish may be eaten. The following supplements are also recommended:

ZINC

Everyone needs zinc, but it is especially crucial for preventing prostate problems, as zinc inhibits the uptake of testosterone into the prostate. Studies indicate that 40 mg of zinc, taken daily, not only lessens the risk of prostate cancer but also helps in treatment. Pumpkin seeds are naturally high in zinc. Other good food sources of zinc are sunflower seeds, as well as eggs, poultry, seafood, peas, soybeans, and mushrooms. As an extra precaution, a zinc supplement should be taken as well, in conjunction with pyridoxine (vitamin B6), manganese, and chromium to help tissues better absorb the mineral. Vitamin A and phosphorus also increase the body's ability to use zinc efficiently.

BEE POLLEN

In addition to zinc, try bee pollen. It helps to reduce an enlarged prostate.

PROSTATE GLANDULARS

Powdered animal prostate is high in zinc and nourishing for the human prostate.

ALANINE, GLUTAMIC ACID AND GLYCINE

These amino acids, combined in equal measure, can help shrink the swelling of the prostate gland. This formula, studies show, reduces nocturia (excess urination at night), urgency, frequency, and hesitation.

VITAMIN C

High doses of vitamin C, and the minerals selenium, copper, and magnesium provide additional support to a body working to overcome prostate cancer. Intravenous vitamin C drips provide a super-saturated concentration of the vitamin in the body, which cancer patients need. This helps to remove toxic materials, mainly heavy metals, and allows the body to repair itself and return to its normal functioning capacity. Vitamin C is a prime antioxidant that neutralizes toxic free radicals.

PROTEOLYTIC ENZYMES

These help with digestion, and when taken on an empty stomach help dissolve the coating around cancer cells so that normal white blood cells can attack them.

OMEGA-3 FATTY ACIDS AND GAMMA LINOLENIC ACID

Borage, black currant seed, evening primrose oil, and flaxseed oil all have beneficial effects.

Herbs

Herbs are effective in treating benign prostatic hypertrophy as well as prostate cancer, and they do so without side effects. The following are especially helpful:

SAW PALMETTO

Saw palmetto is one of the best herbs for prostate health. It produces the same benefits as Proscar but in a shorter time and without PSA repression.

AMERICAN GINSENG AND LICORICE ROOT

These herbs are for prostate problems due to low testosterone and androgen levels. They are safe to take on a regular basis, two to three times a day.

CORN SILK

Corn silk relieves inflammation of the prostate. It is also a remedy for inflammatory conditions of the urethra, bladder, and kidneys.

PUMPKIN SEED EXTRACT

This is an excellent source of zinc and essential fatty acids, both important substances for prostate health. Pumpkin seed extract helps to tone the bladder muscles, relax the sphincter mechanism, and decongest the prostate.

PYGEUM AFRICANUM

The properties of this African evergreen tree help reduce edema and painful, urgent urination. This is because pygeum is rich in phytosterols, substances that inhibit the biosynthesis of prostaglandins, which is the process responsible for prostate inflammation. Once inhibited, prostaglandins return to normal levels, and tissue swelling decreases. Eliminating the swelling helps to normalize metabolism, blood flow, lymph drainage, and nutritional deposition. Some people have ill effects from this herb, but small amounts, used in conjunction with other modalities, usually work quite well.

SIBERIAN GINSENG, WINTERGREEN AND HYDRANGEA ROOT

These may help when there is an overproduction of hormones.

ESSIAC

This is an herbal preparation that is useful in the treatment of all cancers.

UVA URSI

This has antiseptic, diuretic, and tonic properties that target the bladder, kidneys, and urinary tract, benefiting both disorders.

UNCARIA TOMENSOA

This immune modulator from South America may return PSA levels to normal in the case of prostate cancer and help some people when all else has failed.

Homeopathic Remedies

Homeopathic remedies for particular conditions vary according to symptoms. The following remedies may be appropriate for treating prostatic hypertrophy patients with these indications:

APIS MELLIFICA

—Frequent urination with burning or stinging pain, and inflammation.

CHIMAPHILIA

—Urgency to urinate with burning pain; strain to urinate.

CONIUM MACULATUM

—Chronic enlargement; difficult urination, urine flow starts and stops. Helps soften the prostate.

FERRUM PICRICUM

—Frequent urination at night; full feeling and retention of urine.

HEPAR SULPHURIS CALCAREUM

—Dribbling urine or poor flow.

SABAL SERRULATA

—Difficult urination with enlarged prostate; constant desire to urinate.

STAPHYSAGRIA

—Urge to urinate but inability to urinate fully, feeling of bladder not being empty.

THUJA

—Enlarged prostate; sudden desire to urinate; stream is split.

Reflexology

In reflexology, the sides of the feet, below the bony part of the ankles, correspond to the reproductive system. The prostate/uterus points are on the insides of the feet, while the testicle/ovary reflexes are on the outer sides. These areas are extremely sensitive to touch, especially when there is a problem in the corresponding body parts, so proceed with caution.

Walk the fingers along the areas surrounding the ankles, applying pressure to points at every interval along the way. The finger can also be pressed into the bladder point, on the inside center part of the heels. Working these systems increases circulation and helps to speed up the healing process.

Chelation Therapy

A study performed in Switzerland administered 10 chelation treatments to one group and none to another. Follow-up over the course of 18 years revealed that the subjects receiving chelation had only one tenth the cancer deaths of the other group.

Lifestyle Considerations

Patients should exercise regularly, and take in much fresh air and light. Stress management programs may also prove invaluable and can include biofeedback, massage, and meditation.

What to Avoid

Foods to avoid include alcohol, sugar, starch, caffeine, additives and preservatives, impure water, such as water with chlorine and fluoride, hydrogenated fats, such as margarine, and foods prepared in aluminum cookware. Exposure to tobacco should be avoided as well.

Treatment Summary

A low-fat, organic diet is recommended, with emphasis on alkaline foods. Soybeans, lentils, peas, tomatoes, and dried fruits are related to decreased prostate cancer risk.

Zinc is an important nutrient for prostate conditions.

Herbal remedies include saw palmetto, pumpkin seed extract, and others.

Homeopathic remedies may be appropriate for prostatic hypertrophy patients with specific symptoms.

Chelation therapy is proven to prevent diseases associated with aging, such as prostate cancer.

Patients should exercise regularly and use techniques that will help manage stress levels.

Respiratory Illnesses

Most of us take the ability to breathe for granted. But what should be a natural act for all people can prove difficult for some. Respiratory problems range from mild conditions in which a person occasionally experiences slight difficulty breathing, to more severe levels of illness which can impede a person's ability to deal normally in society or, at the extreme, result in death.

One of the most common respiratory problems is asthma. This is a condition that periodically impairs the ability of a person to breathe. Asthma is characterized by shortness of breath, wheezing, coughing, and mucus. According to Dr. James Braly, asthma occurs because airways are irritated, supersensitive, and inflamed—not just during an asthmatic attack, but all the time. A popular misconception about asthma is that it is primarily an obstructive or constrictive airway disease. This has led to the over-prescription of adrenaline-like inhalants to dilate or enlarge these openings. Dr. Braly feels their frequent use may be responsible for the recent 300-percent increase in asthma mortality in the U.S. This distressing statistic, coupled with reports that the incidence of asthma has nearly doubled in the past decade, afflicting approximately 5 percent of Americans indicates that we have to take a serious look at our approach to this disease.

Dr. Braly emphasizes that asthma is a condition that can be caused by allergies to foods and pollutants in the environment. The actual asthmatic attack may occur hours or days after exposure, making the allergenic trigger difficult to identify. He advocates, therefore, increased use of the IgG ELISA delayed-onset food allergy assay and/or the IgE ELISA blood test for airborne allergies.

Asthma can also be triggered by emotional stress, and is associated with a sense of fear or losing control. Sometimes children develop asthma after a frightening experience. In addition, the condition has been linked to the pertussis vaccine, as studies indicate that vaccinated children have far higher incidences of asthma than do non-vaccinated children.

Bronchitis is another common respiratory problem. This disorder is an obstruction of the bronchi, or breathing tubes, that lead to the lungs. It is a condition wherein the mucous membranes of the lungs swell. Bronchitis can be short- or long-term, acute or chronic. Factors leading to the condition include childhood infections, smoking, air pollution, and long-term infections. The condition produces a dry, nonproductive cough that releases mucus, as well as fever and chest and back pain. A person with bronchitis tends to have difficulty walking briskly or with physical exertion. Other symptoms may include lung infections and blue skin, the latter being a sign that there is less oxygen and more carbon dioxide in the blood.

Chronic obstructive pulmonary disease or COPD, formerly known as emphysema, is a lung disease commonly associated with smoking and inhaling chemical pollutants. The condition manifests as the lungs become restricted or obstructed due to blocked bronchial tubes. The onset of the disease is gradual and the patient gets progressively worse. With time, an individual breathes in less and less air. As the disease advances and oxygen levels in the blood become insufficient, medication and additional oxygen are required. Although the disease targets the lungs, complications in the intestines and liver may contribute to the problem.

Treatment

Some of the natural solutions that help to combat respiratory conditions focus on prevention. Should respiratory illnesses develop, they may require medical attention and drug intervention, although natural solutions can provide supplementary help.

Nutrition

Diet plays a major role in the prevention and treatment of all these respiratory disorders. An appropriate diet is, of course, individualized, based on a person's biochemical make-up, although there are some general dietary rules that may help ease respiratory problems. Essentially, the emphasis should be on complex carbohydrates and fiber, with a variety of organic whole grains, beans, fruit, and vegetables included in the diet. Foods rich in omega-3 fatty acids are also encouraged; these include dark-meat fishes, such as salmon and tuna. Diets high in chlorophyll are cleansing. This means juicing carrots in combination with a small amount of celery or parsley. Wheatgrass juice is especially rich in chlorophyll. Radishes, horseradish, and lemon juice are healing to the lungs and should be eaten often. Foods can be eaten raw or lightly cooked. In addition, onion, garlic, ginger, cardamon, cumin, cloves, and cayenne are good herbs and spices to use when cooking.

It is also important to address any food allergies by working with a complementary physician, a doctor trained in nondrug approaches to healing, as well as in traditional medicine. An antiallergy diet can often correct or ameliorate the problem by having the patient eliminate certain foods completely, and eat others on a rotational basis. If the same food is eaten day after day, the body may become sensitized to it, but when the food is spaced four to seven days apart, there is usually no adverse reaction. Three quarters of asthmatic children and nearly half of all asthmatic adults respond to the removal of allergy-producing foods in the diet. Once allergies are diagnosed and addressed, many individuals can eliminate or greatly reduce their dependency on drugs.

Patients with respiratory illnesses may benefit from taking a teaspoon of cold-pressed virgin olive oil first thing in the morning. This helps to eliminate toxins in the intestines, liver, and lungs. Adding flaxseed oil enhances the concentration of fatty acids and can be helpful.

Supplements

A variety of nutritional supplements can be helpful in preventing and alleviating respiratory illnesses:

Nutrients that can help asthma specifically include bee pollen and honey (particularly in attacks brought on by hay fever); bromelein, an enzyme found in pineapples, that alleviates inflamed bronchi; and hydrochloric acid for attacks precipitated by insufficient amounts of stomach acid. Bromelein works even better when combined with quercetin and vitamin C.

Magnesium is an extremely important supplement because it can open the bronchioles, relaxing the muscles inside the air tubes, and stop an acute asthma attack quickly. As a preventive measure, asthmatics can benefit from large amounts of elemental magnesium supplements taken orally. The recommendation for adults is between 1000 and 1500 mg; children and infants can usually tolerate 100 to 400 mg. However, since magnesium has a laxative effect, it is best taken throughout the day with meals, rather than all at once. And, according to Dr. Alan Gaby, when magnesium is combined with calcium, vitamin C, and the B vitamins in an intravenous "cocktail," serious asthmatic symptoms subside within minutes. Magnesium is also excellent for people who are exposed routinely to toxic chemicals and suffer from bronchitis as a result.

Chlorophyll is a supplement that purifies the blood overall, enhancing its oxygen-carrying capabilities. It also chelates toxic metals out of the system. Fresh organic ½/½ dark yellow and green vegetable juices are a great source.

L-methionine, L-cysteine, N-acetyl-cysteine, and glutathione peroxidase help repair damaged tissue in the lungs by counteracting the effects of smoke and other environmental toxins. These substances protect cell membranes from the ravages of free radical damage, lock up toxic chemicals at the cellular level, and speed up the removal of poisons via the liver.

Other supplements recommended to prevent free radical damage and defend against inhalant lung injury are beta carotene (50,000 IU or lower if skin turns orange); vitamin C (up to 10,000 mg divided into five doses); vitamin E (300 IU); and coenzyme Q10.

Some nutrients may be helpful when one is being weaned off prescription medications. These include calcium; coenzyme Q10; dimethylglycine; essential fatty acids; GLA, found in evening primrose, black currant seed, and borage oils; pantothenic acid; and selenium.

Herbs

There are numerous herbs that may be beneficial to people with respiratory illnesses. Garlic, for one, helps fight infections. Mullein tea has historically been used in France to treat inflammatory conditions of the lungs. Easter lily is an old bronchial remedy used to expel heavy stagnant mucus from the lungs, and can be purchased as a flower essence. Yerba santa is a Southwestern herb that grows in semi-desert regions. Its shiny leaf is covered with a resin, an indication of a plant that helps the respiratory system. Resins are sticky substances that pick up and expel mucus, so that the air passages can open up. Yerba santa helps clear out the lungs' membranes and linings, and is especially good for people worn out from a deteriorating cough. For this reason, it has been used for the treatment of tuberculosis.

Other good herbs for respiratory clearing are white pine, spruce, marshmallow root, licorice root, lungwort, and comfrey. Fresh thyme, nettles, and fenugreek are commonly used throughout Europe for treating various lung conditions. Horseradish, taken with more soothing herbs, helps to get rid of lung debris. It can be prepared by scraping, rinsing, shredding, and placing in oil overnight. Ginger is an expectorant herb that clears mucous secretions from the bronchi. One squirt of ginger extract into the mouth will clear the bronchi in a few minutes. For asthma, a hot ginger compress can be applied to the chest to relieve congestion. This method involves soaking a cloth in ginger tea, applying to the chest, and alternating with a cold-water compress several times. Myrrh has also been used successfully for treating lung diseases. However, it should be used in small quantities and only for short periods of time, to prevent toxicity.

For asthma patients, the following are also recommended: cayenne pepper, ginkgo biloba, lobelia, and slippery elm bark. In addition, wild cherry and licorice will work as expectorants to release mucus, while the relaxation of muscles can be achieved through the use of antispasmodic nervines, such as scullcap and valerian, as well as crampbark.

Detoxification

Healing foods and supplements will not work nearly as well in a toxic system as in a clean one, since weak digestion from the buildup of residues in the bowel can interfere with nutrient absorption and trigger inflammatory responses. For this reason, complementary physicians may recommend enemas, colonics, and high-fiber nutrients, such as bran, psyllium, and bentonite. A catnip and garlic enema can be taken twice a week with beneficial results. In addition, exercise and deep breathing of fresh air will eliminate mucus from the lungs.

Aromatherapy

The inhalation of volatile herbs with expectorant properties, such as eucalyptus, hyssop, and thyme, helps clear the lungs of mucus. In addition, a potpourri of lavender, figwort, mullein, horehound, and lungwort can be heated and the steam inhaled. An aromatherapist can guide you in the use of additional essences and techniques.

Homeopathic Remedies

Homeopathic medicines used to restore respiratory health include ipecacuanha, which may be recommended by homeopathic physicians for violent coughing, chest restriction, and choking. Natrum sulphuricum may be suggested for rattling in the chest that gets worse in damp weather, and spongia tosta is prescribed for dry barking coughs, with wheezing, and hoarseness that worsen in the cold air. To open bronchial passages, adrealinum is sometimes used, and ephedra vulgaris is prescribed for queasiness and weakness. Other homeopathic remedies for respiratory problems include belladonna, which may alleviate breathing difficulty, and soidago virgaurea, which aids in stemming heavy mucus, and curbing coughs.

Stress Management

Relaxation techniques are helpful in overcoming feelings of fear and loss of control, which can accelerate a breathing crisis. Deep yogic breathing can immediately replace a sense of tightness in the chest with a calming sensation. Relaxation can also be mastered through biofeedback, meditation, and self-hypnosis.

Magnets

Advocates of magnetic healing report that the negative pole of a magnet can decrease inflammation, and increase oxygen to an area. However, magnets should not be placed directly on the lungs or used on the chest if a pacemaker or defibrillator is present. For best results, wrap three or four stacked plastiform magnets in an ace bandage and place over the chest area for several minutes. Magnets should be approximately 4 x 12 inches. This will bathe the whole area in a magnetic field, providing relief. If constriction occurs, remove the magnets and try again later.

Another recommendation is to drink eight to ten glasses of water that is negatively ionized by a magnet. A magnetic bed pad is also helpful, but should not be used for longer than eight to ten hours; otherwise it is weakening.

Chelation Therapy

The EDTA chelation pulls out toxic metals from the body, such as cadmium, lead, and calcium, and therefore promotes healing.

What to Avoid

A prime consideration for those with asthma should be the identification and elimination of allergens in foods and in the environment. Although any food is suspect, the ones most likely to trigger asthma are dairy products, eggs, chocolate, wheat, corn, citrus fruits, and fish. Preservatives and additives may also be detrimental. In fact, a commonly used food coloring, yellow dye #5, is believed to trigger asthma in as many as 100,000 Americans. Sulfites, preservatives found in many alcoholic beverages and added to salad bar foods in restaurants, are also known to provoke asthma attacks. Monosodium glutamate (MSG), an ingredient used in Chinese and Indian cooking, can also exacerbate symptoms.

In all respiratory conditions, mucous-forming dairy foods, such as milk and cheese, can exacerbate clogging of the lungs and should be avoided. Salt should also be omitted from the diet.

Treatment Summary

A vegetable-foods-based diet is recommended, with any allergy-producing foods identified and eliminated.

Magnesium is one of the nutrients important for those with respiratory problems.

Herbs may be beneficial to people with respiratory illnesses.

Since healing foods and supplements will not work optimally in a toxic system, the following detoxification methods are recommended: colonic therapy, high-fiber nutrients, exercise, and deep breathing of fresh air.

Aromatherapy may help promote respiratory healing.

A number of homeopathic remedies are used for patients with respiratory illnesses.

Stress management is a crucial part of any respiratory health regimen.

Chelation therapy acts as a lung-cleansing agent, and reverses free radical damage.

Sickle Cell Anemia

Sickle cell anemia is a genetic disease affecting over 72,000 African Americans. This painful and disfiguring chronic condition attacks red blood cells, causing joint pain, fatigue, breathing difficulties, blood clots, fever, and long-term anemia.

During a sickle cell crisis, red blood cells lose their shape and elasticity due to an oxygen depletion. The characteristic reshaping of the cells into sickle figures causes restricted blood flow, especially to the pelvic region.

Patients are often hospitalized for weeks, where they are given painkillers and tranquilizers. Repeated crises often lead to physical deformities and severe emotional distress.

Treatment

Drug Therapy

In the U.S., the cancer drug Hydroxyurea has been prematurely approved for use, based on studies showing it to lessen the incidence of sickle cell crisis in patients receiving it. But what has been ignored is the fact that patients given this drug tend to develop bone marrow depression, and that long-term use has been associated with leukemia. The drug is considered too toxic for children, although it is approved for use by adults.

Ozone Therapy

Small amounts of medical ozone, added to the patient's blood, have been found to prevent flare-ups and resolve a sickle cell crisis in half the time of existing treatments, with no adverse side effects. This may be due to ozone's ability to make red blood cells more flexible.

Trials in Havana have led to ozone's approval as a treatment modality by the Cuban Ministry of Health. It is currently available throughout the island, where it is used both prophylactically and during crises.

Sinusitis

Sinusitis is an inflammation of the cavities in the skull, which are found behind the eyes, forehead, nose, and cheekbones. The condition is usually caused by bacteria, viruses, or allergic reactions. Allergy-related sinus conditions may begin as allergic rhinitis, an inflammation of the nasal membranes, and then move to the sinuses. People with compromised immune symptoms are more susceptible to sinusitis.

The combination of inflamed sinuses and thick mucus often leads to pressure and pain. Specific symptoms of sinusitis can include headaches—sometimes even migraines—as well as postnasal drip, a cough, facial tenderness, and occasionally fever. Infections in the sinuses should be immediately addressed; otherwise, they may spread to other parts of the body.

Treatment

Typical treatment for sinusitis involves the administration of antibiotics, which can have dangerous long-term consequences, and decongestants. Fortunately, safer natural treatments and lifestyle changes are highly effective, and without negative side effects.

Diet and Lifestyle

Vegetarian diets that are high in fiber, and free of mucous-forming foods, can help to prevent and eliminate sinusitis. Freshly squeezed raw juices contain beneficial enzymes for fighting infections. An enzyme that is especially helpful is bromelain, found in pineapple juice.

People who get respiratory infections may also benefit from rest, according Dr. Thomas Sinclair. They needn't stop activities completely, but should perform them in moderation for a week following the onset of sinusitis.

In addition to extra rest and a good diet, Dr. Sinclair recommends the following supplements for fighting sinusitis infections: vitamin C—500 mg every 2 hours; beta carotene—up to 50,000 IU 3 times a day; zinc lozenges or zinc picolinate; coenzyme Q10; and quercetin.

Herbs

When a fever is present it is helpful to drink peppermint or elderberry flower tea. For building immunity, echinacea, goldenseal, and chaparral can be taken in tincture, capsule, or tea form. The best time to take these antibiotic herbs is when symptoms first appear. As many as four to six capsules can be taken at first (less if they cause a digestive upset). Symptoms should decrease within 24 hours. At that point, the amount should be gradually lessened. Cayenne and garlic are also excellent for fighting infection.

An effective gargle to get rid of a sore throat and the mucus in the sinuses consists of equal parts of powdered clove, cayenne pepper, and ginger. One level teaspoon should be added to warm water. To clear clogged nasal passages, horseradish, with a drop of lemon juice, can be placed in the mouth.

External Therapies

Moist heat packs applied over the forehead, eyes, and nose three times daily provide relief from sinus congestion, many people report. An herbal equivalent of a moist heat pack is dry powdered ginger and pureed lotus root (available in Asian markets), made into a paste. This should be applied to areas above and below the eye; it heats the area, but does not burn it.

Steam inhalation is also effective and is simple to do. Just heat a pot of water on the stove and add a drop of one or more essential oils. Thyme is antibiotic and antifungal, while eucalyptus and peppermint oil are excellent decongestants. Breathing in the vapors is soothing as well as healing.

Severe sinus infections may need nasal irrigation, which involves the use of warm salt water or boiled water with goldenseal. To do this, towels should be placed on the bed. Then, while one is lying on the towels, with the head extending back off the edge of the bed, either of these solutions should be slowly dropped into one nostril, and then the other. After treatment, the head should be slowly and carefully raised.

Reflexology

To combat sinusitis, reflexologist Diane Rooney recommends working on the tops and sides of all the toes, and the upper part of the left heel that is in line with the fourth toe. Since the toes are far more sensitive than the heel, she notes, work less deeply here. After treatments, more sinus drainage may occur, a sign that the body is healing naturally. Don't take medication to stop drainage at this point, Rooney advises. Just help it along with hot baths and herbs or aromatherapy.

What to Avoid

Common foods that tend to produce allergic reactions include those that people generally think of as healthful, such as dairy products and wheat; both are mucus-forming. Peanuts, corn, and sugar are other common culprits. Smoke is another irritant to be avoided, both through direct and passive inhalation. Other irritants to avoid are air pollutants, such as car exhaust and even perfumes.

Treatment Summary

A vegetarian diet, high in fiber and free of mucus-forming foods, is recommended to alleviate or eliminate sinusitis.

Freshly squeezed raw juices are helpful, particularly pineapple juice.

Recommended supplements include vitamin C, beta carotene, zinc, co-enzyme Q10, and quercetin.

Antibiotic herbal teas may be helpful.

Symptomatic relief from sinusitis can be eased through moist heat packs, steam inhalation, and nasal irrigation.

Massaging areas of the foot, using the principles of reflexology, can provide relief of sinusitis.

See also: Allergies, Headaches

Skin Cancer

In the United States, skin cancers are the leading type of malignant disease. Forty to 50 percent of all people develop the condition at least once by the time they are 65. Most common is basal cell carcinoma, a benign and slow-growing form of cancer that appears as a roughening somewhere on the body, most often on exposed areas, such as the face or neck. Other, more dangerous, skin cancers are squamous cell carcinomas and malignant melanomas. Squamous cell carcinoma is usually a result of too much sun exposure, and appears as a red, painless bump, while a melanoma generally shows up as a flat, dry, brown or black skin patch with an irregular border. The latter two types of cancer grow very quickly, and metastasize to other parts of the body through the lymphatic system.

As with all chronic diseases, cancers have multiple and long-range causes that can be subsumed under the term lifestyle. These include denatured food, air and water pollution, and imbalances brought on by parasites, fungi, bacteria, viruses, toxic chemicals, and heavy metals. Skin cancers in particular are directly attributable to sun exposure. Sunny Arizona has the highest incidence of skin cancer anywhere in the world. In addition to more general concerns, such as nutrition, exercise, and avoiding exposure to toxins, prevention and treatment of skin cancers involve wearing hats, long-sleeved clothing, and sunscreen when out in the sun. Note that sunscreens should be checked for ingredients, as some of these are themselves carcinogenic.

Treatment

Standard treatment for basal cell carcinoma, the benign form of skin cancer, is removal of the tumor through surgery or freezing. When dealt with early, these tumors rarely pose a problem once removed.

Orthodox approaches for malignant skin cancers are not nearly as successful. These spread quickly and usually reappear, even after removal.

Diet

Attention must be paid to balancing the blood pH, as research indicates that maintenance of proper alkaline balance inhibits the proliferation of cancer cells. The blood pH should be between 7.2 and 7.4, ideally. To get the desired effect, the diet should consist of 80 percent alkaline-forming foods. Eating raw fruits and vegetables will create this effect. Many nuts, seeds, grains, and legumes are also good.

Dr. Gerson's diet therapy has demonstrated success in the treatment of all skin cancers. The program involves extensive cleansing using organic juices, coffee enemas and other means. Research shows that in cases where the cancer had spread to the lymph glands, people who underwent operations to remove as much tumor as possible and then used the Gerson therapy had five-year survival rates of 92 percent (early stage) and 80 percent (late stage). This therapy is practiced today by Dr. Gar Hildebrand, who can be reached at 800-759-2966.

Herbs

A classical herbal ointment, commonly referred to as the black salve and made primarily from sanguinaria or blood root, is helpful in treating skin cancers, as it causes the lesion to come to a head and fall off. Blood root extract must be used under the supervision of a qualified physician; skin must be continually monitored and particular attention paid to preventing and treating secondary infections.

Pau d'arco has long been used by the indigenous peoples of tropical America to heal a variety of serious illnesses, including cancer and syphilis. Scientists have found that this herb contains a substance that works against various kinds of tumors by inducing cancer cell death without harming healthy cells. Another herb used for cancer, chaparral, has potentially toxic properties. It can be beneficial, though, when used under the guidance of a qualified health practitioner.

Supplements

Nutrients important in the prevention and treatment of skin cancers include quercetin, pycnogenol, coenzyme Q10, selenium, vitamin A, and beta carotene. Maitake mushrooms are recommended too.

What to avoid

Substances to stay away from include pesticides, synthetic hormones, and antibiotics, including those used in animal-derived foods. Foods that foster acidity should be minimized, and include meat, dairy products, caffeine, sugar, carbonated beverages, liquor, and processed foods.

Treatment Summary

The standard treatment for benign skin cancer is surgery or freezing. Unfortunately, malignant skin cancer is much less responsive to conventional solutions.

A cleansing, highly alkaline diet contributes to success in the treatment of all skin cancers.

Several herbs can aid in the treatment of skin cancer, including blood root, pau d'arco, and chaparral.

Nutrients to use in fighting skin cancer include quercetin, pycnogenol, and coenzyme Q10, among others.

See also: Cancer

Skin Conditions

The skin is a thin layer of tough tissue that comprises the covering of the body. While it protects all of our internal systems, it is also connected to these, so it can react to infections anywhere in the body. Further, if a person is not careful, the skin may also be affected when it is exposed to environmental toxins. Regardless of whether skin irritations originate internally or externally, they are not only uncomfortable, but may cause more severe ramifications, such as scarring and bleeding. Thus, it is important to understand how to prevent and treat the most common skin conditions.

Common Conditions

Acne

This common complaint—commonly referred to as pimples—is caused by bacteria and other irritants embedded underneath the skin's oil glands and hair follicles. It is generally a result of improper hygiene and poor diet, i.e., excessive amounts of processed, fatty, and fried foods, as well as dairy, meat, and sugar. Generally, the liver and kidneys work to cleanse the system of toxins. However, when an excessive amount of germs exist in a person's system, an extra burden is placed on the skin to remove them. If the bacteria are unable to be cleansed from the system, this type of inflammation is the result. Acne tends to develop mainly on the face, chest, back, and shoulders. Generally, the condition is associated with adolescence, but in some individuals, it persists into adulthood and can leave permanent scarring.

Psoriasis

This is a chronic condition whereby the body produces an excess of skin cells, characterized by thick, dry, red, scaly patches over the skin. It affects fewer than 2 percent of all Americans, occurring in people who are highly toxic—particularly those with poor diet and liver function. It is also believed that many individuals have a genetic predisposition to this problem. It is inclined to appear and reappear, but psoriasis never really goes away. Flare-ups of this condition seem to be brought on by stress. While this problem may present itself anywhere on the body, the most common sites are the arms, scalp, ears, knees, and pubic area. It can even cause changes in the fingernails, such as splitting and dimpling. Joint swelling may accompany the disease as well.

Fungal Rashes

These are common rashes caused by infection in various areas of the body. Tinea cruris (more commonly referred to as ''jock itch'') is a reddened, inflamed, and itchy rash found on the groin or buttock crease. Tinea versicolor is a result of excessive exposure to the sun and mainly affects the chest and back. It appears as a dark, flat, scaly rash that can result in areas of decoloration in dark-skinned individuals. Athlete's foot is a red, itchy rash occurring between the toes and in the web spaces. Ringworm presents itself mainly in children and is identified by a red, circular, ring-like inflammation.

Cysts and Abscess

When a sebaceous gland becomes clogged, it will start to progressively enlarge to form a bump under the skin, referred to as a sebaceous cyst. It consists of a fluid that, when infected, causes redness and tenderness. Therefore, if a cyst is not treated immediately, it can develop into an abscess, which is a concentrated accumulation of pus. Another cause of abscess can be skin injuries that are left unattended. This problem generally tends to form on the armpits, genital areas, buttocks, and lower extremities.

Dermatitis

This covers a broad array of skin irritations. It generally refers to a red, inflammatory rash which may include scaling and blisters. It can also be accompanied by an itching, burning, or painful sensation. One type of dermatitis is contact dermatitis, which is most commonly a result of exposure to poison ivy or poison oak. These are plants that produce an irritating oil that, when in contact with the human skin, can cause it to break out in this type of reaction. This same response may also be the result of handling certain common metals, such as nickel, contained in a variety of everyday products.

Another type of skin inflammation in this category is irritant eczema. This is an irritation that is caused by an allergic reaction to impurities or environmental factors (e.g., chemicals in food and soaps; cold weather or heat). Irritant eczema is most common among people who need to wash their hands several times a day and don't allow their hands to dry completely (such as health care and restaurant workers).

Yet another type of dermatitis is seborrheic dermatitis. This is generally due to a genetic predisposition and is typically found in infants and patients with Parkinson's disease. While seborrheic dermatitis produces most of the symptoms common to this category of skin problems, it generally does not produce itching. It tends to occur around the nose, chin, eyebrows, ears, and lips.

Treatment

Conventional treatments for these skin conditions typically deal with the problem once it has emerged. The solutions consist mainly of medicated topical creams and ointments to clear the infected area. However, these may produce side effects, given that the medications often contain antibiotics, steroids, and hormones. Further, since they do not address the cause of the problem, their effects are usually temporary. Natural solutions, on the other hand, are simple, do not produce side effects and focus on prevention so that individuals may lessen their susceptibility to the problem.

Diet

In order to help the system cleanse toxins from the body to guard against infection related to acne, psoriasis, and abscess, a person's diet should be optimized. The best foods for healthy, attractive skin are low in fat and protein, and high in complex carbohydrates. Generally, a high-fiber, vegetarian diet is best. Foods should be eaten as close to their natural state as possible, as opposed to being refined or processed. Good foods for the skin are rich in vitamins A and C, beta carotene, and chlorophyll. They include beet greens, carrots, egg yolk, potatoes, yams, peppers, artichokes, and dark green vegetables. Pure water is also essential for clear skin. At least five 8-ounce glasses are needed daily. Two to three 8-ounce servings of freshly made juice are important as well. Carrot juice combined with a small amount of green vegetable juice contains an abundant amount of nutrients.

It is important to note, when talking about skin conditions, that allergies to certain foods may aggravate these conditions. Common food allergens are corn, soy, wheat, and peanuts. A naturopathic or complementary physician can help you identify these.

Herbs

Herbs can help the skin in numerous ways. Some herbs improve liver and kidney function, thus helping clear the body of toxins that can trigger acne and psoriasis. Other herbs help the skin more directly.

To improve liver function, herbs to consider are agrimony, barberry, dandelion root, echinacea, milk thistle, sassafras, yellow dock, red clover, and sarsaparilla. The kidneys benefit from buchu, parsley, celery seed, corn silk, cleavers, and goldenrod.

To cleanse and nourish the skin directly, one can ingest burdock root, Oregon grape root, or yellow dock. One can also nourish the skin externally through steam treatments or baths that help open up pores and push out toxins. Steam treatments can be made by pouring boiled water over a handful of herbs, placing a towel over the head, and leaning over the container. Herbs recommended for this type of treatment are strawberry leaves, eucalyptus, thyme, and wintergreen. For bathing, herbalist Lynn Newman recommends that hot water be poured over a mixture of chamomile, witch hazel, nettles, echinacea, and calendula. After allowing this to steep for an hour, it should be strained and poured into a tub of water.

Herbs that can be applied directly to the skin to help stop itching include aloe vera, lavender, calendula, and oats. An herb that can prevent the spread of poison oak or poison ivy and can be applied directly to the skin is jewel weed.

Supplements

Nutrients can be valuable in the prevention and treatment of skin conditions and their symptoms. Consider the following:

CHROMIUM

This is perhaps the single most important nutrient for the skin. It balances blood sugar and lowers stress, both of which have an impact on skin problems. In addition to supplement form, chromium can be found in brewer's yeast, complex carbohydrates, and fresh fruit.

ZINC

When taken in the recommended dosage of 30-150 mg daily, this nutrient can prevent acanthosis, which is a thickening of the skin seen in serious cases of acne, eczema, and psoriasis. It is as effective as the antibiotic tetracycline, without the side effects. Zinc's usefulness may be due to the fact that it helps release vitamin A. Good food sources of zinc include eggs and seafood, garlic, onions, and sea vegetables.

VITAMIN A

Taking a minimum of 10,000 IU daily has been shown to cure acne, due to vitamin A's antiviral action The water-soluble form, palmitate, is proven to cure stubborn plantar warts as well. Since there is no toxicity from water-soluble A, up to 100,000 IU can be safely used.

VITAMIN E

In order to heal skin lesions and scar tissue, both internally and on the surface, 200-800 IU daily of vitamin E can be used. This supplement also helps skin stay younger longer.

VITAMIN B6

Pyridoxine, or vitamin B6, protects against infection. This nutrient can help prevent or treat acne, especially in premenstrual women.

LECITHIN

This supplement provides fatty acids needed for healthy skin, and is effective in treating many dermatological disorders. Lecithin helps the body to better utilize the fat-soluble vitamins A, D, and E. Evening primrose oil, borage oil, and black currant seed oil are important sources of essential fatty acids, which work well in conjunction with lecithin.

Detoxification Methods

Bowel detoxification with enemas or colonics is helpful for improving skin conditions, particularly acne, eczema, and psoriasis. When one improves intestinal function and overcomes liver congestion, the skin becomes less burdened, and takes on a more healthy appearance. Colonics can help even long-term psoriasis sufferers resolve itching and sores.

Magnetic Therapy

Removing toxic wastes from the body through magnetic therapy is another approach to improving skin problems. Sleeping on a magnetic bed is used as a way to increase oxygen to the entire system and remove acidity. Additionally, magnets help to eliminate inflammation. Magnets can be placed directly on lesions, but to ensure cleanliness, it is suggested that cotton be placed between the magnet and the lesion. If an area is too tender for magnets, spraying magnetically charged water over the area is a good substitute. Be sure to use the negative pole of the magnet only.

Reflexology

Another way of improving eliminative function to help prevent and overcome skin disorders is with reflexology, a type of massage technique that applies pressure to specific points on the feet that correspond to other areas of the body. To aid the liver in removal of toxins, one can massage the under part of the foot from the ball down toward the middle area. To help the kidneys in the process of excreting fluid from the body, pressure should be applied to the area in the middle of the underside of the foot. The nervous system can also be worked to alleviate stress associated with skin conditions. The area to which pressure should be applied is the inner edge of the foot, starting at the heel and moving upward to the top of the toes. Then, one should massage across all toes. This procedure stimulates the spinal cord and brain.

Homeopathic Remedies

When deciding which homeopathic remedy to choose, consider the one that most closely addresses the symptoms. One of the following formulas may prove useful. But if it does not, seek the guidance of a trained homeopathic practitioner.

CALCAREA SULPHURICA

This formula is indicated for boils and acne when there are pimples at the rim of the scalp that bleed when scratched.

HEPAR SULPHURIS CALCAREUM

This helps moist skin that is very sensitive to dry cold air and touch. Boils can be treated with this remedy.

ABROTANNUM

This solution is specifically used for boils, particularly those that recur on various parts of the body (sometimes as a reaction to antibiotics in the treatment of acne).

SULPHUR

This is for dry, itchy skin that feels worse in heat or after bathing.

BELLADONNA

In some cases of contact dermatitis, where a sudden rash is hot, dry, red, burning, and occasionally itchy, belladonna, given in pellets that are placed under the tongue, may provide relief.

APIS MOLLIFICA

For heat rashes that are bright red and inflamed, this remedy should reverse the condition.

PULSATILLA

This can be used in some cases of dermatitis, where an itchy rash may worsen with heat or when exposed to air.

UTICA URENS

This is another solution for contact dermatitis in which the rash may be itchy and prickly and where red blotches are present. This can either be taken as pellets placed under the tongue or used in a tincture applied directly to the rash.

DULCAMARA

For cases of dermatitis in which the skin reacts to an upset stomach or after exposure to cold, wet weather, this remedy is helpful. Usually, this kind of skin irritation is present on the hands, arms, and face, and is characterized by red spots and eruptions.

CALENDULA

This can be applied directly to the skin for general skin irritations, after the infection has cleared.

RHUS TOXICODENDRON

For the prevention of poison ivy, rhus tox should be used in pellets only and taken prior to exposure to the plant. It can also be used in the very early stages of this rash.

CROTON TIGLIUM

This should be used in the more advanced stages of poison ivy, where there is extreme itching, where burning occurs after scratching, and where there may be blisters that leak.

ANACARDIUM

This is another treatment for extreme cases of poison ivy. While the symptoms are the same as for croton tiglium, they also tend to become exacerbated when warm water is applied. This remedy should be taken in pellets placed under the tongue.

What to Avoid

Avoid refined foods, which are devoid of trace minerals needed for healing the skin. Also, beware of fried and fatty foods, chocolate, other sweets, soft drinks, alcohol, and milk. These contain substances that the body converts into prostaglandin-E2. This, in turn, suppresses the immune system and causes an inflammatory reaction.

Stress should also be avoided, since many skin problems are aggravated when an individual is tense and upset.

Treatment Summary

A diet that is low in fat, moderate in protein and high in complex carbohydrates is recommended to help cleanse toxins from the body and thus decrease the chance of skin problems.

A variety of herbs, taken internally or used externally, can improve skin health.

Chromium is an important nutrient for the skin. Others that are helpful are zinc, vitamins A, C, and B6, and lecithin.

Detoxification methods such as enemas or colonics can be helpful for clearing up skin conditions.

Magnetic therapy and reflexology are additional techniques used to improve the condition of the skin.

Homeopathic remedies are keyed to specific skin conditions and symptoms.

Stroke

Because of the similarity between heart attacks and strokes, the two are sometimes confused. Both involve a cutoff of blood supply: In a heart attack, the supply to the heart—and consequently to all the other organs—is cut off, while with a stroke, blood supply to the brain is cut off, as a result of a clot or a hemorrhage. Once this happens, oxygen becomes depleted and brain tissue dies. This can ultimately result in paralysis, blindness, speech difficulties, loss of function in an arm or leg, and other serious disabilities. There may also be cognitive impairment, i.e., the person cannot think or remember as well as before.

Strokes affect people of all ages. In older people they are usually associated with high blood pressure, elevated cholesterol, and blocked arteries. Younger people can have strokes as a result of congenital abnormalities. Certain drugs, such as cocaine and amphetamines, and the overuse of cold medications containing ephedra, can bring them on as well.

Symptoms

A stroke can produce different symptoms depending upon the part of the brain that is affected and the length of time that the brain is without oxygen. Small strokes may escape awareness and produce slight numbness on the face or another part of the body. Severe strokes can cause any number of symptoms, including paralysis, loss of speech, loss of memory, loss of movement, an inability to swallow, or death.

Prevention and Treatment

The best way to prevent a stroke is to maximize total systemic health. A complementary physician, one who combines traditional and holistic medicine, can determine whether risk factors for stroke are present, and educate the patient on how to lessen them if they are. Such a doctor helps people to lower cholesterol levels, keep blood pressure down, and unblock arteries. Chelation therapy is often recommended for this purpose. A series of treatments can open up the arteries and eliminate the risk of stroke.

Hyperbaric Oxygen Therapy

It was once thought that brain cell damage was irreversible. But this is not always so. Hyperbaric (high-pressure) oxygen therapy can produce a successful turnabout in most stroke patients. When this therapy is used within the first 24 hours of a stroke, aftereffects may never manifest. And even when the treatment is used years later, dramatic improvements can be seen, as many lingering symptoms disappear. In fact, people who have tried every other form of treatment, to no avail, often find success with hyperbaric oxygen therapy.

While this may seem hard to fathom, the reason can be scientifically explained. During a stroke, only a small area of the brain actually dies. This is the part supplied by the blocked artery. Surrounding tissue is injured, but not necrotic. It receives some oxygen from peripheral arteries, but not enough to keep it fully alive and healthy. Hyperbaric oxygen revitalizes this injured tissue, and restores it to fuller function.

Another reason for tissue damage with stroke is brain swelling. During the initial cerebrovascular accident, as a stroke is called, dying tissue swells and squeezes into surrounding areas. Pressure on blood vessels causes loss of oxygen. That, in turn, causes paralysis and other stroke-related injuries. Hyperbaric oxygen reverses the swelling, and in so doing reverses many symptoms, even years later, since brain tissue does not die suddenly. It stays alive many years after the stroke.

Hyperbaric oxygen therapy is more successful when combined with chelation and antioxidant therapies.

Magnesium

The development of a genetically engineered drug called TPA has recently been praised as a significant advance in treating patients who have suffered strokes. But this drug's $2000 cost, and the possible side effect of brain hemorrhage, have hindered its becoming widely used. Interestingly, the natural substance magnesium sulfate, which costs only about $5, is safer and therefore more beneficial than its unnatural counterpart. Not just a treatment, magnesium sulfate is helpful in avoiding stroke as well. Between 800 and 1500 mg can be taken daily as a preventive measure, and the bulk of that should be taken before bedtime.

Other Supplements

In addition to magnesium, these nutrients can help prevent strokes or speed up recovery:

MULTIVITAMIN
Make sure this contains between 3 and 6 mg of copper, as a copper deficiency has been linked to strokes.

B COMPLEX
B-complex vitamins nourish the brain and help the mind overcome depression. B vitamins can be obtained from blue-green algae or bee pollen, 50 mg 3 times a day.

VITAMIN E
This powerful antioxidant helps reduce clotting. Start slowly with 200-800 IU a day and increase to 800-1000 IU.

SELENIUM
Selenium should be taken along with vitamin E to improve its action and to keep tissues elastic, 200 mg.

PYCNOGENOL
Pycnogenol keeps collagen elastic and softens blood platelets so that they can move more efficiently, 400 mg.

COENZYME Q10
This is one of the most important nutrients for getting oxygen into the tissues, heart, and brain. Approximately 200 mg should be taken daily.

LECITHIN
Two capsules taken with each meal help to protect the brain, deter cardiovascular disease, and reduce cholesterol.

VITAMIN C
Take plenty of this vitamin to strengthen arterial walls, thereby preventing a stroke or heart attack from occurring. Vitamin C should be taken along with bioflavonoids, 5,000–20,000 mg.

Herbs

Ginkgo 125 mg a day, is recommended for the brain. Other herbs that help prevent strokes are the same ones used to help the heart. These include hawthorn, garlic, cayenne, and blueberry leaves.

Aromatherapy

Essential oils can play a vital role in the recovery of stroke patients. Oils that stimulate circulation can be highly effective in helping patients overcome the temporary paralysis that often accompanies strokes. In English intensive ward units, essential oils of lavender, lemon, and geranium are used for this purpose. For stimulating a return of memory, rosemary, clary sage, peppermint, rose, or basil can be given. Under the guidance of an aromatherapist, a few drops of the pure essence can be added to water and taken two or three times a day. Essences can also be placed on a tissue and breathed in, or vaporized in the room.

Emotional Support

Depression often accompanies a stroke. The willingness of friends and family to help means a lot to the patient in recovery, and can speed up the healing process. It is important to smile, and helpful to think positively, say affirmations, pray, meditate, or find other ways to keep upbeat.

What to Avoid

When in the presence of a person who has had a stroke, never offer the person anything to drink. If the ability to swallow has been lost, the person could choke.

Treatment Summary

To prevent stroke, a complementary physician can determine risk factors and recommend ways to lessen them.

Magnesium supplementation is preventative.

Other anti-stroke nutrients are the B-complex vitamins, vitamins E and C, selenium, pycnogenol, coenzyme Q10, and lecithin. A multivitamin containing copper is a good idea.

Helpful herbs are ginkgo, hawthorn, garlic, cayenne, and blueberry leaves.

Remedies effective in treating stroke patients are hyperbaric oxygen therapy and magnesium sulfate.

Aromatherapy can aid in stroke patients' recovery.

Emotional support of the stroke patient can speed up the healing process.

TMJ Dysfunction

Temporomandibular joint dysfunction is an abnormal condition characterized by facial pain and problems with the use of the lower jaw. Clicking or popping noises can accompany chewing or other movement of the jaw, and pain may affect not only the jaw itself, but the neck, face, ear, and shoulder. Headaches and toothaches are sometimes part of the TMJ dysfunction picture—even if all the teeth are healthy. There can also be dizziness, difficulty with opening the mouth, and inflammation of the muscles around the mouth, to the extent that they may spasm and prevent closing of the mouth. TMJ problems are widespread enough that Americans spend about $1 billion yearly on treatment and drugs to alleviate them.

Causes

Poor bite is one cause of TMJ problems; typically, new dental work, such as braces, can alter the alignment of teeth, which will then result in TMJ dysfunction. Stress is another common cause of TMJ dysfunction, and the stress caused by hormonal changes, as with premenstrual tension, can bring on or exacerbate the condition.

Indeed, TMJ dysfunction does occur more frequently in women than in men. In addition to premenstrual changes, the physiological changes of pregnancy—i.e., hormonal shifts, weight gain, the loosening of ligaments, and general stress—can foster TMJ dysfunction. And nursing mothers sometimes experience TMJ problems if they throw their bodily alignment out of whack by habitually nursing without proper postural support. The problem stems from the fact that the jaw is not an isolated joint; it's part of the craniosacral system, which extends from the feet upwards and lies along the center of the body. So misalignment occurring in any part of this system, such as the upper back or neck, can get translated into TMJ pain.

Treatment

There are a number of approaches to alleviating TMJ dysfunction, with surgery being the treatment of very last resort. (That's because there is no guarantee of success with surgery and it too often leaves patients with worse jaw problems than they had before they underwent the procedures. Also, most TMJ patients do get better with less drastic remedies.)

One of the less drastic approaches to the condition is craniosacral therapy, usually undertaken by an osteopath or chiropractor. What the doctor does is to try to establish the correct balance between the pelvis, spine, and cranium; breathing techniques may be incorporated into this approach, in order to effect musculoskeletal changes.

Other effective treatments of jaw dysfunction include acupuncture; progressive relaxation training, which has been shown effective both with and without biofeedback; intraoral appliances, especially in combination with biofeedback; isotonic exercises; the use of moist heat; ice; and self-massage. Patient education—regarding proper jaw posture, recommended sleeping position (not on the stomach), and ways to relax the jaw—can be valuable. A healthy, whole-foods diet and nutritional supplements are often suggested. Some supplements that may alleviate TMJ problems are calcium and magnesium—to relax muscles, and the B complex of vitamins. Also, antispasmodic herbs, such as the herbal mixture called Euphytose, can help relieve jaw pain.

Tinnitus

Many of us who live in excessively noisy surroundings learn to acclimate to this lifestyle, not aware of the consequences that could eventually develop. One of these is tinnitus, a ringing or tinkling sound in one or both ears.

Causes

Blaring music, gunshots, explosions, and other extremely loud sound can create ear injury and cause tinnitus. Additional factors are exposures to toxic chemicals in foods, medicines, and the environment.

Symptoms

Tinnitus is characterized by a noise resembling that of a fuzzy television set, and ranging from barely audible to quite loud. The sound may be continuous or heard at intervals. Symptoms accompanying tinnitus can include headaches, digestive disorders, learning disorders, irritability, insomnia, and fatigue.

Treatment

Nutrition

There is a high correlation between tinnitus and poor nutrition. Diets high in fat, cholesterol, and refined sugars are particularly detrimental to ear health. Switching to a diet that is rich in vegetable proteins and complex carbohydrates is, of course, important. In addition, freshly made juices are concentrated sources of healing vitamins and minerals, and of valuable enzymes, all in easily assimilated form. (Unlike store-bought juices, just-squeezed juice contains live, healing nutrients and no chemical additives.)

Supplements

The inner ear contains thousands of specialized sensory cells, which need water, oxygen, and nutrients in order to effectively deliver complete electrical information to the brain. Some of the more important nutrients for this condition are as follows:

> Vitamin A—about 25,000 IU
> Vitamin E—400-800 IU
> Vitamin D—500-1000 IU
> Ionized calcium—500-1000 mg
> Magnesium—up to 500 mg
> Potassium—500 mg
> Zinc sulfate—60 mg

Sometimes an iron deficiency is associated with tinnitus, in which case 75 mg of iron each day for two weeks is recommended. After that period, reduce iron intake to a normal level. Exact dosages of all nutrients should always be given by a physician.

What to Avoid

Avoid excessive exposure to loud noises. Refrain from the damaging chemicals found in alcohol, cigarettes, caffeine, and tap water. Home and office environments should be cleaned up as much as possible. Exposure to copy machines, household cleansers, and common toxins such as formaldehyde can help bring on or exacerbate tinnitus. Medicines known to be toxic to the ear include certain antibiotics, contraceptives, and Novocain. Poor diet is a major contributor to tinnitus, especially a high-fat, high-cholesterol, and sugary diet. Refined carbohydrates should be replaced by complex carbohydrates. Acidic foods, such as meats, should be reduced. In their place, more alkaline foods, such as fruits and vegetables, should be eaten.

Treatment Summary

Switching to a diet that is rich in vegetable proteins, complex carbohydrates, and fresh juices creates an environment conducive to healing.

Supplements of important nutrients can build ear health.

Avoid loud noises and common pollutants as much as possible.

Toxic Shock Syndrome

Toxic shock syndrome is a dangerous condition that affects individuals with jeopardized immune systems. It occurs unexpectedly, as a result of poisoning by a strain of bacteria, called Staphylococcus aureus. This type of staph sometimes creates a poisonous substance called enterotoxin F, which damages cell walls, allowing blood to seep into tissues.

Most cases of TSS occur in menstruating women who are using tampons, although children, men, and women who are not menstruating do sometimes get the disease. Teenage girls and women under 30 have a higher risk of TSS than do older women. Though tampons are implicated in many cases of the disease, they don't directly cause it. Rather, they seem to create a breeding ground for the bacteria that do.

Symptoms

TSS is characterized by headaches, a sore throat, high fever, diarrhea, nausea, vomiting, and rashes that look like red skin blotches or sunburn. These symptoms may then progress to include low blood pressure, fainting, confusion, acute kidney failure, and abnormal liver function. Occasionally, death may result.

Treatment

If you suspect you may have toxic shock syndrome, seek medical care immediately, and if you are using a tampon, remove it. Once a person is diagnosed with TSS, hospitalization may be necessary, depending upon the severity of the case. However, several natural solutions are available once the critical period is resolved; they can also be used to achieve quick recovery in less severe cases. These are also ways to avoid reccurrence of the condition.

Herbs

Dr. Linda Rector Page, author of *Healthy Healing: An Alternative Healing Reference,* reports that the following herbs have been proven to combat toxicity, reestablish a healthy immune system, and restore the patient to health.

GINSENG

This will help to equalize and tone all systems within the body as well as strengthen circulation. However, people are strongly advised to refrain from taking this herb when a high fever exists.

CAYENNE AND GINGER

These aid the body in recuperating from shock. They are nervous system energizers that can be consumed or used as compresses placed directly on the skin.

HAWTHORN EXTRACT

Hawthorn accelerates and regulates the circulation while reestablishing an overall sense of well-being.

Diet

TSS necessitates a diet in which healthful foods can be readily digested and immediately used by the progressively weakening system. Considering this, Dr. Page suggests incorporating the following foods into the diet: high-potency royal jelly, bee pollen, wheat germ, brewer's yeast, and unsulfured molasses. Additionally, important minerals should be included in the diet. These can be consumed in the form of green drinks, such as chlorella, barley grass, spirulina, and wheatgrass juices.

What to Avoid

Women who wear tampons should choose only the absorbency necessary to meet their needs, since tampons present a higher rish of TSS with higher levels of absorbency. Also, women may want to alternate use of tampons with use of sanitary pads. Tampons should be changed no less frequently than every four to eight hours.

Treatment Summary

Any instance of suspected TSS should receive medical attention, as this can be a life-threatening condition.

Some herbs and foods are recommended to combat toxicity, reestablish a healthy immune system, and restore the patient to health.

Trauma

Americans are one of the most stressed peoples on earth. Some of the stress is self-imposed and some isn't, but the bottom line is that most of us suffer from multiple pressures in a given day. There is the stress from unhappy relationships, poor health, working, traveling, or living too close to too many people, artificial time requirements, accepting too much responsibility, and job-related issues. If left unchecked, these stresses can eventually lead to a whole spectrum of physical illnesses, including heart disease, mental illness, high blood pressure, obesity, and insomnia, to name but a few.

Prolonged stress can produce a state of trauma. Physical and emotional trauma can also be induced by an accident, illness, or shocking personal event. Even after muscles and tissues that were injured in an accident are completely healed, symptoms of trauma can manifest.

Treatment

Nutrition

During periods of stress and recovery from trauma, it is particularly important to be kind to yourself nutritionally. Diets should be high in fiber, full of wholesome, organic foods. Stress reactions thicken the blood; therefore, foods with a blood-thinning effect, such as ginger, garlic, and cantaloupe, should be included in the diet.

The best antistress nutrients are B-complex vitamins. One member of the B family, pantothenic acid, is particularly important, as it quickly dissipates during stress reactions. Plenty of vitamin C is important as well in its role as an antioxidant that helps protect the body against stress reactions and many associated diseases. Beta carotene is another antioxidant that will protect the body during periods of stress. Minerals that need replenishing include zinc, potassium, magnesium, and chromium.

While it's a good idea to take supplements, it is even more important to eat foods rich in these nutrients. For example, broccoli and kale are good vegetable sources of pantothenic acid, while red pepper, strawberries, and collard greens are high in vitamin C. When eating or juicing C-rich citrus fruits, be sure to include some of the white inner peel for its bioflavonoid content. Ginger, parsley, and carrots are rich in zinc, while collard greens have lots of magnesium. Bananas, Swiss chard, and spinach contain potassium. Dark green, orange, and red fruits and vegetables are high in beta carotene. More concentrated sources of these nutrients are obtained from juicing fruits and vegetables.

Cherie Colborn, author of *Juicing for Life,* recommends making a mineral-rich juice, with lots of potassium. She suggests combining a handful of spinach and parsley with carrots and celery. To get more magnesium, Colborn recommends combining a clove of garlic with some parsley, carrots, and celery.

Biofeedback

In treating victims of trauma, biofeedback can produce impressive results. Often, a trauma patient will experience decreased muscle flexibility and a tendency to brace the muscles on the opposite side of the body from where the injury occurred. Using computerized EMG instruments, a biofeedback specialist can analyze the muscles for the signs of asymmetrical movement that are typical with trauma patients. Then, with repetitive corrective exercises, the patient can restore the body's ability to function symmetrically.

Purification Lodge for Post-Traumatic Stress Disorder

The purification lodge is a Native American traditional ceremony known popularly as the sweat lodge. Native Americans prefer to use the terminology of purification, though, since men and women who participate do more than merely sweat. Experiencing the devastation of war alienates a person from his spirit. The purification ceremony helps one regain a sense of well-being. First Americans have long used this ritual to help their warriors, and now share the process with others.

That's a reality that George Amiotte, an Ogalala Lakota from the Pine Ridge South Dakota Reservation, knows well. Amiotte served in Vietnam and had a near-death experience there. Upon his return home he searched for ways to restore his own wounded spirit and was guided by Lakota elders to pursue Western medicine and traditional native healing. As a physician's assistant, Amiotte now specializes in helping veterans overcome post-traumatic stress disorder, (what used to be called combat fatigue). Interestingly, Amiotte has been able to achieve success where standard Veterans Administration programs have failed. Puzzled Western doctors have questioned Amiotte on his success. Amiotte points out that healing is more than physical. Healing takes place on the physical, mental, and spiritual levels, and a medical practitioner needs to consider all three aspects for optimum success. This is something Western medicine fails to do.

Another Native American doing similar work is John Joseph, a shaman with the Chinook tribe and a nurse practitioner in Washington state. Joseph agrees that men in war have lost their spirituality and that the lodge becomes a safe haven for them, a place to find it again. Everything said in the lodge remains there. Nothing is repeated outside of it. This gives a person a real opportunity to cleanse the heart, and to place things into the fire. The effects are wonderful and long-lasting, Joseph says, explaining that once people start to get their spirituality back, their physical appearance changes. They start to pay more attention to personal hygiene and to their clothing. More importantly, their thought patterns become steadier, without constant intrusions. Their sleep patterns begin to normalize. The purification lodge, in short, works to make people's lives cohesive and to calm their minds.

What to Avoid

It's important to stay away from foods that deplete the system, such as sugar, which robs the body of chromium, as well as caffeine, alcohol, and over-the-counter drugs. Many medications promise short-term relief, but weaken the system in the long-term, making stress and trauma worse.

Treatment Summary

During periods of stress or trauma, it is especially important to eat foods rich in vitamins, minerals, and enzymes that will nourish the immune system and build health.

Since stress thickens the blood, foods that thin it should be eaten; these include ginger, garlic, and cantaloupe.

After trauma, biofeedback can help the body return to normal functioning.

The Native American purification ceremony helps those suffering from post-traumatic stress disorders move toward normalcy.

Urinary Tract Infection

Approximately six million Americans, most of them women, are treated for urinary tract infection or inflammation annually. Urinary tract infection, known to many as cystitis or bladder infection, is commonly caused by E.coli and other forms of bacteria, which develop inside the large intestine and contaminate the nearby urethra and vagina.

In general, there several categories of women who are at especially high risk for contracting urinary tract infection, with young sexually active women topping the list as the most likely candidates. Young women often acquire UTI after they begin sexual intercourse when bacteria that usually inhabit the vaginal region are relocated further inside the body in the urethra. The female urethra, measuring only about half an inch, facilitates the transportation of bacteria to the bladder due to its relatively short length. Although sexual intercourse may promote the onset of infection, sexually active women should be aware that their partners are not transferring the bacteria from their own bodies; they are merely pushing bacteria that were already present deeper inside the body.

Women who have experienced menopause are also at a heightened risk for UTI, as studies show that 8 to 10 percent of all women over the age of 60 will contract bladder infection at some time during their elder years. Also, people with multiple sclerosis and other neurological disorders are a high-risk group since they often are unable to fully drain their bladders during the excretion process.

Causes

Although many sexually active women contract bladder infection at some point in their life, there are large numbers of females who seem to magically escape this irritating problem. This phenomenon can be explained by the development of hormonal imbalances in certain women. Estrogen and progesterone, which reinforce the urethral cells, attract and entrap bacterial bodies that are propelled into the region. Under normal circumstances the invasive microorganisms are expelled during urination, but in women with hormonal imbalances the bacteria cannot effectively be discharged, leading to recurrent bladder infections. This explains why women who have experienced menopause are often susceptible to this condition; the reduced level of estrogen in the body tends to enhance the adhesive qualities of the urethral lining and, consequently, prevent proper bacterial emission.

Urinary tract infection is often an indication of faulty nutritional habits and a debilitated immune system. Usually the presence of bacteria within the body can effectively be combated by the body's immune system, but when the system becomes weakened the widespread reproduction of disease-producing microorganisms is encouraged, resulting in the appearance of acute symptoms. Prolonged exposure to stress or the occurrence of a traumatic situation, such as a divorce or a family death, can further debilitate the immune system, adding to the chances of illness.

The muscles of the pelvic floor are often weakened after childbirth, causing the bladder to protrude closer to the vaginal region and the rear portion of the bladder to sag below its neck. When this occurs the bladder cannot be properly drained, resulting in the accumulation of stagnant urine and the growth of bacterial communities. This condition is responsible for the multitude of UTI patients who visit the doctor shortly after termination of pregnancy. In addition, a prolapsed transverse colon, which can result from childbirth; aging; poor posture; spinal disorders; and excessive abdominal fat are factors that can contribute to the compression of the bladder, with consequent obstruction of the flow of blood to this organ. Consequently, the bladder, which is deprived of an adequate supply of oxygen, becomes prone to disease-causing bacteria.

Our body eliminates waste products in several ways, including the excretion of feces by the bowels, the expulsion of carbon dioxide by the lungs, perspiration of the skin, and finally, the discharge of urine by the kidneys and bladder. When a malfunction occurs in any of these processes, an excessive burden is placed upon the other systems. For instance, if a person suffers from constipation, hazardous waste that builds in the body must be eliminated by an alternative method. Medical evidence shows that recurrent urinary tract infections can often be correlated with persistent bowel problems.

Practitioners of Asian medicine explain that urinary tract infection results from the presence of damp and warm conditions within the bladder. They say that a weak flow of energy in the spleen and kidney is frequently accompanied by stagnation and a damp environment, which eventually leads to friction and the production of heat. The weakening of the spleen and the depletion of energy is commonly caused by an excessive diet, drinking during meals, and overconsumption of greasy foods. In addition, certain foods, such as dairy and chilled foods or drinks, can exacerbate damp conditions within the organs, while prolonged exposure to stressful situations, including extended periods of studying, promotes spleen damage and continuous energy drainage. According to the Oriental view, the presence of overexertion, anxiety, exhaustion, inordinate alcohol intake, and too much sexual intercourse can hamper the proper functioning of the kidneys.

Interstitial cystitis is a bladder inflammation that's a result of autoimmune or allergic responses, which can result in inflammations of the pelvis and bladder and heightened blood flow in the region. In addition, candida has been found to promote antibody reactions that irritate the bladder.

Symptoms

Urinary tract infections and inflammations are frequently characterized by increased urination, accompanied by a constant feeling of urgency or that the bladder has not been completely drained. In addition, a burning sensation during the excretion process usually develops, along with an intense need to urinate during the later hours of the night. Additional symptoms may include cramps and dark, foul-smelling urine, while more serious cases may involve the presence of blood in the urine.

If you suspect that you suffer from urinary tract infection or inflammation, be sure to seek medical attention so that the problem can be effectively treated before it becomes compounded. The examination for an infection is relatively simple, consisting of having a midstream urine sample analyzed for bacterial infection. The presence of an inflammation is more difficult to assess due to the lack of bacterial evidence in the urinalysis.

Treatment

The traditional medical approach to treating UTI involves the administration of antibiotics. Prolonged exposure to these drugs can have adverse long-term effects due to their tendency to attack microorganisms that actually aid the body. A major problem is that the undiscriminating nature of antibiotics often results in the destruction of helpful gut bacteria, which in turn allows the propagation of harmful bacterial strains, including E.coli and *Candidia albicans*, in the gastrointestinal region.

Ideally, then, reliance on prescription medication should be avoided in favor of alternative modalities. If the holistic approach repeatedly fails, the condition may necessitate a small dosage of bacteriostatic antibiotics. This form of treatment is less severe than traditional antibiotics because bacteriostatic agents simply restrain bacterial development, rather than kill these organisms. Thus, bacteriostatic antibiotics do not provoke yeast infection and the resultant gastrointestinal disorders. Some members of the medical community prescribe surgery, hormonal therapy, and antidepressant drugs to treat more severe cases of chronic urinary tract infection. However, these therapies should only be used under extreme circumstances, when all else has failed.

Nutrition

There are a variety of natural remedies that can alleviate urinary tract disorders without the risk of harmful side effects. To begin with, the consumption of one 8-ounce glass of water per hour can aid in the treatment of an infection, and is especially helpful in ameliorating severe pain. Unsweetened cranberry juice or cranberry capsules contain natural antibacterial agents and increase the acidity of urine, creating an unpleasant environment for bacterial communities to develop. Recent studies have demonstrated that 15 ounces of cranberry juice can hamper bacterial growth by up to 80 percent because the bacteria are no longer able to adhere to the urethral wall and, consequently, are excreted during urination. Other research has demonstrated that the consumption of vitamin C along with the cranberries can further heighten the acidity of urine. Some other beneficial drinks that tend to alter the pH level of urine are lemon juice mixed with water, buttermilk, and a mixture of two teaspoons of apple cider vinegar and water. These concoctions should be consumed three to four times a day.

Severe UTI symptoms can also be alleviated by temporary changes in diet. Increased intake of acidic foods, such as certain grains, seeds, nuts, fish, dairy products, and bread, and reduced consumption of fruits and vegetables, is recommended during acute attacks, but it is important to remember that this dietary modification should be short-term only. Usually, foods that are low in acidity, such as whole grains, vegetables, flax oil, fish oils, and beans, are recommended to prevent irritation.

Supplements

Vitamin C, which is ascorbic acid, can intensify the acidity of urine and aid in the expulsion of infectious bacteria. For maximum results it should be administered to bowel tolerance, or when the stool becomes soft and almost diarrhea-like. When fighting an infection, the body can require up to 15,000 mg of vitamin C daily, and sometimes even more intravenously. Since it is water-soluble, vitamin C should be taken every two to three hours to prevent nutritional loss during excretion. People who do not suffer from an infection but wish to use vitamin C as a preventive agent should take between 2000 and 6000 mg daily. C serves as an effective combatant of urinary tract infection because of its antibacterial attributes and its ability to enhance the operation of the immune system by encouraging the production of infection-fighting white blood cells.

During acute attacks, a daily dosage of 50 mg of zinc can assist the body in white blood cell production and the elimination of bacterial intruders. In addition to zinc and vitamin C, vitamin A can fortify the mucous membrane lining of the bladder, prevent irritation of the bladder, and improve functioning of natural antibodies and white blood cells. Note, though, that pregnant women, or those who may be, should substitute vitamin A supplements with risk-free beta carotene, as studies have correlated high maternal dosages of vitamin A with birth defects. Other people can receive sufficient quantities of vitamin A by consuming up to 25,000 IU in halibut or cod liver oil capsules daily. Some additional preventive agents that can be used daily include 100 to 200 mg of vitamin B6 and four to six capsules of evening primrose oil.

Herbs

Antiseptic herbs, including buchu, goldenseal, uva ursi, juniper, and garlic, are helpful in curbing the onset of cystitis. Marshmallow root, juniper berry, and corn silk, which are classified as demulcents, soothe the mucous membranes of the urethra and bladder, while diuretic herbs, such as parsley and goldenrod, encourage the production of urine and the elimination of bacteria. A mixture of equal quantities of burdock, fennel, and slippery elm can be effective when a teaspoon of the mixture is added to a cup of boiling water and allowed to sit for 20 minutes. This herbal solution should be consumed after each meal and before retiring for the evening. Other efficacious natural remedies include flaxseed tea and uva ursi/buchu tea, which should be prepared in a similar fashion to that described above. These solutions should also be consumed three to four times per day. Although they may have an unpleasant taste, herbal teas can often produce dramatic results in the battle with UTI. In addition, the homeopathic remedy cantharis can be used to alleviate irritations of the bladder and urethra. A final suggestion for preventing urinary tract infection: After having sexual intercourse, women may want to gently cleanse the opening of the urethra with a dilute solution of Betadine or a potent solution of goldenseal tea in order to remove harmful bacteria that may have been pushed into the region during intercourse.

Exercise

Participation in aerobic exercise, including jogging, walking, swimming, and bicycling, can enhance circulation and aid in the elimination of blood congestion in the pelvic area. Inverted-position exercises, such as yoga headstands and shoulderstands, and rotating the legs in a bicycle-like motion, are also beneficial for improving circulatory functioning. If you suffer from back or neck pain and are unable to perform these exercises, you can use an old door or a couple of wooden boards to support the body by bracing one end on your couch and the other on the floor. The slanted position of the body facilitates the transport of blood away from the pelvic region and toward the head. It is advisable to limit such exercises to three to five minutes at a time because remaining in a slanted position for extended periods can cause dizziness.

Additional Treatment Modalities

Sitz baths and hot compresses enhance blood flow, allowing for the removal of hazardous waste in the pelvic region. In addition, these natural remedies can alleviate some of the pain of urinary tract infection. The preparation of a hot compress consists of dipping a small towel into a tub of hot water, squeezing out the excess, and applying the towel just above the pubic bone. When the cloth eventually cools, prepare another compress and reapply. After applying approximately eight or nine compresses take a rest for several hours, and then repeat the procedure two or three additional times later in the day.

What to Avoid

There are numerous preventive measures that will hinder urinary infections and inflammations. First of all, after urination, women should wipe from front to back, rather than vice versa. Also, before engaging in sexual intercourse your partner should clean his hands. In addition, try to avoid the transportation of bacteria from the anus to the vagina during intercourse, and remember to change pads or tampons frequently during menstruation. Tight-fitting jeans and nylon pantyhose can facilitate the spread of bacterial infections, so try to wear clothes that will allow ventilation, such as loose-fitting cotton pants or skirts and stockings with garter belts. Chemical irritation to the urethra can be prevented by avoiding perfumed and artificially colored hygiene products. Women susceptible to infections should substitute use of birth control pills and diaphragms with condoms or fitted cervical caps to avoid further infection. Those with urinary tract infection brought on or exacerbated by spinal disorders should seek the guidance of an osteopath or chiropractor.

The consumption of seven to eight glasses of water can dilute the urine and discourage bacterial development. Urination should be encouraged because it rids the system of harmful bacteria. Women who neglect their need to urinate are at an increased risk of infection. It is important to urinate after sex in order to eliminate bacteria forced into the urethra, so avoid urinating before sex. In addition, drinking a glass of water prior to intercourse will increase bladder content, allowing more bacteria to be eliminated during post-coital urination. If you suffer from persistent infections you may wish to cleanse the vagina with a direct stream of water from a shower massage prior to sex. This technique will eliminate a significant portion of vaginal bacteria, hence reducing the quantity of bacteria available for transportation to the urethra.

Excessive consumption of tea, coffee, alcohol, and soda should be avoided. Furthermore, intake of red meat, dairy products, citrus fruits, and shellfish should be limited because prolonged exposure to these foods can increase the acidity of the body and promote bacterial infection. As discussed earlier, acidic foods and drinks can sometimes aid in combating UTI, but only when the body is experiencing acute symptoms and needs to be immediately flushed. Long-term acidic dietary modifications can have adverse effects and so should be avoided.

Treatment Summary

The conventional medical approach to treating urinary tract infection generally involves antibiotics, which tend to produce adverse side effects. In the case of chronic UTI, hormone therapy and antidepressant drugs may be prescribed. Natural solutions present excellent alternatives in both cases, although, if they do not work, a small dosage of bacteriostatic antibiotics may prove beneficial.

There are a variety of drinks and foods that can alleviate urinary disorders. These include cranberry juice, and acidic foods (for acute attacks).

Herbs will prevent UTI as well as alleviate symptoms. Some useful herbs are uva ursi, goldenseal, buchu, juniper, and garlic.

Exercise can enhance circulation and aid in the elimination of blood congestion in the pelvic area. Inverted-position exercises are helpful.

Among supplements recommended for UTI are vitamins C, A, and B6, and zinc.

Sitz baths and hot compresses are recommended.

II.

Treatments and Patient Experiences

There is more than one way to heal from a disease. This section describes a variety of nontoxic noninvasive therapies that permit the body to heal itself.

Usually, in a book like this one, the scientist's or doctor's view is presented and the patient's outlook ignored. But here, patient stories are included to elucidate the benefits of the treatment modalities. We feel this perspective is valid and can offer valuable information and insight.

Acupuncture

Acupuncture has been used successfully for thousands of years to heal the body of specific diseases, relieve pain, and enhance well-being. During treatment, hair-like needles are placed into the skin on specific points along a series of lines known as meridians. Exact placements are determined by pulse diagnosis. Needles open up congestion and allow energy to flow freely into these areas so that healing can occur. While not a cure-all, acupuncture is remarkably effective when used in conjunction with other therapies, such as diet, herbs, and homeopathy.

Patient Stories:

Cathy on seasonal allergies

I was first diagnosed with allergies about seven years ago. It got to the point where I was suffering for over half a year; I had allergies from March to the first frost. . . . It got to the point where I had to sleep with an air purifier on at night and take medication first thing in the morning. Despite all this, I was absolutely exhausted. I was sleeping a lot and had trouble getting through the day. Last year, I was so physically drained that I lost about two weeks of work.

Last summer I became fed up and decided I could not take it anymore, especially after the allergist said that this would get worse as I got older. The diagnosis was not encouraging. I basically felt that I had two options. One was to get allergy shots. The other was acupuncture. I decided to try the acupuncture.

As a journalist, I have written some articles on asthma and acupuncture. The research I did impressed me. I spoke to several acupuncturists in Boulder last summer and learned that I should try the acupuncture before the allergy season started, so I waited until February. It's been remarkable.

When I went in to see the acupuncturist, at first we talked about my main concern, which was allergies. He explained a little bit about the philosophy behind acupuncture and about energy patterns in the body. Regarding allergies, he basically said that most people do not have a reaction to pollen in the air but for some reason my body was reacting to it. There was something out of alignment with the way the energy flows were working in my body. He told me that the first treatment would get my body into alignment and that the second one would get rid of negative energy.

I was comfortable with his explanation and said I wanted to get started. On the first treatment, he placed one needle on the inside of my elbow. I didn't really feel anything. When he hit the meridian point there was a flare of intensity but it was very brief, maybe 10 seconds. I was surprised and asked, "Is that it?" He said a lot more happened than I realized.

Leaving the office, I felt giddy. I couldn't decide if it was my excitement at having done something for myself or if something was happening in my system. By the time I got home, I was completely exhausted and decided to take a nap.

The next week I went back and he did the treatment to release negative energy. This involved a number of points on my back and was quite intense since the needles remained there for a longer time. I asked him to cut the treatment short since it was painful. He said that it was not pain but an intense sensation. I thought that was funny and said, "You can call it what you want but it hurts." He cut the treatment short and I had to have it repeated at another time.

Since that time, I have had a series of treatments, about 12 in all, and it has never been as intense as the second one. At most, I would feel a flare sensation where the needle would go in and come out. I would never come away from it feeling sick.

After the first three or four treatments I became really tired afterwards but that shifted. Now, I usually come away feeling very energized.

The reduction of my allergies is amazing. Every day I look forward to getting out of bed. I still have a little bit of an allergic reaction where my eyes sometimes are bloodshot in the morning. And sometimes I get a little bit of a headache. But it in no way compares to what I had to put up with over the last five years.

For the first time in five years I have actually enjoyed spring. I didn't realize that I hadn't been enjoying it until this spring when I was looking at the grass growing and the trees blooming and saying, "Isn't this beautiful" instead of wishing for snow.

Joe on allergies

My allergies that I had gotten in my mid-20's were getting worse and worse. I was gradually losing weight. I was physically cold a lot of the time, even in the summer heat. Different types of foods were increasingly bothering me. I had strange body odors that came and went that were obnoxious to me and other people. I had unreasonable levels of fear that just didn't seem appropriate to the circumstances. My thinking was foggy and I needed to concentrate to get things done on the job.

I went to a number of doctors and chiropractors and found little bits of help here and there. Finally, I found a physician who said that I had indications of problems but that she did not know what to do for them. She suggested that I try some other types of healing paradigms as some of her other clients found help from alternative forms of therapy. I finally decided to try acupuncture in the fall of 1993 and have been receiving treatments now for the past two years.

This is the best I have felt in 15 years or more. I am seldom cold. I think better. I have what I believe to be excellent energy levels. I no longer have unreasonable fears. I see great changes.

I am absolutely convinced that my condition was not psychosomatic and that the therapy is not a placebo. I kept journals and logs where I measured and tracked my condition. I can go back and pull stuff out and tell you what I did and ate on certain days, what my responses were, and how bad I felt from my allergies. I have an engineering and computer background and am very analytical. Since then, I have given up tracking because my condition has improved so much. There is no question that I am better.

Joanne on allergies, skin problems, and candida

I had a terrible case of allergies where I would break out in rashes and hives all over my body. This went on for a number of years, and I tried all kinds of treatments. Acupuncture and Chinese herbs were the only treatments that helped me. I was going to my acupuncturist for less then a year when the skin rash disappeared. It has never returned.

I'm still getting treatments but I don't need to get them every week anymore. Now, I just go to stay healthy, energized, and in balance.

The cost is very little. The other treatments I tried were much more expensive. . . .There is no question in my mind as to whether acupuncture works. After using the treatment, my allergies and candida have completely disappeared.

Michelle on Cushing's disease

Once my pituitary tumor was diagnosed, the doctor recommended surgery. I had the surgery but was also taking herbs. I attribute the lack of any dire side effects to the herbs I was taking. I never got the diabetes that the doctor predicted I would get, and I didn't have to live on hormones.

However, I still had a lot of residual hormonal discomfort. I was tired most of the time, and I had sleep disturbances that kept me awake during the night and made me want to sleep during the day. That was difficult because my daughter was two years old. I was still very overweight and with the adenoma I gained 30 pounds in three weeks. I still had a lot of hair that you get from this illness.

After awhile, I found a doctor who did acupuncture. The acupuncture seemed to assist me further in balancing. He recommended herbs, homeopathic remedies at times, as well as the acupuncture. Together, these treatments have been very helpful in alleviating my symptoms. I lost some weight and, as a result, my whole body looks and feels better. Also, I have more energy. Whenever I get a flu or cold, I bounce back very quickly and am never out for more than a day.

The acupuncture also assists me emotionally. When there are deaths in the family and other upsets, acupuncture helps to calm me down. I also go to my doctor's wife for private mediation and yoga classes. One thing we have to remember is that a person is not just a body but a mind and spirit as well. When you address all three spheres, the healing, joy, and potential for growth are enhanced.

Acupuncture has helped my whole family. My husband was diagnosed as having a hernia and was supposed to have surgery immediately. Instead, he went to the acupuncturist and worked with herbs. As a result, he has not needed surgery. Acupuncture and herbs have also helped my daughter when she tested positive for TB. The doctors wanted to place her on an antibiotic regime. We were very anxious about this. We brought her to the acupuncturist instead and to a doctor who uses homeopathic remedies. She is tested every six months to make sure that her TB does not become active.

I feel that acupuncture has benefited me on two levels. It has had a preventive effect because I never manifested the side effects that I was expected to get from Cushing's disease—the heart, liver, and kidney problems. I also think it has helped with some chronic issues. For instance, when I had a gallbladder attack, I didn't need to take any medicine. The acupuncture relieved the discomfort. So, it has alleviated chronic conditions and acute conditions at the same time.

Maxine on skin problems

It started with an itch on my foot. There was nothing there to see, and yet, it was persistent. I was in a Feldenkrais training at the time so I was aware of the depths of changes I was going through. One of my classmates recommended acupuncture. Originally, I began with herbs because I was a little nervous about the needles. At some point, my doctor said that it could go a lot faster if we had acupuncture as well. I lost my fear after the first session. The symptoms disappeared within a month.

I continued with the sessions in order to deal with chronic, long-term issues, particularly issues around a certain pattern of pain. It had never occurred to me to approach this through acupuncture but once I started to know more about acupuncture as a way of looking at the human being as a system, it made perfect sense that this could be useful. So, it evolved from being about relatively superficial symptoms to becoming about how I could be more of who I really am. It helped me to work through all of the different compensations that I had adopted over the years.

In the past, any small change or trauma caused me a lot of anxiety. One of the things that I have been learning through all of this is how to ride with the waves more comfortably. I may have a reaction of anxiety or a reaction of joy and come back to a kind of more comfortable neutral.

I firmly believe that disease is an outcome of many small decisions that we make, many refusals to take chances, and many refusals to look at certain issues. So, for me, the idea of a medical system that deals with the whole person—the spirit, the body, and the intellect—and deals with it in a way that can help you through the process, makes perfect sense. I always felt that, in Western medicine, they were all so quick to give you an antibiotic or to make a particular symptom go away without looking at . . . what the role of the symptom is in the whole picture.

I feel that acupuncture is, first of all, truly a preventive medicine. Second, it makes the quality of life much better. I am much more out there in the world and out there in a way that is comfortable for me.

Ruth on yeast

I went to a Western doctor because I was quite tired. I was given an extensive blood test and the results indicated that I was positive for yeast. After that, I went to see an acupuncturist. At the end of three months, I went back to the doctor to be retested and was negative for yeast. Actually, my doctor was surprised to learn that she completely cured the problem with a combination of acupuncture and cooking herbs.

I have been going for acupuncture treatments for about a year and a half. Although the yeast cleared up in a three-month period, I find that ongoing treatments continue to help me with my whole life. I feel much stronger and calmer and better able to deal with issues. It has returned me to me. I also find that acupuncture works as an immune system booster. I have two small children and tend to get every virus that comes down the pike. Now, when I do get something, it moves through my system faster. My body is definitely more on the offensive.

Lorraine on hepatitis A

I got very frightened one day after going to the bathroom and discovering that my urine was completely orange. I called the doctor, who said that I had hepatitis. I went to see him and he confirmed this with some blood tests. There was nothing I could do, I was told, but to wait it out. Months later, the worst was over, but my liver enzymes were not dropping back to normal. I was having terrible mood swings and could not pull myself out of them.

I decided to give an acupuncturist/Chinese herbalist a call. After the first session, my mood swings stopped and my mood stabilized. That was such a relief. She told me that certain things would happen along certain timetables, and they did. She said my liver enzymes would go down in a couple of months and that is exactly what happened.

I am positive that this is from the treatment. After the acupuncture, I would feel a release under my right rib cage, which is where the liver is. I also took a lot of herbs in the evening before bedtime to cleanse the liver. Then I would switch to herbs for building it up.

Acupuncture, combined with herbs and diet, cured me of hepatitis. Now I am absolutely in the normal range.

Donna on pain

Two years ago, out of the blue, I had excruciating, relentless pain in my left shoulder. I can't describe how bad it was. I couldn't do anything. I couldn't sleep or eat or function in any way. I was aware of nothing but the pain.

This went on for several days before I sought medical help. I didn't want to go to a doctor, but I did. I was x-rayed and the doctor told me that I had calcium deposits on my shoulder, which were pressing on a nerve. He said that there was really nothing that could be done other than surgery. The surgery might impair the use of my arm slightly. I consulted a few other doctors to see if there was anything else that could be done. The general consensus was that there was no other way.

Fortunately, someone gave me the name of an acupuncturist. I called and he said he thought he could help. When I went to see him, I was literally bent over from all the pain. The treatment consisted of placing a few needles in my shoulder, hand, feet and other areas. I left there with an 80 percent reduction of pain.

It wasn't just an anesthesia to get rid of pain; the treatment got to the cause of the pain. Once a week, I would return for treatment. I went back four or five times. In between treatments I noticed myself getting slowly but steadily better. It's more than two years now and I've been fine ever since.

Alexander Technique

The 19th century actor Frederick Alexander created the Alexander technique while attempting to overcome a physical problem that no doctor could cure. The problem was that Alexander would lose his voice whenever he needed to perform a long recitation. After several physicians said that nothing was physically wrong, Alexander decided that the problem must reside in his presentation. So, he began to observe himself in a three-way mirror as he rehearsed, and noticed that his nose and chin lifted in such a way as to place pressure on the back of his neck, which cut the wind off from his vocal folds. He also noticed that by lifting his chest and pushing his lumbar spine forward, he was narrowing his back and imposing on his diaphragm. Alexander's self-observations continued for 11 years, during which time he discovered a more natural way for the body to be in space.

Alexander developed a system wherein the whole person, not just the body, is involved in movement. His technique particularly looks at the relation of the head to the spine. When the head is out of balance with the spine, negative consequences can result. Too much pressure is placed on the internal organs and there is interference with breathing, as the diaphragm is not free enough to move.

The Alexander technique helps people rediscover their natural ease and balance. Through simple verbal and hands-on guidance, students get in touch with patterns that they naturally had as children, but lost. Students are made aware of their styles of movement; then, they are taught to release incorrect patterns, and to organize new ones that are in line with their center of gravity.

Alexander work is profound in that it is a psychological, physical, and neurological reeducation. Some people feel it has a spiritual quality as well in that it takes an enormous amount of trust to give up old ways of sitting, standing, and moving and to form new ways of being.

Patient Story

Mimi on back injury

I have been studying the Alexander technique for about 20 years. When I started, I had just had a child, and I would get tired a lot, with no particular symptoms. But within a short time, I injured my back, and it helped me enormously in that area.

When I started, I was in my early 30's. I needed help for working long hours standing up. Now, 20 years later, this is the same technique that has made it possible for me to work well all the time and feel strong. It's a balance, an ease. The better you learn the technique—and anyone can learn it—you learn to do what you do in everyday life with less tension and better balance.

Applied Kinesiology

In the 1960's, chiropractic physician Dr. George Goodheart founded the practice of applied kinesiology after observing that muscles correspond to specific organs and weak muscles indicate organ weaknesses. Applied kinesiology is a system of diagnosis that uses manual muscle testing to identify various organ dysfunctions in the body. The technique does not necessarily replace conventional forms of testing, as it can be used in conjunction with standard procedures, such as x-rays and blood tests. It is particularly valuable when a patient has symptoms of a problem that are not explained by medical tests. Applied kinesiology can be used to treat problems in a very early stage or to treat problems that conventional methods often fail to find, like chronic fatigue or environmental illness.

Besides manual muscle testing for organ weakness, the health care provider may place certain foods, vitamins, minerals, herbs, or homeopathic formulas under a person's tongue and test for muscle strength. An immediate improvement indicates that the remedy will help correct the person's condition. Conversely, sustained weakness indicates that the remedy will not work. Applied kinesiology can also be used to test the effects of other noninvasive modalities, including acupuncture, biofeedback, and chiropractic adjustments.

Patient Stories

Ellie on environmental illness

I thought I might have had chronic fatigue or Lyme disease. I was always tired and depressed, and unable to keep up with my life. I had joint pains, digestive problems, depression—severe unwellness, as I put it. I started going to a lot of different doctors trying to determine the problem because I knew there was something wrong. I went to many traditional doctors who told me that my tests were good and that everything looked okay. They pretty much were saying that the problem was all in my head. But I was really in bad shape. And I was very frustrated and becoming desperate.

I had heard about Dr. Silverman through a local health food store. I spoke to some of his clients who told me that they had chronic fatigue or Epstein-Barr and that Dr. Silverman had helped them. I made an appointment to see him because I was getting sicker and sicker.

Dr. Silverman has a holistic and environmental approach. First, he would have me come in twice a week for three or four months and he would muscle test me for all my foods. Each time I would bring in 10 to 12 foods and he would muscle test me to see whether or not the foods strengthened or weakened me. If the foods weakened me, I would eliminate them from my diet. In addition, he would have me bring in all of the products I used—face creams, deodorants, etc.—and he would test these as well. Right away, he tested the drinking water and determined that I must stay away from tap water, and drink only good filtered water. That made a very big difference because I actually had an accumulation of toxic metals in my system from the water. Another thing I learned was that my digestion was very bad, which prevented me from assimilating food properly.

Homeopathic remedies worked very well for me. They helped to leach out the metals in my system and improve my ability to assimilate foods. Within a few weeks, I started feeling an improvement. That really lifted my spirits because I was feeling like nobody out there would be able to help me. With Dr. Silverman, I started to feel more and more encouraged and life just got better and better.

One of the most important things Dr. Silverman does, in my opinion, is go to your home and work environment, and muscle test you in that space. You could have a rug next to your bed, or you could be sleeping on a pillow or a quilt that outgasses chemicals and adversely affects your health. Don't forget, you're sleeping 12 hours a night in your bedroom, and if your surroundings are hurting you, it can have a severe impact on your system. Dr. Silverman helped me out with that.

I started making more and more improvements to the point now where I feel that my health is good. If I feel I am slipping a little, for whatever reason, I go in for a tune-up. If I am beginning to use some new products, I go to Dr. Silverman and he tests me. He says this is good and this isn't. I just feel that I am on a much, much better track. My outlook is much more positive now. I am encouraged about facing the world in a dynamic manner. And it's just great. I have more energy, no more joint pains, better digestion, just general, all-over improvement.

Elaine on chronic pain and Lyme disease

I have been bothered with chronic pain for many years. It started when I was 17 and I'm 47 now, so that's 30 years. I've spent many years going to a lot of different doctors. They did the traditional things—x-rays and lab work—and everything always came back negative. I went for years without knowing what was wrong. About five years ago, I went to a rheumatologist. After ruling everything else out, he came up with a diagnosis of fibromyalgia. That's where a whole list of medications came in. I was taking loads of medicine which weren't doing much good. They helped a little, but not very much. Somewhere around four years ago, I started to develop a lot of new symptoms other than just generalized body pain. New things like headaches and a sleep disorder started to come into play one at a time. My doctor suspected there might be Lyme, so he tested and it came back negative. From there, we just kept on treating the symptoms of fibromyalgia.

About January of this year, my pharmacist started to become very concerned about all the medications I was taking. They really weren't having a very big effect. He had seen an ad for Dr. Silverman's lecture, and it mentioned fibromyalgia, so he asked me if I would like to go to the lecture. You get to a point in time where you think, I'll do anything. So we went to the lecture and listened, and most of the things he talked about were kind of foreign, like kinesiology, and homeopathic remedies. But he does a demonstration at the lecture. And that kind of convinced me that there were possibilities there.

I made an appointment for that night, and I started to see Dr. Silverman twice a week. A couple of weeks after I started to see him, he kept reminding me that one negative Lyme test really doesn't mean that you don't have Lyme. And I really had the classic symptoms of Lyme disease. So we decided to test again, and this time it came back positive.

So right now, I'm being treated for Lyme disease, and I'm continuing to see Dr. Silverman two times a week. He realigns my spine. Each time I go, I take 10 items with me to find out if they are making me weak or strong or whatever. And as you go along, you take out the things that make you weak. He gives you things that makes you strong. I'm taking nutrients for bone and tissue repair, arthritis and muscle pain, and liver detox. I'm also taking a multivitamin and mineral supplement. And I do aerobic exercise every day, which really seems to help the pain a great deal. I'm about a month into treatment for Lyme, which is Doxycycline. And I'm continuing to feel better. Compared to how I felt when I first went to Dr. Silverman, there is less pain and few symptoms. I would say that probably the best thing is that I have a very dramatic increase in my energy level. I used to wake up in the morning and just drag through the day. Now I'm at a point to where I'm getting up and living each day. I expect that it's bound to get better if I continue.

Aromatherapy

Aromatherapy is the application of essential oils for healing purposes. Essential oils are volatile materials, which means they evaporate. An example is a peppermint leaf, fresh out of the garden. Squeeze it, and you smell an aroma. That smell is the essential oil. These oils differ from cooking oils, which do not vaporize.

Over the centuries, aromatherapy has been a part of various civilizations. Ancient Egyptians, who are considered the fathers of medicine, prized essential oils and incorporated them into religious rituals central to their culture. The oils were also valued for their everyday uses, and utilized in the treatment of emotional and physical ailments, such as diabetes, cancer, ulcers, and depression. Early Greeks and Romans respected the therapy as well. In the first century, the Greek physician Dioscorides praised the essence of onion for its diuretic and tonic properties, and its effectiveness against infection. Fortunately, thousands of plant oil recipes were recorded and are being rediscovered today. In France, where the therapy is used widely, many physicians never resort to antibiotic prescriptions, using aromatic substances instead.

Research confirms that essential oils have many advantages over antibiotics. First, the patient does not acquire a resistance to an oil; essences remain efficient for long periods of time. Second, there are no negative side effects. Third, aromatics successfully treat a number of diseases that pharmaceuticals have little success with.

Aromatics are widely available and fun to experiment with. However, a few guidelines should be followed:

Only use oils that are pure and natural.

Use oils sparingly. They are highly concentrated, powerful substances.

Learn to use oils properly. Some should be ingested, some should be applied topically, and some should be dispersed into a room with a diffuser. Although oils are generally safe, some oils are contraindicated for certain conditions. It is wise to begin aromatherapy under the guidance of an aromatherapist or other health practitioner well-versed in this field.

Ayurvedic Medicine

This medical system has been used for thousands of years in India, and has recently gained popularity in the United States through lecturer and best-selling author Deepak Chopra. Ayurveda means the science of life, and this practice uses various modalities, such as herbs, diet, exercise, aromatherapy, and massage, to overcome sickness and enhance well-being. Disease is treated as an imbalance of the elements (earth, air, fire, and water), and specific recommendations are made according to an individual's constitution. Individuals are classified into one of three types: pitta, vata, and kapha. Pitta types tend to be excessively hot, vata types tend to be restless, and kapha types tend to be lethargic. Getting well is a matter of correcting imbalances in these types. More than a medicine, Ayurveda is a knowledge about how to live correctly for optimal health and longevity.

Patient Stories

Lavonn on idiopathic pulmonary fibrosis and fibromyalgia

I had been seeing doctors for about seven years and they had yet to diagnose me according to their tests. Everything is by tests. If they can find a test to diagnose you, then that's what you have. Diagnosis was a long process. There was a six-week wait here, and a six-week wait there. I was going down and had to sell my business. I couldn't work anymore, and I felt that the doctors were looking at me as if I was nuts. In fact, one prescribed Prozac. Needless to say, I was depressed, because at one time I had worked 70 hours a week with my business and now I could hardly take a shower and get dressed in less than a couple of hours.

I was in the bookstore one day looking at the health books when I came upon *Perfect Health* by Dr. Chopra. I read through it and thought that it sounded very interesting. I tried one of the recommendations, boiling ginger root, and found that it helped clear out mucus. I wondered what more Ayurveda could do for me. Three to four months later, I went to their clinic in Lancaster, PA. It's a very interesting program that involves cleansing toxins that build up in the body and cause illness after many years. The system is guided by the seasons and the time of day. It works through natural processes rather than a lot of pills.

My father was ill at the same time. By the time he passed away he was on $500 of medication a month. I felt that I did not want to go down that road. I really feel your physician needs to be behind you 100 percent. And I found that this was very true with Ayurvedic medicine.

When I arrived home from Lancaster, I started seeing some differences within two months. Four months later, I went down to Fairfield, Iowa, and went to the clinic there for another week. They recommend you do it twice a year, but the first year I needed to go three times.

The whole idea of Ayurvedic revolves around the digestive system. If the digestive system is not working, the body gets ill. This is very important. What nourishment you put in your body is vital. Schedule is very important, and the main meal should be eaten between eleven and two.

The first thing I learned about was meditation, and that has been very helpful. The mind is a positive force you need in your life because what you think about comes about. This is where the medical doctors have been so wonderful.

They prescribe many combinations of Indian herbs. I eat fresh basil leaves three times a day and that is helping to balance the body. Licorice powder and ginger root boiled together takes care of a lot of the mucus too. Before doing this, I was using aloe vera, which I also recommend highly.

Ayurveda works on balancing the elements or doshas in the body. Once they get balanced, you get well. They don't really like to talk about the fibrosis or fibromyalgia because these are just symptoms in the body.

The doctors are very supportive and call to check on me. I never had that with my regular M.D. It's a wonderful program. I could not say anything more positive.

Bema on maximizing energy

I was a competitive athlete in college and I wanted to continue playing basketball and soccer, and weight lifting. Of course, working full-time in New York, it takes a lot of energy to continue sports. I have been a vegetarian since 1970 and have studied meditation since that time as well. This goes right along with my interest in natural foods and meditation. It has given me a lot more energy to pursue sports. I'm not sick, but I use it for my training.

The therapy consists mainly of herbs and natural foods. You go to an Ayurvedic store and you get the proper herbs from the people there. They try to balance you depending on your constitution. That's what I did. I went for an interview where they questioned me about the different foods I eat, my energy, and other things. Then they would prescribe depending upon my nature. The herbs they gave me really increased my energy level, which I put into sports as well as my work day.

Matt on psoriasis

I had a severe case that began in 1987 and peaked in 1990. Ninety-nine percent of my body was covered. There were not too many places that were not. What wasn't red and inflamed was white and flaky and falling off. I couldn't even sleep at night. I went to western doctors, and they told me it was incurable.

Then I went to an Ayurvedic doctor. I was introduced to him through a friend who was a registered nurse. According to Ayurveda, just about anything is curable. It's just an imbalance somewhere in the system. So I opted for the system of medicine that said it was curable. And it worked!

Ayurveda just nicely said, it's toxins coming out of the body. They can't find any other way out. Ayurveda is very big on proper digestion and proper elimination. They recommended a specific diet for me, a specific exercise program, and a cleansing program.

I grew up on a very tough meat diet—meat and potatoes, meat and fries, you name it. I don't think I touched a vegetable until my mid-20's. Then I started transcendental meditation. It took me 10 years but I slowly became vegetarian. Today, I don't eat any meat at all. Apparently, for my particular constitution, it was a blessing. I couldn't digest the things that were in that meat, and that was coming out through the skin. I weaned off meat to fish and turkey for a couple of years, and then less and less of that.

Also, according to Ayurveda, there are three particular doshas, or predominant qualities in the body. And that is pitta, vata, and kapha. I was diagnosed with a particular tendency toward one of those called pitta, which is hot and moist. So, I should stay away from those foods. No salsa, no onions, no garlic—nothing that would inflame the internal because that was being reflected through the external, through the skin. . . . And if you buy into the concept that what comes in has to eventually come out, I was then, through Ayurveda, put on this road of taking in less and less that was bad for me. I was going through purification techniques as well.

I literally woke up one day and 80 percent of it was gone. As quickly as it came, it left. It was amazing. Nobody has to sell me in Ayurveda. I'm a firm believer in it.

Hubbard on chronic sickness

I tried a number of other approaches. I did acupuncture and I also tried Western medicine. They couldn't find anything wrong with me and it was very frustrating. I had horrible hay fever. Nothing was life-threatening, but I had one cold after the next. Six months out of the year I was sick. I didn't know what it was, only that I felt lousy and that I couldn't do anything for it.

A friend of mine went to the Raj in Fairfield, Iowa, and had had miraculous results. His cholesterol dropped 50 points in seven days. He told me to go and I was so desperate that I did.

It's truly amazing. As I said, I tried all these other ways of going and nothing has helped like this. I have not been sick once in two years. It is such a restful experience.

I have changed my diet a little bit, but not as much as some other people. So, I really think it depends on the person. But what I can say is that this technique works. I learned about cycles of rest and activity. I used to live in New York City, where I was a night bird who would stay up all night long. I would paint and work all the time. Now I go to bed before ten. For my physiology, it's really important that I get sleep. I also meditate, which I never did before. And I eat my biggest meal of the day at noon, because it's when the digestion is the strongest.

I would say that everyone should start with where they are at. You make the adjustments slowly. The whole philosophy is to be gentle and to do it in your own time. It's not at all a rigid thing.

What they do is they unblock. They feel the reason you get sick is that things get blocked up. They give you massages. You lie on these tables. The temperature in the room is body temperature. If you are a woman you will have two women working on you. You are massaged with warm sesame oil. And it's all done in silence. I think a combination of going there, changing your diet a little bit, taking some supplements, and just living a natural life, exercising, and getting enough sleep, can make a difference. It's not all that difficult or demanding. It's really quite a natural process.

Sharon on Epstein-Barr virus and menstrual pain

I was getting sick every two weeks when I found out that I had the Epstein-Barr virus. I also had severe menstrual problems. Conventional medicine did not help. I even went for a laparoscopy just to determine what was causing all of this. Nothing was found. I also had irritable bowel syndrome.

All this led me to seek out alternative ways of healing. I discovered Ayurveda at a health fair and started taking one of the formulas, which helped me a great deal. That led me to find Dr. Chopra's book. As I read it, the whole concept made a lot of sense to me. So I decided to go to the school and become a practitioner. I have seen tremendous success, not only with myself, but with a lot of my clients and family members and friends.

I used to eat raw broccoli and cauliflower, but I learned through Ayurveda that this was the worst thing for me because I'm a vata type, an air type, and this increases air. I realized that if I only knew how to cook these vegetables, using various digestive spices and herbs, it would be a lot easier on my digestive system. Cardamom, ginger, coriander, fennel: These are all things that I have learned to cook with that basically help my digestive system to work a lot better.

Epstein-Barr is basically related to a very stressful life. That's where meditation helped me a lot. It brings the body into focus and helps calm the mind down. It keeps you in touch with the higher self. If you just take the time to meditate, two times a day, 15 to 20 minutes, it is very beneficial, as is yoga, massage, and aromatherapy.

David on maintaining nervous system balance

There are a lot of different things you can do in your daily routine to help keep your nervous system in balance. They include keeping regular hours in terms of when you eat, when you get to sleep, and when you get up in the morning. When I get up in the morning, I have a routine that I follow. In terms of the Ayurvedic practices, one thing I do every morning is an oil massage. Usually it lasts for about five to ten minutes. This is a routine that I learned the first time that I went to the Ayurvedic clinic. I also take an herb called amrit kalash, which is free radical scavenger.

I probably would be a lot more stressed if I didn't meditate. That I do every single day, twice a day. It is part of my Ayurvedic routine in terms of preventive medicine. I am not someone who has any particular illnesses. I have some minor things that bother me occasionally, but overall, I would consider myself a very healthy person, and I would like to stay that way. The way I look at it is that there are a lot of things that one can do to preserve one's health, and Ayurveda is one of those things. It's an ongoing process.

Biofeedback

Biofeedback teaches relaxation skills to patients with a variety of problems in which stress plays a role. The modality uses instruments to measure certain functions of the body, such as blood pressure, muscle tension, and brain wave activity. The patient is taught how to recognize different physiological states, and how to alleviate signs of stress through relaxation techniques. If a person has tension headaches, for example, he may learn how to relax the muscles of the forehead, neck, and shoulders. At the same time, the person hears a tone or sees waves on a screen that indicate the physiological changes taking place. In time, the person learns how to differentiate between tension and relaxation and how to create the latter state. Biofeedback is used to help alleviate pain and to correct a variety of conditions, including high blood pressure, insomnia, and migraines.

Patient Stories

Julie on patients with hypertension and low back pain

I'm working with somebody right now to lower his hypertension. Learning diaphragmatic breathing, and learning to warm your hands—which is getting some control of your cardiovascular system—can help in lowering blood pressure. It's important to apply those skills in situations where you tend to get tense.

I've also done a lot of work with patients with low back pain. The pain can come from an accident, like an injury on the job, or it can appear just all of a sudden. The back pain appears one day, or little by little it creeps up. Very frequently, much more frequently than people realize, there's a muscle tension component to back pain. A lot of physicians just look for disc problems or pressure on a nerve. But much more often we find that back pain is related to muscle tension. So again, using biofeedback to learn specifically to relax the muscles of the back in the area of discomfort can help people to control their pain.

Another very interesting aspect of the physiology that we can look at now with computerized biofeedback is to look at whether people recruit the muscles of their back say, when they're moving or when they're standing still, whether they recruit the muscles in a symmetrical or an asymmetrical pattern. If you think about it, if you're just standing straight and then you bend over straight forward and then bring your head back to center it ought to be the case that the muscles on the right side of your back and the muscles on the left side of your back do an equal amount of work if you're standing centered.

In a lot of cases with muscle pain in which the amount of muscle tension that appears on one side will be 20, 40, 50, 100 percent greater. Sometimes what we do that helps is to teach people to deliberately tense the side that's too relaxed, and then, when they learn to do that, the muscles on the other side don't have to bear such a heavy burden. That can result in a reduction in pain.

Affrine on severe migraines

I've had migraines for about three years now. So far, I would say that biofeedback training has been the one thing that has helped me. . . .

We did a lot of the hand warming and the surface electromyography and relaxation techniques. What I've learned is basically that your whole body is disposed to respond a certain way after many years. Biofeedback helps you to take control of how you are going to respond to certain triggers. Sometimes, with me, just being on the subway will trigger a headache. I've learned that the trigger is not necessarily the cause. Just getting a hold of these triggers has actually helped me tremendously.

At the very beginning when I started this I was not successful at all. It took a lot of practice; it's a lot of work and a lot of time. But nothing else has helped me.

I do it every day and I have different techniques. I have a comfort cycle tape which features a type of relaxation. I also have hypnotherapy and imagery. That's another tape that I listen to. I'm in the pain program at Lenox Hill Hospital and so I do those three things every single day. I think it's worth the effort because I used to get headaches all the time. Sometimes I'd get three a day, and sometimes I wouldn't get one for three days. I haven't had one in two weeks, so I think the success is really high for me.

Biological Dentistry

Your mouth is the gateway to your entire system. It is involved in every part of your total well-being. Biological dentistry takes this into account and is guided by the philosophy *do no harm*. This is accomplished by paying attention to what type of work is performed on teeth and gums, and what substances are placed in the mouth. Dental work is meant to last a lifetime. It is therefore important that it has no ill effects.

One of the biggest concerns are metals used in fillings. Most people receive amalgams, which contain a high percentage of mercury. Nickel, beryllium, and other metals may be placed in the mouth as well. These can be harmful for a number of reasons. People may have sensitivities and develop allergic responses. Also, metals can give off ions and cause damage throughout the body; they can depress the immune system, overstimulate the cardiovascular system and affect the nervous system, causing a variety of disorders. There can also be energy disturbances from different metals, where a battery effect is created. Electrical currents are formed that are much stronger than the body needs for nerve transmission. Consequently, the metals become interference fields along the acupuncture meridians in the mouth, which flow to every organ, muscle, gland, and tissue in the body. Biological dentists test the effects of metals, and recommend replacement with biocompatible materials. In the past decade, thousands of people have chosen this route and have reported substantial health improvements.

Attention is also paid to infections, known as cavitations. Bacterial pockets can form under the teeth, and fester silently for years. The person may be totally unaware of the problem; yet gradual damage goes on.

Just as the teeth affect all areas of the body, so does the health of the entire system affect the teeth. Health-centered dentists may therefore advise patients on the importance of a healthy diet and supplementation. In addition, patients are taught how to participate in their own dental health so that their need for dentistry diminishes.

Patient Stories

Kasha on mercury poisoning

I'm 40 years old now, and I was in good health until five years ago, after the birth of my second child. I was always getting headaches and feeling tired. I was fatigued no matter how much I rested. I started to get other symptoms too. There was numbness and pain in my legs, pain in my joints, irritability, depression, memory loss, insomnia. And my immune system was low. I also got a lot of colds and flus.

I saw an M.D. in 1991, who diagnosed me as having arthritis, which didn't seem right. In 1992, I found a naturopathic doctor, who thought I might have chronic fatigue syndrome. I tested positive for Epstein-Barr virus, low adrenal function, and abnormal intestinal flora. The doctor started me on a lot of vitamins and supplements for my immune system and intestinal tract. I took colonics too. My condition stabilized, but I did not improve a great deal. I still felt ill a great deal of the time. I was also seeing a chiropractor for sciatic pain.

Another year passed. In late 1993, I saw a Dr. Chan in Manhattan. He looked into my eyes and said that he could see a heavy metal toxic ring around the iris. He tested me using bio-energetic analysis, which is an FDA-registered device that measures electrical factors in the body with the help of computer mathematical analysis. It assesses the most stressed part of the body. That testing also showed metal toxicity. So, it was Dr. Chan who discovered the underlying source of my problem as mercury toxicity from my amalgam fillings.

I was really in shock. I couldn't believe that that was causing my problem. I hadn't heard much about it, so I had to do a lot of research. In early 1994, I found out about the work of Dr. Huggins in Colorado, and I read his book, *It's All in Your Head.* Then I came across some other bulletins from the Foundation for Toxic-Free Dentistry. I found out that the so-called silver fillings in my mouth were really 50 percent mercury, and that mercury is more toxic than lead, cadmium, or arsenic. Contrary to what the American Dental Association puts out, there's a lot of research stating that mercury is not stable in the mouth. It will migrate to other parts of the body.

In February 1994, I found a holistic dentist in Orange, Connecticut. He and his staff were terrific in helping me to understand this. He tested me using an acupoint testing device, which showed elevated metals in my body. He also ordered a standard urine mercury test, which is used in cases of industrial mercury exposure. Even this test showed elevated mercury levels. Then and there I decided what had to be done. All these fillings had to come out. I had 11 teeth with major fillings. All my molars were metal.

Before he did the work, I was placed on a diet which excluded all seafood. I ate foods that were high in sulfur, such as eggs and garlic. Sulfur binds with the mercury and aids in its elimination. I used supplements such as digestive enzymes, coenzyme Q10, super blue-green algae, a lot of things to help detoxify.

In April 1994, I had all the fillings taken out in two three-hour sessions. I was given an IV drip with vitamin C during the process.

It was not particularly uncomfortable, and I managed to get through it. I felt I was doing the right thing getting all this stuff out of my mouth. That kept me going.

Once all the metal was taken out of my mouth, the sciatic nerve discomfort that I had felt for three years almost disappeared right in the chair. From what I understand, the metal fillings can create minor electrical currents in the body, which interfere with the nervous system. By the second session, after all the fillings were taken out, I felt the tension in my leg immediately go away.

About three days after that, I started detoxifying, and needed almost total rest. I had lots of headaches for almost two weeks, and a strange metallic taste in my mouth. I drank lots of fluids to get this stuff out. My urine was dark and it had a strange odor. This was all a part of the cleansing process that was going on. I had faith that this was all working to my benefit. And it did.

About two weeks later, I woke up one day feeling great. I couldn't believe it. I didn't have a headache. I felt clear and energetic. And my body didn't hurt. It was just wonderful. Over the year, I had several more periods of cleansing, mostly lasting three to five days, with similar symptoms. There were headaches and the strange, metallic taste in my mouth. After every round of cleansing, I felt even better. I felt a new sense of wellness.

Now, it's almost 14 months since the removal of the mercury, and I really feel great. I feel like 18 instead of 40. I'm not sick and my health and energy are reliable. I can really get a lot done. As supplements, I still take coenzyme Q10, 60 mg a day, and super blue-green algae, 3 g a day. I am grateful to have found out what was making me ill, after nearly five years of looking.

Eric on mercury fillings

My initial awareness of another possibility in dentistry goes all the way back to Carlton Fredericks, who used to say in his program that based upon the admonition to dentists by the American Dental Association on how they were to handle mercury, the only apparent safe place for the mercury was in your mouth. He made me aware that there were other possibilities. But moving from that to actually finding a holistic dentist at that time was something else. I investigated, and quite frankly, found some that talk the talk but don't walk the walk. In other words, they appeared holistic until I got in there. It was a gradual learning process that involved the gathering of more and more information.

I found myself that I prefer a one-on-one situation with a dentist. I went to a group office and it seemed to me that the partners were placing their economic returns before the interests of the patient.

I finally found a woman dentist, named Elmira Godall. There was an instant rapport. She presented options. She made her recommendations very clear, but she empowered me to take responsibility for the choices I made. She, herself, went to the trouble to learn Huggins's protocol. She went to Colorado to learn about mercury removal, and essentially followed his protocol.

When she removed mercury amalgam from my teeth, she simultaneously administered a vitamin C drip. She put a composite filling in a tooth that had an awful lot of mercury amalgam in it. My previous dentist insisted that the only option was a crown. The composite is holding up very well indeed.

She happened to be so sensitive in her skills with the drill that I have never had to have Novocain. With my previous dentist, I found that after leaving the office, I always ended up with a bunch of canker sores in my mouth. I haven't had a single canker sore since [switching to this] dentist.

In general, I found that being able to deal on a one-to-one basis with a person who respects you and who considers your ability to take responsibility for your own care to be an important factor. She is not lording it over you, but you are making a joint decision. That seems to be the critical factor here. I will conclude by saying that I am exceedingly pleased with the results I have attained.

Patricia on periodontal disease

I went to a dental hygienist on a referral from my dentist. She told me that I had periodontal disease and suggested a vitamin protocol, an herbal rinse, and a particular toothpaste with no sugar. She showed me how to floss all my teeth, including the ones that have crowns.

At that time, my gums bled whenever I brushed my teeth. I had bad breath. I had pockets with trapped food. I had never been informed about ways to clean my teeth.

Now when I brush my teeth, they seldom bleed. I no longer have bad breath. I have an awareness about dental hygiene that I never had before. I think that she's a very good hygienist and I have seen major improvements in my own dental hygiene.

Patty on candidiasis

I've had years and years of the traditional approach and I've had lots of mercury put in my mouth. As a kid, I lived on sugar, which gave me major cavities. At 16 I had my first root canal, and two years ago, I had another one.

I have been suffering for about 10 years with chronic candidiasis and chemical sensitivity from a lowered immune system.

I have been seeing Dr. Levin for about two years now, and he recommended that I have the root canal taken out, as well as the mercury. I just had the root canal removed about eight months ago and I'm in the process of removing the mercury. I need to get eight or nine more fillings taken out. I know that it's good to get vitamin C drips along with the treatment, but since I can't afford that right now I take lots of C orally, and sometimes charcoal tablets, to help absorb the mercury that otherwise might go into my system.

My dentist uses a dental dam. She is extremely conscientious. She herself has suffered from candida and knows a lot about holistic healing.

When the root canal was removed, they found an infection in that part of the gum. I'm glad that I had it taken out, because I think in the long run it is a healthy thing to do. I've read a lot of literature on the disadvantages of root canals and I will never have another one. . . . I believe that they have definitely contributed to my lowered immune system.

Marjorie on sinus problems, arthritis, rashes, and high cholesterol

I had been having rashes and allergies for over 30 years. I had hay fever, I was lethargic, I had chronic arthritis, and my cholesterol was high.

A nutritionist, who was also an M.D., started me on the macrobiotic diet about five and a half years ago. That helped me a lot, but I still couldn't tolerate certain foods. I had lost weight and couldn't gain any back.

I went to Sherry Rogers, up in Syracuse. She was the first to introduce me to the idea of getting the mercury amalgams out of my mouth. My initial reaction was how could something so prevalent, that everybody has some of, possibly be a problem? So I let it go for a couple of years.

And then a year ago, another doctor also recommended it. He sent me to Dr. Bryner. I did have the amalgams removed and the composites put in. At the same time he tested me for mercury toxicity and my measured level then was 9, which borders on a toxic level, consistent with industrial exposure, because the expected range is less than 2.

At the same time he did an electric test to see what organs were harboring the mercury, and recommended the DMPS treatment. And that's used for the treatment of heavy metal toxicity. It binds, I guess, to the heavy metals, and washes them out of your system.

So I've had three of these DMPS treatments following getting the mercury out and I've never felt better in my life. I'm more alert. I've gained back a few pounds. Initially I went from 135 down to 99, and I'm back up to about 106. I can now tolerate more food.

Nancy on pleurisy and pneumonia

I was unaware of the fact that my jawbone was being eaten away. I had a little tingling in the spot where I had a root canal previously done, four five years earlier. I'd think, "Gee, that's funny," and then I wouldn't think any more about it. I think maybe one of the dangers of root canals is that without a nerve there, you cannot sense the pain, and pain is nature's signal that something is wrong. So it's kind of a scary thing when you can't tell that there's something wrong.

I went for a regular dental check-up and had x-rays. Dr. Bryner said, "We've got a major problem here." This root canal was apparently infected and was eating away at the jawbone. And I was what I considered to be healthy at that time. So I went home and scheduled an appointment to have this root canal taken out—I mean remove the tooth.

Before I could get back for my next appointment, I came down with pleurisy, and that developed into pneumonia. So I had to delay my appointment a couple of weeks. Eventually I did go in. I had two root canal teeth right next to each other, on two lower molars. The one farthest back was the one that was infected. I decided to have him take both of them out. Why wait until the next one has a problem?

In the meantime I had read a book on root canals which really opened my eyes to the problems. Apparently, there are bacteria there all the time. When a root canal is performed, they can't ever get it totally sterile, so they do their best. Then they close that area off. We assume that these bacteria die when they are cut off from oxygen. But what in fact seems to happen is that they mutate and become anaerobic, which is really scary because then they can live anywhere in your body and you don't know it. They can gravitate anywhere, maybe to a weaker organ.

Anyway, when I went back for my appointment I had both of those root canals taken out. Dr. Bryner had told me some time before that that every tooth is related to an internal organ. I originally went to Dr. Bryner because I had had twenty years of chronic headaches and I had heard that amalgam removal could possibly help that. When he took out my two root canal teeth I said, "I'm just curious. What are these teeth related to?" These were two lower molars that happened to be on my right side. He looked it up on the chart and said, "The lower molars are related to the sinuses and the lungs." I was amazed. I had had sinus headaches all those years, and sure enough, with this infection and these anaerobic bacteria gone, I had no more problems in my lungs.

Dr. Bryner was good enough to give me a homeopathic remedy to follow up with that. I went back to my walk-in clinic where I had had the original x-ray and my lungs were clear! I hate to think what would have happened had I been going to an ordinary dentist. They probably would have tried to save the tooth, which is what dentists always try to do. I think I would have made a trade-off to keep the tooth and lose my health. I'm grateful that I found Dr. Bryner because although I may have lost a tooth, I have my health.

Sherry Dodson-Puziss (dentist) on mercury poisoning

My story is a story of being poisoned through my work, but I hope it talks to people who are also poisoned through their fillings and their lifestyles because it's really a story of poisoning.

I worked in an old, old dental clinic. The room had lots of mercury spills— five times higher than what the U.S. laws allow for mercury vapor. The mercury was not vacuumed out of carpets; it just stayed. It's odorless and tasteless and you absorb it through the lungs and your skin. That's where I got my exposure for about six years.

I probably went to 10 or 15 doctors who felt I was just stressed from having a baby and working. They never got the diagnosis right, and they wanted to give me phenobarbital and things like that.

Instead, I went to the medical books, read up on the symptoms, and found out that I had the classical symptoms of mercury poisoning. We had someone come in and test the air, which was highly toxic. We got rid of the carpeting.

I worked for a large, traditional clinic where it was not politically proper to do further reading on mercury toxicity. There was a political move to keep this rather quiet, and so I let it go and continued to practice my dentistry, thinking that the problems were taken care of. I wanted to keep my job because I had a family, and I was supporting a husband through school back then. So I didn't do too much reading on mercury toxicity at that time.

Over the course of 18 years, I got sicker and sicker. What happens is your liver gets killed. So do your organs of digestion. It's like a slow starvation. I became more and more ill without knowing why, and didn't realize it was still the mercury until I finally totally broke and fell apart in 1991.

I was in bed for two and a half years with immune system problems. During that time, I began reading. I got access to the Library of Congress, where I was able to read abstracts on mercury research dating back up to 30 years. I learned that both my children were born poisoned with mercury. A lot of these poisons pass the placental barrier and also come through the nursing milk. Children are far more susceptible to the effects of the toxins than adults.

Basically, I realized that you have to remove environmental toxins. You have to look around and that's what I did. I stopped spraying my lawn with insecticides. I stopped bringing poisons into the home, like laundry fabric softeners. I got my drinking and showering water filtered. Water filters on the shower absorb tons of chlorine, a toxin that adds to the mercury. You've got basic mercury poisoning and then everything else added to it makes it worse.

After this is where you need professional help from complementary physicians, naturopaths, chiropractors, clinical ecologists, somebody who understands toxins. You have to get your liver restored. The liver is the organ that cleanses the body and so it gets all the poisons, and it backs up. You get too much poison. So the liver's got to be cleansed and healed and get healthy. Then after that you have to go after the stored body toxins, because these things stay in your fat cells and in all your body cells, your brain cells, your bone cells, everything.

I went through chelation therapy. . . . You may need as many as 15 IV or IM treatments, after you've had your fillings removed. And you have vitamin and mineral supplements in between because mercury depletes these from the body. At the same time, the supplements pull mercury out of the body. Chlorella is a green algae supplement that removes mercury from the body. We know the foods cilantro and asparagus do as well.

. . . We know that sweating works too. If you take a dry sauna, sweat profusely, and shower afterwards, assays on the sweat find metals coming out. Baking soda and epsom salt baths can also help. You can take two cups of baking soda and two cups of epsom salts in a hot, hot bath and soak. That helps pull out the metals.

So I did that. Had I not done the alternative complementary route I feel I wouldn't be alive today. Experts in this field say that. I think it's extremely important to self-advocate. The prognosis for mercury poisoning is generally good, I think, although you may be left with some central nervous system damage, including numb fingers and toes. I don't know if the ability to memorize fully comes back or not, because I'm still in the process of healing and getting better.

I implore people to self-advocate because nobody's going to do it for them. In my case, I saw 25 doctors, and nobody picked this up.

Nancy on headaches

I had had incapacitating headaches, the kind where you just have to go lay down. I guess you could call them migraines. I had visual disturbances and I would get nauseous. After my amalgam removal, I had fewer headaches and they were less intense. But I still would get some.

Following the root canal removals, I have far fewer headaches, and the ones I have are very mild. I guess you call them tension headaches. They're sort of the run-of-the-mill things that everybody gets. I don't have to stop what I'm doing with a headache now.

Let me just give one little detail on the headaches. I tend to get them at the approach of a storm. I think I'm sensitive to barometric changes. I had my root canals removed in December of 1993. That was a terrible winter with storm after storm here in the northeast. Where I live, in Connecticut, we had 17 major snow storms. Yet I did not get a single headache the entire winter. Now, that is phenomenal, because for 20 years I had been getting headaches whenever a major low pressure system came through my area. That's probably the most significant improvement for me.

Flip on periodontal care

I'm in my 40's, and I've been going to my childhood dentist for years. He is a very nice fellow but he paid very little attention to my gums over the years. I don't hold that against him because back in those days nobody was really talking about that. Anyway, he discovered some pockets and asked me to have them checked out by a periodontist. I went to a periodontist who dipped little needles down into the pockets that I had between my teeth. He asked me to come back a couple of days later for the diagnosis.

When I returned, he said that I needed about $5000 worth of gum surgery. At the time, I was not inclined to do that, and I didn't really want to spend money I didn't have. Then he added that I needed a root canal for a problem tooth before he could do surgery. Not knowing anything about the ill effects of root canals I went ahead and got it.

I went to a new dentist, who gave me a perfectly fine root canal. While I was sitting in the chair, I said, "I've had surgery recommended, and I wonder if you know of any alternative hygienist that I could talk to." That's when he told me about someone in the next-door office. I made an appointment with her, which is what changed my—I can't say life, but I can say that it certainly changed my mouth.

She gave me a deep cleaning and talked to me, saying that this was not about my mouth, but about my stomach, my intestines, and my entire system. She recommended that I transform my diet and my nutrition, which would both cleanse my system and boost my immunity. That, in turn, might help to reverse the bone loss that I was having and actually improve my periodontal condition.

I started in on this, although I was kind of skeptical at the time. It involved something I had never heard of before called coenzyme Q10, and an entire regimen. To cleanse my system, I stopped drinking coffee and cut dairy out of my diet. I'm kind of addicted to pasta so I never did get the wheat out of my diet entirely, but I drink a lot less coffee and I am almost completely off cheese.

In addition to the coenzyme Q10, I started to take a group of minerals and vitamins that included lots of vitamin C with bioflavonoids, zinc, B complex, and vitamin E. I began drinking water with half a lime or lemon every night to help my liver. I still do this, and it is quite pleasant.

After she cleaned, she sent me home with an herbal rinse made from echinacea, goldenseal and cayenne and a couple of other things. At first it was kind of a bitter brew but I got used to it, and after about a week I began to think that this was the most delicious thing I had ever taken.

Over the course of a few years, with a lot of flossing, my bone loss never got any worse and my mouth has completely changed. I feel comfortable with it, and my gums don't bleed anymore.

Now this has become a daily routine for me. When I'm under a lot of stress I might boost up my vitamin C intake and possibly take another Q10 or something like that because I find that when I'm under a lot of stress it affects my gums. And I really notice a difference. Anyway, that's my experience. My mouth feels very healthy right now.

Karen on husband's heart condition and her clinical depression and menopausal problems

It started about seven years ago. We were given an Ayurvedic preparation that came into the country, probably not in a kosher way, you might say. Anyhow it was given for indigestion and we didn't know that it contained mercury at the time. He took it for indigestion and he experienced low atrial fibrillation. And he was quite symptomatic. His pulse was about 40; he was ashen; he was nauseated. Blood pressure was about 50 over God knows what. He was hospitalized.

The medical profession didn't understand why he was low atrial fib. He was about 32. It was Christmastime, actually Christmas Day. And so they allowed me to bring him home from the hospital since I was a cardiac nurse, and we just monitored him. We were kind of wondering, what did we do different? You know, why is this happening?

And so one of the things we decided was to stop taking some of these Ayurvedic preparations that we had gotten. We called a friend, and she did identify, in some formula that she had, that the preparation that we had had mercury in it. It was commonly used in India with no problems, but it did cause my husband a problem. We stopped and four days later he converted on his own, and he was in normal sinus rhythm. We had done a little chiropractic work in the meantime to help his body cleanse, but that's all we did. That's all we knew.

About two years later he went into atrial fib again. And this time . . . we didn't know what was going on. It was again even more serious than it was the last time. He had to be cardioverted and he was on all kinds of cardiac drugs. He had terrible reactions to them and I really thought he was going to die once. It was just awful. And then he was on a drug—a heavy-duty cardiac drug—for about four years. But it was really giving him a very difficult time with his intestines. So we felt we've got to go off this. The cardiologist agreed. He didn't like it, but he agreed, and he tapered Gary off his drug.

Gary was good for about a year and a half. Then he went into slow atrial fib again. Again, extremely symptomatic. Absolutely no energy. He would be exhausted just picking up the telephone and saying hello and, you know, we're only talking 40 years old now, so we were really concerned.

We went to an alternative M.D. She dealt in other things, other than just your standard medical fare. She did a couple of tests and discovered that indeed, there were a lot of mercury problems in Gary's system. She suggested that Dr. Bryner could help him. We went to Dr. Bryner. He did some testing on Gary, and felt that he was a good candidate to have his mercury out. We did it, and his digestion got stronger. Before, he wasn't absorbing magnesium or calcium, which is essential for good cardiac function, and they thought the mercury was interfering with that because of his intestines. . . . To make a long story short, it's been a year for Gary, a little over a year. He's on no cardiac drugs. He did not have to be cardioverted.

Nine months into that process, because I saw how wonderful he was doing, I did the same. I had some menopausal problems, some clinical depression, which was just awful. I had the mercury taken out of my mouth and right in the chair, like somebody turned a light switch on, while he worked on my teeth my depression left. I mean I wasn't even thinking that was going to happen. He told me that my intestines were going to get better but he said nothing about depression whatsoever. And I just got so happy and I've been happy ever since. So my husband's got a good heart and I have a happy mind.

Sharon on dental problems

I've gone to several dentists in the last eight years who let me know that I had a potential problem, that the pockets in my teeth were increasing. I really didn't understand what that meant until my present doctor told me that if that continued the bone underneath would melt away and disappear. I let these dentists know that I wanted to participate in my own healing. They always gave me certain exercises to do, but unfortunately it didn't get better.

This past January, my former dentist, a very nice person, said that there was nothing else to do but surgery. I let him know that that would be the last thing I would do, and asked him if he could tell me about something else. He couldn't, but he gave me the names of other dentists. I was in a quandary because I had the feeling that the people he told me about wouldn't know how to do anything except surgery.

But I asked around and learned of a dentist in Brooklyn. I started treatment with her . . . on a holistic regime. Basically the first thing that had to be done was amalgam removal. That was difficult because it was expensive, especially since vitamin C drips were given at the same time. But I decided to do it anyway. I think there were about seven to eight treatments. In addition to that I started to use magnets in the evening. I had magnets on either side of my cheeks.

I saw her a few days ago, and what's been happening is very, very interesting. It seems that clinically I regained this is what she said—extra attachments in the pockets. My pockets are shallower. This is really interesting because I've asked all over and everybody has told me that that's absolutely impossible. It just can't happen. But it's happening to me.

Claire on periodontal disease

I've had periodontal disease for quite some time, and I was told by a dentist, at least 10 or 12 years ago, that I needed to have periodontal surgery, which I wasn't very happy about.

By accident I discovered the International Dental Health Foundation. Since I was having so much trouble with my teeth, I decided that I might as well go. So I beat my path to the foundation, which is located in Reston, Virginia, and there I saw Dr. Keyes and Dr. Watts.

First they took a culture of my gum which they studied under a microscope and at the same time projected onto a large screen. This enabled me to see what was going on in my mouth. There were a lot of bacteria at that time.

Dr. Keyes taught me how to use a peroxide and baking soda paste. He instructed me on making the paste to the consistency of honey and using it twice a day with a small toothbrush.

In addition, Dr. Keyes sold me a Swiss irrigator, called the Porpoise, and told me to use it twice a day with a salt solution or diluted peroxide. That seems to work very, very well. Here in New York the dentists have told me not to use the irrigator because it pushes the food particles under the gum, but Dr. Keyes laughed at this and said it is not so. The irrigator helps to control the bacterial population in the mouth.

I have been using the irrigator for the past 11 years, and have been able to maintain my natural dentition. I've been having problems on and off, but I'm able to control them. These Swiss-made irrigators are not available in the United States, but they are available all over the world. The Colgate company is producing their own brand of irrigators in Hong Kong, but they are facsimiles of the Swiss machine. They work for a while, but they tend to break down a lot. The public is not aware of the Swiss type.

Recently I went to see a Dr. Resnik in Edison, New Jersey, who is on the board of directors of the Dental Health Foundation. Through him I obtained a Swiss machine which is the latest of the irrigators, called a Hydrofloss. This Hydrofloss comes with three different picks: the regular pick, the perio pick, which has a smaller opening and is able to deliver the solution deep under the gum, and a third irrigating device, called a cannula. I call it a needle. This really delivers the antimicrobial solution deep under the gum. And what I'm using is chlorhexadine. This is very effective in controlling the bacteria and in just helping me to maintain my natural teeth.

And it's really unfortunate, but our society seems to ignore dental health issues and it's quite a [problem] because a person cannot chew their food properly without teeth. Poor chewing causes malabsorption and this causes all kinds of diseases. I consider myself extremely lucky that I was able to maintain my natural teeth. . . . If you need information about the Dental Health Foundation, their telephone numbers are 703-471-8349 and 800-368-3396.

Bob on periodontal disease

I neglected my mouth for years, sort of thinking of it as something that would just disappear, a separate entity. In the meantime, my gums had been receding and bleeding. I was horrified at the expense of gum surgery.

After a number of years of feeling more and more tired and sluggish from the overall neglect, I decided to start looking at the factors contributing to my poor state of health. I was persuaded by a homeopath that I see to go to a dental hygienist. I went to a great one, who was horrified by what she saw in my mouth. After a few minutes, I became ashamed of my condition, and that shame would have kept me from doing anything, but her attitude was extremely positive. She assured me that my condition could be reversed and that gum surgery was absolutely not necessary provided that I followed her protocol. This sounded much better than gum surgery. . . .

I basically followed a whole regimen, relearning basic habits that I had never really integrated as a kid. I started flossing morning and night. She literally showed me how to brush my teeth correctly. Since old habits don't change overnight, there was some backsliding, but seeing her a few times would reinforce some of the basics. It all sounds very primitive and it was. she also told me to brush my tongue because it is a great repository and breeding ground for germs and gum disease.

She gave me an herbal rinse to use after flossing. Then I got on a protocol of multivitamins, calcium, coenzyme Q10, beta carotene and so on to boost the immune system.

In a nutshell, it took me two weeks to stop the bleeding in the gums that had been going on for years. That, in itself, was a great incentive to keep going with this. I have noticed some regrowth of the gums, which feels miraculous to me. But it's no miracle. What's happening just makes sense. By following this regimen, my mouth is refreshed and it makes a difference head-wise.

Annette on silver and mercury amalgam extraction

Well, first of all my mouth feels entirely different. It's so much cleaner, which is not the most important thing, but I'm aware of it every day. The really big thing is that in these three years I haven't been sick. I haven't had a cold. I haven't had a sore throat. I haven't had the flu. I haven't missed any work because of sickness. It's been absolutely amazing, and there's been no other change in my life. I eat the same way, I live in the same place, I have the same job.

Prior to the mercury coming out, I had nothing out of the ordinary. But every year I had at least one or two colds or the flu. That wasn't the reason that I went to Dr. Bryner, but that was certainly an unexpected benefit.

Marcia on fatigue, allergies and headaches

I had my mercury fillings removed about four years ago. My symptoms were tiredness, allergies, headaches, and a metallic taste in my mouth. After removal of the fillings, it took approximately six months to a year until all of these symptoms went away. The metallic taste naturally disappeared right away. Then I found that the headaches and allergies took a longer time. So did the fatigue. But they all did disappear.

I believe this is all due to the mercury being removed from my mouth. I went to a holistic doctor who specialized in this. He tested me and they found that I had a high mercury level. Mercury was being released when I chewed at a much higher rate than was acceptable. So, I would attribute my results to that, since basically I hadn't done anything differently. I was taking vitamins and I had a good diet before that. But I still had those symptoms and they did seem to gradually go away.

Chelation Therapy

Chelation therapy is one of the most exciting healing therapies available. If it was used more widely, it could be saving hundreds of thousands of lives each year, and improving the lives of millions more by treating conditions such as strokes, cardiovascular disease, diabetes, peripheral vascular disease, memory loss, and damage due to long-term smoking, drinking, and exposure to toxic metals.

Chelation therapy is an intravenous treatment for the removal of toxins and metabolic wastes from the bloodstream. The process involves the slow drip of a drug called ethylene diamine tetraacetic acid (EDTA) and various nutrients into a vein in the arm over the course of approximately three hours. The word chelation stems from the Greek term "chela," meaning claw, and implies that heavy metals and excess calcium bind to carrier molecules after they are picked up in a pincer-like fashion. Substances exit the body through the kidneys, preventing the formation of stones and hardened tissue. Generally, a series of 30 treatments is initially given, and a smaller number are given each year thereafter as maintenance. This, of course, can vary depending on the patient's state of health.

It was in 1948 that the benefits of chelation therapy first became apparent, when a group of Detroit physicians who were employing the modality as an antidote for lead poisoning noticed positive side effects in their patients. These included better vision, better hearing, loss of or decreased angina, less pain, an ability to walk farther, and a reduction of intermittent claudication. They related these improvements to a reduction in arteriosclerosis.

In 1950, Norman Clark, M.D. confirmed these observations in clinical research when he found the therapy effective in removing calcium deposits from the human body. He reported in the medical literature that EDTA might dissolve plaque and improve blood circulation. As a result, pioneering doctors began using chelation therapy for the treatment of arteriosclerosis, with great success. The holistic medical community now considers chelation therapy a

454

safe, alternative to coronary bypass surgery and angioplasty, and one that is actually more effective than those invasive procedures.

Chelation therapy also acts to reverse the aging process in three senses. First, chelation keeps free radicals in check, resulting in slowed cellular destruction. Second, oxygenation to the heart and blood vessels is strengthened, so that organ systems are revitalized. And third, osteoporosis is prevented or diminished as excess calcium is transferred from the arteries and joints to the bones. Many health practitioners recommend that chelation therapy be used by everyone over the age of 30 to slow down the aging process and to prevent the onset of disease. The treatment is not a ''magic bullet,'' but rather works best as part of a comprehensive program that includes proper diet, supplements, and exercise.

Patient Stories

Lee on heart disease

I had two bypass operations, one during Christmas 1975 and a second in July 1981. In September of that year Social Security forced me to go back to work at the Post Office once a week. Even though I was working with great constant chest pain, they removed me from Social Security because I looked so healthy. They had a local clerk say that, as far as they were concerned, there was nothing wrong with me even though I had blocked arteries and constant pain shooting throughout my chest.

A year and a half later I ended up in the local VA hospital. While there, they told me I had four arteries blocked 100 percent. I was only able to get from my bed to my bathroom. That was it. I was given a handful of pills and told to go home. Three weeks later I had a real bad spell where I had to sit up in the chair the whole night because I couldn't catch my breath. My arms, legs, my whole body, swelled up like a basketball and I turned just as blue as the car that I drive. I had to concentrate to get every breath. I felt like I had one foot in the pine box and the other one on a banana peel. I promised myself that if I woke up in the morning I would go to see Dr. Sessions, whom I had known for about 10 years.

I did start to see Dr. Sessions who gave me chelation treatments. I can't tell if it was psychological or physical, but the very first bottle I was given removed the shooting-star chest pain that I had for over five months.

I have learned from Dr. Sessions that previous to treatment I had an unbelievable amount of iron, zinc, cadmium, and lead in my system. Now I have changed my diet. Previously I was a heavy beef eater, but I no longer eat red meat.

Claude on intermittent claudication

I had a blockage in the bend of my leg. My leg circulation was so bad that I could hardly walk. After running an arteriogram on me the doctor said I should take an aspirin a day. Then I went to Dr. Sessions, and I have had no trouble since. I have had 95 chelation sessions, and I can now walk. My legs don't hurt me like they did and I can do almost anything I want to. I believe that Dr. Sessions's chelation therapy kept me from having my leg amputated. I was also right on the verge of a stroke when I went to him and he straightened that out. I am over 81 years old.

Randolph on advanced arteriosclerosis

I am 66 years old. Back in 1989 I had artery blockage for which I had an operation. After the operation I still had blockage in my main artery because it was that bad. A friend of mine told me about chelation. I have had 40 treatments; a treadmill test given by my cardiologist shows no sign of blockage anymore.

Chelation therapy has made a substantial difference in the quality of my life. Before I took chelation I couldn't walk a block. Now I have no problem walking. I can walk two miles three times a week. Also, my eyesight has gotten better. In fact, I hardly have to wear glasses at all, even to read, whereas before I had to have them with me all the time. I would start chelation all over again if I needed to.

Mr. H. on diabetes, heart disease, glaucoma, and kidney stones

Approximately 12 years ago I suffered from diabetes, hypertension, high blood pressure (250/110), glaucoma, and kidney stones. There were weeks of time where I did not get out of bed. Evidently my condition was terrible. My kidney stones were so large that I was told they could not be removed except surgically. Dr. Sessions suggested that he might have a treatment for me and I started taking it right away. After the 20th treatment I began to feel better and I have continued to take chelation ever since once a month. In all, I have had 300 treatments.

I am 83 years old and currently I have no kidney stones. This morning my blood pressure was 130/60 and I feel great. . . .

In addition to chelation treatments I have changed my diet. I take vitamins and do not eat animal fats. I exercise as well.

If it had not been for chelation treatments I do not believe I would be alive today. I intend to take one treatment each month for as long as I live.

I have seen many, many people come through Dr. Sessions' office, and almost everyone, including those who were facing amputation, have suffered no ill effects.

I think this is a treatment most of us need since all of us have been contaminated in some manner with lead and other chemicals that chelation removes.

Dr. B. on arteriosclerosis

I was going through a period in life where a lot of my friends, who are in the over-50 age group, were experiencing heart attacks, angina, and associated symptoms. That prompted me to think about my own condition, so as a precautionary move I took a thallium stress test.

To my surprise, they found a blocked major coronary artery. The hospital recommended at that time that I do an angioplasty where they open up the artery. I felt that that was an invasive procedure which should be used as a last resort.

I discussed this with Dr. Corsello, who suggested I try chelation for a year or so. She said I could always have the angioplasty done later because it was not yet at a serious stage. I agreed. In fact, I had wanted to take chelation therapy for another reason. As a dentist I had been exposed to a lot of heavy metals over the years.

I went through a year's chelation therapy. During that year I had a tremendous increase in my energy level. I had younger-looking skin and I felt younger and everyone said I looked great. A year later I went back for another thallium stress test and to the doctor's surprise the blockage was no longer there. I have had two successive thallium stress tests since then with the same results. I have maintained a schedule of having chelation therapy once or twice a month since that time and my heavy metal level has decreased almost 80 percent. I feel great.

Some of my patients have used chelation and the results are equally positive. It alleviates tiredness and it restores the immune system. I have even seen people suffering from Lyme disease have equally good results. And I have seen other people who were intoxicated with heavy metals who have all had favorable experiences. We had one person with Epstein-Barr who was walking around with a cane for years because nobody was able to ascertain what he had or give him a definitive treatment. He calls me up every month to thank me.

Don on lead poisoning and carpal tunnel syndrome

When I first came to Dr. Corsello I had lead toxicity that measured in the upper 300 category. She brought it down during a period of less than a year to about 77 or so, at which point I decided to stop chelation for a while. One of the curious byproducts of the treatment was that it has a remarkable effect on alleviating the bilateral carpal tunnel syndrome that I was suffering from for almost 10 years. After chelation, it disappeared.

Chris on angina and bursitis

I am 75 years old. In 1975, I had a massive heart attack that left me practically a cripple and forced me into early retirement. I could hardly walk even one city block; the pain would get so bad that I would have to stop and wait approximately 15 minutes before going another block. I went to see one of the famous cardiologists in New York and the diagnosis was that if I lasted five years I would lose both legs. I didn't like those odds at all.

In the meantime I heard of something called the Dr. Rinse formula and I started with that. It seemed to help a bit but I still had no pulse in either ankle.

Then I finally heard about a Dr. Levin at the World Health Center and I went to him. I went through his course of chelation and I suddenly realized that I was able to walk as many blocks as I wanted. My angina disappeared. My bursitis, which had made it very painful for me to get into or out of a shirt, just vanished. At the end of the treatments with Dr. Levin I was able to walk several miles with no leg pain and I have a pulse in both ankles. It has worked wonders for me. I am positive I would not be alive today if it were not for chelation.

George on arteriosclerosis

Before therapy I had a heart attack. They found that two of my blood vessels leaving the heart were restricted, one 95 percent and one 45 percent. After leaving critical care, I was not able to walk without experiencing pain. They had me on a couple of drug programs to control my blood pressure and heart action and they told me I should take nitroglycerin for the pain. I couldn't walk more than a half mile without pain after my heart attack.

After I had 9 or 10 treatments of chelation therapy I was able to walk without pain. I could walk 3 miles in 45 minutes. My cardiologist is monitoring me and my injection fraction (which is the cardiac output), has gone from 49 to 54 percent. This astonished the cardiologist, who still to this day will not acknowledge the fact that my progress is due to the chelation therapy.

Originally, I was a fire-fighter and I built houses in my spare time. Since the chelation therapy I have been able to maintain activities similar to that. In fact I recently helped a friend put up a building. I have done carpentry work in my own home and I have completely finished my basement.

Paul on high blood pressure

My blood pressure was elevated all the time so my doctor suggested I take a stress test; it showed that I indeed had some problems. I ended up having a catheterization and they found some blockages in my heart.

Having had 28 years of experience in the pharmaceutical field, and having heard of chelating agents, I started inquiring about them. Dr. Scarchilli was recommended to me by my family physician. He took tests prior to my treatment and there were several things that were wrong other than blockages in the heart. He put me on a program of chelation therapy and diet and exercise. I rode an exercise bike all winter long, 45 minutes each night, while doing some weight-lifting exercise and maintaining a very rigid diet.

I have made progress. I notice my memory has improved. I do power walking now at the doctor's suggestion and I can walk one and four tenths of a mile in 18 minutes. I take my pulse immediately afterwards and it is 88. That is excellent and indicates that my blood flow and overall physical condition is good. I have stopped using my heart medications almost altogether. I carry them with me just in case I need them, but I'm going to stop carrying them pretty soon because I feel a whole lot better.

Ziegfried on blocked arteries

I had a massive heart attack that left me in the hospital for months. One artery was 100 percent blocked and the other two were 60 percent and 40 percent blocked. Of course, the doctors recommended a bypass operation, which I was not very keen on doing. I thought I would try other possibilities, with chelation being at the top of the list.

Since that time I started taking chelation therapy and am now on my 23rd treatment. As a result I feel a lot better and I have increased my walking ability. When I first started I couldn't even walk 100 yards without getting chest pains. Now I can walk three to four miles every morning.

I changed to a completely vegetarian diet and cut out all my fat intake. It took a little getting used to but after three to four weeks I was able to adjust. I have lost 42 pounds in the last three months just from changing my diet.

Leo on blocked arteries

Approximately two years ago, I was suffering from dizzy spells, which at times were just unbearable. I went to see a few physicians who couldn't find out the cause of my trouble. Finally, one suggested that I go to a vascular surgeon and I did. He gave me a thorough examination with all his technology and equipment and then told me that my condition was very discouraging, as one carotid artery was 100 percent blocked and the other was blocked 75 percent. He said my condition was inoperable and that I would have to wait for the inevitable to happen. That was in February 1990.

I then heard of chelation therapy through a friend of the family who gave me the name of Dr. Dan Roehm in Florida. I have since received between 75 and 80 treatments, and as of March 1991 the results have been remarkable. My right carotid artery has gone from 100 percent to 83 percent blocked and the left one has gone from 75 percent to between 44 and 48 percent blocked.

All in all, I have found that this has done me a world of good, as I am able to get around and do my work. I can highly recommend the treatment to anyone in the same position as myself. I am 85 years old and feel that chelation therapy has added quality to my life. In fact, I feel I would be dead today without it because they couldn't operate on me and I was going downhill at the time.

Steve on heart attacks

I had a couple of heart attacks about six or seven years ago and I pulled through those in fair condition. Then I had a bad one where I had an infarct and I checked into a hospital with that. After that I couldn't walk too far or do too much work because I would get angina and a heavy chest.

I accidentally heard about Dr. Schachter on the radio. I went to see him and after several chelation treatments, I began to feel a lot better. It took a little time, but after a couple of years, I could reduce the treatments from two a week to one a week, to once a month.

Now I am feeling fine and can do a lot of work around the yard. I do gardening, I walk better, and I don't have the angina the way I used to have it. I used to walk half a block and take nitroglycerin. Now, I'm doing pretty well on the supplements that they instructed me to take plus the treatment. I recommend chelation highly to anyone with a problem of the vascular system.

Charles on angina and arthritis

In 1984, I was diagnosed as requiring a quadruple bypass. My left ventricle was 85 percent blocked and the rest of my body wasn't too good either.

I was barely able to walk when I started out. Now I am 71 and can walk two miles without any great sweat. Also, I can exercise for 45 minutes or more every day, and I do. I also found that what little arthritis I had left me and I am free from pain. I hardly ever have any angina now.

I have had over 80 treatments by now and I still continue maintenance treatments once a month. I would say that chelation, coupled with exercise and supplements and keeping control of your diet, is pretty much the path to success.

Mrs. K on strokes

Two years ago, at the age of 70, my husband had many strokes which affected his mental capacity. He couldn't remember things and was having difficulty in general.

We took him to our local doctor, who gave him an MRI test and sent him to a neurologist. The outcome was that they decided he had atherosclerosis. When I asked what could be done for that, he said there was really nothing except medication for high blood pressure. We had him on five pills a day until one day I decided that perhaps, since both my husband's parents had lived well into their 90's and had been well and sharp, I should try to do some research to see what I could do with diet and other means.

A year ago last May I found a book on chelation in the library and read about what it could do for the brain. I called medical establishments in Nassau County but they gave me no information on it at all. They thought I was talking a foreign language. Then I found out about Dr. Yurkovsky through a friend and we went to see him.

My husband has had about 40 half treatments and I have seen major improvements in his condition. On a scale of one to ten we have gone from about three to eight, and that makes life much more comfortable.

Florence on blocked carotid artery

My problem was a clogged carotid and I think that chelation therapy saved me from having a stroke. I went for chelation after the Mayo Clinic wanted to put me on Valium for the change of life. I asked the doctor there what tests they took to show I had a Valium deficiency and we were downhill all the way from that point.

My husband had severe rheumatoid arthritis and after five treatments he improved tremendously. We had no idea this would do anything for arthritis. He also started to go for treatments after the Mayo Clinic told him to take 15 aspirins a day and that he would be in a wheelchair in six months to a year. Since the treatments, he has worked 11 years without missing a day. . . .

I can't praise this enough and I just can't believe that the doctors and insurance companies are not allowing this to be spread and accepted.

Mitch on heart disease

I started chelation therapy in March 1987 after having had three open heart surgeries from 1975 to 1987. In all, I have had a total of 11 bypass operations. In March 1987, I went to my cardiologist and he told me to have a heart transplant. I would not hear of it and he just said that I should go home and get my affairs in order.

I heard about chelation therapy from Dr. McDonagh's book *Chelation Can Cure* and got an appointment the day after talking to my cardiologist. By the way, I am 54 years old and was 50 at the time. I had my first heart attack at 36. By the time I got to Dr. McDonagh's office I was taking 29 heart pills a day and my total bill for medication was $394 a month.

In January 1988, Dr. McDonagh began taking me gradually off all my heart pills. Since that time, I have had 100 chelation sessions; I no longer take even one heart pill, and I have never been in the hospital. I work between 12 and 15 hours a day and I travel over 80,000 miles a year making my own deliveries. I do carry nitros but I do not use them. I go back to Dr. McDonagh three times a year for maintenance and I take three bottles every time I go back. I never get a cold or flu or anything like that.

Ed on arteriosclerosis

I started with Dr. McDonagh in 1978. Previously, I had a history of severe leg itching where I would scratch my leg so much that it would sometimes bleed. And I would get out of breath from walking 15 minutes or longer.

I finally decided to do something to help my body so I made an appointment with a well-known physician in Kansas City and had a physical. He diagnosed me as having hardening of the arteries and said that I was 50 to 60 percent blocked. After some tests, he recommended that I have bypass surgery.

I gave it some thought and decided it would be better to get a second opinion so I went to another well-known cardiologist who likewise diagnosed my condition as being 50 to 60 percent blocked in the left femoral artery. He suggested immediate bypass surgery as well. A third opinion was the same.

I decided instead to try chelation therapy. That was in December of 1978 and since that time I have had about 60 chelation treatments. As a result I have never in my life felt better.

Chiropractic

Chiropractic is one of the most important and universally available therapies. It is based on the principle that there is an innate wisdom in the body, which promotes health and healing. Chiropractic's founder and developer, B. J. Palmar, describes it this way: "The master maker of the human body did not create you and then run off and leave you masterless. He stayed on the job as the fellow within, as nerve transmission, controlling every function of life."

The goal of the chiropractor is to unblock energy so that inner intelligence can work better. This is done by determining the state of the musculoskeletal and nervous systems. Then, physical imbalances are corrected by manipulating the spinal column to correct partial dislocations known as subluxations. These adjustments allow the brain's messages to flow freely down the entire spinal cord. This, in turn, can promote self-healing of numerous afflictions.

There are approximately 20 different chiropractic techniques. Chiropractors try to fit the technique to the patient's needs. Some chiropractors integrate nutrition and lifestyle counseling into their therapy. Accounting for individual needs and combining various approaches makes chiropractic an excellent form of preventive care.

Though this modality is widely accepted today, this was not always the case. For decades, chiropractic care was maligned by the orthodox medical community. In its darkest hour, the American Medical Association made a concerted effort to completely eliminate the profession, and employed over 70 people full-time for this sole purpose. Fortunately, they were found guilty of violating the Sherman Antitrust Act, and chiropractic survived.

Today the specialty not only survives, it thrives. Chiropractic is widely accepted as a legitimate science and is the largest alternative healing profession in America. Chiropractors are highly trained professionals. Several years of premedical training followed by specialized education results in a D.C. (Doctor of Chiropractic) degree.

463

Patient Stories

Ben on psoriasis

I had a severe case of psoriasis. In addition, I had headaches and stomach pains of unknown etiology. Allopathic doctors tried all kinds of medications but were not able to help me. It was so bad that I almost committed suicide.

I went to see a chiropractor who helped educate me about nutrition, exercise, and stress management. I was worried and upset about my problem and what I learned helped me to calm down. Little by little I have been able to overcome my problems. Recently, at the age of 47, I was able to run the New York City marathon.

Now my psoriasis is under control. It's not gone yet but it is much better than it was. My stomach pains and headaches have disappeared. I feel like a new person and feel like I belong here once again.

I believe my success is due to the fact that chiropractic medicine specifically and holistic medicine in general helps. Chiropractic care works with you and doesn't cause problems.

Elaine on ear infections

When my son, Alexander, complains of pain in his ear, our chiropractor, Gary, adjusts him. Sometimes the earache leaves immediately; other times, it takes a couple of adjustments but he always helps to break down the congestion that causes the inflammation.

I'm certain this is not a placebo effect because you cannot trick children. I've witnessed Alexander getting onto the table with a lot of pain and getting off with none.

Fernando on overcoming physical handicaps

Ever since I was a teenager, I have suffered with lower back pain and a knee problem. For 20 years, I was convinced that I had a physical handicap and that I would have to live with my condition for the rest of my life. Thinking this way rationalized my avoidance of physical activities.

Three years ago, I met a podiatrist who began to educate me about my physical weaknesses. I started to learn about my body structure and how I did not have to suffer or avoid physical activities. I also learned that I had a misaligned right hip and that I would have to seek chiropractic care.

At first, I was skeptical. I'm the type of person who needs proof that something will work. Actually, I was looking for someone to tell me that I needed an operation or medicine. Luckily, I met people who recommended holistic care.

Out of curiosity, I went to a chiropractor. At first, I didn't feel any benefit.

After a few months of treatment, I started to lose interest because I didn't think that this was going to work.

Then one day, I went to see him with a really bad stiff neck. This was a turning point for me because he was able to help me. In a matter of hours, I was feeling great. In the past, I had suffered from stiff necks that ruined my days and weekends.

This was proof for me that chiropractic care works. Because of that, I decided to continue treatments, hoping that one day I would feel the same effects on my lower back. I decided to give it about two years or so.

At the same time, I was seeking help from the podiatrist and changing my diet. My chiropractor helped me to improve my nutrition. I was actually knocking down a lot of old walls that kept me from being physically active for so long. I started running for exercise.

One day, I realized that I running better than longer. I was becoming a marathon runner and decided to run the 1994 marathon. Being able to prepare for and race in the marathon is what ultimately convinced me that chiropractic care works. Before treatments, I never thought I would be able to run 20 miles in my training. I kept my appointments when it got close to the race and stayed with the treatments.

Finally, the day arrived when I was lined up with some of the best runners in the world because I pushed my way to the front of the line. Here I was waiting for a 26-mile race to begin. What's interesting is my chiropractor is also a marathon runner so he understands what I was going through. The support he gave me was great. He even gave me a final adjustment before the gun went off. This was a blessing for me which left me fully prepared to race and helped me finish the race. At the 25th mile, my knee gave me a little problem, which just showed me that I needed to do more work.

I definitely attribute [my success to] a program that includes chiropractic care. This treatment helped me to break through the old walls that I had built around my life and allowed me to let out the spirit of a runner.

Bill on headaches and a liver disorder

Over the years, I was in a lot of car accidents. The worst one was in 1978. As a result, I lived with severe headaches for a number of years, up to four times a day. Sometimes I would scream at the top of my lungs. The pain was so severe that at times I became suicidal.

At first I went to orthopedists and neurologists who gave me a bunch of pills that just worked for short amounts of time. Then, luckily, through a friend, I found chiropractic and I have been getting better. I haven't had a bad headache in seven months. All liver problems have subsided. The tests have shown the improvement. I feel chiropractic care has saved my life.

Besides chiropractic care I actively take care of my health in other ways. I exercise and have become a vegetarian. I also seek out homeopathic care when I need it.

Alma on skin problems

I never believed in holistic medicine until a friend of mine referred me to a holistic doctor back in 1989. One of the most serious problems I had throughout my life was a dermatological problem where my scalp would break out in sores and scabs. I spent thousands of dollars seeking help. As a child, my mother did the same. All the treatments ever did was make my head greasy. They never healed the problem. After just three sessions with my chiropractor, the sores went away. I never had to use anything on my scalp. I have stopped seeing a dermatologist for my scalp because there is no need to see him. Three adjustments took care of the problem, which turned out to be allergy-related.

Then, in June 1991, I was caught in an armed robbery on the job. The robbers really did a number on me. My chiropractor is now treating me for herniated discs in my neck and lower back. I also have other medical problems. He treats me for high blood pressure and for allergies. Treatments relieve me of stress. I see him on the average of three to four times per week. He is wonderful and has convinced me that holistic medicine really works.

Donna on complications during pregnancy

Initially, when I found out that I was pregnant, I had gotten very bad sciatica. My leg was drawn up; I couldn't put it down. I went to my chiropractor for a couple of visits. I still was uncomfortable but I was able to walk around and get around.

He also helped me during my pregnancy with carpal tunnel syndrome. Initially, I was told by my medical doctor to get surgery on my neck to see if it was coming from the neck. Then they would check the elbow.

Overall, it helped improve my well-being during my pregnancy. It helped everything move and go much better. I had a 100 percent wonderful pregnancy. Now, I'm on my second pregnancy and at this point I am really doing fantastic— a little uncomfortable here and there but I keep getting adjusted and I'm doing great.

Sherry on neck and back pain

I suffered for many years and was on all kinds of medication. When it got to the point that medication didn't help anymore, and they wanted to put me in traction, a friend suggested that I see a chiropractor. Not knowing too much about them, I wasn't that willing to go but I spoke to the doctor on the phone.

He said he couldn't guarantee that I would run out of his office but he could guarantee that I would walk.

I went and it certainly helped. I'm off medication. I have arthritis in the neck and it's quite painful. When it gets bad, I start my treatments again and it helps so much. I couldn't bear being without a chiropractor.

Before getting treatment, I never believed that chiropractors could be this helpful. You could have never convinced me because it's not something that's talked about. A doctor tells you to take pills to feel better. Of course, you do these things because a doctor tells you to. But when I went to the chiropractor I soon learned that I did not need these pills. All the pills did was upset my stomach. As soon as the medication wore off the pain was back again. With chiropractic treatment, you do get helped and the pain stays away.

Eileen on Bell's palsy

Last year I began to have seizure-like symptoms. I had an MRI done because I had what appeared to be Bell's palsy on the right side of my face and I tended to walk to my left side. The hospital found nothing wrong and said it was Bell's palsy. That was the end of it.

The episodes continued. I finally sought the care of a holistic doctor who gave me some supplementation. The episodes didn't completely go away so he referred me to a homeopathic doctor who referred me to a chiropractor. I was a little skeptical in the beginning about going, but willing to try anything. The doctor did some adjustments on me and amazingly I didn't have any more episodes. When I stopped going, the episodes began again. I went back to him and after my adjustment the episodes dissipated. Thus far, they have not returned. I am very grateful that I don't have them because they're a little on the scary side. I think holistically between the chiropractic work and a combination of a lot of other modalities, I have been helped a lot.

Pat on knee pain and sciatica

About a year ago, I was actively exercising and taking dance classes about three or four times a week. Unfortunately, I injured myself in class. The injury resulted in pain and numbness in my leg. I had difficulty walking, going up and down stairs and driving. Also, I felt that the strength in my legs was gone. If I tried to run, it felt as if my legs would give out underneath me.

At this point, I went to see several doctors. I was in an HMO at the time. The doctors tested me but couldn't find anything wrong. A neurologist ordered a couple of very painful tests. Basically, I was given electric shock for about 45 minutes on and off. Also, a needle was inserted into my leg and I was told to flex my muscle. The test came back normal and they could draw no conclusions from them. Basically, all they did was put me on Motrin for some time. I found it not to be helpful and discontinued that.

In the meantime, from about June to September, I found that the traumatic part of my injury got better. I could function okay but I wasn't back to my normal self. From about October to April, my leg was achy on and off. I also had numbness on and off. I was not exercising.

Finally, in the spring, someone suggested that I see a chiropractor. I went to a chiropractor who suspected that I had sciatica. The improvement I saw over those six weeks was significant whereas the six months prior to that did not show any major change. He said I should visit twice a week for four to six weeks. During that time, I noticed subtle but significant differences in my leg. I also started exercising very, very gradually. At this point, I am doing a lot more exercise.

There were a couple of other positive side effects which I did not expect. I noticed immediately after the first visit that I had a lot more mobility in my neck from side to side. After adjustments, I could also feel energy flow throughout my whole body. Overall, I have had a very positive experience with chiropractic.

Suzanne on knee, hip, and neck pain, and hormonal imbalance

I'm a runner. Last March, I had to stop running due to pain in my right knee and right hip. My neck had been giving me problems for some time as well. The movement in my neck was more and more constricted. It felt like it was constantly misaligned. I heard about Dr. Gary Deutchman through the running club. I saw him giving other runners ankle and knee adjustments. I was very impressed so I started to him last March. He suggested a program for me to correct the curvature in my neck and inquired about my overall health.

I take very good care of myself regarding diet and exercise and the taking of supplements. I also have an excellent physician who has helped me a lot. Still, I had a low thyroid condition for about two years that I had been unable to correct and very, very painful menstrual periods practically my whole life.

Dr. Deutchman suggested I take an herb called wild yam to help balance my diet's hormone systems. He also gave me special adjustments for the menstrual pain.

Last month, for the first time in my life, I had no menstrual pain. I saw my regular physician last week and he told me that my thyroid condition was normal for the first time. This is a remarkable, major change for me. I have more energy and I've lost some weight. My complexion is better and people are commenting on the way I look. Gradually, I've been able to run again, little by little, with no pain. Now, I'm in training for the New York City marathon.

This weekend I did my first race since my injury in March and set a personal record. I'm very pleased about all these changes. I feel the adjustments have helped my body to correct and heal itself.

Ann on torn cartilage

About three years ago, I tore the cartilage in my knee. Several surgeons suggested that I have surgery. I heard about Dr. Robbins and consulted with him. He said that surgery should be the last alternative and that we should try other things first.

First, I tried placing an orthotic device in my sneakers. That worked fine. The only problem was that I became a little overconfident and twisted a knee in my aerobics class.

When I went back to Dr. Robbins, he suggested that I go for chiropractic treatments with Dr. Proffman because my knee was locking three or four times a day.

I liked that Dr. Proffman explained the chiropractic treatment. He analyzed my posture and my walking, and told me that I was out of alignment, and trying to compensate for the pain. He adjusted my back and that seemed to help. That first weekend was very active. It wasn't until Sunday evening that I realized, not once did my knee lock. From then on, I was sold on the chiropractic treatment.

I have been going to Dr. Proffman twice a week, and I have had no problems with my knee. I feel it saved me from surgery. I feel much more energetic now that I am in alignment.

Dorothy on pain and general health and wellness

I began chiropractic care late last year with a desire to improve my overall health, but also for specific discomfort in my neck, lower back, and hip.

I feel that chiropractic treatment has significantly lessened the frequency of the pain I was experiencing. It specifically improved the strength of my arms and legs by relieving the interference on my nerves. I feel that it has improved my energy level as well. I racewalk for exercise and find that the chiropractic adjustments help my ankles and hips when they feel strained or out of position.

Chiropractic care has also helped me to increase my awareness of my body. I find that I am more diligent about attending to stress or injury. I pay more attention to my posture and to my position while sleeping.

I find the entire approach to healing helpful. The lifestyle recommendations, the atmosphere of the office, everything about it has made me very happy.

Some time ago, I had a few chiropractic adjustments with a different health practitioner and it was not the same experience at all. The other individual's approach was to use only chiropractic. He treated me for one subluxation in my lower back area, and that was the extent of the treatment. There were no discussions of lifestyle, nutrition, or stress. It was just more of a mechanical adjustment rather than a holistic approach.

Elise on headaches

I have been seeing a chiropractor for about two years now. I started going because I was experiencing daily tension headaches. The conventional route didn't appeal to me because I had the feeling that my headaches would be treated with medication.

The results were not immediate. I would like to emphasize that because many times people think a treatment is going to work like magic. After awhile, there was a significant decrease in the number of headaches that I was experiencing. Before I began the adjustments, I had a headache every day. After two months, I could go for seven or eight days without a headache. This was a new and wonderful experience for me.

At the same time, I started examining my diet. I worked with my doctor to see if some of the headaches were caused by food allergies. The change in my diet, which was a gradual elimination of meat, dairy, sugar, and salt, contributed to a further decrease in headaches.

My son, who is three, started this journey with me, two years ago. He gets adjusted right along with me. As a result he is very, very healthy. I believe that the combination of our weekly adjustments and good diet has contributed to my headaches going away and to the good health of my son.

Maji on degenerative arthritis and sciatica

I became a disabled Vietnam Veteran after receiving an overdose of Thorazine for a nervous breakdown after the war. I was very toxic and later developed painful arthritis. I started to use medication to relieve the pain, thinking that this was the only alternative. I believed that arthritis was a totally irreversible, terminal condition. Every medication I was given for pain gradually wore off and left me with more pain.

I thought I was headed for the wheelchair because I had sciatica as well. I even bought a ground floor apartment so that I could have wheelchair access. I was using a cane for four years and reached a point where I could not go up stairs at all. I had to quit a job in real estate which required stair climbing. Two months ago, I started going to a chiropractor on the recommendation of a friend. I was skeptical but desperate. When I first met the doctor, he told me that the adjustments would release subluxations. As a result, nerve energy would flow more freely and my health would improve. At the time, I had several subluxations. All my joints were affected. It was up and down my spine, especially in my neck and low back.

After my first adjustment, I went to a restaurant to have lunch. When it was quiet, I was aware of a tremendous feeling of activity in my neck. It was as if a little river was flowing through it. I realized that it must be the nerve energy my doctor had talked about. When I saw him again, I asked about it and he confirmed my thoughts. He said my neck was really subluxated and that the treatment released nerve energy.

Now the healing process has taken hold and my body is running more efficiently. In two months, I've lost 10 pounds due to improved metabolism. I am also walking better. In fact, I'm fast-walking and climbing stairs a little bit. My knees feel stronger and no longer shaky. I can sleep well, whereas before I had insomnia. My headaches are gone.

I still experience some pain and realize that it is going to take awhile to reverse a lot of my problems. The Thorazine overdose caused tardive dyskinesia and made one leg shorter than the other. Fortunately, this is beginning to release. My sciatica pain has been cut down to a third of what it was.

I am trying to get the Veterans Administration Hospital to introduce chiropractic into their program as part of their physical therapy. I have met a lot of vets in my physical therapy program at the VA who could really use it. When I was in physical therapy, the difference from before my chiropractic and physical therapy and after was really noticeable. My therapist at the VA even noted that I was a lot stronger.

Before chiropractic care, I was using the yellow theraband, a stretch band that exercises the muscles. The yellow is the weakest and the blue is next to the heaviest. I went from the yellow to blue in two days after my first adjustment.

I'm very grateful for chiropractic and would advise anyone to try it to see if the treatment works for them.

Sonia on multiple sclerosis

It started about six years ago. I had extreme fatigue, nervousness, and panic attacks that escalated to the point where I couldn't leave my home. I saw many doctors who said that I was undergoing a lot of stress. They prescribed Valium.

My symptoms progressed; after a year, the doctors suggested that I see a psychiatrist. In my heart, I knew that there was something physically wrong with me. One day, I awoke with paralysis of my right eye. It was at that point that I knew that there was something wrong.

I saw a neurologist, and he suggested that I have an MRI. This revealed that I had the beginning stages of multiple sclerosis. My doctor told me that there was no cure for multiple sclerosis. There was nothing that he could do. My husband and I left the office feeling very upset. In our hearts, we knew that there had to be something that we could do. My husband was listening to the radio, and came across a program one afternoon. He became encouraged by what he heard when he realized that there was some things that we could do. He heard of a Dr. Schwank, who did a lot of research in multiple sclerosis. We decided to go to the library and take out every book that we could find on multiple sclerosis. We started to apply some of the protocols that were in the books, and we realized that these alternative treatments were really helping.

We saw a homeopathic doctor who was also a chiropractor. Those were two methods that we were going to concentrate on. We found a chiropractor who spent a lot of time with me. He suggested that I eat organic foods, that I go on a detox program, that I have regular and strengthening exercises, and also a stress management class. . . .

After trying his protocol, I saw a remarkable difference in my health. I became stronger; I had no more fatigue; I was able to leave my home and go back to work. I had no more limitations. The doctors told me that I would get progressively worse and probably wind up in a wheelchair. But as a result of his treatments, I'm able to continue in my profession as a physical education teacher working with special education children. I have no limitations and was even able to have a child a year and a half ago, which the doctors told me I would never have. I feel completely excellent as far as my health goes.

Mary on osteoarthritis

I have had a bad back since I was 29 years old. Over the years I saw many orthopedic doctors who only prescribed drug therapy to deaden the pain.

One day, I decided to see a chiropractic doctor. In addition to the adjustments, he gave me vitamin supplements, and showed me how to change my diet and exercise habits. Now I take lots of vitamins. I eat lots of green vegetables, lots of fruits, and no red meat. I drink lots of water, up to eight glasses a day. My exercise includes walking and playing tennis.

This has helped immensely. Now my pain is gone. I am able to sit, whereas before I was never able to sit without very bad pain. Now I can sit and watch TV, and I can sit to knit and sew. For those who do not believe that they can reverse arthritis naturally, I am here to say that after 40 years, you can. I am living proof. Now I can play tennis without the pain.

Robert on osteoarthritis

I was experiencing stiffness in my shoulder, lower back, and hip area. After I had x-rays taken by a chiropractor, I learned that I had arthritis. I received chiropractic treatments and started eating more fruits, vegetables, vitamins, and juices. I take magnesium, potassium, vitamin E, garlic, a lot of herbs, echinacea, shark cartilage, bovine cartilage, and chondroital sulfate. I have stopped eating a lot of red meat and a lot of dairy. And I exercise more.

All this has given me a tremendous surge of energy. I don't have stiffness anymore. In damp weather I used to have quite a few cramps as well as cracking and popping of the bones. But I don't experience that anymore.

Chiropractic care, a vegetarian diet, and the other changes have made quite a big difference. I'm glad I started listening to people who said that chiropractic worked. That's something that I will continue to do for the remainder of my days on earth.

Barbara on osteoarthritis

I'm no stranger to chiropractic. I've been using it for 20 or 22 years, but I always used it for a crisis because I had an extremely bad back. Later I learned that I had arthritis. I finally decided to use chiropractic regularly as a preventive measure. I just decided, "Let me go see if this is going to make a difference." And it's made a tremendous difference in just weeks.

Before, I couldn't walk two blocks without pain. I would have to stop and sit down. I would stay home because walking was too uncomfortable. And I was really upset because I went from being 5'10" to 5'4½". I was startled by how much I lost in height. I knew some of it came from aging but that some of it had to do with accommodating for my pain.

Chiropractic has given me back some of my posture. Now I'm 5'7½". I don't expect to regain my full height from when I had no arthritis and was far younger, but I'm hopeful that I will feel far better. The pain is diminished. It's wonderful to be able to lean over quickly. The difference is quite stunning. People I know have commented on the change these past weeks. One neighbor chased me down the street, saying, "I almost didn't know that was you. I didn't realize you were so tall." That's no kidding.

Colon Therapy

Colon cleansing is an ancient and time-honored health practice, initially used by the Egyptians and the Essenes thousands of years ago, and later recommended by Hippocrates, the father of modern medicine. It works on the principle that disease starts in the colon, since most foods, drugs, and other chemicals that do not leave the body are stored there. At first, there are few or no symptoms, but after years of putrefaction, subclinical signs graduate to disease status. This is because several pounds of fecal material laden with millions of bacteria can attach itself to the colon walls. This toxic waste can generate all kinds of havoc with the system. By cleansing the large intestine, colon therapy restores the organ to its natural size, shape, and correct function, thus preventing disease.

During treatment, water is gently infused into the large bowel so that it is thoroughly washed. This allows old encrustations and fecal material to loosen, dislodge, and be swept away. As body pollution is eliminated, many conditions are alleviated, including severe skin disorders, breathing difficulties, constipation, depression, chronic fatigue, nervousness, flatulence, bloating, and arthritis. As people become physically unstuck, they become emotionally ligh

ter, freer, and better able to express their feelings. Colonics provide great relief, especially when accompanied by dietary changes.

A qualified colon therapist uses pure water that is administered at body temperature and a sterilizing device known as an autoclave. The person knows reflexology, as massaging points on the body that relate to the colon enhance the therapy. The practitioner should also test the ileocecal valve, the small valve between the small and large intestines, using kinesiology. If this is jammed open or closed, the therapist can correct it, which will make the session more comfortable.

Patient Stories

Edwina on aging

This is something that I believe in very strongly and have had really good results with. It's wonderful for the skin as well as the colon and all the organs. It also is good for cellulite because oftentimes cellulite is just an accumulation of toxins. So you see, this really works in a multitude of ways.

I found someone who is really quite good through an advertisement. The name of his company is Nature's Path. He's extremely clean and very, very thorough, and not rushing people is really important. It's important to have a full treatment, which could be up to 45 minutes for the average client.

All it really is is water going into the colon and water going out. And of course, when water goes out, waste also goes with it. It's important to do, even if you are going to the bathroom; you can be going two to three times a day, but your body still might not be cleansing properly. . . . Even if a person has a really good balanced diet, there are certain stresses involved that can take away from a full cleansing process.

Not only did it help my body, I felt that my mind also was clearer and more focused. I felt happier and lighter, not just physically, but also mentally. It's wonderful. I would call it the fountain of youth and the greatest thing known to man.

Jill on allergies

I was feeling quite miserable. Then I was lucky enough to find the treatment I'm presently in. In just two days, I'm already feeling a thousand percent better in that my stomach is not distended, gas is eliminated, and my runny nose is gone. I'm no longer walking around with tissues in hand. This treatment is pretty new to me and I was a little apprehensive, but I'm a believer right now.

Once I'm finished with this treatment, my allergies should be gone if I change my eating habits. I am really trying to learn how to eat healthier to avoid this problem again. I may always have this problem, but at least I will be able to avoid the severity of symptoms that I have been feeling up until now.

Dorothy on diverticulitis

Prior to colonics, I tried laxatives and other drugs. Nothing seemed to work. There was no real bowel movement. It was all building up inside of me and I was constantly bloated. It was very discomforting.

Then I got my first colonic. I was a little leery but I was anxious to get it because I figured it would work. And it worked. After all this time.

I only had two treatments and I only took about a quart of water each time.

I couldn't hold more. But I had a bowel movement each day for the last month and four days, a total of 60 inches throughout the day, heavy. Unbelievable.

In addition to the colonic, I was taking bentonite and psyllium. I was told to avoid half and half and carbonated drinks and processed foods. By eliminating all of that, I've really improved and feel like a million dollars now. I am 76 years old and feel like 36.

Linda on eczema

I had a really severe case on my hands on feet. I went from doctor to doctor, trying to clear it up, but was really never successful at it. This winter, when I was in Florida, I showed it to my brother who had been doing colonics for the last ten years. He said, "Your body is toxic. You've got to get to a colonic therapist and have this procedure done." I wasn't really thrilled about doing it, but he's a wise person and I listened to him. I also had no energy and was not able to lose weight. I kept gaining weight even though I was exercising my brains out.

Well, I went through a colonic series. I had 15 done. I have lost 20 pounds and my eczema is almost totally cleared up. I have energy again. I think this is one of the best things that I have ever done for my health.

Jerry on congenital conditions

I was born with twisted intestines. In my early days, I was deathly ill. Even getting up in the morning was painful, and my mother had to put drops in my eyes to get them to open due to the toxins forming all night long. I could not physically open them until the drops were put in.

Ultimately I became a naturopathic physician. And I can let people know that good health is achievable but that it just doesn't happen overnight. Part of my early studies included being sent by Dr. Bernard Jensen to a clinic outside of Guadalajara, Mexico, up in the mountains. There I learned not only proper eating methods, but the cleansing principles of using colonics and enemas and so forth. I learned what to mix in there to help break up the impacted matter, as well as have proper elimination.

Interestingly, they had their own version of a colonic board. Everything was made out of marble because marble in Mexico is very inexpensive. They had a large table that a patient would lay upon to have a tube inserted. The tube came down from a marble 5-gallon holding tank with the turnstile for the water down at the base. Patients could virtually turn on the water themselves, fill the bucket, and go through the process. Everything was easy to clean therefore. It was a remarkable idea.

I got used to the use of this kind of method instead of the normal small enema, which is a bit uncomfortable, and eventually was able to correct my condition, in spite of the many impactions and surgeries that I had at a much earlier age. To this day, if I am fairly careful, I have no major problems with my digestive system anymore. I'm much older now but it has held up very well for all these years.

I would like to tell people that anything less than two or three bowel movements a day is not normal. Even once a day is holding too much waste material and can become very dangerous. To those of you who are getting on in years, I would like to say from my own experience, that the use of an enema or colonic once a week, whether needed or not, can be a very good insurance policy.

I have a colonic board at home with a 5-gallon bucket. I add in a chlorophyll and comfrey mixture, as well as some red clover and a tablespoon of an electrolyte solution to help maintain the electrolyte balance of the soft tissue, as well as restore the peristaltic action of the bowel muscle. I try doing this every Sunday afternoon or Saturday evening, and I find this clears out dangerous waste matter from the week before.

I think it is absolutely critical to do upon return from a trip. Taking an enema or colonic immediately will remove all that excess waste matter. I have known of a number of cases of people who return from trips to Europe, who come back with very poor bowel habits. Within a month many of them develop a heart attack and pass on. I find that totally unnecessary. You can take an enema with you, perhaps some herbal laxatives, and get one, upon returning. If you don't want to set up an enema at home, by all means, make an appointment with a colonic expert, and get your digestive system cleaned out. This is critical in today's world with all the additional chemicals, pesticides, and toxic material that can accumulate in your system.

An interesting article from the old *Saturday Evening Post* of April 1982, was titled "Constipation and Breast Cancer." The authors pointed out that women who only have several bowel movements a week have at least a four times higher risk of breast cancer than women who have at least one bowel movement a day.

Regarding the bowel problem itself, one of the important things I learned down at the clinic outside of Guadalajara are that modern toilets are a nemesis in that the bowel was meant to be in a squeezable position so to speak, as we squatted to the ground for hundreds of thousands of years if not millions of years as an upright human. That allows for a total elimination. I remember that as a child being sickly and sent to the farm and not wanting to use the outhouse that much. I used to go in the field very often, and when I went in the field, I did feel better and was healthier. So we recommended in the clinic, in Guadalajara, the use of a footstool to raise the level of the feet for more of a critical v-shape for the bowel track.

The only other nation I know of [besides the U.S.] that is so far behind with digestion and bowel constipation is England, which has a highly refined diet. It is also known that during World War II, when England could not get processed foods shipped to it, they increased the amount of fiber in the diet by grinding grains less, and there was very little sugar or other refined products available. The incidence of heart disease and cancer dropped rapidly. It's ironic, but right after World War II, disease figures went up tremendously.

The use of the enema, in the evening particularly, before going to bed on a full stomach, I think is very important for those who have not moved their bowels that day. Statistics show that most heart attacks occur late at night or early in the morning. And a number of naturopathic physicians, myself included, feel that the end digestion food turns into a toxic gaseous substance, which produces quite a strain on the heart, to make a long story short. Statistics show that a large incidence of massive heart attacks occur late at night or early in the morning, which are usually fatal.

In order to get that peristaltic action back in the bowel muscle, we were taught to give patients flaxseed and/or flaxseed oil every day, as well as psyllium seed. Flaxseed serves two purposes. One is as a fiber and a second is as a lubricant. For bowel health, it is probably one of the least expensive and best ways of keeping things moving along.

Ann on breast cancer

I was diagnosed with breast cancer, two years ago. I knew that my problem was that I didn't go to the bathroom often enough. Throughout my whole life, I only went twice a week. I was told by many, many doctors that that was normal for me because I had a nervous stomach. And unfortunately, I accepted that.

When I look back now, I realize that I had food allergies all my life. That stopped me from ever being normal in the bathroom.

This year, I decided to really attack it. Things were getting better and better over the last few years and I wanted to do colonics. I found someone here in New York and had a series of 15 colonics.

It really made a difference for me. Now I go to the bathroom six to eight times a day. I have a complete emptying feeling. . . . And I feel great.

Charlotte on heart attack

I had a heart attack and I was six blocks from the hospital so I survived it. Two weeks later I was home, again six blocks from the hospital, when I developed a hole in my heart, they tell me, and I got there just in time to have emergency open heart surgery, which they didn't think I'd survive.

It's been about three years of recovery, which I never would have made without . . . colonics. Since that time, I've probably had over 100 colonics and herbal cleansing. And I'm an entirely different person. In fact, the doctors want to know what my secret is. They just can't believe that I've survived these particular situations.

Last year, I was back in the hospital with right-sided heart failure because after having a piece taken out of my heart on the left side, the right side was trying to compensate. The fluid backed up like any plumbing problem. Eventually, it was pumped out of me. . . . This could not be done naturally. I lost 65 pounds of fluid in 16 days. It was the colonics in the end that saved me.

The material that came out of the colon has been photographed. It was remarkably awful. It was black, tar, putrid-looking material. At one point, I had terrible pain in my left side, near the place where I had the surgery. And I always used to say to doctors before and after the surgery, if you could fix this terrible pain, I'd be very thankful. During a colonic, the hygienist was massaging that area and the final debris came out of it. Then that pain was gone forever. So there you are.

Charlotte's son, Matthew, on mother's heart attack

It was just interesting in that if you picture the letter "U" and you picture the top of each side as being good health and the bottom as death, I basically saw mom deteriorate before me, going down the left side of the letter "U" and then having her heart attack in which they had to shock her and bring her back to life, and then build up her on the medications. She started going up the other side. But then she started getting the allergic reactions to the medications, and slowly sank back down to the bottom of the "U" again, or near death, it seemed.

That's when she started to get colonics. It was at that time that she got all that residue out of her system and started to assimilate good health. Then, instead of going back down to the bottom again, she was able to eclipse it and come across the top and work her way back up to the other side of the "U" and back to good health. It has been an amazing experience for me.

I have decided to get a head start, so I started colonics and began to change my eating habits.

Barbara on constipation

I was constipated my whole life and the doctors never thought that was a problem. I guess I was about 19 when I started working. I became lazy and stopped working out as much. I had a desk job and my health became affected.

My fatigue started getting very, very intense. I became lethargic and started getting really run down. Then I got into that health craze as far as working out more and doing as much as I could, but I just wasn't getting any better. At that point I was running 18 miles a week. My weight kept going up and up and up. I got up to about 194. Nobody could figure it out. I went to doctor after doctor. I had a lot of female problems. I had no periods and was just a mess. No one ever said anything about the constipation.

I went on a Fit for Life health diet. It was a very healthy diet and was great for helping me to lose weight. But I never felt better. I never got my energy back. Then I was rushed to the hospital and my colon was totally impacted. Their solution didn't sound good.

My husband heard about colonics in the past so we went for a series. I was in my early 20's when I went in, and I felt that if I lived to be 35 it would be a miracle. The colon therapist would tell me to stick to the program and that I would be able to go on my own every day. I told her that I could never do that. The doctor said a lot of people are just naturally constipated. The hygienist said, ''No, they just don't know how to tell you to get it to work right.'' I just stayed with it.

After a long period of time, I got my colon to start working on a daily basis. My female problems totally went away and all my energy returned. I started having regular periods. I can't imagine it's like that for everybody but it totally fixed that problem without me even realizing it was going to do it. It just was outstanding. To this day, I go in for maintenance just because I believe it gave me my life back.

Susan on chronic fatigue syndrome

I had pneumonia and afterwards I was so weak that I couldn't stand up. I had chronic fatigue for three months before I could even crawl. I went to a holistic doctor, who gave me supplements, IV vitamins, and nutritional advice. I was gradually getting back my strength and was able to go to work for an hour a day. By the time I went to Anita, I was working about three hours a day for five days a week. That was the maximum time I could actually work. I was sleeping 12 to 13 hours a night. I couldn't walk up a flight of stairs and I couldn't walk more than half a block without having to stop to catch my breath.

I asked my doctor if I should take enemas because I was constipated. I was going to the bathroom about once a week. He said he didn't believe in enemas and that I should take different powders instead. Meanwhile, I had been on a natural foods diet for 12 years and I didn't eat processed foods for years. But it didn't have any effect on the constipation. In my mind, I was thinking that I should get enemas even though the doctor said not to.

I heard about the Healing Center on Gary Null's shows. I thought I would go there and try it. I went over there for colon therapy, and after the first visit, I felt very, very good. Anita was wonderful and she made me feel relaxed. As soon as I walked out of the office, I felt great. I was able to work the rest of the day without fatigue. That night, I slept seven hours. After that, every single day, I slept seven or eight hours, which was a tremendous difference from what I was going through before.

I have been to her nine times. Every visit made me feel even better. The chronic fatigue is gone. My energy is still not optimal, but I don't feel that terrible drained feeling that was dragging me down. The constipation is gradually starting to go away. I had acne my whole life, and that disappeared. My eyesight cleared up. I didn't think there was anything wrong with my eyes. According to my exams, it's 20/20. But after the first visit, I noticed that the colors looked bright and clear. I used to have menstrual cramps, and after my visits, I no longer feel any cramps. I have lost about 8 pounds. My appetite has changed. I used to crave sweets and caffeine, even though I tried desperately to stay away from it. But I would give in to sweets just to keep going. Now I have no desire for sweets at all.

Gary on lack of energy, constipation, and baldness

I didn't really have any pre-existing conditions that I was aware of at the time. I just went to the therapy to detoxify my body from things I had eaten over the years that I felt needed to be cleaned out of my system. I have been to Anita four times.

I have seen a lot of results already. I have more energy and less sluggishness. I don't need as much sleep. I used to need seven or eight hours, and now I need four or five hours and then generally, I'm fine. Then I used to have a noontime nod off, and I don't need that anymore. That was one of the conditions I wasn't aware of that the colonics corrected.

The other thing is I have more frequent bowel movements. I used to have one movement every two or three days. So, I was relatively constipated and didn't know it until after the treatments. It's also much quicker. It used to be a big ceremony type thing, 30 or 40 minutes at a time. I would have to take the magazine or newspaper. It almost became a reading library to try to get through. Now that situation is kind of cleared up.

The other thing I found interesting is that I feel my hair is starting to come back. I'm in my 30s right now. I have a small bump right above my left temple. That's been almost like a benchmark as to where my hair has been going. When I was in high school, that bump was completely covered with hair. When I went into college, it was right at the edge. And when I got out of college it started pushing further beyond. The past couple of weeks, I've noticed that the hairline has been starting to push forward. That bump is now starting to be covered with small fine hairs. I believe that is because the intestinal walls are free of debris so that the vitamins, minerals, chlorophyll, everything I've been taking in now has a greater effect to start maintaining my body where it should be. I think the hair growth is a part of it. I find it a little amazing.

Enzyme Therapy

Enzyme therapy may be the best-kept secret in medicine today. An enormous body of research credits enzymes in the prevention and treatment of a variety of conditions, including circulatory problems, cancer, premature aging, skin problems, damage from injury, digestive disorders, back pain, immune deficiencies, arthritis, bursitis, multiple sclerosis, and viruses, including herpes and HIV. Their wide range of effectiveness is due to the fact that enzymes are essential to all life processes. They work as catalysts. Without enzymes, there would be no cellular activity.

Critics of the therapy say that enzymes lose their potency after they are digested. But this is contradicted by studies showing that when enzymes are orally ingested, blood levels of enzymes increase remarkably. As we age, we need more enzymes. In fact, research shows enzymes to be a key factor in staying young.

We get enzymes from live foods, such as raw fruits and vegetables. Some people have difficulty breaking down food enzymes and need to take them in tablet form. The best mineral supplements are plant enzymes in crystalloid form with electrolytes. These penetrate cell walls, strengthen the body, and help the complete digestion process.

Patient Stories

Marianne on yeast infection

In 1990, I had exploratory surgery for endometriosis. Because I had previously been diagnosed with mitral-valve prolapse, it was suggested I take antibiotics for this surgery. Ten days following the surgery, I had a wicked yeast infection, which my doctor gave me vaginal medicine to help cure. Three months later, it recurred. Every month thereafter, just prior to my period, I would get an infection. I was experiencing such pain and discomfort, I didn't know who to turn to. My gynecologist, of course, found no yeast in my culture, and told me there was nothing he could do.

One day, while at the drug store, I came across a book called, *The Yeast Syndrome.* One of the coauthors happened to practice close to where I lived. I called his office to find out he was a podiatrist. However, he was able to recommend another doctor who might be able to help me. . . . This doctor had an allergist in his office test me for all kinds of allergies. It turned out I was not seriously "allergic" to anything. At this point, my doctor said he really had done everything possible and didn't feel a need for me to continue as his patient. His allergist did, however, tell me about a person who might give me additional help. This person was Robin Keuneke.

Robin did an initial phone consultation with me and felt she could help me with proper diet and nutrition. I met Robin to further discuss my situation. Below are Robin's recommendations to me and what eventually helped me clear up the infection and get back on track:

1. The first thing she said was to immediately stop taking any further medication. She felt this was only driving the infection deeper into my gut (medication kills enzymes).
2. She put me on a strict diet, requiring me to eliminate soda, coffee, commercial teas, dairy, eggs, sugar, any meats with hormones.
3. She had me add tofu, more fish (lots of salmon), grains, more vegetables.
4. I bought everything organic and drank only filtered water (pesticides and chemicals kill enzymes).
5. I learned how to use miso correctly (don't boil—boiling destroys enzymes). Initially, I used only dark miso and was able to later add the lighter miso.
6. I used more fresh garlic, ginger, herbs, and spices in recipes.
7. I added more seaweed, kabocha and delicata squash, and very lightly cooked dark leafy greens with umeboshi vinegar and lemon.
8. I had pressed or fresh salad daily.
9. I drank kukicha tea with umeboshi concentrate.
10. Since frying kills enzymes, I eliminated this type of cooking. Robin taught me how to "water saute" my vegetables, which requires much less oil. I use olive and sesame oils sparingly.
11. I later added chicken and lamb which contained no hormones or antibiotics, and was minimally processed, and organic eggs sprinkled with flax oil.

Initially Robin added a very few important supplements to my diet: liquid chlorophyll, a strong probiotic, vitamin C, a dry vitamin E, chromium picolinate, sea vegetation tablets, and garlic. My present supplements are acidophilus, chlorella (which contains chlorophyll), a multiple vitamin, vitamin C, a dry vitamin E, chromium picolinate, Evening primrose, calcium/magnesium, and garlic. I also use flaxseeds and flax oil daily.

It probably took about one year to get 100 percent, with Robin's guidance. Remember, I had this ongoing infection (not just before my period) for a few years. Robin was honest with me in saying it could take this long for me to be able to add new things to my diet, like shoyu, tamari, rice vinegar, etc. I am presently able to eat a much wider variety of foods, and even enjoy a glass of wine on occasion. I continue to buy as much organic foods as possible, drink kukicha with ume concentrate, and have my dark greens with ume vinegar. This helps to keep a healthy amount of good bacteria in my intestines. I still avoid dairy and fried foods. Robin has suggested I buy a juicer to take my improved health one step further. I hope to do so in the near future.

Herbal Therapy

Herbs have been used as medicine long before recorded history. Generations of trial and error taught prehistoric people which plants to use when treating injuries and diseases, and this life-saving knowledge was passed down through the ages. In China and India, the study and use of herbal medicine has evolved over 5000 years. In ancient Greece, the father of modern medicine, Hippocrates, used hundreds of herbs in his practice, many of which are still popular today. In short, the healing properties of plants are time-tested, which is why herbal therapy is respected in cultures around the world.

As the limitations of modern medicine become increasingly apparent, the medical profession is once again looking to the plant world for help. Scientists around the world, in a desperate search for answers to AIDS, cancer, and other conditions not cured by standard medicine, have begun to study the properties of herbs, and are amazed at their immune-enhancing effects. Astragalus, licorice, and panax ginseng have powerful anticancer properties, for example, while echinacea and goldenseal taken at the first sign of a cold or flu will often stop the disease in its tracks.

How do herbs help us? Some are like super foods whose nutrients are building blocks for the entire body. Others have drug-like actions, and exert specific strengthening or stimulating effects on certain physiological functions. Still others help to detoxify the system. Some herbs perform more than one function; for example, they may cleanse to a degree, but predominantly build up the system.

While herbalists know that specific herbs are helpful in correcting certain disease states, other factors are taken into account as well. The herbalist considers the whole person, and this is especially true in Chinese medicine, where an herbalist will look to see which symptoms are the most outstanding. If a patient is diabetic, for example, a person can exhibit great thirst, hunger, or urination. The herbalist also considers the state of the overall system: the digestion, sleep patterns, energy. In this way a basic formula for a condition is modified to meet the individual needs of the patient.

486

Herbalist Christopher Trahan sums up the value of plant remedies: "Herbal medicine works very well because they are biological entities which have evolved simultaneously with human beings. When we use herbs, we are using foods that are molecularly and energetically a part of us."

Homeopathy

Homeopathy is a system of healing based on the law of similars. In the late 18th century, homeopathy's founder, Dr. Samuel Hahnemann, discovered that like cures like: Administering a substance that causes a disease in a healthy individual can cure an illness in a person who is sick. So, for example, if someone with rashes is given a substance that creates rashes, it helps to neutralize and thus end the problem.

Homeopathy uses natural substances that are prepared by a process called dilution and succussion. This means that remedies are diluted over and over until they are no longer detectible. When the final product is viewed through a microscope, there appears to be nothing there. Frequently, homeopathic remedies are highly toxic substances in their natural form, and might include snake venom, arsenic, or harmful bacteria. But after being diluted, they are completely nontoxic. In fact, there appears to be nothing left but water.

If nothing is there, how does homeopathy work? Although no physical substance remains, the vibration of the material endures, and stimulates energy systems of the body to address both subtle and obvious causes of disease. Emotional states such as fear, anger, anxiety, and depression, which may underlie physical diseases, are dealt with, as well as physical symptoms. By rebalancing the whole person, emotionally and physically, homeopathy can make a big difference.

Homeopathic medicine differs from the allopathic tradition in that symptoms are viewed as an expression of the body attempting to heal itself, not something to be masked. The body is always faced with numerous stresses, and people are always reacting emotionally, physically, and mentally to regain balance. Covering up symptoms only pushes them to a deeper level, causing more serious consequences in the long-term.

Homeopathic remedies are either taken orally on placed onto the skin. Health food stores sell remedies labeled 12X or 30X, 12c or 30c, to indicate the number of dilutions that the formula has gone through. The X signifies that the formula has been diluted to a proportion of 1:10, while the c potency means it's been diluted to a 1:100 level.

Patient Stories

Lillian on liver cancer

Three years ago, I was diagnosed with a cancer below my rectum for which I received chemotherapy and radiation. That got rid of it for a while but in time it reappeared in my liver. I received 50 chemotherapy treatments but had I known what I understand today, I would never have had any.

I was very sick and waiting to die. I could not hold food or water down and lost a lot of weight. My bowels were totally paralyzed and I could not go to the bathroom at all. The nurses told me I only had a short time to live, and I wanted to die. The pain was so bad that I had to live on morphine and a narcotic pain patch.

Thank God my daughter introduced me to a homeopathic doctor who gave me a new lease on life. My doctor has done an awful lot for me. My therapy consisted of a lot of natural herbs and vitamins. I juiced and ate a diet high in healthy vegetables. Red meats were eliminated. He gave me medicine to alleviate edema and to lessen acidity. In addition, I received colonic therapy to detoxify my bowel.

When I got home, I had renewed strength. I could walk around and even drive, whereas before I needed a wheelchair. In six months, I have been able to gain some weight back and have no more bowel trouble. I had a myelogram last month. The doctors were shocked that I was able to come this far. They can't believe it. My blood pressure is down, and I have no trouble with my blood. I am a totally different person. I am amazed and my whole family is amazed as well. I feel that if I didn't go there, I would be gone. If I had to do it over, I would not have chemotherapy or radiation at all. I would go the homeopathic route.

Patty on accidents

I was introduced to homeopathy by my husband, 17 years ago. I married a man from a little town in Pennsylvania where 80 percent of the people use homeopathy because in the 30's, 40's and 50's, the hometown doctor was a medical homeopath. When I got married, his father handed me belladonna and arnica and said, good luck.

I didn't pay much attention to it until six or seven years ago when my husband put his hand underneath a lawnmower and almost severed a decent-sized piece of his finger. We went to the hospital where they did a lot of surgery and reattached it. He was told that he would never have any sensation there again because the nerves had been severed. They recommended plastic surgery.

I called a very wise old woman from my husband's home town and asked her what she would do. She said hypericum was the remedy that helps regenerate nerve endings. If anything could help, that would be it. We started giving him hypericum. Now, five years later, you would never know that anything had ever happened to his finger.

In my own case, the value of homeopathy was clearly demonstrated one Thanksgiving Day while I was baking the turkey. My daughter was about three months old and it was a lot of effort to make the dinner. I wanted to do everything perfectly and was very anxious. I put the pot holder on my right hand and took the turkey out of the oven with my left hand. I pretty much melted four fingers. They were pink and shiny and the fingerprints were pretty much gone. They were blistering in a matter of seconds. I remembered that the remedy for burns is camphorus. I only had a 30x, which is not incredibly strong, but camphorus is effective at any potency. In homeopathy, the indications on the bottle sometimes say to take it and wait four hours. In an emergency situation like the one I was in, it's important to take it as often as you need it. I was taking a little pellet of camphorus every minute. Then, it got to the point where I could take it every three minutes, every five minutes, every ten minutes. It got better and better all day. By night time, I was able to wash dishes and take a hot shower. Usually the pain is so phenomenally excruciating that you can't be near hot water. The next day, there was only a little bit of melted blistery stuff on one finger. The other fingers had totally healed. That amazed me. Not just that the pain was relieved, because that in itself blew my mind. But the fact that my fingers healed, and that quickly—that was amazing.

One of my favorite remedies is arsenicum for food poisoning. This is homeopathically prepared arsenic. When I've had food poisoning in the past, I probably would have voluntarily taken the substance arsenic just to get rid of the pain. I was lying in bed on a heating pad doubled over with horrible, horrible stomach cramps from food poisoning I had gotten that day. I also knew that in the refrigerator was something that I wanted to eat very much from the day before. It wasn't the thing that had caused the food poisoning but I knew that there were oysters and black bean sauce in the refrigerator and that if I didn't get them, someone else might.

As I was lying in bed, I looked up at the bureau and saw my remedy kit, which, at that point, I hadn't used a lot. I thought, wait a minute, arsenicum is a remedy for food poisoning. I took a dose. Again that was 30x. I got back on a heating pad and about 15 minutes later I took another dose. Within an hour I was eating the oysters and black bean sauce. I have never ever had a recovery from food poisoning that quickly in my life.

Alan on infections

About five years ago, I had a serious infection in my tooth. The doctor said I would have to take antibiotics or else I would end up in the hospital. The problem was, the last time I took antibiotics, I almost died from it and ended up setting off all types of alarms in the hospital. I was caught between a rock and a hard place.

A friend suggested that I see a homeopathic doctor. I didn't know what that was but I didn't have a choice so I went. The doctor gave me little brown pills to put under my tongue. The remedy was called hepar sulfuris calcareum. It is very good for infections around the teeth and gums. In a couple of hours the pain was gone. In two days, it completely disappeared.

I was amazed that you could treat an infection without antibiotics and started reading about homeopathy to learn more about it. Since then, I have many different remedies for lots of different things.

My wife had a headache that was so intense that she asked me if I would take her to an emergency room. At the same time, she was very, very angry. She was angry and complaining about unendurable pain at the same time. I remembered that those were the characteristics associated with a remedy called chamomilla. I approached her very gingerly because she was in a very angry and nasty mood and I put a few grains of chamomilla on her tongue. I walked out of the room and came back a few minutes later. She was sitting up and she said, ''Do we have any ice cream?'' We were walking the dog about 20 minutes later. She was okay. It's amazing how fast it works, especially in an acute situation, when you hit on a remedy.

I have learned that homeopathy is prescribed on an individual basis. While hepar sulfuris calcareum was the appropriate remedy for my infections, someone else might benefit from mercurius. This is another remedy useful for infections, especially in the mouth or gums, but for other places also. What characterizes the need for this is a very bad odor coming from the mouth and a tremendous amount of saliva, yet at the same time, a great thirst. There is also a creeping chilliness.

Another remedy called puirogenium is very good for septic infections, the kind of thing people are rushed to the hospital for. I've known people who have used that remedy and then were fine in a couple of days.

Thomas on multiple sclerosis

I was diagnosed as having multiple sclerosis at a major university teaching hospital. The M.D.'s did not give me a very optimistic prognosis. It's the old thing that if you don't like the message, shoot the messenger or change messengers. I sought out somebody who would tell me what I wanted to hear.

All this transpired about four or five months ago. I am 56 years old. What brought me to the M.D.s in the first place is that I had developed some M.S. symptoms. My balance was very poor and I had great difficulty in speaking. I would say that my balance was about 75 percent of what it should be and my speech was about 50 percent of what it should be.

After going to Dr. Ken Pitoway, a homeopathic doctor, I've seen considerable improvement. My balance has gone up to about 95 percent and my speech is back up to about 80 or 85 percent. That's my own subjective evaluation.

I feel homeopathy has made a big difference. I feel better and people tell me how good I look. I'm sure it's how good I look in comparison to how I looked before. My color used to be very pale. I was almost like death warmed over.

When I was with the M.D.'s, in essence, there was no hope. They implied that I should start shopping for a motorized wheelchair. Since changing to homeopathy, I'm jogging 25 miles a week. That's better than a wheelchair!

Before homeopathy, I was not jogging. I was a couch potato and I was letting myself deteriorate. Even though homeopathy didn't suggest that I jog, my general well-being improved to the point where I felt I could jog and wanted to. I believe that had I not started this program I would probably be in a wheelchair today.

It can be argued that whenever you have an MS flare-up, you're always going to improve from the worst point. But I feel that I've improved more than I would have because my general health is better. I'm still under treatment, and I look forward to a complete recovery.

Sandi on carpal tunnel syndrome and other problems

I suffered with carpal tunnel syndrome for three years. This caused me great difficulty at work. I owned a restaurant and had trouble holding onto things. At first, I was on some very bad drugs to control the inflammation and pain but the drugs began to bother my stomach. My orthopedic surgeon was going to perform carpal tunnel surgery.

At that time, a friend of mine encouraged me to call a homeopathic physician. I had never been introduced to homeopathy before and was hesitant about going. She kept telling me I could always have my surgery if the homeopathy didn't work. So, I went.

I was put on a homeopathic remedy called rhus tox. Within a couple of weeks, my hands were completely well. It has been five years since I took that homeopathic remedy. I never again suffered from carpal tunnel. I was saved from surgery on both hands and I saved my health because my stomach was beginning to bother me a great deal. I was also starting to have cardiovascular problems and those have also been relieved. So, I have had great success with homeopathy.

Since then, my family has used homeopathy over and over again and has had nothing but success. I have a grandson who was born with difficult breathing problems. Soon afterwards, he developed a hernia of the testicles. The pediatrician wanted to perform surgery immediately but my daughter wanted him to see a homeopathic physician first. Within two weeks of starting the homeopathic remedy, there was no sign of the hernia left. He too was saved from having surgery.

After a cesarean birth, my daughter's blood count went down to 7. The doctors wanted to give her a transfusion but we talked him into waiting at least 24 hours so that she could be administered a homeopathic remedy. She was given ferrum phosphoricum, which is a remedy that helps increase oxygen in the body and raise the blood count. Within that 24 hours, her blood count raised significantly and she did not need a transfusion.

Another daughter had toxemia related to pregnancy. We administered a homeopathic remedy called apis which took all of the poisoning and swelling out of her body within a very short time.

I can't talk enough about our successes and how it has kept us away from surgeries time and again. It just does wonderful things. Our bodies are much more capable of healing than we give them credit for. I'm all for allopathic medicine when other things won't work, or for diagnosis, but it is not needed as much as people think.

Helen on muscle and joint pain, emotional trauma, and sequential homeopathy

I had terrible muscle and joint pain that kept me incapacitated. I tried acupuncture, Chinese herbs, diet, intravenous vitamin therapy, just about everything, and they all helped. They got me about 50 percent better. But then nothing else worked. I got to a point where I was at a standstill; it stayed that way for a few years. I was relatively happy because I was much better.

Then a friend of mine died of AIDS. Two weeks later, my cat died. That sent me right back down the drain and I could no longer get back up. That went on for about two years. I tried a lot of things but nothing worked.

Then I decided to try homeopathy. The person I found does sequential therapy, which treats emotional wounds and removes repercussions from all life traumas. It starts in the present and works back to when your mother was pregnant. I've been doing this for ten months now. It's a slow process and will take about two years to complete. As a result of this therapy, I feel drastically better. I can drive again and do just about everything. At this point, I still have my problems and I still have pain, but, emotionally, I am 100 percent better.

Now, I'm treating my animals sequentially from all the little traumas that they have had from being strays. I treat them the same way a human would be treated. If they've been outside, you have to assume that they've been abused in some way. I give them opium for fear, natmur for grief and staphysagria for anger. It's definitely working. One cat wouldn't get out from under the bed for two months. We treated her and within a week she started coming out. Another cat of mine was biting and doing all kinds of strange things. We treated her this way and she's also much better. It doesn't happen overnight but it works and it's wonderful.

I also treat them with homeopathy for acute problems and it works wonderfully. Also, it is far more economical than going to a veterinarian. Vets have gotten so outrageously expensive and this is a very inexpensive way to treat them.

I just think it's a very dynamic and very wonderful way to heal. If you're going to get to the basis of where most illness come from you need to address emotions. Traumas certainly affect us for the rest of our lives and need to be removed. Sequential homeopathy can do that.

Dory on asthma

Pre-homeopathy, my oldest daughter was four and my youngest daughter was a newborn, less than a year old. Both of them had severe asthma. We tried the usual medical treatment with the bronchodilators and frequent runs of steroids. On the average, we visited the hospital's emergency room once a month for shots of epinephrine. They were also on nebulizer treatments three times a day.

A friend recommended that I take my children to a homeopath. I basically had nothing to lose because they weren't getting any better on any of the medications. On the contrary, they were getting worse and deteriorating rapidly. Our trips to the hospital were much more frequent. It was very frightening because my children would turn blue three o'clock in the morning.

We went to a homeopath, an M.D. Within six months, my oldest daughter was weaned off all medications. She has had no asthma attacks since that time. Previously, allergy tests showed that she had severe allergies to cats. We could not even go near a house with a cat. We now own a cat and she has had no allergy outbreaks and no asthma.

My youngest daughter's course of treatment took about a year. Same story. No asthma. We've had the lung function test repeated. It's perfectly normal and shows the lungs to be functioning 100 percent.

I absolutely know that homeopathy saved my children's lives and it gave them quality of life to boot.

Kim on ear infections

My son was taking antibiotics for chronic ear infections. It ended up being a dependency relationship. He would get better initially, but then it was really just a back-to-back-to-back series of 10-day courses of antibiotics. Sometimes, he would be on his tenth and final day of antibiotic therapy, and that afternoon, his ear infection would be back again. That would happen after taking my son to the doctor to make sure that his ear was okay. It really was just a Band-Aid effect, and not a long-term healing situation.

With homeopathy, once the remedies kick in, he's fine. His ear infections have dropped to maybe one or two a year instead of six or seven. He had one ear infection in February and another one last month. We treated them with pulsatilla over-the-counter eardrops from the health food store and he's fine.

Virginia on multiple sclerosis

First I tried the allopathic medical route but they could do nothing for me. They chose to really downplay what I was already doing, trying to eat right and exercise. I knew there had to be something else out there.

I turned to homeopathy and got tremendous results through a doctor in the Detroit area. He gave me natural homeopathy remedies and taught me how to eat right. I also was taught how to go inside myself to learn how to become well and to want to be well. Through this combination, I have been able to reverse some of my MS symptoms and feel basically well.

Hypnotherapy

Hypnotherapy can alleviate a wide variety of problems by quieting down disturbing and nonproductive thought processes in our conscious mind, and tapping into our subconscious where suggestions and insights allow us to change our perceptions. Among its many uses, hypnotherapy can help increase energy, manage chronic pain, and overcome addictions, such as overeating and smoking. It can also help one build confidence, and get over anxieties and phobias. Women can use hypnotherapy to subdue PMS, cramps, and other pain. Athletes can use it to enhance performance.

Hypnosis is not a total loss of consciousness, as most people believe. A client is aware and relaxed, almost as if his body is asleep but his mind awake and alert. A typical session begins with an interview, in which the patient communicates his or her problem to the therapist. Then the patient is guided to a peaceful state of mind, referred to as a trance. In this state, imagery is much more powerful than usual. The therapist makes suggestions and the person uses his imagination to shift his view the world. Some changes are substantial. An example would be a person who does not stop smoking because of a deeply ingrained belief that she is unable to do so. By changing that core belief, smoking can be stopped.

Hypnotherapy holds great promise for life-threatening diagnoses. In these situations, a person has often been led to believe that he has no future. By coming into contact with all his beliefs about death and illness, doctors and hospitals, and then creating imaginary situations in which health has returned and he is surviving long into the future, a patient can shift from a point of no return to a turning point, a new beginning.

When hypnotherapy does not work, the failure may at times be attributed to resistance. As illogical as it seems, the problem may be doing something for the person on a subconscious level. It is creating a benefit, perhaps keeping the person from working, or putting the person in a situation where he or she gets more attention than usual.

Generally, the time invested in therapy is brief, and effects are immediate.

Three to six sessions are usually all that are needed, and sometimes only one is sufficient.

While hypnotherapy is a wonderful modality, there are a few words of caution to heed: A client takes in the energy as well as the suggestions of another. It is therefore imperative to work with someone whose intentions are pure, based on references and intuition.

Patient Stories

Cynthia on psychological blocks

For most of my childhood and part of my adult life, I was in traditional psychotherapy, trying to handle issues around my father's death, which happened when I was a child. I always felt that this was a major albatross stopping me from having the life I really wanted.

I met a hypnotherapist who felt that he might help me. We worked on my particular issues, and the results were truly amazing. I had a good job as a corporate recruiter, but I wanted a better one. I would stop myself from going after my goals because I was frightened that no one would hire me. I thought I wasn't smart enough and that I didn't deserve it. Negative ideas kept blocking me. Soon after the session, a company sought me out and I accepted a great job. Now I have an incredible position, something I only dreamed of before.

Other good changes came of this as well. I always wanted to have great relationships with people, but couldn't because I was afraid that they would leave. Now people gravitate toward me without my seeking them out. I have good, strong friendships, and a great relationship with my mother. These were tremendous issues for me.

Susan on multiple sclerosis

I went to sleep perfectly normal one night, and woke up the next day physically unable to move. I lost my vision, was unable to dial a phone, and was in severe back pain. I didn't know what was happening until going for an MRI, which confirmed that it was multiple sclerosis.

I have always believed that the mind has tremendous power. I knew that I had my work cut out for me, but that I would overcome this condition. Unfortunately, I shared this belief with my first doctor, who told me that I was in denial, and who added that I would be in a wheelchair. That made my situation more of a challenge because I certainly wasn't going to buy into a defeatist belief system.

I found a neurologist who understood holistic health and who believed in me. At first I had to take a drug to get my eyesight back. Otherwise there could have been permanent damage. After that I decided not to take anything. I did lots of affirmations at night, where I would say, ''I'm getting better and stronger.'' I visualized myself healthy again, seeing myself exercising and in better shape than I ever was. I kept writing down my thoughts, telling myself that I was bigger than the disease. I was not in denial; I knew what I had, but I wasn't going to let the disease own me. I was very strong about that.

Now it's five years since my diagnosis. And I'm fine. I've had my bouts and moments, but I have always been able to get back on course because I realize that the mind has tremendous power. Whether it's remission or hypnosis or positive of thinking or the combination of all three, I don't know. But it's working.

Today, I practice hypnosis and help other people with MS to realize that they don't have to give their power away to doctors. They can heal themselves by having a positive mindset, a good diet, exercise, and surrounding themselves with positive people. I try to show people that the mind has tremendous power, and that a crisis can turn into an opportunity. I show people how to erase negative thoughts and make new tapes in their minds. I'm not claiming that I have a cure, but I can help people to get to the root of the problem, negative thinking, so that they can stop feeling sorry for themselves and rise above it.

Anthony on obesity

I went to the Hypnosis Institute and worked with Barry Seidman. And I have lost a substantial amount of weight, 46 pounds in six months. Although I'm a strong individual, I still did not believe I could lose weight because I was quite obese. His suggestions taught me how to think, and how to become more confident.

Alicia on resentment

I had been in therapy for many years and had made many improvements in my life, but I still was stuck in a cycle of resenting my mother and other people I knew. I sought hypnosis to try and alleviate the problem, and found that it vanished after one 2½-hour session with George Bien, a really marvelous hypnotherapist.

As far as the session goes, I am not really sure how it helped. I believe that hypnosis starts a process of organic change within body and mind. Over the course of a few weeks, I was simply able to drop it. I found that indeed I loved her again.

I feel that part of it is simply that you go into an altered state of consciousness. The conscious mind quiets down, and the subconscious mind opens up. One thing that happened to me in the course of the session is that we did a visualization in which I spoke to my mother and asked her why she did not love me. It became very clear to me that she would have loved me if she could. At that moment, the realization was so intense that when I came out of trance I suddenly knew and understood her limits as well as my own. I was able to simply accept the situation and move on from there.

I was fortunate to be in the hands of a gifted therapist. That's very important. George is gifted and astute and able to perceive an individual's problem. It's not simply going in and doing some unilateral technical magic play. The therapist has to understand your situation and be able to use techniques of regression so that you, personally, can be helped.

I think that out of the experience of working with George and simply having this moment, this intense physical and emotional moment of realization and recognition, I was able to simply pass through the problem because it affected me on an emotional, physical, and spiritual level. Before, when I was in therapy, I was cognitively aware, and I could do a little word dance. I would say to myself, "I know I should feel better about this," but it never worked. Hypnosis, on the other hand, was a transformative experience.

Maryanna on confidence

About two years ago, I took the Barry Seidman certification course in hypnotherapy, and it really changed my life. I really thought that hypnosis was about mind control and I wouldn't let myself try it. But Barry changed my whole perspective. He was so personable and warm that he was able to convince me that it was the other way around.

I am finally getting someplace now with my acting career. Not only that, I am working with him at the Hypnosis Institute as a hypnotherapist. So you can see how it completely changed my life.

I use it before auditions. As a matter of fact, it helped me land a principal role in a movie before becoming a member of the Screen Actors Guild. Everybody was telling me that I needed to be an extra in a film before I could get into SAG. I said, "No, I don't have to do that. I can get a principal part." Just like that. I was able to get to my higher intelligence through hypnosis, and get the audition without an agent. I got a small part in *Little Odessa,* and now I'm in SAG. I'm also working with Barry. Everything is so wonderful.

Michael on tumors

This is a case of a physical challenge that was tremendously aided and abetted by George Bien's gifted hypnotic skills. Several years ago, I was in Florida, when a healing crisis ensued. Literally overnight, a gigantic tumor appeared on my spine and another near my rectum. I woke up the next morning terrified and extremely upset. These were not small bumps. They were as big as half a tennis ball. I went to the emergency room, where I was told that this was extremely dangerous. I needed surgery and a barrage of x-rays. But I didn't go that route because of a prior incident.

Twenty years earlier, I was told that I had a brain tumor and that something was wrong with my spine, by three different specialists at three separate hospitals. My leg completely withered up as well. I didn't have any money and I was scared stiff. So I went to Weiser's book store and found a book called *Your Mind Can Heal You,* which came from the Christian metaphysical tradition. That led me to the mountains, where I remained alone for five months. I lived through a Canadian winter eating raw grains, and repeating positive affirmations.

Fortunately, that ameliorated the condition without any allopathic remedies, though I really didn't understand why until much later. I didn't understand that the subconscious, like a genius or brilliant inductive child, receives suggestions. I was doing meditation to empty my mind and giving myself strong self-suggestions that my body and leg were healed and whole. The subconscious, according to some schools of hypnotic thought, receives these suggestions uncritically. Because I was isolated, I was not getting the propaganda from society or from the medical profession telling me how dangerous everything was. I was less frightened and my leg came back to full strength.

I returned to my doctor who examined me and looked at the results of my test before telling me that I was 90-95 percent healed. He asked me how it happened and I told him in very sincere, but apparently naive terms. His face was a mixture of contempt and disturbed uneasiness, as he asked me to leave his office. He wanted me out. The power of my experience, combined with the neurologist's reaction, opened my eyes to the nature of Western medicine.

This time, I was told that I needed surgery at once, and that this was tremendously dangerous. Although I was in great pain, and really quite frightened, I went to Chinatown to see a really good traditional Chinese doctor. He also said that I had a tumor and told me that I should begin taking herbs. I did but there wasn't much of a change. Meanwhile, I got sicker and sicker to the point of being bedridden with tremendous sweats.

I had trained with George prior to this and had always loved hypnosis. I had done self-hypnosis before, but in this case, I was not capable of dealing with this problem alone. I went to see George, who I would call unique. He is a genuine healer. He saw me the next day. And for a fee, which I can only call beyond reasonable, I had a three-hour session.

The experience was profound. I can only liken it to an exorcism. The man literally had my jaw open at one point. There was dry heaving stuff that had been so ancient, so toxic in me. I can't even give you a map of what took place during that session, but the next day, this thing broke and drained. This took place literally within 24 hours. The whole psychological situation that I had endured for over 40 years, immediately went into a healing modality, and it has remained that way. There has been no recurrence.

People need to know that their body would not do anything to hurt them. They need to know that their own mind is not their enemy. In fact, quite the opposite. With some loving, conducive suggestions, proper, clean, healthy diet, and a few other things, healings happen very quickly.

Vicki on weight loss and chronic back pain

I went to Barry Seidman for weight loss back in January, and since then I have lost a total of 46 pounds. Now the weight is just falling off, and I have much more confidence and self-esteem. I can't buy clothes small enough fast enough. It's just been a wonderful experience. I got so interested in this that I took a certification course in it.

I was a compulsive eater, big-time. After my three back surgeries, food was my salvation. It was my way of making myself feel better about myself, and it was my way of rewarding myself.

I went through the hypnosis, which gave me more self-confidence and esteem . . . but also helped me to know that these fattening foods were bad for me. The suggestions were that I would eat healthy foods and I would eat what was good for me and only enough for my normal body weight. He just suggested that I eat healthy foods and drink plenty of water. I can't get enough water now. I don't drink soft drinks anymore, just water.

Barry also taught me self-hypnosis, so that I can manage this on a daily basis or as needed. Now it's not a daily basis, but as needed. I just don't want the fattening fried foods, and, as you know, down here in the south we eat fried foods continuously. I no longer eat anything that's fried. It's mainly salads and vegetables. In fact, I don't even eat meat anymore.

I have so much energy because I exercise now, whereas before I wasn't able to physically exercise. This hypnosis has helped me tremendously, and I would advise anybody to go for it.

My son brought a pizza home and I had been a pizza fanatic. I looked at it, and I knew it tasted good, but I just didn't want it. It's as simple as that . . . I talked to Barry last week and I've lost another pound since then.

I was bedridden for three years with chronic back pain. Barry did a private session with me to change the energy through forgiveness. That was a big part of it, a very big part. To forgive you just have to mentally visualize the face and the name of every person who has hurt you in your entire life. You just mentally have to say, "I forgive you," and move on. You just move on until your list is complete. The last person you need to forgive is yourself. That's very important. When you do that, it feels like a weight is lifted off of your shoulders. You actually change the energy in your body from negative to positive, and you can actually feel something going on inside of your body. Then you feel even lighter. When I left there I was on cloud nine.

Before I would try to go to the track to walk, and it would take me forever. I mean the little old ladies were passing me two and three times on my one time around. I would have to get back in the car and go home because I couldn't take it. Now I'm doing two miles and it's wonderful. I love it. I don't hurt anymore. My pain was from a botched surgery and I had nerve damage in my right hip and leg, but I don't hurt anymore. And if there should happen to be a little twinge or something all I do is go into self-hypnosis now. We put a switch up there and I just turn the switch off so it doesn't hurt. A lot of people might think that sounds crazy, but it works. My husband cannot believe the change. He says I'm a totally different person.

Peter on combined therapies

Hypnotherapy has clearly illuminated some of the things from my past that have made an impact on my present life. That was through the combined modalities of regression, Gestalt therapy and psychodrama while in the state of hypnosis. Through that, I have some very clear explanations of some of my present behaviors and how I arrived at that position.

I had been in traditional therapy for about two years and that was helpful, but in hypnotherapy, using Gestalt and psychodrama, I reached better insights because traditional therapy is all talk, while these other processes are more emotional. I could really feel what had occurred and how it was affecting my present situation. I saved a lot of time because I was in traditional therapy for about two years, but in hypnotherapy this was all accomplished in a matter of four or five sessions. I have a lot of faith in hypnotherapy, when it is done with a very skilled practitioner who also employs psychodrama and regression.

Dorothy on sugar addictions

I was a sugar addict, eating a quart of ice cream a day, and putting four to six teaspoons of sugar in each cup of tea. My cholesterol and my sugar were high. And even though I was concerned about my health I just couldn't stop.

A friend finally convinced me to try hypnosis. She gave me the name of Barry Seidman. She felt he could help me, and he did.

I've stopped eating sugar. My blood values are now normal and my cravings are gone. I haven't used sugar in a year. I eat ice cream very occasionally at parties only. I was so impressed with my success that I studied hypnosis at the Hypnosis Institute. It's done wonders for me.

One thing that you learn is self-hypnosis and that is the most wonderful tool. Anyone can learn it, anyone can perfect it. I am now healthy. I am a vegetarian. I use self-hypnosis every day to relax. I feel good about myself. My confidence in myself has increased. I'm positive about my future. I now have a five year plan whereas before I didn't know what I would do five years from now. I am going to have my own practice in a year.

I always wanted to fly. It has been a fantasy of mine for a long time. Now, I know I'm going to achieve it within five years. I am going to learn to pilot a helicopter.

Anyone out there who feels that they are held back should try hypnosis. It does wonders. I'm so much happier with myself since I stopped eating sugar.

Dorothy on self-hypnosis

[In self-hypnosis], the first thing that I do is breathing. I breathe to relax. Then I look at an object, usually above eye level, with focused attention, and just concentrate on that until I feel very relaxed. My eyes become heavy. I say one, two, three, relax, and access my subconscious mind. That's when I give myself positive suggestions: "I am confident, I feel good about myself, the world loves me, I love the world, I can be a hypnotherapist, I will get that doctorate in hypnotherapy, I see myself learning to pilot a helicopter."

I was not always a very confident person. I was very insecure. Self-hypnosis has really been wonderful. I repeat these positive affirmations to myself, which only takes about three minutes. Then I just say, "One, two, three, awaken, emerge."

I do this often during the day—when I'm washing my hands, doing the dishes, walking. I'm now walking anywhere from two to four miles a day, except when it rains.

Joe on overcoming obstacles to success

About a year and a half ago or so, my wife became interested in self-hypnosis. I saw some changes going on in the way she approached her life. She's Japanese and it's taken her quite a while to get used to living in a different country.

Very soon after that, I found Barry Seidman, who was giving a course in certification in hypnotherapy. I really didn't know much about it, but it seemed like an opportunity to get started and to do something that I had always wanted to do, which is work in the field of health. So I took Barry's course and did a little work with some people. I realized at one point that I probably needed to undergo some sessions of my own to understand a little more about it and get the feeling of the person who is having the sessions.

So I had some sessions with Barry and many things in my life began to change. Success seemed to come even more quickly. My wife and I had been involved in various ventures. We publish a magazine in Japanese, and the opportunities that have been coming in since then are just incredible.

I have an offer to publish another magazine on natural health in the near future, and we're working with a health product and beginning to export it throughout the world. This is something that I think came through those sessions because for a long time I believe I've been hesitant to use my abilities fully to reach for a certain level of success, for whatever reason. I feel that I have a greater access now to my subconscious mind. The work with Barry, I'm sure, is a large, large part of that.

This is the feeling that I have. It connects you not only with yourself but with other people on a special level. You become more open to things. I feel like now I have an edge. There's a certain level of confidence and a certain demeanor that I think I've acquired that goes beyond what I had expected of myself before, and I really attribute it to the work I've done. The work actually gets done on yourself by yourself, although there's an impetus that comes from someone else. I think that the beauty of it is that you're working with someone to unleash the powers within you, and eventually you're in control of those powers.

Massage Therapy

Swedish massage, a method of manipulating muscle tissue using specific strokes, movements, and pressure, has several therapeutic benefits: relief of pain, relaxation of muscle tension, improved blood and lymph circulation, better absorption and elimination, greater mobility of muscles and joints, and assistance in the repair of injured and damaged tissue.

Massage can help a wide spectrum of individuals. Athletes can relieve over-exhausted muscles after a race, while the bedridden can alleviate muscle fatigue brought on by lack of exercise. Injured individuals heal faster, while average persons function better all around from a reduction in stress. Massage can help relieve sciatica and common backaches, speed up the healing of fractures and sprains, and even alleviate some of the symptoms of diabetes, multiple sclerosis, cardiomyopathy, hypertension, and fibromyalgia.

Many therapists combine massage with aromatherapy. Inhaling sage or lavender can calm a person, for example, while peppermint can get more energy flowing. Oils open up various meridians, or energy pathways, so that greater healing takes place.

Patient Stories

Sonia on car accident

I had a car accident about four years ago which left me with severe whiplash in my neck, and back problems. I started going for massage with a woman named Susan and it was a wonderful experience. At first, I went once a week for three years. Then I started going every other week, and now I go every third week. I have to say that I ended up feeling better than before the accident.

I'm a painter. I spend lots of hours standing at an easel and painting. The tendons going through my neck would affect my shoulder, and that would affect my painting ability. Because everything got loosened and freed up, I was able to be more comfortable when I was painting. That was definitely an advantage.

I even felt that the massage helped me to feel better than going to a chiropractor. I think that's because the total experience was so comfortable, rewarding, and pleasurable, and that she did such good, deep tissue work.

Linda on dance injuries

I used to train and dance professionally. Later on, after having a child, I continued just to stay in shape. I had a couple of injuries and went to Sarah Vogler, who is a neuromuscular therapist. The first one was a knee injury. I saw her for about four months and she helped with the patterning of my knee. I don't know what she did technically, but she relieved my symptoms a lot. However, I later had to have surgery on that knee.

The other thing that happened is that I had a strain of the psoas muscle. This was a dramatic injury that happened during a class. I couldn't walk out, and left on crutches. I thought of Sarah again, who agreed to barter with me since I had no insurance. I went to Sarah on the crutches and after one session didn't need them. I saw her three more times and was well.

Diane on spasmodic torticollis

This is a condition that affects the neck muscles, causing them to spasm and twist. If it is not treated, it can progress and get worse. The neck muscles tighten into a knot, and it is very painful. After awhile it shortens and twists. I tried several ways of treating it. My most successful way was through massage.

When I go for my massage, my therapist works into the muscles to elongate and relax them. There are several different techniques that she uses. Her fingers can tell an awful lot. She does Swedish message, which is very relaxing, but a lot of times to work into the knots in my muscles, she does more of a deep tissue therapy with her thumbs and knuckles. It's a matter of upkeep because it does help.

As you know, when you get nervous or upset, the first thing to react are your muscles. With people who do not have problems with their muscles, over time or overnight they relax again. The problem is that my neck muscles don't relax on their own. So massage therapy is definitely a blessing. I have been going about once every two weeks for about three years and it really has helped a lot.

Jerry on car accident

I was involved in a motor vehicle accident. . . . I had severe injuries to the neck, shoulder, and arm on the right side of my body. I was being treated by several physicians, who recommended that I see a massage therapist also.

When I saw my massage therapist, she first took a complete medical history in order to individualize the type of treatment that was required for my type of injuries. The emphasis, in my case, was the neck, shoulder, arm, and leg. When you go into the room, it's dimly lit with soothing music to relax you.

There was limited range of motion in my arm and neck. She massaged certain muscle groups and the injured areas by finding the pressure points affected. She worked out the knots, tightness, stiffness, and soft tissue injuries, and relieved a lot of the pain that I was in.

As a result, I was able to increase some of the range of motion, relieve a lot of pain, and improve the flexibility and mobility of the affected areas. She took away a lot of the stress, which was causing me to be irritable and moody. I was completely relaxed after the treatment. I highly recommend massage therapy.

Wendy on tightness

I practice yoga, which gets me more in tune with my body. I basically know where I need to have releases done. I love body work. It's just wonderful.

Sarah Vogler is my body worker. She does some craniosacral work with me, which is a subtle approach. It's mostly a very gentle touch that works with the neck, the bones, and the head. I go in feeling not too bad, thinking, "I don't really need this today." Then I come out feeling much better.

Janine on stress management

Unfortunately, I lost my parents and my brother within a two-year period. I witnessed illness, and obviously the stress that goes along with that is very high. I felt that I needed to start doing things for myself so I began massage therapy. The therapist started treating me with a technique called AMMA therapy. I don't know much about the scientific end of it, only that she applies pressure to certain points while I am on the table. She will hold a certain spot on my head or my foot or other areas. I don't know exactly what she's doing. All I know is that after I finish I feel a new energy and I feel that physically something does occur. It is helping me a lot.

Laurie on cystic fibrosis

Cystic fibrosis is a lung disease like asthma but a little bit worse. Basically, it causes me coughing and digestive problems. I have found massage to be terrific. It definitely helps because I can feel the difference before I get a massage and afterwards. I feel that my lungs are a lot clearer. I start coughing and I know that it helps to bring everything up.

Pam on insomnia

I was experiencing a lot of fatigue and stress from work obligations. There were also problems with muscle spasms and sciatic nerve. It was all getting compounded because I would drag myself through the day and then fall asleep for two hours. Then I would wake up with a lot of pain in my hips. A bad problem was getting worse.

I thought massage would be a good way to start getting myself back in shape. I went for Swedish massage, which helped me alleviate the aches and pains. Right away I started feeling relaxed and better able to work and sleep. Muscles stopped aching. And the results would last a whole week. Another side benefit was that I realized that I needed to focus on what I needed to change in my environment to be less fatigued. So, there were many benefits that came out of the massage treatments.

Lynn on chronic muscle tightness

I first started having massages when I was traveling as a flight attendant. When you are working those long, hard, stressful hours in toxic conditions, it's a great release to wake up in a foreign city and head to the gym. So, I'd have a workout, a sauna, and a massage.

Because I'm kind of a hyperactive person, it was good to have deep tissue massage. I found shiatsu to be the most effective although I have had Swedish and aromatherapy with crystals, and that was very interesting as well. I understood that it helped to detox because they're stimulating the lymph glands. In particular, my neck and shoulders were always full of these toxic knots. So, usually Japanese ladies would walk up and down my back for twenty minutes or half an hour and then work on my neck for 15 minutes alone. That, in itself, was amazing. Later on, I discovered a masseur who also did acupuncture. He specialized in athletic injuries, so I would have a massage and acupuncture which was amazing. I would be up for 12 hours by the time I got to Japan. After a massage I would wake up revitalized and go out dancing for the evening. So I think it had some very positive effects.

I noticed that when I did that crystal aromatherapy, I would feel euphoric afterwards. I literally felt an electric shock-like feeling go through my head when she would release something by using what she called a sulfur crystal. So there are some amazing things that a masseuse can do to energize the body by releasing blockages and breaking up toxic knots.

The therapist would massage me with oils of various scents that are geared to trigger particular emotional responses, depending on what she felt I needed. She would place the crystal on various parts of my body or adjacent to it. I remember one time, in particular, she said she couldn't determine exactly which crystal I needed until she got to the sulfur. That's when I felt this electricity go through my head. It was just a "ping" moment. That's when I realized this wasn't hocus pocus. Then afterwards, I always felt euphoric for at least an hour. I think it must be similar to the neurological responses that get set off when people listen to chant music.

Seth on sports injuries

Race-walking taxes the hamstrings quite bit. I decided to combine massage and physical therapy, which worked out very well. Usually, I would get the physical therapy first and follow it with the massage.

I found that my shoulders would loosen up. As a matter of fact, it felt as though they had broadened. And it helped my hamstrings tremendously. I think massage is an excellent way of getting out the knots and the aches and pains. Typical shoulder and leg problems are helped.

I saw my massage therapist a few weeks ago, and I got a terrific massage in a nice quiet, peaceful room, with some meditative music in the background. You really need the quiet. I think the benefit was really tremendous. I certainly do want to come back and get massaged more.

Tom on stress

I had a lot of job-related stress and tightness. Massage helps me to release a lot of the emotional stuff that I tend to hold onto. Since I have been going for massages, I have been able to relax. I do not feel as tight, and I do not feel a lot of pain in my body. Liz is great. She is strong but gentle. She goes in deep, yet she doesn't leave you screaming. Also, one of the things we work with is breath and I try to carry that with me through the week. I tend to hold a lot of stuff in and close up tight, particularly in my shoulders and lower back. By staying with my breath and breathing longer and deeper, I can release a lot of stress.

Gil on hamstring tear

I went to an orthopedist and paid $175 to hear that there was nothing he could do about this for a year and a half, so good-bye and good luck. Since I was nearly at the point of walking with a cane, that was unacceptable. So I decided to try massage to get at least minor relief. Within two weeks of having massage three times a week, there was improvement. Within five weeks, I was pretty much pain-free. And by the end of two months, it was normal.

Nutritional Therapy

Comedian and social activist Dick Gregory says people commonly confront him about his vegetarianism, insisting that meat is necessary. There is a lot of protein in a steak, he agrees, but cow's don't eat steak. Many plant-based foods provide the right vitamins, minerals, and enzymes to help our bodies manufacture everything it needs.

While a strictly vegetarian regimen may not be the answer for everyone, the idea is that many people are uneducated in their nutritional understanding, and do not realize how the foods they eat relate to every variety of chronic, degenerative illness. They may become depressed from a common food to which they are allergic, or hyperactive from sugar, and never make the connection because they have eaten this way all their lives. Most people can therefore benefit from nutritional counseling, which incorporates supplementation and dietary changes for optimal health.

Patient Stories

Mary on hepatitis B

I used to eat any and everything. I became so sick that I didn't think I was going to make it. I didn't know what was going on but then I found out what I had. I must have had it for years. I had a test for something else. Through that, I found out about the hepatitis.

Then I saw a nutritionist and I learned what I was supposed to do. I needed to eat well and to rest. I think rest is most important. So I became more careful. I started taking a whole spectrum of nutrients for strength. I drink soups and eat green vegetables and sometimes fish. I stay away from the red meat as much as I can. I do take a little beef once in a while.

I had a couple of ozone treatments. That helped too. My blood tests looked much better than they did before. With the ozone therapy, I felt much better right away. So, I assume it's a combination of the ozone and the nutrition. All this has helped me. I'm hoping that I'll stay this way for a long time.

Rabbi Jeff on obesity

I have lost a total of 140 pounds, and I have never felt better in my entire life. Before I was lethargic. I was always tired and needed to sleep 12 hours a night. I had trouble walking a flight of stairs. I had trouble walking around the block. I had difficulty breathing. I had difficulty living. Now I walk five miles a day. I exercise vigorously and regularly. I eat voluminously, but I eat totally differently. I have become a total vegetarian. I have even given up eating fish. My sources of protein come from beans, legumes, and rice. I feel invested with a tremendous sense of energy, a very vital dynamic, and have literally never felt better in my entire life.

Years ago, I would go on a diet for three weeks, and the only thing that I lost was 21 days. This time, I did not go on a diet. I completely changed the way in which I think about food, prepare food, consume food, and apparently, the way I now absorb food and deal with it in terms of my nutritional well-being.

I had reason to see a proctologist for a leftover problem, and he was amazed at the cleanliness of the colon. It was just absolutely marvelous. I feel an invigorated sense of vitality. I saw Dolores, my nutritionist, about eight months ago, and she instructed me in terms of various vitamin, mineral, and herbal supplements. I read voraciously and have found the information inspiring and informative. I have become a kind of local focal point for people in my religious community. People who might not otherwise have access to this information have now begun to call me with some degree of regularity. And I refer them to nutritionists.

The most important element of this entire protocol is the fact that I feel wonderful. Having given up meat, chicken, and diary products, and a whole variety of other foods, I don't wake up with headaches anymore. I used to think that it was appropriate to wake up in the morning with a headache. I now wake up with a clear head. I have a wonderful sense of vitality, a sense of purpose and direction that is literally inspirational. If someone would have told me two years ago that I wouldn't be a carnivore, I would have laughed hysterically. I was the most carnivorous human being on this earth! If it had four legs and rabbinic supervision, I ate it with great glee and in great quantity at all the wrong hours of the day. Today, I feel refreshed and revitalized, in all aspects of my life. I feel a tremendous sense of joy and vitality.

My total cholesterol used to be 297. Without any medication whatsoever, it is now 171. All the other blood work is much improved: kidney function, liver function, blood pressure, everything, is right down the middle now, whereas before I was a major bomb ready to burst.

It has gotten so good. In fact, I recently had a circumcision to perform on a Sabbath when I'm not allowed to drive. I walked 6½ miles there, did the circumcision, standing at all times, and walked 6½ miles back. I felt great, and realized, "My God, I've just walked half a marathon."

I was all excited and called Dolores. She suggested that I enter the New York City marathon, and I'm pursuing this. For me, to have watched the marathon 140 pounds ago would have been a tiring experience. Now I am at the point where I am entering the marathon. This is a 180-degree change in my life. I owe it to the brilliant science of good, old-fashioned, basic, fundamental nutrition.

Gay on hyperthyroidism

When I first came to the Healing Center, I saw Dolores Perry. She was very helpful in determining whether I had hyperthyroidism or hypothyroidism, and as it turned out I did have the symptoms for hyperthyroidism. I have the bulging eyes, the irritability, the increased perspiration, and things like that. Hyperthyroidism is a disorder where the thyroid gland produces too much of a hormone, which results in overactive metabolic states. Body processes, including digestion, speed up with this disorder. My husband would make fun of me sometimes because I would always be hungry and eating. I guess that was from the hyperthyroidism. Needing to eat so much was unnerving.

Dolores Perry helped me to design a proper diet. I learned how to eat the right foods and to stay away from foods that caused my thyroid to produce too much of its hormone. This helped me with my weight. I was telling Dolores that I was have a problem filling out my jeans. Now I no longer have to wear my leggings underneath my jeans to fill them out.

All the medical establishment wants to do is pump chemicals into your system. And chemicals are not natural. They treat you like a guinea pig, saying, "If that doesn't work, come back and we'll prescribe something else." That's ridiculous. The best thing for the body are natural foods in their natural state. I would definitely recommend that anyone, even people who think they are healthy, go on a natural diet.

Jean on post-polio syndrome, hypoglycemia, and fatigue

I contracted polio when I was very, very young. Then, in the late 80's, I was had some weird, weird symptoms, and I was tired all the time. The medical doctors used that six letter word, stress, and put me on a lot of tranquilizers. I knew that wasn't working. Then I began to have a lot of other symptoms, which as far as I was concerned, were not related to my post-polio syndrome. A friend of mine said that I might have hypoglycemia. I went to a health store and got some paperbacks, specifically, Carlton Fredericks, and realized, "Yes, that's what I have."

I was hospitalized briefly for a rapid heartbeat. They started to pump me with heart medications. But I told the doctor I wanted a glucose tolerance test. That proved that I was hypoglycemic. . . . I found an endocrinologist [but] he made me worse because my body needed a very restricted diet.

When I finally found Marilyn, who I call my guru, I found that I had to be careful of complex carbohydrates. My intake had to be very, very low to avoid symptoms. An added bonus was the supplements that she ordered for me. They helped my muscle tone and bone density in my right legs and hips. That was something I didn't expect.

Right now, I'm not going to say that I'm 100 percent better. I do get fatigued and I do have to pace myself. But this is nothing like what I had prior to 1989. I make sure I eat a correct diet. I eat all natural foods and buy a lot of my stuff in the health food store and make sure that I take my supplements.

The doctor is very pleased, even with the pulse in my right leg. I had been wearing an elasticized knee brace, which had absolutely no movement in it. After the supplements, I started going for days without the brace. I realized, "Oh, my God. I don't need it." I have discarded it and only take it with me when I go away or go out, in case I should fall. But it's also affected my hip and arm. I find that I can grasp better with my right arm now. These changes came on gradually. I never realized that those supplements were going to help with that also.

Valerie on dizzy spells and fatigue

I had a lot of dizzy spells and fatigue, which made it difficult to get out of bed. My normal, daily activities were very limited. I also had a lot of infections: upper respiratory infections, sinus infections, yeast infections, and so forth. In general, my health was very poor.

I went through quite a few doctors, but nobody was able to help me. I was tested to see if I had an autoimmune illness. They thought it might be a variety of things, but nothing ever showed up. Nobody could really help me. Meanwhile, I couldn't even get out of bed. Everybody realized I was sick, but they didn't know what to do for me.

For a year, I was on antibiotics, almost constantly. I was also on other medications, like meclizine for the dizziness, and decongestants for the sinus infections. I think I had about 16 different medications that year. And they were pretty potent. At this point, I am not taking any of them.

It all began to change for me after I saw Gary Null at a seminar held through the Learning Annex in Manhattan. He was discussing diet and supplements.

It was the only thing left that I could really do at that point. So I went to see a nutritionist.

I saw a nutritionist who told me specifically what to eat, and what not to eat. It was a very limited diet, but there was enough of a choice for me to still eat normally. At the same time, I cut out things that had been bothering me, but that I didn't know were bothering me. For example, wheat flour and dairy products where things I had been eating all the time that I didn't realize were having an effect on me until I cut them out. Then I had a total reversal of most of my symptoms.

The first was difficult. I guess I was addicted to a lot of foods. I felt very depressed and weak, but once I got past that point, I gained strength. I did a lot of journaling and that helped me to see the progress that I was making. In the beginning the notes read, "Today I was able to get out of bed, and do some light housework." At this point, I am able to do light jogging. I'm more active for an extended period of time.

When I began seeing a nutritionist . . . I saw the results right away. The first week, I noticed that a lot of the mental fogginess I was having was gone. I was alert. My eyes were very clear. These were things I didn't realize until I changed the diet. Then, all of a sudden, I improved.

I think the main problem was that I was eating a lot of wheat and dairy. Now I'm on a vegetarian diet, except for fish. I have a whole list of what I am able to eat and I try to eat everything as natural as possible. I follow the advice in Gary's books. I study them to make the diet more interesting.

I take a variety of supplements too. The main thing helping me is the Green Stuff. I used to have a lot of hair loss. It was becoming very noticeable. I'm only 28, so that was really upsetting me. My skin and hair were dull too. Since I have been taking the Green Stuff, that's totally changed for the first time in a very long time. I also take choline, inositol, antioxidants, and aloe vera juice.

It feels good to know that it's in my control, whereas before I felt like everything was taking me over. So this has helped me mentally as well.

Nina on digestive disorders

From the time I was in my late teens to my early 20's, I had severe digestive difficulties. I would get debilitating abdominal pain from severe gas in response to eating foods. I would get together with friends to eat Chinese food and go out to a movie. Afterwards, I would have to be literally helped into a taxi to get home.

Eventually, I started getting very fatigued, because if you're not digesting food well, eventually, that's what will happen. I experienced depression from having low energy.

I thought my diet was quite good. In my early 20's, I stopped eating dairy, and I started eating a vegetarian diet. But I still had a lot of problems with food allergies.

I started seeing a nutritional doctor in the late 80's. That helped a bit. Then I worked with a chiropractic nutritionist. She suggested digestive enzymes and that helped even more. But I still had chronic constipation. So about a year and a half ago, I started working with Dolores Perry. She suggested a real high level of supplements and herbs.

It's one thing to have food allergies, but do you have food allergies because your digestive system doesn't work or does your digestive system not work and then you get food allergies? You've got to both work with food allergies and energize your system. So that's what the supplements have done for me.

Now my digestive system works pretty well. And if it doesn't, I can bring it back into balance with supplements and herbs.

It took just a few months to see an improvement. Now, I'm a very happy, outgoing person. For a number of years I was an unhappy and depressed person. A lot of that was due to the fact that I wasn't physically feeling well. It's made a big difference.

I value working with Dolores because I really work with her. I bring in research articles, we discuss them, and she makes suggestions. I'm really working with her and treating myself. I'm in charge, and I really appreciate that.

Greg on brain tumor

I was on chemotherapy for about four and a half months, when I asked to be taken off it. This was about three and a half years ago. I had had a craniotomy, and they resected the tumor from the brain. Then I went through a regimen of radiation. I was led to believe that that was that. Suddenly an oncologist came in and said that I was to go through chemotherapy. I was having some bad reactions to either the chemotherapy or one of the antiepileptic drugs they were giving me. I had scar tissue remaining in my head and it was causing me some minor seizure activity.

I started the chemotherapy in Chicago, but moved out to San Francisco. I was at the University of California, San Francisco, where I was reading a lot of articles from the American Brain Tumor Association about the permeability of the blood brain barrier. I went to the radiologist for an MRI, which at that time was every three months. I asked if they could do an enhancement to show the permeability of my blood brain barrier. They assured me they could, but upon giving me back my films they could not.

I went to my neurologist and asked him to please show me how permeable the blood brain barrier was. He really couldn't show me either. I asked, "What evidence do I have that the chemotherapy is actually going after these cancer cells and eliminating them?'' I would go there every month, and all my blood counts would be very high. Then a month later, after the chemotherapy, everything would crash; my platelet counts would crash, and my white blood cell count would crash. That's my immune system. It didn't make a lot of sense to me that no cancer cells were being chased around in there but good cells were dying. I wanted to build up my immune system, rather than tear it down.

I said, ''If I were to stop today (which was actually two and a half cycles short of what was recommended), and I were to have a recurrence, would it be because I stopped taking chemotherapy?'' The neurologist said, ''Absolutely not. In fact, we really don't even know how much chemotherapy you should be getting. All we do know is that after six cycles we could start doing some damage to your other organs.'' After that, I said, ''We're through today.''

The other alarming thing about it is that I had asked the oncologist what I should be doing nutritionally, regarding supplements. The first oncologist said something strange, and I quote her: ''I really don't think you should be taking supplements while you are on chemotherapy. The object is to make you sick.'' I thought the object was to make me well. I asked her to explain it further and she said that with the supplements I could be weakening the effectiveness of the chemotherapy by strengthening my cancer cells. I didn't follow. I had some problems with her and stopped going there.

I went to another oncologist who had no problem with me taking supplements. But in the end, when I was out in California I just decided to stop.

From the very beginning, when I was diagnosed in Barcelona, I began studying what the disease was and the little that was known about it. I started studying about nutrition because nobody could ever answer a question about what I should be eating and avoiding. My cousin had the same exact brain tumor at the same exact time that I did. She was in the same chemotherapy protocol that I was, and we were both given lists of foods to avoid. But our lists were very different. I asked the neurologist and oncologist about it. They didn't have an answer. I said, ''I have a feeling that some people on chemotherapy call after a bad reaction. You ask them what food they've eaten and it ends up on that list.'' They said, ''Yeah, I think that's what happens.'' At that point, I started not trusting conventional medicine.

I started to look at how my nutrition can help bolster my immune system and also how I could eat foods that would not detract from it or harm it. At first, I was doing it on my own. It was a long process of reading a lot of materials. I started reading about a lot of supplements and learned what vitamins and minerals are contained in which foods. I learned how much I would have to eat in order to get an amount that would be effective.

I actually did go to one doctor whose book I had read. I told him that I had gone on a strict organic foods diet and that I had quit all forms of caffeine and processed foods. He told me that the whole idea about organically grown food or food without pesticides or growth hormones or whatever is all a bunch of nonsense. He said his daughter and son grow their own food because they believe the same thing, but the stuff can't harm you. This man wrote a book about nutrition for chemotherapy patients. I became skeptical and didn't know if anyone knew anything about nutrition.

Fortunately, I ended up doing some volunteer work at a natural foods store, which happened to be the first collective or food co-op in San Francisco, years and years ago. I was educated well there by people who had been working there for 15 or 20 years. And also by a lot of people who shopped at the store, some of whom were writers. That's where I got my first quasi-professional advice.

Finally, last year I was able to secure some health insurance in New York. That's when I was told about Gary Null from a taxi driver. I went to see Gary. He found my case to be very interesting because I had just run the New York City Marathon. Part of my regimen for getting well was nutrition. I have a pretty strict diet. I seldom eat out; I prepare most of my food and buy only organically grown food. I pay attention to what kind of oils I use. He explained to me how some supplements can help me out. My metabolism really sped up as a result of training for a marathon. I was having a hard time keeping weight on. He introduced me to some products that would help balance my weight. I was complaining about a lack of energy. He said I was putting a lot of stress on my body and that a B complex would really help. The local health food stores have people who can also answer questions. They're pretty well informed.

I think the greatest testimony to nutrition being very helpful is that last week I had my five-year MRI, and it's fine.

Charles on chalazions and allergies

The specific problem I had was something called chalazions, which was something I would get on my eyelid. I had a history of getting these cysts for 14 years. I would try things like hot compresses. But they would often develop into infections. The doctors would give me antibiotics. When that didn't work, they had to be surgically removed, so I had about four or five surgeries. They were treating them, but they just weren't going away.

Imagine having to go to work like this. My eye would be partially closed. And I would be uncomfortable, even in pain sometimes.

It started getting worse. Not only would I get chalazions, but I would also have infections on the eyeball itself, for which they would give me topical antibiotic drops. Sometimes it would clear it up and sometimes it wouldn't. I wasn't getting any answers. All they told me was that it was related to stress and that I needed to calm down.

I picked up Gary's book, *No More Allergies,* and realized that this condition, along with many others that you wouldn't normally associate with an allergy, could be related to an allergen. After that, I went to see Dolores Perry, who told me to stay away from certain facial washes and scrubs that I was using. She told me to use a specific type of soap and natural cream. More importantly, she told me to avoid wheat and a few other foods. She also told me to use aloe vera in the eye, which helped me tremendously. When I went to see her I was in the acute phase of another attack, and the aloe vera did a much better job of clearing it up than any antibiotic would have done.

Now, there is nothing wrong with either eye whatsoever. Before seeing Dolores, I had never gone for more than 30 days without redness in my right eye. But I have gone now for seven months with no problem. I think it was the wheat because once I stopped, my eye immediately cleared up.

At first, I found the change somewhat difficult because everything I was used to eating had wheat in it. But I learned how to go on a rotation diet and substitute other grains. One day I will eat spelt, the next day barley, and the next quinoa. For breakfast, I might have amaranth with bananas and peaches and coconut milk. There are just so many grains out there and so many wonderful dishes to prepare.

Since following this diet, I have noticed other changes in my health. By eating more complex carbohydrates versus refined carbohydrates, I find that I have a tremendous amount of energy.

Bob on hypoglycemia and lipoma

I became interested in nutrition about 20 years ago. After being an art dealer for 16 years, I had a mentor who got me involved in the health food industry. That led up to my present position of owning a vegetarian restaurant in New York City.

I had many personal miracles that helped my own health in the early days. I got into the field because I was suffering from the classic low blood sugar. I was having the usual mood swings. At the time I was smoking cigarettes and drinking black coffee. Slowly, I weaned myself away from all that and found out that a wonderful, steady energy came up which has stayed with me since.

About 10 months ago I had another personal miracle. We were constructing a restaurant, and working 16 to 18 hours a day. Suddenly, I felt some fatty tissue under my armpit. I had it diagnosed and it turned out to be a lipoma. End of story. It's gone. Completely vanished. As I speak to you, I am touching the area, and it's flat now. That I attribute to my own whole grain diet, which

I have been eating for a year now. I've been eating tons of greens and no dairy.

I'm feeling fine now. I'm in my 50's but still dancing around like a 30-year-old.

Joy on increased energy

I just began eating vegetarian food and have noticed that my weight has begun to come down. I was quite lethargic before, but have much more energy now.

I am a nutritionist. I was counseling people and working many, many hours. I was exhausted. Then I started eating at a natural foods restaurant and noticed how good I was feeling. I would finish a meal and say, "Wow, I feel so good. I don't understand why." Then I figured out that it was the food that had been making me lethargic and the food that was making me more energetic than ever. It's amazing. I had an education in the field, and even graduated magna cum laude, but I had to experience the effects in my own body to really understand the power of the food.

Renata on polio and migraines

I had polio, many, many years ago, when I was 40. When it began, I was having terrible, terrible pains. My husband thought I had the flu and didn't call a doctor. When I got my head back, I called the doctor, who asked me to come in as soon as I could walk. But for about six weeks, I was completely bedridden. I couldn't walk at all.

In the meantime, I had dreadful pain and didn't know what to do about it. Everything ached. My older daughter worked in a health food store and told me to take calcium. I did and the pain immediately went away.

It took about three months before I could walk. And it took me the whole day to get dressed. To this day, it amazes me that anyone thought I had the flu. I was completely paralyzed. I couldn't even lift my head.

Somewhere in that period, I started reading Adele Davis and started taking the sorcerer's potion. It was her own mixture of lecithin, vitamin E, garlic, and a whole lot of other stuff. Then in 1975 I started going out to concerts again. To make a long story short, I met my soul mate at one. Then I wanted to live again and really started getting into life again.

Years later, after my mother died I had become depressed again. . . . My daughter always listens to Gary. She said to me, "You know, Mom. You really should go and see a nutritionist." So . . . I found a nutritionist and found me a new friend.

I have changed my diet. Of course the wheat is out. And coming from

Germany, that wasn't easy. Germany has got the most wonderful breads, absolutely sublime. And to come here and eat spelt bread didn't exactly thrill me. But I don't get headaches anymore. I have had migraine headaches frequently. Barely a day would pass where I didn't have a headache. The headaches are now 99.99 percent gone. (If the weather changes I still get them.) She put me on a diet, starting off with watermelon. I have lost 20 pounds on it. It was wonderful because you can eat as much watermelon as you like. I'm on all sorts of supplements and they're doing something.

My joy for life is back.

John on malaria and rheumatoid arthritis

In the late 1970s, I was working as a war reporter, traveling with soldiers in a war zone for about 10 months, when I got very ill. My weight dropped from about 180 to 120 pounds from not having much food. I had been faithfully taking the prophylactic medicine that is supposed to prevent malaria the whole time. But we were in an area that was highly infested, and I came down with malaria.

At the time, I was out in the middle of nowhere. It was several months before I got to an area where they could do a blood test. At that point, you can't tell what type of malaria you've got. You have to diagnose it in the first couple of days.

About the third day, they gave me injections of the normal treatment. About two months later, I got back to Sudan where I was able to see a doctor and get blood tests. I was still very ill. My weight had dropped to 100 pounds. Every week, I would have three or four days of vomiting, high fevers, delirium, extreme muscle weakness, anemia, visual distortion. The medicine I was taking just wasn't working.

The doctors said it was no problem. They had injections for resistant strains, which was what I probably had. I took that treatment in Sudan and it didn't clear it up. I got to Egypt on the way home and got very ill the next week. I went to another doctor and he said the same thing. He said the medicine they gave me in Sudan was the normal backup, and usually does the trick, but when it doesn't, he has something else. Well, this went on and on. I went to Egypt, Lebanon, Rome, Paris, London, New York, back to a special hospital in London for tropical diseases. I went through seven different backup treatments. Each one promised to cure the malaria and didn't.

They finally said that there was nothing more they could do for me. My condition was so bad that they thought I would probably get black water fever and die. Or I would have a miracle where my body would just figure out how to solve it on its own. They said there was nothing more they could do.

I came back to New York, and lived for about 18 months like that. Every week, I would be extremely ill for about three or four days. Often, I would be in delirium.

One day, I met a painter who was working in my building. He saw me in the elevator and we talked for a few minutes. When he realized what my condition was, he said, "Come to my girlfriend's house, Friday night, eight o'clock, and I'll show you what to do." I was kind of startled. He said, "Just trust me."

I went. Turns out these people were into raw foods. It's the first time in my life that I had ever seen a juicer. They gave me a little book by Dick Gregory, and they explained fasting and cleansing. That night, they sent me home with a jar of juice, and instructions on what to do in the morning. They basically put me on raw juices for the next two weeks, a half a day on citrus juice, a half a day of vegetable juice.

For the first time in about 18 months, the malaria didn't come back. It didn't come back the first week, and it didn't come the second week. It hasn't returned since in 17 years. That's important because they tell you that malaria is something that always recurs. Once you get it, you never really get rid of it. It's never come back.

After those first two weeks of doing juices and taking enemas to help with side effects, I noticed that all types of other symptoms in my body were better. My hair looked better, my skin looked better. A lot of residual problems that I had from arthritis disappeared as well.

I had developed arthritis when I was 13 or 14, which left me with quite a few deformities. I had bumps on my hands and elbows. There was extensive calcification between all the vertebra. So, I had quite a limited range of motion. I noticed that all the stiffness felt much better. I mentioned it to them and asked if the treatment for the malaria could be helping the residual arthritic damage. They said that it definitely could, and advised me to stay on the program.

For the next two years, I ate a largely raw foods, vegetarian diet. And I did lots of fasting and cleansing. I did two fasts of 120 days, and four fasts of 90 days. About half of each year, I would be in a juice-fasting state. I would go through gallons in a day.

After two years, all the arthritic damage completely disappeared. A couple of times since then I have been x-rayed for injuries. Doctors always say that they don't believe that I had arthritis when I was younger. They say they know the disease and that I should be totally crippled by this point. They also point to the x-rays, saying that there should be evidence of it. But the arthritic damage is totally gone from the body.

As years have gone by, everybody comments that I look much younger than my age. Here I am at 47 now, and people are always guessing that I'm 10 years younger than that. Often people say, it must be my genes, but I have 10 younger brothers and sisters, most of whom eat a conventional meat and white flour diet. About half of them look older than I do. It's very clear to me that the main change is diet, eating really good, healthy food, and fasting and cleansing.

I also noticed that as I did this, especially the long fasts, my frame of mind really changed. I had been a depressive personality and had done therapy for that. I noticed that the longer I could stay on fresh, live, whole food, the better I felt. So, it really affected me from deep in the bones, to a consciousness, to my skin.

Dorothy on periodontal disease and other conditions

About two and a half years ago, I converted to a natural foods diet, and began to take vitamin supplements. I was always fatigued at that time and I was overweight. I had my allergies identified by blood tests, and I stopped eating those foods. At the same time, I began walking regularly for exercise.

Over a period of a few months, I lost about 25 pounds. I slept better, and I woke refreshed. I had much more energy. My digestion and elimination improved. Also, my cholesterol level dropped about 45 points, and my thinking became much clearer. I used to have vertical splits in some of my fingernails and I had cracks at the corners of my mouth, both of which indicated vitamin deficiency, and they're all gone now. The condition of my nails, my skin, and my hair improved, and I regained a pinker color in my cheeks and lips.

. . . Some years ago, I had several surgeries on my gums due to periodontal disease. I wasn't familiar at that time with nutritional approaches nor holistic dentistry. I also had several back teeth extracted at the same time because of the gum disease.

Since improving my diet, taking supplements, getting vitamin drips, my gums became much healthier. In fact, recently my dentist showed me x-rays that I had regrown bone partially in one part of my jaw and completely in another area. These had been two areas with very significant bone loss.

I suspect that had I been knowledgeable about nutrition and holistic dentistry at that time, I could have avoided the surgeries and not lost those teeth.

Overall, I am very pleased because I feel and look much better. I attribute these changes to eating natural foods, getting rid of alcohol and caffeine, and taking vitamin supplements. The vitamins and minerals particularly helpful for the gum disease were coenzyme Q10, vitamin C, vitamin E, calcium, and magnesium. I know that without nutritional changes, these improvements wouldn't have taken place.

Chris on athletics

I went to a nutritionist just to supplement my diet. I was a rower and I do a lot of in-line skating. I train fairly hard. I just wanted to make sure that I was getting everything that I needed in my daily intake of food. I went to a nutritionist, who gave me a great balance of supplements to my diet.

I sense that I am gradually discovering what my body needs and why I need to take these supplements in order to perform and just feel better during the day.

Ron on headaches and runny nose

My whole life I spent with tissues in my hand. Now there are no tissues, no runny nose, no headaches.

I learned more about nutrition and what my body needed in order to improve my whole life. I stopped eating dairy and animal products. After that, I had no more headaches, no more colds. I never get sick.

That made me feel so good that I'm out there helping others now. I opened up a group of organic health food stores and restaurants so that everyone else can eat as well as I do.

Oxygen Therapies

Oxygen therapies are extremely effective in treating a variety of conditions because oxygen creates optimal function in every cell in the body, whether it be muscle, bone, skin, or brain. Inside the cells, mitochondria become activated, and energy increases. Outside the tissues, oxygen mobilizes immune cells to engulf and kill foreign substances. In fact, harmful germs are less abundant in the presence of large amounts of oxygen.

Oxygen therapies are administered in several different ways. One is hyperbaric oxygen therapy. Hyperbaric, or high-pressure, oxygen first became popular in the United States in the 1920's and 1930's, when clinics with metal oxygen chambers were built, and people from around the world sought treatment. Despite its success, oxygen therapy was all but forgotten during World War II, when metals were used by the military to build submarines, rather than oxygen chambers.

Today most doctors are not schooled in the amazing benefits of high-pressure oxygen. But it has many vital uses. Hyperbaric oxygen can be given to treat diving accidents, carbon monoxide poisoning, gangrene, wounds that do not heal, and flesh-eating bacteria. The effects of serious injuries and strokes can be greatly minimized by this modality especially when it's used within the first 24 hours of the accident or stroke. It is excellent for overcoming viral problems, including chronic fatigue, HIV, and Hepatitis B and C.

Intravenous peroxide therapy is another way the healing power of oxygen can be used. Many people know the benefits of applying peroxide externally. Some use it to brush their teeth and gums, for destroying harmful plaque. Others use it to dissolve wax in their ears. But it has other therapeutic uses as well. Complementary physicians administer small amounts of pharmaceutical-grade peroxide intravenously to supply extra oxygen to tissues and to kill germs throughout the body.

Ozone therapy is another way oxygen is used. Many regard ozone (O_3) as the safest, most effective, and most promising treatment for a wide spectrum of diseases. The therapy has benefited numerous patients over the years and is widely used in Europe, as well as Cuba. Ten million patients have been treated with ozone in Germany alone since the early 60's. Unfortunately, it is currently illegal in most American states.

Medical ozone differs from the atmospheric type in that it is pure and concentrated. This is an important distinction because atmospheric ozone, produced from ultraviolet radiation, is combined with different nitrous oxide and sulfur dioxide products and is harmful. It is not used in medical practice.

There is a strong argument for its legalization. Consider that in Germany it is routinely used for treating hospital patients after every major operation. When small amounts of ozone are introduced into the bloodstream, it kills harmful microorganisms. This helps prevent secondary infections, which are a leading cause of death in the United States. It is estimated that between 10 and 50 thousand Americans die each year due to complications from post-surgical infections.

Not only does ozone kill microbes; it improves blood circulation. Hence, think of all the people with coronary heart disease, pulmonary disease, strokes, clogged arteries, diabetic neuropathy, intermittent claudication and gangrene who can be helped with this mode of treatment. Better circulation means more life-giving oxygen going to the body's tissues. Doctors report particular success with the different types of hepatitis, as well as with candida, allergies, and bladder infections. Other disorders treated with ozone therapy include herpes, arthritis, respiratory conditions, multiple sclerosis, sexually transmitted diseases, and parasitic conditions. Ozone is especially impressive in its effect on frequently debilitating conditions, such as AIDS, HIV, sickle cell anemia, and cancer.

Doctors administer ozone in several ways. A small amount of a patient's blood may be removed from a vein and a small amount of ozone added to the blood, which is then reinfused into the patient. This process, known as autohemotherapy (AHT), is used throughout Europe, where it is reported to have therapeutic value in circulatory disorders, viral diseases, and cancer. Tiny amounts of ozone can also be given to patients in the form of an enema in a process known as rectal insufflation. The mixture is absorbed into the blood through the intestines. Sometimes a plastic bag is placed over the area to be treated, and an ozone/oxygen mixture is pumped into the bag and absorbed into the body. This method is often used to treat skin diseases, diabetic foot problems, and gangrene. Ozone can also be used topically to treat burns. It accelerates wound healing, induces enzyme production, and activates immune system response. Additionally, there is a procedure known as polyatomic aphoresis, which uses O4 instead of O3. Proponents of this method report that it is highly effective, even in end-stage disease.

Healthy people can become more healthy using ozone to rejuvenate cells. Because ozone increases the effectiveness of the antioxidant enzyme system, which scavenges excess free radicals in the body, ozone therapy helps people stay younger longer.

Clinicians usually recommend ozone as part of a larger holistic protocol in the treatment of seriously ill patients. Dr. John Pittman, of North Carolina, explains: "I rarely give ozone treatments unless they are combined with some other supportive therapy. Admittedly, the shortcoming of doing this is that you don't always know which component is most beneficial. But I certainly know from experience which things generally help the most. Combining ozone with proper dietary therapies and addressing other cofactors, particularly in the GI tract, results in tremendous changes in a person's constitution. Their blood work can turn around, and it definitely can improve the quality and length of life."

Patient Stories

Richard on prostate cancer

Before discovering that I had prostate cancer, I had severe pains, especially during sexual relations. I was passing blood and had an awful time urinating. I went to see a specialist. After taking tests, he told me I had a solid cancer and that he needed to operate.

Fortunately, I learned through someone else about a doctor in Mexico. When I got to the clinic, my prostate count was 78. I began ozone treatments and after three weeks, my count was down to 37. I continued treatments at home and after six months, my count was down to zero.

I continue using ozone to this very day. I take it in different ways. I have an ozone machine, and I use it when taking a bath and I ozonate my drinking water as well. I use it a lot because I feel if I don't the cancer will come back.

Since my treatments, I feel better than I have felt in years. Now I can pass water without a problem. I can work and feel very well. I am more than pleased.

If it hadn't been for the ozone treatments, I wouldn't be here today because that cancer would have had me. Surgery would have done no good.

Brian on viral infections

I first found out about ozone from Ed McCabe who directed me to a conference in South Carolina which, in turn, directed me to a conference in Germany. There, I learned first-hand, from the people who had been using this method the longest, how it should be done. I learned about major autohemotherapy.

The reason that I did this is because I am a nurse. I got a needle stick from a patient who was infected with HIV, Epstein-Barr, CMV, hepatitis B and C, and several other things, and became very sick within months. I had night sweats, severe diarrhea, and I lost a lot of weight. I couldn't live that way and wanted to be healthy, so I started ozone treatments.

I had 16 treatments over a period of six weeks. By the end of that time, my health was back to normal. I was gaining weight, feeling better, and my symptoms were disappearing. My T-cell counts did some amazing things. At my lowest point, it had dropped down to 371. Two weeks after the ozone treatments, I was tested again and they went up to 671. They more than doubled.

I'm excellent today. I have no symptomatology at all, no night sweats, and no more weight problem. I am very physically active and able to enjoy life. I actually feel better than at the time I got the needle stick. My health is excellent.

I couldn't have done it without the ozone. That's what made the difference. I tried vitamin C therapy for a while and that helped, but I still had the chronic diarrhea four or five times a day, and I still had the weight loss from not being able to keep food down. Then I started the ozone therapy and that brought me back to normal health.

Angelo on colorectal cancer with metastases to the liver

I was feeling tired every day and coming home to take a nap in the afternoon. That wasn't me. I had been a real active person all my life. My wife suggested that I take a blood test to see if anything was wrong. I did and my doctor found that my blood was low. He suggested that I wait another week before taking another test, which I did. My blood was still low so he suggested a colonoscopy. I went and had it done. The colonoscopy found a tumor in my colon. I had it operated on and taken out. The surgeon told me that he successfully removed it and that there was no more cancer there.

About three months later, I had a CT scan done that found spots on my liver. The cancer had metastasized to my liver. I received chemotherapy treatments for approximately six months. After the first set of treatments, another test was taken which found that the chemotherapy hadn't done any good. I continued with the chemotherapy for another three months. When that didn't help, the doctor said that there was nothing more he could do for me. I asked if I should continue with the chemo or just sit and die. He shrugged his shoulders as if to say there was nothing more he could do for me. I asked the doctor how much time he thought I had and he said three to four months.

My son, who was there with me, had heard about a holistic program at Santa Monica Hospital utilizing ozone and vitamin therapy. He said I should take the treatments there, and I did. I received treatments for 21 days. They asked me to wait for eight weeks before having a CT scan. When I finally took the CT scan, the radiologist called my doctor and told him that he had never read a CT scan like mine before. It showed that the cancer cells in my liver had become capsulized. That prevented them from spreading.

The cancer cells have remained encapsulated and I've been in remission for a year and a half. There is no question about it. The ozone treatment saved my life. In fact, I have so much faith in it now that I plan on going there every year and a half just to make sure that it stays that way.

Philip on chronic active hepatitis B

It was a long process getting diagnosed. I had flu-like symptoms, diarrhea and fever, and was not feeling well at all. They initially diagnosed it as arthritis. Finally, a rheumatologist thought to do liver work. He did a liver biopsy, and it came back chronic active hepatitis B.

They suggested interferon. . . . That only had a 40 percent efficacy. I had heard a program on vitamin C drips and began with that. I decided to go further. I started ozone treatments. Once I started that, my liver SGPT came down dramatically. I am waiting today to get results and hoping to hear that it has cleared up entirely.

Jane on breast cancer

I was diagnosed in 1989 with breast cancer, for which I had a modified radical mastectomy. I had numerous surgeries before that time as well. I wasn't really having any life at that point in time. I was a sick person waiting to die. They had cut out some of the cancer but I wasn't well. A friend of mine finally advised me not to have any more of those treatments because they were killing me.

I had the book *Third Opinion,* which had something in it about Dr. Donsbach. I called Santa Monica Hospital and went down there. I was astounded by the humaneness at Santa Monica Hospital. In other hospitals, I had some negative experiences where I felt totally robbed of all dignity and where I was treated like a specimen.

Santa Monica had a program that I could tolerate. I had decided that I was not going to have any more cutting, any more radiation, or any more chemo. There would be no more invasive procedures.

The first week I felt really, really sick because I was detoxifying from all the chemicals in my system. I had been on 10 different medications for multiple problems. Besides cancer, I had ulcers, asthma, everything you could possibly imagine. The cancer had set off a systems reaction and I was having problems in every part of my body.

After about the tenth day, I started to feel like getting out of bed. I began to participate in the therapies and started beach walks. I continued to get better and better.

I have been there six or seven times because I had some tumors in the other breast as well. I received ozone, hyperthermia, and thymus injections.

I don't have any tumors now. Most of all I have a life. I work full-time and I play an active role in the lives of my granddaughter and daughters. I am able to go to church. I participate in library programs. I walk on the beach every day. I follow my program.

I learned some things in the hospital that I need to be real careful with. Santa Monica Hospital will be the first place I go to if I begin developing symptoms. I don't think I will, though. I think I'm cured.

Charles on prostate cancer

I had a needle biopsy roughly a year ago which indicated prostate cancer. I never believed in the orthodox approach and sought another method of treatment. Finally, I decided that I would go to Mexico and get treatment which was not available in the United States. After doing a certain amount of research and checking with other people, I decided the Donsbach clinic in Rosarita Beach was the best place to go. I had been familiar with Dr. Donsbach for a number of years and felt that he offered the best options.

I feel that the treatment has been very satisfactory. At present, my prostate has substantially improved. I'm not free of cancer yet nor was there any promise that I would be that quickly. I am on continuing outpatient care. But I feel it has most definitely made a difference. The PSA, for example, has dropped very substantially, which is probably the best measure of prostate cancer. I certainly feel a great deal better than when I first went to Rosarita Beach.

Madge on arthritis

In 1993, I had been in the hospital five times. I had severe pain in my legs and excruciating pain in my back. In addition, I had fever, sweats, and tachycardia. I would go to the hospital and they would send me home not knowing what was wrong. They said that the next time I came back they would do exploratory surgery just to find out what was wrong.

In the meantime, I found out about Dr. Donsbach and went to Santa Monica Hospital for a month. When I left I had to be helped onto the plane. I came back a month later turning cartwheels. A miracle happened to me and I wanted everyone to know.

So now, I'm fine. I seldom take anything for pain. I dance three times a week and play tennis. I was ice skating and broke my shoulder, which gave me a little setback, but I'm getting better now. I believe the ozone insufflations saved my life and that Santa Monica Hospital is a fantastic place.

Debbie on Hodgkin's Disease

I got sick in December 1985. At that time, I had a lump in my neck, which the doctors removed. They diagnosed me as having Hodgkin's disease and gave me radiation treatments. They radiated me from the chin area to the breast area for six weeks and from the breast area to the pelvic area for another six weeks. After that, they told me I needed to come back every three months for a chest x-ray.

About eight months later, they found a tumor on my lung and said that I needed chemotherapy. I got chemo for a year and a half. A year and two or three months later, the tumor started to grow while taking the chemotherapy. They had to change my chemo twice.

They didn't know what to do anymore so they sent me to the Mayo Clinic in Minnesota. There, they said that the only thing I could do was get a bone marrow transplant. That was in February 1988. For three months, I was given massive doses of chemotherapy to prepare for the transplant. That's when terrible things began to happen. I had seizures for three months straight and had to remain in the hospital all that time. I couldn't walk anymore and was like a zombie. They damaged my right hand with chemotherapy and I could no longer use it.

My husband and I finally met with the doctor. When he walked into the room, he wouldn't look at us. We knew that something was definitely wrong. He finally said, I'm sorry, but due to the shape your body is in, you'll never live through this bone marrow transplant. I started to cry. I said, "You guys said this is the only thing left to save my life. What am I supposed to do? I'm only 30 years old and I thought I had a little more time left." I had two small kids at home.

My husband heard about a hospital in Mexico but I couldn't believe that they could do something in Mexico that they couldn't do here. Being brought up in the Midwest, you think that if your doctor can't help you, you can go to the Mayo Clinic. If the Mayo Clinic can't do it for you, that's it.

On our way home from the Mayo Clinic I listened to the tape that my husband had on oxygen therapy. It just sounded too simple. I thought I was doomed.

My husband continued to stay excited about all of this material that he found. He even went to the library to do more research on oxygen therapies. He kept bringing these things home for me to read and I kept telling him that he was crazy.

Finally, one day, I was sitting at home having a pity party for myself. My mother called and advised me to go. She said that I had tried every avenue possible and that she didn't believe they were going to hurt me.

I finally agreed to go to Mexico. We went there in September 1988 and stayed for three weeks. During that time, I had hydrogen peroxide, DMSO, multiple vitamins, ozone, a lot of different therapies. I was always afraid that doing this would make me sick, like the chemo and radiation, so I would finish my treatment and go back to my room. I would lay down expecting to get sick but I never did.

Instead, I got back on my feet. After my therapies, I would walk on the beach with my husband. I felt that I was on a vacation instead of in a hospital. I also was put on a machine that helped with my hand and arm that was numb from the chemo. The feeling, which had been gone for over a year, started to come back. My hair started to grow. I was up and around and not laying around in bed feeling like I was sick and dying. That was back in 1988.

When I came home, I continued to stay on a home program. I would go back to my doctor every six weeks, then every three months, then every six months. Now I go once a year. A year after I was at the hospital, I had scans and blood work. I had been on medical disability while I was getting ready for the bone marrow transplant and had been out of work for a year and a half. After the scans, my doctor said that he couldn't keep me on disability any longer. He couldn't see any tumor growth. He said I was doing fine and that I could go back to work.

It's been six and a half years now and I'm doing great. I feel wonderful and my blood chemistries are completely normal. If not for the treatments, I might have had a year left. I believe that I was dying from the treatment, not the cancer. The seizures were secondary to the massive doses of chemotherapy.

Harold (medical doctor) on circulatory problems and ulcers

I had very bad circulation in my legs, especially varicosities. My legs were very swollen, especially on the left side. I also noticed that they were increasingly discolored and becoming bluish. At times, I had cramping in my calves and legs and I would feel coldness there. It was very, very painful. I also had an ulcer. Nothing was helping and everyone was saying I couldn't do anything about it. One time, my leg was all blown up. I went to a surgeon because I wanted him to drain it but he would not touch it.

I started to take large amounts of vitamins A, C, and E, but that didn't help me. I thought there must be some other answer. I heard about ozone and I started to go to a physician for it. First, my ulcer healed. Then, the pain in my legs gradually began to go away. I started to feel warmth in my feet and the discoloration started to leave.

Now, I am able to walk better. I used to limp and I don't limp anymore. I don't have the pains like someone is crushing my ankle with a noose. I have very good circulation there and I feel like I almost can run. I was even playing a little bit of basketball with my son the other day. I am beginning to get the feeling and strength back in my legs. My energy has also increased tremendously and my clarity of thinking is much better than before.

I have also seen other patients who were very ill. Some of them had hepatitis. The physician, knowing that I am physician, showed me their lab values and I was astonished to see how much they changed. I could also see improvement in their appearance. When they first came in, they looked half dead. After a few weeks, they left with improved color and energy. There were also tremendous decreases in the enzymes of these patients.

I myself am doing very, very well with this. I want to continue this and I am looking into doing it myself, as I feel that people should have this treatment readily available. I am always, of course, afraid of someone coming down on me, like the FDA, but I feel that if I can do it for myself, why shouldn't I be allowed to do it for others?

Preston on hepatitis

In February of this year, I was very sick. I was about 60 percent bedridden and barely able to function. The liver specialist I was seeing essentially told me that he was at the end of his rope. He said there was no hope for me and that he could perhaps help to keep me alive until some miracle cure appeared. That was February 28.

On March 9, I began ozone therapy twice a week. Within six weeks, my enzyme levels had dropped dramatically. Other blood scores also improved. More important, my quality of life improved immeasurably. I was able to actually get on an airplane and take a three-day business trip to California in the early part of May.

When I went to see my liver specialist again, he did not accept the improvement. He looked at the blood scores and said that it didn't show anything. The analogy he used was "the bees are in the hives," meaning that the virus was still there but not visible. I got the impression that he would be happiest if I died. If I want my insurance company to pay for my blood test, I have to have them ordered by one of their approved physicians. I continue to have only as much contact with that doctor as I need to for insurance purposes.

Gay on colon cancer

I was diagnosed with colon cancer in 1989. After they gave me 18 months to live, I opted to find other alternatives and did so. I never received standard treatments even though they wanted to do surgery and chemotherapy.

Right now, I'm sitting on an IV of hydrogen peroxide with DMSO and all kinds of supplements and vitamins. That, along with a good diet and the help of a good friend, has gotten me this far. According to their predictions, I should have been dead in 1991 by the latest. In 1991, I made my second visit to the Hospital Santa Monica in Rosarita Beach.

Now I am in remission. When I am checked by the M.D.'s they are amazed. I have no more cancer in my colon. I have literally passed tumors through the rectum. The latest test showed that I have no tumors.

Ricardo on chronic active hepatitis

In 1990, I was diagnosed with hepatitis C and cirrhosis of the liver. I went to a specialist at one of the biggest hospitals in the city. He put me on alpha interferon for six months and told me that if that didn't help, nothing would.

After that, I started researching milk thistle and other remedies for the cirrhosis but I didn't really know what to do for the hepatitis. I drank a lot of fluids to try to flush it but I was basically ignorant.

In March of this year, I had an attack and was hospitalized for five weeks. They told me that I needed a liver transplant and that the cirrhosis was running rampant throughout my body.

I heard about ozone therapy and was wondering how to get it. A neighbor called and I found out that it has been available in this country.

I've been taking it since May and what it has done for me is unbelievable. When I came home from the hospital, I was lethargic and did nothing but sleep. I started treatment on May 4 and took blood tests that same day. My bilirubin count was 12.4. That Tuesday, on May 9, I went to my gastroenterologist and took another blood test. In those five days, my bilirubin fell from 12.4 to 9.42. I'll take another blood test in June again.

I feel like I'm coming back and I believe the ozone has made a difference. I've been able to stop taking all the medications I was on which were causing my liver to become inflamed. I was on five different medications and they weren't doing anything for me.

Now, I'm out and about. I'm even wrestling. I don't even take a nap during the day. My appetite has returned, which is conducive to getting better. I really believe in this thing and I'm going to stick with it because I don't want to go under that knife.

John on foot infection

I started getting direct injections of ozone in February. Just two injections of 5 cc of ozone eliminated the infection I had been fighting for months.

Before that, I had orthodox physicians who wanted me to go on massive doses of antibiotics, who were worried about my foot having to come off because I am diabetic. I took antibiotics for a little while and they were doing nothing. I did some hydrogen peroxide, which was helping to get it under control.

But ozone is what really did it. It totally eliminated the problem. The infection is no longer in my foot. I don't feel pain from it anymore. I can now start working on rehabilitating my leg.

Qi Gong

Qi gong translates from the Chinese as energy cultivating. It is a system of refining, purifying, circulating, and storing energy. Over time, the practice yields many benefits. Health challenges are overcome as positive energy is mentally and physically directed to all systems via meditation, posture, breathing, and relaxation. As blockages are released and abundant energy flows freely, body systems rebalance, stamina improves, and the manifestation of illness disappears.

Qi gong is an integral part of Eastern cultures where several styles are practiced; many forms have been developed by different lineages and handed down from teacher to student since before recorded history. In China, the value of qi gong is acknowledged by the medical establishment. But the practice is largely unknown to westerners, as information about it has been largely unavailable and highly esoteric. Recently, with the availability of more and more understandable information in books and classes, many Americans are turning to qi gong, and finding that it improves the overall quality of their lives.

Patient Stories

Octavio on nervous disorder

This year, I was very, very bad, and in the hospital because I had nervousness, depression, and paralysis on part of my face, which the doctors called Bell's palsy. My condition was very severe.

After that, I started to do qi gong, and began to feel better and better. In five days the Bell's palsy disappeared. Now I practice almost every day. It's really fantastic. I recommend qi gong to everybody, especially for stress.

Bob on eye disease

A year and a half ago, I developed a rare eye disease called ischemic optic neuropathy. This is a swelling of the optic nerves that progressed quite rapidly.

Each day for two weeks, I would wake up and see less than I had the day before, with the potential of blindness. I had nearly exhausted all the medical assistance that I could get. I had seen some neural ophthalmologists, and I had been to Will's Eye Hospital twice in Philadelphia. I was given little hope. They knew very little about the disease, but they knew the outcome.

I spoke to a friend in Hawaii and he suggested I see a qi gong master. . . . I needed someone to go with me that day because I couldn't see well enough to bring myself down there and back.

What he did was quite remarkable. The first thing he did was diagnose me by looking at me. Through an interpreter, he described that I had a swollen optic nerve and said that he would work on it. What he did with a series of movements around me is he extracted the bad energy (qi) from that area and implanted good qi. He literally reached out with his hand as if he was grasping something very close to my eye and he would pull it away. He would do this any number of times. Then he would hold his hand up to the sky and reach down. It looked like he was pushing energy into my eye. He also gave me some herbs.

I had had a previous doctor's appointment the very next morning with one of the neuro-optomologists I was seeing. She said, ''Bob, you have turned the corner on this. The nerve has stopped swelling. It will not get worse even though there is not much chance of it getting better.'' I continued seeing Master Lee for several months, sometimes two or three times a week. I also contacted a client of mine who taught me qi gong. It's a movement like yoga only there is no stretch involved. I went to see him and I did it on my own. And I learned how to harness that energy and bring it into my eyes and body.

I love happy endings and this is one. Today I am able to drive, read, and work on my computer with no difficulty at all. I do wear glasses, but you would never suspect for a moment that I had had this problem. It took just three to six months to see significant improvement and as I continue to bring qi into my eyes, they continue to heal.

Miriam on joint problems, fatigue, and partial hearing loss

I've had a lot of problems with my joints—chronic aches and pains in my wrist, knees, and elbows. I have been doing the movement form of qi gong since September and find that it increases my circulation, which helps the joint pain clear up faster. It generates a lot more energy because I've also had a lot of problems with constant fatigue. It basically irons out all the kinks in my body so that the energy flows a lot easier. It also gives me a sense of emotional well-being from stress. I tend to be able to deal with my emotional problems in a much more balanced, easy way.

I have been dabbling with energetic healing work and I have taken a couple of introductory courses on that. I never really felt anything, even though you are supposed to feel energy emanating from your hands. I imagined that I felt it but never really felt it in a strong way. Over a period of time from doing qi gong, I have developed a strong sense of energy emanating from my hands, which was really interesting.

One more thing that came as a result was the correction of a blockage in my right ear. I had a partial hearing loss and there was a lot of sloshing around of liquids and stuff. From doing the work and using the energy that I was able to generate from my hands and placing that over my right ear, I was able to start to heal myself in my right ear. Now the blockage has pretty much cleared and the hearing has returned.

In addition to qi gong there are other things I do as well. I see a chiropractor and I take super blue-green algae and I do Feldenkrais movement techniques. All this has contributed to a more energetic and healthy me.

Dan on stomach cramps and anger

I started learning qi gong about two years ago. I learned to feel the energy movement in my body and to accept that everything is energy-based.

This weekend I had some stomach cramps. I went through an affirmation and breathing and was able to shift energy in myself. I found it very effective. The first thing I do is to realize that it's energy-based. I raise my awareness and accept whatever is going on instead of judging it. I tell myself, "Whatever emotion this is I accept it." Then I state my intent, which is to heal and shift this energy. Sometimes I tap into an anger there and am able to move it. Along with mental focus is breathing, which is the physical aspect.

Whenever I get angry, qi gong helps me to shift away from that state. I have learned not to get involved with it because I see that it is energy in motion. First I had to feel it and actually experience it in my body to get it mentally. Practicing the qi gong, I kept saying, "This is energy. This is energy." Then when I felt the shift in my body, my forehead got hot or all of a sudden I had tingling in my hands, and I wasn't really doing anything to facilitate that. But all of a sudden I was sweating and really not moving. When I really started experiencing qi gong physically, that's when it started clicking in.

Another example is where a store clerk gave me the wrong change the other day. It was just a few cents difference. Normally I am a calm person but all of a sudden I became upset and ended up walking out. Standing outside the store, I did my breathing. The first thing I did was to say, "Okay, I'm emotionally upset right now. And for me to confront or throw anger at the person wouldn't be useful to me or to them." I realized I was upset so my awareness went up. Then I moved to acceptance by saying, "I'm allowed to be really angry. Anger is not bad. It's just an emotion." I did my breathing and I continued mentally saying, "It's okay. I'm allowed to do this." And then I released this energy. I stood and I may have put my hands on my stomach or on my heart chakra, just to say, "It's okay, it's safe," and to bring in the energy and state the intent to release this anger coming up without judgment. Or if I am in judgment, saying, "It's bad to be angry," I accept my anger and accept whatever is coming up as I state my intent to release it. I say that I don't choose to hold onto it anymore, without a lot of stuff behind it, like making myself wrong. That, along with the nice, slow breathing made me feel just fine. I looked around and I said, "It's a nice, sunny day." As soon as I noticed that, I knew that I had shifted the energy.

There is no one right method. A lot of what you do is intuitive. Sometimes I will go to a qi gong class and start the exercises and then be physically exhausted. I will sit in the back and do a meditation and work with the energy as it is coming up with me. Sometimes I will need to do the movements. It's different every time. There is no pat answer. It's learning to tune into me. It's learning also the acceptance and stating my intent. That's what qi gong is.

Diane on thyroid cancer

I had radical neck surgery for a thyroid cancer six years ago. Of course, that entailed the loss of half of my left, upper shoulder muscle and the musculature on that side of my neck.

Now I have no cancer left in my body. I have maintained myself very well. But one of the residual things I was left with was some nerve loss, which made me feel very off balance. Of course, I had a shoulder slump on the left side of my body because of the loss of muscle. I was very upset about it and went to physical therapy. I knew there was a good deal that was not going to return to me.

I had taken hatha yoga many years ago and I thought that I would go back to that, but discovered that because of the loss of musculature that I couldn't do any of the inverted poses. Just by chance, I walked into a qi gong class. I started to go and realized after about a month and a half that my balance was returning. The discomfort that I was feeling on my left shoulder was subsiding. Any time I have a problem with it, if I just go through some very basic qi gong exercises, I have relief for a good period of time.

What I think happens to me is I tense up and get myself blocked. This side is much more vulnerable because of the real physical blocks from the surgery. What the qi gong has allowed me to do is find new nerve endings, a new way to connect with the loss and to compensate. It's a very accepting process.

Barbara on insomnia

I had sleeping problems for years. I had a pretty significant sleep disorder and I was diagnosed as having a chronic sleep disorder, etiology unknown. I went to neurologists, psychologists, psychiatrists, internal medicine doctors, even a specialist in the field of psychopharmacology (it cost $500 an hour). But I was desperate. At one point I was awake for six weeks. I tried many different Western medications, but they only exacerbated the problem. I never got any relief. I went to sleep disorder clinics and was wired up with all kinds of machines. But no one was ever able to help me.

I tried several acupuncture doctors and finally hit upon one in Rhode Island who also used diet and Chinese medicine and herbs along with acupuncture. He was the one who told me about qi gong. I went to a conference at his insistence. He said that this would be the thing that would really cure me. So I went to the qi gong conference in Boston and met a qi gong master. I practiced the qi gong there.

It really helped when I went to the prescription seminar that he held during his conference. He was able to give me a prescription for Chinese herbs which I had filled in Chinatown. It's probably about 27 Chinese herbs and it comes in big, brown paper bag. A certain amount of each herb is measured out for my particular prescription. I take it home and boil it in water for a period of 15 to 20 minutes, each time straining the water off. I have been drinking the tea since about November and I have not had a problem sleeping since that time. I have since decreased my tea intake and now only take it as necessary. I, for one, am a firm believer in qi gong and Chinese herbs.

Vicki on becoming centered

I learned qi gong about a year ago on the recommendation of a friend. I had practiced tai chi about 15 years ago for quite some time, but found the form quite complex, and didn't stick with it to learn it well. I became drawn to qi gong because you could learn the form in a much shorter period of time.

Mostly I take classes where I work with other students. I will practice parts of the form at home as well. I find that it helps me to become more centered, more clear about wherever I am at that time, more clear in myself, whether that means realizing that I am tired and need to rest or that I need to make a decision. The practice facilitates a sense of wholeness, which is very important.

Allison on centering

Last year, I learned the eight routines of soaring crane qi gong in a class. I find it to be a very useful technique for centering myself. I think it also gives improvement flexibility and tone. The centering is very important because it helps you pull energy in and blend your own energy with what's out there in the world. There's not a line delineating you from the outside world, which I find very helpful. It helps me move through life a little easier.

I use qi going as a way of starting my day and as way of getting my body warmed up. It also helps me to deal with whatever projects I have on hand. I am an actress, so I often use qi gong prior to a performance. I find that even using one or two of the routines in the soaring crane method helps me to generate my own internal energy and to have greater focus. Because it's a standing meditation, I don't space out. I actually keep a very sharp focus and the energy just sort of flows. Because of that, I feel energized and very clear. My mind is no longer a jumble. I benefit a lot from it.

Bob on relaxation from stress

I have been helped by qi gong in a lot of ways. It really helps me to relax after a stressful day of work. It gives me greater stamina for physical activities. The list goes on an on. More specifically, after doing qi going, I find that I am in a certain relaxed state and that I have a very clear thought process. It allows me to approach my work with new energy and insights. So it's very helpful in that way.

The benefits are difficult to put into words because the effects are personal. It is something that allows me to really relax.

Reconstructive Therapy

This little-known therapy has great potential for healing painful joint conditions, even after other modalities have failed. Reconstructive therapy actually builds new joints, ligaments, and tendons. By doing so, it gets to the root of the problem and provides freedom from pain.

Our bones and muscles can place undue stress on our ligaments, tendons, and cartilage. Joints in the knees, ankles, neck, wrists, and elbows and the entire spine, can become damaged as a result. Sometimes people are born with joint weaknesses; their joints are loose and unstable, causing them to be hypermobile or double-jointed. Reconstructive therapy helps either scenario by creating tighter joints. Ligaments become larger, stronger, and attach more firmly to bone.

During the course of treatment, low doses of nutritional substances are injected into the ligaments. The exact nutrients given differ, depending upon the needs of the area involved. These agents stimulate a slight irritation that promotes healing. New blood vessels grow into the area. More blood means greater oxygen and nutrients. Tissues heal as fibroblast growth factor puts more fibroblasts and collagen into the ligament, tendon and cartilage. As a result, ligaments become stronger, and better able to hold vertebrae and joints in place. This, in turn, eliminates pain.

Reconstruction therapy differs markedly from the conventional approach, which addresses symptoms only. Usually, doctors begin by giving anti-inflammatory medications, which only help temporarily. These drugs cause inflammation of the GI tract, and inhibit collagen formation, which prevents true healing. The next step is often exercise or physiotherapy. If that does not work, cortisone shots are given. Next in line is an arthroscopy or mini-surgery. Then more cortisone and more anti-inflammatory treatments may be given. Finally, joints are replaced. The person gets a new knee or hip. Or a laminectomy may be performed to remove a disc from the neck or low-back area. This type of operation adversely affects structure, and makes the person weaker and more prone to pain.

With reconstructive therapy, by contrast, ligaments actually strengthen and results are permanent. This therapy is used to treat any number of musculoskeletal conditions, including low back pain, arthritis, bursitis, carpal tunnel syndrome, disc problems, sciatica, tendinitis, frozen shoulder, and athletic injuries. Reconstructive joint therapy is also useful for people with torn ligaments and cartilage problems. Candidates for treatment are people on anti-inflammatory drugs, such as aspirin, cortisone, Motrin, and Naprosyn. Also people who have joint sounds—grinding, pops or clicks—when they move their neck or knee may benefit. This technique is also for people who continue go to chiropractors because they can't stay in alignment, as well as for people who feel worse with exercise, and people who have undergone surgery. People who are not candidates for reconstructive therapy are those who have a marked impairment in their immune system. This includes those with cancer and AIDS.

A big advantage to the treatment, as opposed to surgery, is that there is no down time after treatment. A person can return to work immediately. Also, there is an amazingly high success rate: 88 percent of patients respond, and the results are permanent.

Patient Stories

Al on knee injury

Approximately eight months ago, I suffered a fall which resulted in a completely severed, interior cruciate ligament, several other partially torn ligaments, and injury to the medial meniscus. Within three to four weeks of that injury, I came to Dr. Calapai for reconstructive therapy injections into the area. This resulted in almost immediate relief of terrible, severe pain.

Now my knee is almost normal. As a matter of fact, a result of having a completely severed interior cruciate ligament is that one can no longer straighten out the knee unless one has surgery to sew the interior cruciate back together. Miraculously, after a number of reconstructive therapy injections, I can almost completely straighten out my knee without any surgery whatsoever.

George on back injury

I have been in construction all my life, and somewhere along the line, I injured my back, although I didn't realize it until I started getting aches up the back of my left leg. I heard about reconstructive therapy, so I started getting treatments for my back. Then I treated my hip, knee, and shoulder. All these areas improved and feel great at present.

Ann on sprained ankle

Over a period of years, I sprained and resprained my ankles. I tried lots of therapies, including massage and orthotics, but nothing helped.

Then I came to Dr. Calapai, who diagnosed me as having hypermobility of the joints. He treated my ankles with reconstructive therapy. Now I am able to participate in most activities without pain or stress. The podiatrist said he never saw anybody heal so fast. He called me his phenomenon.

Terri on arthritis

For years, I have been suffering with arthritis, and have been in severe pain most of the time. It really put a damper on my life.

Then I discovered reconstructive therapy. I'm starting to walk normally again, and there is a tremendous relief from pain. I'm looking forward to a complete cure. I'm 60 percent there already.

Reflexology

Reflexology is an ancient technique based on the premise that there are reflex points on the feet and hands that correspond to every muscle, nerve, organ, gland, and bone in the body. Pressing on these points breaks up congestion and helps the nerves to relax. This, in turn, reduces vascular constriction so that the blood and nerves flow more freely. As circulation improves, toxins are released.

There are roughly 7200 nerves in each foot. When the body becomes imbalanced, through the course of daily living, nerve impulses can become blocked. This means that nerve impulses to the muscles, organs and glands of the body are impeded to some extent. Reflexology stimulates nerve endings and starts up nerve communication. Reflexology also promotes endorphin release, enhancing one's sense of well-being.

The treatment can be performed by a therapist or it can be self-administered. There are several books on the subject, as well as workshops and courses that offer certification. After learning the basics, a person begins treatments with gentle finger pressure. Tenderness means there is a problem in the area corresponding to the reflex point. After resting for a day or two, the area can be reworked again. In time, there will be less tenderness as the problem heals.

Practitioners of this modality assert that performing reflexology once a week can catch most problems early and quicken recovery. This is because reflexology gets the circulation flowing so that the processes of nutrient absorption and waste elimination are improved. This is not to say that reflexology is a panacea. If symptoms are serious or prolonged, a doctor should be consulted.

Patient Story

Rochelle on ulcerative colitis

A while ago, I was in a bookstore, and I saw Laura Norman's book, *Feet First*. I read it through and it sounded very interesting. I decided that this might be something I should try, so I started seeing Laura.

After some months I started to notice some positive changes. My colitis symptoms abated—the diarrhea and bleeding have completely stopped—and I believe that reflexology has been a very, very important factor in accomplishing that. Laura also helped me to change my diet. All this has opened up my life magnificently. This has been the most positive step I have ever taken for myself.

I continue to get reflexology weekly. It helps to keep me healthy. It helps to reduce my stress levels, which I think is a factor in ulcerative colitis.

Reiki

Reiki is the Japanese word for universal life force. It is an ancient hands-on healing modality originally developed by the Tibetans and rediscovered by the Japanese in the 19th century. During treatments, energy is channeled and amplified from the universal life force through the Reiki practitioner to the client for the revitalization of body, mind, and spirit. Reiki can also be self-administered. By releasing physical and emotional blockages, and increasing energy, Reiki promotes total relaxation, which, in turn, enhances the body's ability to recover from stress and injuries.

Reiki is easy to learn and relaxing to both practitioner and recipient. It is usually taught in a one-day workshop where a Reiki master performs a series of attunements on students. Once the four upper energy centers, known as chakras, are opened, the student can channel energy.

Reiki can facilitate healing in a variety of circumstances. It works, practitioners explain, on the principle that the body recognizes this universal life energy and uses it to promote balance and total health.

Patient Stories

Nilsa Vergara on her clients's experiences

My first example is a 59-year-old woman, who came to our healing circle feeling old and tired. She suffered from aches and severe pain in her neck and knee from car accidents. She was also going through job changes, and her relationship with her adult son was estranged.

Each week, she received a 15-minute session and quickly began feeling better. She released a lot of emotional toxins via crying and verbal expression of what she was feeling. She decided to take a Reiki class so that she could give herself daily treatments.

Within a month, her changes were quite dramatic. She had a tremendous increase in energy and vigor. She told me she now feels like she is 28 years old. With the Reiki, she now has very little pain. She feels emotional and vital. Her attitude has changed. She feels self-fulfilled and in control of her life. Her relationship with her son has greatly improved. To quote her, she says, "I feel like my whole life is as it should be."

As far as other modalities, she takes vitamin supplementation, food-grade hydrogen peroxide in her water to help oxygenate the body, and is about to receive acupuncture for her neck.

My next client is a 65-year-old woman. When she first came to see us, she was depressed. She had been in therapy for years but nothing seemed to lift the depression. She felt tired all the time and would catch colds easily. Emotionally, she felt like a victim, and others treated her as one.

After her first 15-minute session she felt immediately better. She knew that something powerful was happening. She returned and eventually studied Reiki. Today, she reports feeling much healthier. She has more energy and an optimistic outlook. She no longer feels like a victim and if anyone tries to put her in that role, she is no longer afraid to set limits. In addition, she is much better able to tolerate the cold weather, which indicates that her body has improved its oxygen intake.

My next client is a 60-year-old woman, who was feeling emotionally devastated when she first came to our healing circle. She had had cancer on her vocal chords, for which she received radiation therapy. Even though she was told that she was cured, she was still feeling pretty awful. She had lost her job and was feeling hopeless.

She had Reiki for five months and took a class. Now she feels totally different. Her hope has been renewed and she feels empowered. She is picking up a better sense of who she is internally. Her identity is not tied up with her job. She also has gotten better at eliminating physical toxins as well as people who tend to use her. On the physical side she had had a back problem with one of her discs, which she says is improving with Reiki. She says that Reiki has been a wonderful discovery for her.

This woman has an 83-year-old mom who fell and broke her hip bone as well as the bone in her wrist and arm. She decided to give her mother Reiki regularly and her mother responded quite well. She began feeling stronger and stronger. Within four weeks, she was out of her cast, walking with just the aid of a cane, and not a walker. This is pretty remarkable for an 83-year-old, because having a broken hip does not always hold a good prognosis. So, as you can see, Reiki really enhances the body's ability to recuperate.

A 45-year-old woman was diagnosed with lymphatic cancer in December 1994. She was feeling disconnected from herself, and working at a job that she hated. She had been given chemotherapy, which made her lungs less elastic. Then, she was given steroids to increase the flexibility in her lungs.

She heard about the healing circle, and she came to us in August 1995. She received 15-minute sessions about three times a month. Reiki was the first alternative healing method she ever tried.

She feels that Reiki helped her to reconnect with her inner self. It also helped her to slow down and not be such a hassled A-type personality. She is starting to pay much more attention to herself. Becoming conscious and aware of the self is one of the most important parts of healing. She is also more aware of her breath. She is beginning to investigate additional modalities, such as diet, exercise, and food supplements.

My next client is a 53-year-old woman who had some serious memory problems. Her thinking was scattered, she was fearful and guilt-ridden, and she was estranged from her adult children.

I recommended Reiki to her to see if we could work through some of these emotional blockages and change these negative patterns. She took a Reiki class. Six months later, her memory improved tremendously. She was much more focused in her thinking and her job performance improved greatly. She became more insightful, much less fearful. Now she can speak with her adult children, set limits, and no longer feel anxious and guilt-ridden. In addition to using Reiki, she uses herbal teas for detoxification, drinks vegetable juices, fasts, and gets colonics.

An 83-year-old friend of hers was terminally ill. He was suffering from severe respiratory problems and had been hospitalized. He was in intensive care for two weeks. After leaving the IC unit, she gave him Reiki every day for a week. A nurse who was observing her commented that the patient who had been agitated, miserable, and in a great deal of pain became quiet, peaceful, and pain-free. The nurse told her, ''Please, whatever you are doing, keep on doing it.'' He passed on very peacefully.

Reiki is very effective in helping those who are close to death by releasing pain and fears. My client felt a great sense of empowerment that she could do something for him to ease his passage and to connect with him in a very caring way.

Rolfing

Rolfing is a bodywork technique that aims to realign the body through deep work on soft tissue and fascia surrounding muscles. The premise behind Rolfing is that people lose symmetry between the right/left and back/front planes of their bodies, and that these discrepancies get worse with time, and result in dysfunctions. Rolfing works to reduce these discrepancies. Also, people tend to lose touch with their natural centers of gravity, which Rolfing works to correct so that standing and moving become more comfortable and efficient.

Once structural changes are made, the system works to improve itself. Treatments follow a pattern and a whole series is usually 10 sessions long. Every part of the body is addressed, not just the area that hurts, so that lasting changes can be made. Sessions vary according to individual needs. And effects are cumulative. With each session, resultant changes last longer and longer. An aspect of this practice is that Rolfers often help clients improve their work habits, e.g., the way they sit at a desk or work on a computer, in order to ensure long-lasting health.

Patient Stories

Elizabeth on body trauma

When I was two years old, I had bad pneumonia and I was in the hospital for about three months. I just about died. As a result of that, my body had a lot of trauma. I was very weak when I was growing up. I had a collapsed chest and rounded shoulders.

Initially, I started to go for Rolfing at age 20. Then I met Beth a bit later. Although I had 10 different Rolfers work on me, when I started working with Beth, it was the first time that I really started to experience a lot of changes. At the same time, I was working with some equestrian instructors, trying to make some progress riding. It was a marvelous thing to be able to work with Beth while I was also working at this new physical skill, learning to jump horses.

We worked a great deal with my hips and the rotation in my femurs, the rotation in my legs, also with the chest and shoulders, and a great deal with my back. Her work is hands directly on the body, going deep into the tissue, doing basically the Rolfing movements.

I found it to be extremely helpful. I found that I was able to move out of movement patterns and go into using my arms and legs in ways I could never do before. My coordination increased a great deal as well.

Jeanne on lack of flexibility

I had gone for several years without an enormous amount of exercise. I had some pain in my lower back. And basically, the problem was that I was very stiff. I had some tendinitis and some problems with my knees. I started to work with a personal trainer, but my flexibility was really awful.

I had known about Rolfing for a long time. I remembered reading about it long ago. I saw Beth's name in a magazine that listed practitioners so I called her.

I have had eight sessions with her now. The first session, she worked all over my body. Then she did my lower legs, my knees, my hamstrings, my shoulders, my back, even my head actually. Some of the changes have been really dramatic. There have been dramatic increases in the flexibility in my legs. When my trainer and I stretched out after a session of work on my hamstrings, I got a 3-or 4-inch increase in the stretch in my legs. The week after that, she did my lower leg, and the alignment of my knee changed dramatically. I normally was knock-kneed. When I bent my leg, my knee went out over the arch of my foot. It now tracked straight over my toe, which is where it is supposed to be. That hasn't changed back since I have been going to her. I had very tight trapezius muscles around my neck. Since Beth has been working with them, they have notably started to relax down. I don't have the bulging around my neck that I used to have. The changes have been dramatic and beyond what I expected to have happened.

Shiatsu

Shiatsu is a Japanese system of bodywork that translates to mean finger pressure. During treatment, various degrees of pressure are used to balance energy along energy pathways (meridians) of the body. Different styles of shiatsu use varying degrees of pressure.

Shiatsu is both a diagnostic tool and a method of treatment. Practitioners diagnose from the abdomen, where centers representing each of the meridians are present. During a typical session, a client will come in and give the therapist an idea of how he or she is feeling physically and emotionally. The person then lies down on a floor mat or a massage table, with clothing on. The session begins with palpations to the abdomen to feel energy imbalances. Then the therapist works different meridians throughout the entire body that correspond with imbalances in the abdomen. Shiatsu practitioners look for tsubos along the meridians; this refers to points that either have too little or too much energy. By applying a certain type of pressure, shiatsu either brings energy to those points or disperses energy, thereby bringing the body into greater harmony. In sum, the therapist's role is to observe the way energy moves in the body and to guide energy to make the shift toward greater balance. At the end of a session, the therapist will once again palpate the abdomen to see if any changes have been made.

Shiatsu realizes that each person as a unique entity; therefore, different people with the same symptoms may respond differently to a session. Some people will experience great benefit right away while others will need several sessions in order to feel better.

Shiatsu is similar to acupuncture in that it works with meridian systems; however, the main difference is the use of hands and finger pressure in the first therapy, and the use of needles in the latter. Shiatsu is also less concerned with specific points and more involved with the whole meridian. Shiatsu is even more dissimilar to Western allopathic medicine, since shiatsu is a holistic, noninvasive therapy. Also, shiatsu also realizes that getting ill is a process and that getting well must take time, whereas western medicine often takes a quick-fix, silver-bullet approach.

Patient Stories

George on hypertension and emphysema

My wife was at a bookstore in Greenwich where she saw Ken giving someone a partial treatment. She was impressed by his talk and by what he did, and thought it might be good for me. So three years ago I went to see him. Shiatsu helped me in so many ways that I just continued.

In general, I feel much, much better. Ken has a technique of working on the lungs to increase their capacity. I also become more relaxed, which helps the blood pressure go down for a while.

I find Ken a truly sincere guy who cares about how you feel, unlike a doctor who can't get you out of his office fast enough. I look forward to my weekly shiatsu sessions. It makes me feel good in many, many ways. My wife tells me I look better, which makes me feel better too. My blood pressure went down, but not enough to get off medication, although my dosage is lower than it was. My breathing capacity is much improved, too. I'd recommend it for everyone.

Lilly on stress

My desire for shiatsu was not due to any medical condition; I just carry a lot of stress in my body. I work in the television business, which is stressful and has long hours. I went for shiatsu hoping to alleviate some of the stress so that I wouldn't feel so tense. I began to go once every 12 days.

The first time I went, I honestly didn't notice anything. I also happened to have a cold and was really out of it. The third time and the remaining times, I began to feel much more relaxed throughout my whole body. It's not just relaxation, like regular massage; this really works on the meridian points in the system. After this, I felt less fractured. I felt like my head and my body were connected and I was calm and relaxed. But it wasn't as though I was sleepy. It was as if all the energy was flowing better throughout my whole system.

Now, I don't carry tension in my body in the same way. If I was under a lot of tension, I would hold it from my neck down. With the bodywork, I don't carry it there. It really releases the stress in my back. My body is a lot more aligned.

Tai Chi Chuan

Tai chi chuan, usually called tai chi, is a Chinese martial art and meditation that combines a choreographed series of slow movements with mental concentration and coordinated breathing. Practitioners learn how to align their bodies with gravity, which creates a profound sense of relaxation that benefits the individual on all levels: physically, emotionally, mentally, and spiritually.

On a physical level, tai chi improves health as gentle movements massage internal organs and enhance their functioning. This deepens breathing and gets more blood and energy flowing throughout the whole body. One way in which tai chi helps circulation is through shifts in weight. With each posture, the weight of the body alternates between the right and left side, causing the leg muscles to contract and expand. That helps pump blood back up into the heart, making tai chi a wonderful practice for people with heart disease. Tai chi also increases joint flexibility, making it an excellent practice for arthritics. Also, by aligning the body with gravity, tai chi helps the spine straighten, which alleviates tension, especially in the lower back. This is why many chiropractors and other doctors who deal with pain recommend tai chi to their patients. Many other conditions can be ameliorated in that tai chi releases stress, and most diseases have a stress component.

Tai chi can provide greater emotional stability and a better sense of self. When you practice this art, everything slows down and you see your life in a different perspective. Tai chi allows people to see the big picture, to step away from anxieties and irritations, immersing themselves instead in something quiet and slow. Breathing deeply fosters relaxation as well.

People who practice tai chi report that as the mind becomes balanced with the emotional and physical centers in the body, it stops dominating their awareness with plans, calculations, details, decisions, and worries. As greater awareness moves into the body, the mind empties and calms down enough so that clearer thinking prevails.

On a spiritual level, tai chi can be a beautiful meditation in movement that takes you on a journey of self-discovery. It helps people to improve awareness and let go of blocks. As one works in silence, the spirit has the opportunity to open up and grow.

Finally, tai chi can be used as a nonaggressive form of self-defense. When one can relax in the face of danger, one becomes more alert and better able to deal with whatever is happening in the moment. Tai chi teaches practitioners how to overcome muscular strength with softness. So, without resisting or running away you learn to yield to incoming forces by listening and interpreting energy rather than opposing or fighting it. This is called cultivating strength through softness.

Patient Stories

Carol on Crohn's Disease

My condition hasn't gone away, but tai chi is one of the things that helps me to manage it and reduce stress without any toxic side effects. I can't say whether or not there is a physical difference in my intestines before and after beginning tai chi. I can only tell you that my experience of it is that the complete concentration that it takes to do the form helps to get rid of all the junk in my head. It gives me a vacation from concern. Tai chi is one of the things I do in my life where I'm not aware of myself every second as a person with an illness. That's a tremendous gift.

Christiana on aggression

I was introduced to tai chi by a Chinese friend of mine about a year ago. We were talking about the meaning of suffering, violence, and aggression and I told her that I didn't want to react to aggression with aggression because I believe that gets you stuck in a vicious circle. Physical violence doesn't happen every day, but verbal violence is something that concerns me a lot. I was looking for a way to get out of that.

My friend does tai chi and he introduced me to a form. I realized there was something more there than just intellectual knowledge. There was something that went through his whole being. That fascinated me because it showed me a side of him I had never seen before. It was so serene and serious and deeply human that I yearned to have this experience myself also.

Since starting tai chi, I accept life more and I live more through my body than my intellect. It has also influenced my body posture. I realized that I used to often carry my shoulders up and now I am able to relax them. Just because of that, my presence has changed, and people react differently towards me. I have become more aware of my surrounding. I watch animals and children more, and they are more dear to me now, because I realize that they are doing tai chi all day long. They have this basic life force in them, and I am trying to learn from them. Tai chi has brought more spirituality into the most ordinary things, for instance house cleaning, and being with strangers on the subway.

Eric on creativity

I am a creative artist who was in a certain space when I was being creative, and I wanted to have that feeling of creativity more throughout my life. What I found with tai chi was that it allowed me to have creativity in my everyday actions. So, I went from a place I was creative for short periods of time in my artwork to a place where everything I did became connected. Tai chi is a moving meditation. When you meditate, you see yourself more clearly; there's more energy available. Doing tai chi in a group helps you become more aware of energy. You can feel everyone moving together, even if you are not seeing them. You become very aware of everyone being connected. That feeling stays with you after class, when you go outside.

Vitamin Drips

A vitamin infusion usually combines measured amounts of vitamin C, with other nutrients such as B-complex vitamins and botanicals, to improve the immune system and overall functioning. Much higher dosages of vitamins are absorbed intravenously than orally. Optimal vitamin dosages help reverse many serious conditions, including AIDS, cancer, and chronic fatigue syndrome. Well people benefit from the therapy in that it keeps the body functioning at its best.

Patient Stories

Mildred on fractured nose

My problem started on New Year's Day 1994 when I skidded on some ice coming home from work. As I was stopping for a light, I hit a tree head-on. I had multiple bruises but my main injury was a nasal septic fracture, telescope septum, a deep vertical laceration, and a piece of the nose was just gone. The fracture was so comminuted that the doctor had to press the splinted pieces of bone in place. It was probably the only time in my life I was glad I had a big nose.

The surgeon had one other patient in his practice with a similar injury. He didn't mention the outcome or follow-up treatment, but he did say that if the integrity of the cartilage was compromised that it could be replaced with a synthetic material. That didn't sit too well with me. It put up a signal for me to do something more aggressive.

I did get some supplementation. I got some collagen, homeopathic medicine, and magnets, but somehow I felt I could do more.

Then I saw Dr. Robbins for a podiatric routine examination. He suggested that vitamin C therapy could help. . . . I've continued on a fairly steady basis with a hiatus of about six months. I have resumed treatment and am now up to about 100,000 units.

It was during my last visit that the doctor showed me photos of my face right after the accident. It was swollen and deformed. He seemed somewhat pleased and surprised at my progress and took follow-up pictures.

I really think that he didn't want to frighten me earlier on but is now confident enough to show me the earlier pictures because he feels that the healing process is sufficiently on its way. I really feel that a miracle happened. The scaring is hardly visible, which I wasn't even concerned about. It can be smoothed out in the office next visit and there will be no visible signs of the accident.

Sam on mercury poisoning

I had a car accident and chipped my tooth. This was just before the New York City marathon. I ran the marathon and was absolutely drained.

I went to a holistic dentist, Eli Stern, and discovered that I had mercury in my mouth which was weakening my immune system. I was very surprised.

I gradually had the mercury removed. After each dental visit, I would have chelation therapy to get the mercury out of my body. Then I would take 100,000 mg of vitamin C and other nutrients in a drip to build my immune system. I did this religiously three days a week for a month.

I think it is important for athletes to know that silver amalgam fillings are draining to the immune system.

I plan to continue taking vitamin C drips after races to keep my immune system 100 percent strong and to make sure that nothing weakens my immune system and that no illnesses happen. This is one way that I can do it.

Marisa on HIV, cytomegalovirus, Epstein-Barr virus, and herpes 6

I didn't know I was in such serious shape. I thought I just had colds. The cold that I had prior to taking the drips stayed with me for about a month and I was very sick with it. I was totally nonfunctional, but I thought it was just a cold.

I watched a program on alternative medicine and called up to make an appointment. I went to Dr. Calapai who put me on a diet and vitamin C drips. The protocol he put me on called for drips three times a week in the beginning. I could feel my body getting a lot stronger. It didn't stop me from getting colds but if I got a cold, it did not stop me from being able to function.

He also took a blood test. My blood work showed that I had CMV, EBV, and herpes 6. After a series of vitamin C drips, all of these decreased to normal levels. I am definitely an advocate of alternative medicine and vitamin C drips. I think everybody should take them, especially those of us who get a "death sentence" when they are HIV-positive. To me it is more of a wake-up call to take care of your body.

I feel great today. I have two jobs and take care of my three-year-old son. My son is also HIV-positive. I can't give him drips but I do give him large amounts of vitamin C. As a result, he is very stable. I don't want the doctors to suggest that he go on anything. So far, they are very pleased with his blood work. One day, the nurse said to me that his health is nutritionally related. He hasn't dropped down and doesn't need to go on any toxic drugs.

I have preached about vitamin C drips to quite a few friends. A very close friend of mine did not go the alternative route. She chose to take AZT, DDI, and some other toxic drug, and has since died.

When I went to Dr. Calapai, I met a friend there. When I first met her, they literally carried her in. She was like a stick. She has been taking the drips and has since moved into her own apartment. She takes care of her daughter, is working at a job, and is in excellent health now.

Aaron on asthma

I started taking vitamin C drips almost a year ago. At first, I was very consistent and would go about three times a week. Then due to business, I went less consistently but as often as possible. I began to notice improvement immediately. As the dosage increased, so did the improvement.

I can't say that I've cured asthma yet, although I believe I will. I have had a lot more relief. In general, I have a lot more energy. Specifically, regarding the asthma, I don't have as many attacks as I used to have, and the severity of the attacks is much less than it used to be. That alone has been tremendous. It's a great change and a real important part of my life. I believe in the vitamin C drips and continue with it, as well as an improved diet and exercise.

Lynn on chronic fatigue syndrome

Chronic fatigue syndrome is a nightmare. You have viral symptoms, swollen glands, mental confusion, memory loss, paranoia, and no one in the medical profession knows how to help you.

Fortunately, I had a holistic physician in 1986 who diagnosed it and started me on low-level IV vitamin C drips. I followed that protocol for a few years and it helped to stabilized me. I was able to continue working at a reduced level.

Because my immune system was so compromised, on a trip to Mexico, I ended up picking up three parasites and candida in one fell swoop. My doctor had me on Flagyl for two years, and that debilitated me even more. Eventually, he didn't know what to do for me. I developed a terrible cough and was continually coughing green phlegm. My muscles were so sore that it felt like I had broken my ribs on three different occasions.

I came to the Healing Center in March 1993. That's when I tested positive for four viruses. Before I didn't even know what I had other than chronic fatigue immune dysfunction. The doctors started me on an IV vitamin C protocol. The vitamin C drip also included glutathione, liquid vitamin A, and glycyrrhiza. I continued the drips three times a week. At first I received 100,000 mg and eventually worked up to 200,000 mg because I wasn't really getting that much better on the lower dosage. I was functioning but I still had colds. Without the higher dosage, I would still be sick today. There is no doubt in my mind about that.

I also take [supplements]. I eat organic vegetarian foods. I took ozone a few times. I had the silver removed from my teeth. I took colloidal silver, which helped my pneumonia tremendously.

After almost two years of drips, I definitely feel significantly better. The virus has abated or been reduced. I no longer have swollen glands, mental confusion, skin funguses, body aches, or arthritis. My pneumonia is minor. Now, instead of having colds for two to three months, they last only a few days. I am mentally clear and much more productive. I'm a happy person and I'm able to exercise three times a week, as I was prior to this illness.

The male ego in the medical establishment is very frustrating to work with. When I first told my physician about the vitamin C/glutathione therapy, he screamed at me. He said I was crazy and that the treatment was dangerous. As I said, if it weren't for the 200,000-mg IV vitamin C program with all the extra things in it, I'd still be sick today. There's no doubt in my mind about that. . . .

Toni on Epstein-Barr virus

I was a very energetic person until six months ago. Then I could hardly walk to my chiropractor's office, which is about a mile away. I told her that I was extremely tired and she did a blood test. Epstein-Barr showed up.

The regular medical establishment just doesn't want to deal with it because EBV has such a mishmash of symptoms. You have a sore throat, a stiff neck, tiredness, swollen feet, diarrhea, and muscle aches. They tell you that you are just working too much or that you have the flu and need antibiotics. They basically ignore you because they don't want to deal with it.

Then I heard you talking about a doctor at the Healing Center. I went to him and got a very thorough blood test which demonstrated four viruses, not just the Epstein-Barr.

He started me on vitamin C drips with the glutathione. I didn't have an immediate result. I got disgusted with it and almost decided to quit. I stayed with the treatments and am glad that I did. By the time I hit 100,000 units I started to feel great. It was like a light switch going on. I had 15 symptoms and 80 percent of them are totally gone. The remaining symptoms are alleviated. I am almost 100 percent back to normal. It's just wonderful.

One pleasing effect is how dramatically my skin improved. I'm 48 years old and beginning to get lines and wrinkles like everyone does. The lines around my mouth, which had started to appear, totally disappeared from the treatments. My skin is as soft as a baby's skin.

Ethyl on metastatic breast cancer

I was originally diagnosed in November 1987. Since that time, it spread to my bones and liver. I was on chemotherapy for two years, on and off, and was experiencing tremendous fatigue during and after chemotherapy. I had reactions where I had sores in my mouth, bleeding in my nose, and general malaise.

Since starting direct ozone and vitamin drips, I have no more bleeding, no more sores, and no fatigue.

The last time I was in the hospital for chemotherapy, my doctor said to me, "We'll probably have to give you a tranfusion." I replied, "I don't think you're right." He did some blood work and then told me that I was much stronger than he had thought I was.

I really feel a tremendous, tremendous difference. I can't wait until tomorrow to get my vitamin C drip because it is very healing for me. When I start getting ozone next week, I'm going to be a new person.

Patients Speak Out On Cancer Therapies That Work

To demonstrate the power of natural approaches to healing cancer, this section offers firsthand accounts of people who have used them. Approaches to treatment vary, but one factor remains constant: these people, who had life-threatening illnesses, are now alive and well.

714-X[1]

Susan on son's Hodgkin's disease

Last summer, Billy was diagnosed with Hodgkin's disease. We didn't know any better so we went with chemotherapy. Billy had five treatments from August until October. Although he did fairly well compared to some people, he did have the typical side effects. He got nauseous and tired, he lost his hair, and he had some jaw pain. His main concern with the chemotherapy was that it was poisonous. He would look at the drugs dripping into his body and realize how toxic they were. That, in a nutshell, is why he ran away.

When we started to talk about using other forms of treatment, the doctors began to use scare tactics on us. They told us that Billy would die if he went off chemotherapy and they described to Billy, in detail, exactly how he would die. They said that in addition to the chemotherapy, Billy would have to have radiation at the end of the treatment program. Billy refused any more treatment.

We were contacted by many people about many therapies. One of these people, Charles Pixley of Writers and Research in Rochester, New York, told us about a therapy called 714-X. Initially, he sent us a booklet about the treatment. Eventually, Billy, my husband, and I, decided to use it. That was in January and he has since flourished. His cancer is gone. Last December,

---

[1]Author interview with patients, 6/12/95

he was tested and there was some cancer at that point. In March, he was tested again and the cancer was totally gone. He continues with the treatment. They recommend a six month minimum treatment. We're almost at the end of that.

Billy is flourishing with this therapy. His hair has come back. He has gained weight. He has grown. He is like a vacuum cleaner as far as his appetite goes. He is a very active young man. He loves skateboarding, and skateboards every day if the weather permits.

The doctors who originally said he would have been dead more or less pat us on the back and say, that's nice. Instead of expressing an interest, they tried to force us into continuing with chemotherapy by reporting us to the Department of Social Services. However, no action was ever taken and we were able to pursue the treatment of our choice.

I have informed the media about our story in an attempt to get on national TV again. I want to tell them about 714-X and where to get it because we get hundreds of calls from people all over who have searched for it. The media is apparently afraid because they all appear interested when I call them but I never hear back from them.

Harry on massive tumor outside the colon

I was given six months to a year to live. The surgeon said for me to live it up, eat and do anything I wanted to do. He sent me to the oncologist who told me that they could give me treatments but that I had about a 15-percent chance of being helped, and even if I was helped, the treatments would only increase my longevity by a couple of months. I was discouraged with that so I made some trips to Mexico to study various alternative treatment approaches. Then I got a newsletter from a friend of mine about 714-X and I decided to try it because it was something I felt I could continue on.

My son gave me the injections, which were painless. We followed this program for six months. The total program consisted of 168 shots. Right after I started taking the 714-X I felt better. I feel just fine now.

When I started on this program, my son turned my way of living around 180 degrees. He prepared an organic diet for me. I cut out alcohol and cut down on cigar smoking to one in the morning and one at night.

Since then, I have felt much better than I have in years. The 714-X stimulated my immune system back to normal.

I went back to my doctor two years later and was given a colonoscopy and some other tests. Tests showed that the tumor had not enlarged and that the growth had stopped. It became dormant. The oncologist wanted to see me, I guess, out of curiosity. He told me that I have a 60-percent better chance of survival. He said that, eventually, the tumor will shrink and then disappear.

Rick on leukemia

At first, I tried chemotherapy, but it failed to work five times. After each treatment I would experience a relapse because my leukemia was so aggressive. I was working on my next option, a bone marrow transplant. Iowa City had a few matches for me. The first one they tested was almost a perfect match so I went in and had the transplant done. They gave me a 5-percent chance of actually making it through the transplant. Even if I made it through the transplant, I only had another 5-percent chance of cure. I survived the transplant but, three months later, my blood tests were really bad. My platelets never did recover completely.

I continued looking for answers. I was very familiar with Reich's technology and felt strongly that something along those lines could help me. The only problem was that nobody was using or dealing with this technology.

I had a live cell blood analysis done, which tells you more than a CBC or any test given in conventional medicine. According to my test, it was obvious that I was relapsing from the transplant. My relapse wasn't documented by conventional medicine but, of course, they don't use this method so it doesn't matter. I knew and other people knew.

Eventually, I found a group that was duplicating what Reich did with his ray tube. I found this machine, got the 714-X again, and went back on these alternative therapies. Three weeks after getting this machine and getting back on the 714-X, my blood counts, every single one of them, returned to within the normal range. It was amazing. Everybody was astounded by it. I don't know what to attribute it to but I do know that something helped me. I had my transplant in January 1994. I relapsed around April, and here it is May 1995. I've had normal blood tests ever since.

Combination Therapies and Lifestyle Changes[2]

Ed on prostate cancer

I had a radical prostatectomy. Afterwards, my PSA kept going up. It got to 9.1. They thought it would be in the lymph nodes and they wanted to do chemo and radiation. At that point, I was pretty disgusted.

I wanted to try some alternative approaches. I went for hypnotherapy . . . I also started working with a dietitian to change my diet. I started eating whole foods: fruits, vegetables, foods that weren't processed. I ate more organic foods.

---

[2]Author interview with patients 6/21/95

This was a big change for me because I was brought up on meat and potatoes. It was also difficult for me because I grew up not liking vegetables. As a child, my mother forced us to eat what was on our plates, which included spinach and Brussels sprouts and broccoli and I didn't even like being in the same room as a Brussels sprout. So, I had a lot of changing to do.

I also started Essiac tea. When I started on the tea and the diet, it started moving my PSA down. It's down to 0.1 now, the normal range. I feel as healthy as a horse.

Cathy on stage IV Hodgkin's disease

I was in such bad shape that I couldn't lay down or walk. There was fluid in my lungs and tumors around my heart, which advanced into my abdomen. I had been on chemotherapy for about 10 months. At first, the chemo got me back on my feet but after awhile it stopped working. That's when the doctors recommended a bone marrow transplant. They said it was my only hope for long-term survival.

At that point, I simply could not tolerate any more chemotherapy and the thought of a bone marrow transplant was out of the question. I had heard about 714-X from a very well-respected physician in British Columbia and I decided to start it. At the same time, I began to follow a holistic program.

I made quite a few changes. I always thought that I had a healthy lifestyle but I learned that, in fact, it really wasn't. I started doing everything that I could do to strengthen my immune system. That included a completely chemical-free lifestyle and an organic diet, with no white sugar or flour and very little dairy. The little dairy that I did have was unpasteurized and organic. I also had a lot of fresh vegetable juice and used only distilled water. I was very also careful about using chemical-free skin and hair products and about avoiding toxins such as household cleaners and pesticides. Along with that, I was on a very strict detoxification program which included cell cleanses, gallbladder flushes, and coffee enemas. I exercised using a trampoline and took pancreatic enzymes and glandulars that were specifically prescribed for me by a holistic physician. All together, it did the trick, and now I'm completely clear.

I began to notice improvement two to three weeks into the program. My energy level increased and I had less pain. The best way to describe it is to say that I started to feel like my old self again. Two months after starting the 714-X, I had a CT scan done and it showed marked improvement so I knew I was on the right track. I was very excited. On my latest scan, which I just had last month, it showed that there was no sign of disease at all. I feel wonderful.

The most important thing is to have hope no matter what your physician tells you. You have to believe that there is more out there. You can fight for your life. I did and it worked. It's just a matter of getting the right information. I think it's important to get information from both the medical side as well as the holistic side and find out what is best for you and what you believe in. Then go for it. Put everything into it that you can and it will work.

Orville on lymphoma that had metastasized

I am 66 years old and had always enjoyed good health until two years ago when a bump appeared over my right temple. It started growing fast and was about the size of a marble. It was removed and I was told that I had aggressive non-Hodgkin's small cell lymphoma.

I was interested in alternative medicine and that's the route I took. First, I went to Mexico for treatment and it disappeared in about three weeks. I thought that was fantastic since I had arrived with cancer all over my body.

A few months later it began to appear again. I went to Dr. Michael Schachter's clinic in Suffern, New York. After a couple of weeks of treatments there, it vanished again.

Then it came back a third time, months later. At one point, the cancer got as large as a golf ball on my jawbone. It was pulling at my cheek and I could hardly talk or swallow. It was just a bad-looking thing and a bad-feeling thing, and it caused me a lot of pain.

This time I combined the therapy Dr. Schacter had me on with homeopathy. Basically, the therapies I used included eating organic foods and adding such things as laetrile, shark cartilage, homeopathic remedies, and a well planned, well thought out vitamin and mineral program.

The bottom line is, it worked. Utilizing all the different therapies made the cancer shrink and vanish. My medical records show that it disappeared in two months and 11 days. That was little over a year ago. Any time I get an examination, everything is clean. I don't seem to have any sign of cancer. There is nothing like the alternative way of treating cancer.

Lucinda on advanced breast cancer

I had severe breast cancer that metastasized to my ribs and throughout my whole spine. My prognosis was poor. Basically, I was told there was nothing they could do for me. Still, they wanted to try by putting me through the trauma of chemo and radiation even though it wasn't going to cure me. It could only possibly prolong my life a little bit. I refused treatment and they just sent me home to die with a box full of drugs.

Something inside of me said, no, wait a minute, I choose not to do this. There's some other reason I'm supposed to be here. Through the grace of God, or the universe giving me another chance, I was put in contact with a clinic down in Mexico called Genesis West. I went down in a wheelchair on just about every drug you could possibly name. I was totally nonfunctional, mentally and physically.

In the clinic, I received a wide variety of treatments. A few of them involved ozone therapy and hyperthermia. Of course, diet and supplementation to build the immune system were used. The whole basis of this is that the body is built to repair itself and that it has that capability.

I came back a total fighter. Now I'm walking, talking, and living my life completely and fully. I'm fighting every day and I'm determined to beat this.

The change is nothing short of miraculous. In fact, the medical doctors are amazed. Of course, they don't want to admit it but it's real concrete proof for them. I haven't gone in for any tests, like bone scan or MRI or anything like that yet but they look at me and can see that I'm clear-eyed, walking, and functioning. Nobody can tell anything is wrong with me. Obviously, something I'm doing is working.

This experience has been a blessing for me. I want people to know that they have a lot more power and control within themselves than they know and they need to learn that because there is always hope. You've got to always keep fighting if that's what you want.

Leslie on metastatic breast cancer

I have been treated at Dr. Schacter's office for a little over a year. I came from Sloan Kettering in Manhattan where I was treated with radiation and chemotherapy. I was there for nine months. None of those treatments worked and the cancer kept spreading. It finally spread to my liver and I was given six months to live.

When I came to see Dr. Schacter, I was in pretty bad shape. When I started on his oral supplements, and later on his IV supplements, I started to get better. At the same time, I cut out dairy products and red meat and increased my intake of fresh fruits and vegetables. I made sure that I had no refined foods or sugar. If I did have something it would be from the organic food shelf rather than from a fast food chain. I started juicing and that gave me a tremendous lift in energy. My body was telling me that it was very happy. That was a turning point for me in knowing how important nutrition is in battling cancer.

I started to lose the cancer from my body. The tumor markers improved and I started gaining weight. I had much more energy. At this point in time, my blood tests are back to normal. If you looked at me, you would not know I was a cancer patient.

What happened to me is amazing. I feel that it was a combination of the right treatments for me and a lot of prayer, creative visualization, and meditation. I continue to live that way now.

Essiac Tea[3]

Marilyn on breast cancer

My husband brought home an article out of the newspaper about Essiac tea just before I had my lymph nodes removed. They figured for sure that the lymph nodes were invaded with it. I started on this tea 10 days before going back into the hospital. I went in and the lymph nodes and the rest of the surrounding tissues were clean. Three specialists were very surprised and kept remarking what a miracle it was because of the stage III cancer that had already broken free of the tumor and was already invading the rest of the breast.

Although I opted for a traditional approach to treatment, I attribute the lack of hair loss and the ability to handle radiation and chemotherapy without side effects to the benefits of the tea. I feel wonderful today. I've got a new lease on life. I drink the Essiac tea twice a day faithfully. This has been two years now.

Lynette on bone cancer

The prognosis was really bad. I went to see a bunch of specialists and they basically all said the same thing: If I lived I wouldn't want to because everything was just disintegrating. It was a big old mess and I wasn't real happy because I wasn't able to get any answers.

I went to the health food store and started reading different books and talking to some people. That's how I learned about Essiac tea. I was kind of skeptical but got a number to find out what the deal was on this tea. I spoke to someone who told me that she had come across an all-natural herbal tea that doesn't affect any other medication that you're on. I said, what the heck. I'll try it.

At the time, I could barely walk. I have total shoulder replacements and a hip replacement. They tried doing bone grafts but that didn't take. The disease was in my ankles, wrists, and knees. They wanted to do knee replacement surgery on me. In my situation, there is no stopping the disease and there is no treatment for it. What they do is cut out the dead bone and try to put metal in there. I'm basically all bionic.

---

[3]Author interview with patients 6/21/95

When I started taking the tea, I could barely walk. I was on crutches and my legs were swollen. I had them wrapped. I drank the tea three times a day. Within three to four days, I didn't have any pain.

I had some x-rays done before starting on the tea and afterwards. Before the tea, they were really bad. My bones were fractured and broken and that all the ligaments were eaten away. Four weeks later, I had x-rays taken again. The doctor was amazed. The x-rays showed some bone damage, but not as much as before. A week later, I went to another doctor and had x-rays taken again. This was six weeks after taking the stuff. All the bone damage was gone. There was nothing there. They thought they mixed up my x-rays.

Today I'm great. I go biking and study martial arts. This stuff is great.

Hippocrates Health Center[4]

Mike on kidney cancer

I'm a high school teacher from Los Angeles. In February of 1993, I had a kidney stone. After some x-rays and a CT scan, I was diagnosed with kidney cancer in my right kidney. I had two or three tumors. My doctor told me bluntly that if I didn't have a radical nephrectomy, which meant the extraction of all my lymph nodes underneath my arm all the way down to my hip, if I didn't take out my adrenal glands and kidney completely, and if I didn't have that operation by November of that year, I would be dead, no question about it. I told him that I wanted to get a second opinion and he told me that it would be useless because it's cut and dried; there was no other thing that I could do.

My brother, Ronnie, was diagnosed as having cancer of the bone marrow by Sloan Kettering and Johns Hopkins University. I called him to say that I had cancer too. He told me to do what he did. He went to the Hippocrates Center and went on a fast. I went on a 32-day water fast. Then I went on a 7-day juice fast. After that, I became a vegan. In other words, I didn't eat any meat, chicken, fish, or dairy products. I maintain that diet.

I go in for a CT scan every six months. The last one showed that the smallest tumor shrunk a very small amount. I've had every kind of blood test and analysis that you can possibly think of. I just recently had one, and I sent it over to the Hippocrates Center because I'm going back there. They found that everything with my blood is 100 percent normal. I'm in great health.

The Hippocrates Center looks at you as a whole person. They don't threaten you; they just treat you like a human being. They use a natural diet. In other

---

[4]Author interview with patients 8/22/96

words they don't heat anything up. Everything is raw food and raw grains, slightly cooked.

From that, I have maintained a phenomenal lifestyle. I'm active. I have three children. I'm not dead. I teach every day and it's pretty hectic teaching in the barrios of Los Angeles. Yet I maintain a high activity in life. What can I tell you? Things look great; I'm alive and I'm here.

George on prostate cancer

I went to a Hippocrates program for three weeks. about two years ago, and as a result of that my prostate cancer went into remission. It was a program which consisted of organic, fresh, raw vegetables. It also consisted of green drinks which were taken twice a day. In addition to that, there was a great deal of wheatgrass, which I drank—also enemas. I did that for three weeks, and then I stayed on that program after I left the group. I went to the doctor about a week ago, and the doctor said that my cancer has disappeared; it is no longer there.

Patients of Dr. Nicholas Gonzalez[5]

Edmund on kidney cancer

Four-and-a-half years ago, I had major surgery. The doctors removed my left kidney, a large tumor, and one lymph node. I followed this with an interferon program for nine months to prevent any recurrence of the tumor. Unfortunately, this did not work for me because a second tumor came back. At that time, the doctor said that even though kidney cancer does not respond to radiation or chemo, we should try radiation. The radiation stabilized the second tumor but it did not make it disappear. At that time, I realized that the interferon was not going to work.

A friend of mine was on an aggressive nutritional program with Dr. Nicholas Gonzalez, in New York City. I started this program in January 1992, which was three-and-a-half years ago. Three months after I began the program, the second tumor disappeared. My weight, which was way down to 105, is now back to normal at 135. I'm feeling good. My color is back. And recent CT scans and bone scans have been negative. I'm 70 years old.

Henrietta on breast cancer with metastases to the lung

My original cancer was discovered in 1988. I had lymph node involvement and went through surgery. After six months of chemotherapy, I had a 50-

---

[5]Author interview with patients 6/21/95

percent chance of surviving five years. They never say anything about getting totally well, just five years. After three years, it metastasized around my left lung. At that point, the prognosis was not good. I was told that my life expectancy was two to three months.

At that point, I found Dr. Gonzalez in New York City. His treatment is a three-part program consisting of supplements, diet, and detoxification. I have been going to Dr. Gonzales for three years and nine months.

The program has been very successful for me. I can't say it is an easy program. It requires a lot of self-discipline because the diet is rigorous. I'm not saying that you just start on this program and feel great. You don't. If anything, I felt worse before I felt better because of the toxicity that was built up in my body. But it has worked for me and I believe so strongly in the program that it has taken the fear of cancer away. I think this may be a major key because when you believe in something that strong it takes fear away.

At this point, I am stabilized. My cancer level is down to a safe zone and I am functioning normally. I feel great.

The clinic I went to originally was contacted. My oncologist said that if indeed I was still alive, I was a very lucky woman. They didn't give me any hope of living with the traditional medicine.

Dr. Max Gerson's Therapy[6]

At the beginning of the 20th century, Dr. Max Gerson was a specialist in internal medicine living in Germany. Early in his career, while working at a sanitarium, he made a link between food and illness. He noticed that on Mondays, patients would have a gross exacerbation of their symptoms. Having a curious mind, he wanted to find out why. He found that patients ate diets from home rather than the hospital during the time their families visited them. These foods were high in saturated fats, salt, preserved, pickled goods, and alcohol. During the week, by contrast, they were on a bland diet.

He started looking for an ideal dietary approach for patients with lupus and tuberculosis. There was no treatment of any value for lupus at that time. Yet, he was able to reverse a lot of the disease process by putting people on a diet of grasses and vegetables that he would juice. In fact, he became so well known for his success in treating these conditions that the German physicians made him director of the clinic. Later, he would go on to write several textbooks on the subject of natural approaches to reversing conditions previously considered irreversible. Dr. Gerson was something of a superstar in Europe until the 1930's.

---

[6]Author interview with patients 7/11/95

He later came to the U.S., where he started using the same therapy, but for cancer. He found he was able to successfully treat many people by giving them 13 glasses of fresh vegetable juice a day, and by eliminating from the diet extra sodium and all animal proteins except for yogurt and a cultured buttermilk. He also gave potassium supplementally. He was able to provide treatments for cancer that no one else could match. In fact, so impressive was his work that early on in his career the *Journal of the American Medical Association* published an article of his. This very same journal later attacked Gerson and called him a quack.

By the time he reached the height of his career, there was a special Senate investigation of his work headed by Senator Claude Pepper of Florida. Pepper invited Gerson to bring forward medical documentation and patients. Gerson brought forth 50 patients who had suffered from what had been considered terminal illness but who, five years after Gerson's treatment, were alive and well.

Pepper and his committee were so impressed that not only did they not condemn him, but they actually commended him.

Today, his work is continued in Mexico by his daughter Charlotte Gerson Strauss.

Tom on skin melanoma

In March 1982, I found a mole on the right side of my forehead. It didn't concern me much because it wasn't big; it was about half the size of my little fingernail. I talked to my family physician about it, not thinking much of it, but when he saw the thing he was concerned. He said, we'd better take this off and biopsy it.

They did that and the report that came back really shocked me because I had been eating organic foods and a right diet for many years. The news was all bad. It was malignant, it was Clark Level 4. . . .

After the surgery, the cancer returned within 10 days to the site of the incision. I guess that was because they didn't get it all. Then I began to have tumors appearing all over my upper body, chest, and arm. This all happened within a matter of days.

Initially, they wanted to do extensive surgery at the site of the original appearance, but when the thing spread, four different doctors started giving me different advice. Basically, they were all saying that nothing was going to cure this cancer.

At that point, I declined the radical surgery that they wanted to do on the site of my head, and I started looking for different approaches. I knew something about alternative methods, but nobody was at all hopeful, until we talked to the Gerson people. We called the Gerson Institute, and they said that the Gerson therapy was very effective with melanomas. They said that the fact that I hadn't had other treatments which would tend to suppress the immune system was in my favor. Also, the fact that I was fairly young, 42 at the time, was in my favor. I knew something about the therapy, so it wasn't a complete shock. I had some belief in Dr. Gerson and his therapy, so I tried it.

I talked to Charlotte [Gerson Strauss], and she said that melanoma patients detoxify rapidly. She said my chances of recovery were good, but that I would have quite a bit of nausea in the beginning. Everything she told me came true. I got quite ill initially, the type of illness that you'd have if you had a stomach flu. But I was nervous enough about my situation that after I had been on the therapy for a week or so, I thought, my God, I'm not going to be able to do this.

The family had a council of war. We all talked it over with the Institute. They calmed me down and told me they'd cut back the juices a little bit, and cut back the medicine a little for a few days, and just keep trying it. We got through that period and I felt better again.

The heart and soul of the Gerson therapy is that every hour of the day, from 8 in the morning to 7 at night, you have an 8-ounce glass of fresh-squeezed vegetable and fruit juice. It alternates. Basically, one hour you have a juice that's half carrot juice mixed with apple, and the next hour your have green juice, which I think is three different types of lettuce, plus green pepper, red cabbage, and then apple with that also. The juices are laced with potassium salts. In addition, you have three meals. The Gerson therapy is not a fast at all, but your diet is specified.

In the beginning of the therapy, you start digesting the cancer and putting it out of the body in the form of metabolic toxins. If your body is full of cancer, the way mine was, you're going to have a lot of toxins to process. To help that out, in the beginning . . . you take a coffee enema every four hours when you're up: 6 a.m., 10 a.m., 2 p.m., 6 p.m., and 10 p.m. The coffee enemas put the drug caffeine directly into the portal vein. That enables the liver to detoxify a lot more efficiently than it could otherwise. The coffee enema is a great help. It relieves pain, it relieves digestive discomfort, and it is a crucial part of the therapy. That's basically how it went in a day.

Within two months, every visible tumor on my body had regressed. It had shrunk, dried up, and fallen off. It all happened so quickly. I started out in March 1982 thinking I was a healthy guy. Then, in early May 1982, I was told that I had cancer and very little chance to live. In July 1982, I was on the Gerson therapy and everything cancerous that could be seen had regressed and disappeared.

The Gerson people said that even though everything that could be seen was gone, there was more of a problem under the surface. They recommended that I stay on the therapy for 18 to 24 months, which I did. I stayed on the therapy for 20 months, and in the subsequent 13 years, I've had no recurrence of the cancer.

Over the years, I've talked to hundreds of people with cancer of various types and I try to share my experience with them. You can pretty much see who will succeed with this type of therapy and who will not. People used to the passive mode, where professionals do things to them—they cut, they burn, and they put chemicals in, and the patient sits there and it happens to them—are generally horrified when they find out the extent to which the patient has to cooperate in his own recovery on one of these metabolic programs. But people who can take that aboard have a very, very high success rate on this therapy. The exceptions are people who have been bombed with chemotherapy before they get on it. In order to do the Gerson therapy you have to be motivated and open to a radical change in lifestyle that a diet change like this imposes.

Joan on breast cancer

I had a radical mastectomy. One year later, I had a recurrence. It was not biopsied, however. The surgeon said that he would monitor this mass.

My husband and I did a lot of research and decided to try the Gerson therapy. I began the program in August 1977. By May 1978, when I saw the surgeon again, the mass was gone. Since that time, I have remained completely clear. It has been 18 years, and I have never had any recurrences. I have had myself closely monitored over the years by surgeons and lab work.

The Gerson therapy is intensive and comprehensive. It consists of nutritional treatment through diet and 13 juices per day. It consists of medication: potassium, niacin, thyroid, lugol solution, pancreatin, acidol pepsin, and liver and B12 combined as daily injections. It also consists of detoxification in the form of coffee enemas to help the liver. It's a very comprehensive therapy.

I still continue with my diet of organically grown fruits and vegetables. I also continue with almost daily coffee enemas. I have not eaten meat, except for poultry and fish, for these 18 years. That was a decision I made on my own. Some people go back to their former diets, but I realized that my former diet was too high in fats, and could be a possible problem again.

I did not tell the surgeon that I was doing the Gerson therapy. Nor did he ask me any questions. I wanted to keep the surgeon monitoring me, so I decided not to make him angry by telling him what I had done.

At that time, there was not the knowledge and the education about any options as far as treatment was concerned, except for the orthodox establishment options. I had been told at the beginning about the American Cancer Society's statistics and what their thoughts on treatment were. I was an RN who saw that much of this treatment was ineffective with the cancer patients, so I did not feel that the American Cancer Society was credible. Having seen this in my profession, I decided that I was going to do a different therapy. I had read about Gerson's therapy in Dr. Gerson's book. I felt it was credible and the thing to do for myself.

George on pancreatic cancer

I went to the Gerson therapy center in February 1983. Prior to going there, my wife and I were on the way to Hawaii. We were in Seattle and preparing to leave for Hawaii the next morning. I got very sick and had a lot of pain in my stomach and back. We phoned the doctor who was listed in the hotel directory, and took a taxi to the hospital. I had a blood test, an x-ray, and examination by a doctor there. The doctor said that he wasn't sure what the problem was, but he suggested that we not go to Hawaii. He said we should go home instead and get further tests done. That's what we did.

My doctor sent me to a specialist in Victoria. I went through a lot of tests that I never heard of before. On January 21st, he took some blood tests and said that the amylase in my blood was high. A normal level was between 70 and 320, and mine was 627. It proved that there was a very bad infection in my body.

I finally took a CT scan, which showed a mass in the head of the pancreas. The specialist said that there was absolutely no question about it. I had cancer of the pancreas.

We had heard about Gerson's therapy through somebody that my daughter knew. We phoned the Gerson Institute and went down there in February 1983. We spent one month there.

Afterwards, we stayed in our condo in Escondido for eight months because that was the only place we could get organic foods. We had our organic vegetables delivered by a lady who got her vegetables from the same source as the Gersons.

When we came home, I had put weight on and I felt good. My blood tests were also good. I took another CT scan and it showed no tumor. I phoned the head doctor at Gerson's in April 1984, and he told me to stay another four months on the program . . . That's 11 years ago, and I have had absolutely no problem since.

Patricia on pancreatic cancer

I had pancreatic cancer that spread to my liver, gallbladder, and spleen, and was told that I had less than three months to live. My doctors were doing nothing. They said that chemotherapy and anything else would not help me, and that I should prepare my family and get my affairs in order. I was in the process of doing that. Then one morning, my husband and I heard about the Gerson clinic in Mexico. My husband got up and said, "That's it. Pack your clothes. We're going."

We went down on March 7, 1986, and started the therapy that day. Before I started the therapy, I had been throwing up mouthfuls of blood. I was just about finished. Ten days later, I stopped bringing up blood and the pain was gone. I said to my husband, "I don't know if I'm going to live, but I feel better than I have in a year."

Six months later, I went to see my doctor, who wondered why I was still around. He asked if I would have a CT scan, which I did. The test showed that the masses of cancer had gone. My doctor said, "I don't know what you're doing, and I don't want to know what you're doing, but just keep doing it." I think he was shocked to see that I was still around.

Another six months down the road, he asked me to take another CT scan, which I did. He said, "Patricia, there's no sign of cancer at all." That was nine years ago. Today, I feel wonderful. I have no sign of cancer at all.

I took the two Gerson books to my doctor, and he read them, but he said that it was just too deep for him. He just calls me his miracle now.

Marilyn on melanoma and cervical cancer

I developed these conditions in 1979 when I was 36 years of age. My prognosis from my physicians was not good. The melanoma, in particular, was very virulent. They didn't come out and tell me how long they thought I had to live, but they tactfully tried to tell me that my chances weren't good. I read and did some of my own research and found that with stage 4 melanoma, the patient tends to expire in one to five years. It's now been 15 years. I'm not a typical patient.

I did a lot of research and picked Dr. Max Gerson's therapy because I felt that it was the hardest and the most curative. It had the best results with melanoma. I was inspired by the fact that Dr. Gerson had worked with Albert Schweitzer, and that he was a pioneer. He just was an incredible physician with a wonderful answer, but not many people were willing to use this therapy for their problems.

I found after the first six months of the therapy I began to feel really normal. I didn't have reactions and feelings that come when you do a metabolic therapy. I started to feel intuitively that I wasn't going to die, that I was never going to have a recurrence. I know that the mind has a great deal to do with healing. I just knew because this diet was building my cells that my mind was stronger. If felt that I had turned the corner. It's been almost 16 years, and I feel better than I ever have in my life. I attribute that to his work and, of course, my participating in it.

Sharon on non-Hodgkin's lymphoma

I did not have chemotherapy. I went directly to the Gerson Hospital. I was there for two weeks, and in five days I lost 28 pounds of fluid. I had been very swollen with edema. When I got back, I continued on the therapy, and in six months I went back to the doctor. I had an MRI, and my tumor was gone. I am not on a modified therapy. It's been three years.

For more information call 212-787-2404.

Dr. Emanuel Revici's Therapy[7]

Dr. Revici, a man who has hit the century mark, has practiced medicine for over 70 years. In that time, he has saved numerous lives and has been acknowledged by some of the world's greatest scientists. Dr. Revici has received many rewards for his unique and spirited approach to science. He has also been slandered by the American media, who have no knowledge of the thousands of patients he has cured. As a result, he was put on trial, but he was completely exonerated. To date, Revici is totally acquitted of every charge made against him.

Norman on colon cancer

Over six years ago, I had surgery for colon cancer. The doctors didn't have any recommendations; they said I was on my own.

I heard about Dr. Revici and decided to see him. It's probably the best thing I have done in many, many years. I went on his program which consists mostly of minerals. At first, it was rather intense in that I had to use them four times a day, but like everything else, you get used to it.

Now I'm on a maintenance program where I use his prescribed minerals one month on and six months off. My CEA test, which is the test that they use for colon cancer, comes in below 0.5. I only need to have a colonoscopy every two years because I've been clear for several years. I'm just happy to be here. I only have praise for him.

I personally feel Dr. Revici's therapy has made a difference in my life. He's so positive that when he tells you something you almost walk out feeling you have a white shield around you that will protect you. I wouldn't think of not using his program. I wouldn't consider it. In point of fact, I recommended it to one person who was very far gone, and he helped that person. I can't say enough about him.

---

[7]Author interview with patients 7/10/95

Charlotte on ovarian and oat cell lung cancer

My story started in 1980 when I was diagnosed at New York Hospital with oat cell lung cancer. I walked out of there not wanting to take their treatments. A little while later, I went to Mt. Sinai Hospital and was diagnosed with ovarian cancer as well. I had a hysterectomy there and was put onto the lung cancer ward where I received chemotherapy. I took two more chemotherapy treatments after that.

During that time, I got on the Kelly nutritional program, which was available at that time. I started to make a lot of changes in my lifestyle. I had a clean x-ray after the first chemo and thought that was it. I shook hands with the doctor to say good-bye. He held onto my hand and said that this happens to 50-percent of the people who use chemo. Unfortunately, he said, it's not a cure. He told me that if I didn't continue to take chemo every month, the disease would be back in three weeks, and that I'd be dead within six months. That was frightening, but I also felt that chemo was not going to help me live a long time. He wanted me to take chemo for two years. I asked him if at the end of two years if I would be free of cancer and cured. He said, if I lived that long we would talk about it then.

I got help from a psychiatric nurse who got me some statistics, and I found out that I had less than a 1-percent chance for survival. I figured that that wasn't a very good record. I wanted to look around and thought I could do better myself if that was all that they were going to be offering me. Also at that time, they were telling me that they wanted to radiate my brain because oat cell lung cancer usually metastasized to the brain, and I would die a horrible death.

With that prospect looming on the horizon, I figured I had to make some changes. I went to see Dr. Revici and explained my situation to him. I said that I didn't want to continue with the chemotherapy because I didn't believe it would help me. He gave me a complete examination, and said that he thought he could help me. My impression of Dr. Revici was that he was a pure healer, innocent in spirit. He is a lovely individual. When you meet him, you feel complete trust and sincerity, and you believe that you can do well in his hands.

I took his medicine which I understand is toxic except for the way that he delivers it. And being delivered on the lipids, that it goes directly to the tumor. I went along with his program. It really was not devastating in any way. It was just one capsule a day.

After three months, I had another x-ray taken, and it was clear. I stayed on his program for a year. I've always had clear x-rays since I've been with him, and have never had any signs of disease since that time. I go for a lung x-ray from time to time, and the doctors ask what I am there for. I say that I'm checking up to see how my lungs are doing. They look at my lungs and say that I have absolutely no sign of ever having had lung cancer. Now, I do have my former x-rays and my pathology slides, so I can prove that I did indeed have lung and ovarian cancer. I have no doubt that it was Dr. Revici's treatment that helped me.

What a shame that people go at the end of a disease rather than at the beginning when they have a better chance of getting help. They tend to think that alternatives should be saved as a last-ditch effort. I've seen people even at the end do very, very well indeed with him, but I think we need to let people know that for best results they should seek out alternative therapy at the beginning when they have the best chance to support their own innate healing ability, rather than going against it with chemotherapy, surgery, and radiation. If people would like to reach me, I am at 212-777-0111.

Robert on angiosarcoma

In early 1987, I discovered that I had a lump in my jaw. I went through a series of extensive tests, including two biopsies, one in the hospital and one outside. It included MRIs, CT scans, x-rays, and that sort of thing. Out of that came the diagnosis of angiosarcoma. Basically, the doctor who was associated with Georgetown Hospital told me that with this diagnosis I had about one chance in 10 of being alive in five years. He said that that particular kind of cancer was not treatable by any of the usual techniques, namely surgery, radiation, or chemotherapy.

Given that kind of prognosis, and given the lack of treatment options . . . I decided it was time to look elsewhere for treatment. My wife had worked with a lady who was a former patient of Dr. Revici, so I knew of Dr. Revici through her, and contacted the doctor. I became a patient of his in 1987. I was actively under his care for about six years. By that I mean I went to see him in his office approximately once a month. The treatment consisted primarily of capsules that I took orally. He put me on a number of different medications.

What struck me about his treatment is that he tailors it to the person. He would sometimes have me on two or three medications. He would tell me to call him in three or four days, and he might change the medication, depending upon how I was reacting to it. Over that period, he probably had me on a couple dozen different things. I have not been receiving treatment for a little over a year.

His office asked me to have an MRI done, which I did a couple of months ago. I sent them the results. Basically, the MRI shows that in the last three years, there has been no growth at all in the tumor.

Jay on squamous cell carcinoma

I had a squamous cell carcinoma in the throat and was given two to six months to live in 1982. They wanted to operate and remove my entire voice box—my vocal cords and everything—and give me chemo, which I wouldn't allow.

I immediately got on Dr. Revici's therapy, and studied his entire program relating not only to his medication, but the nutrition, vitamins, minerals, enzymes, even some bioactive frequencies later on.

That was 13 years ago. Today, I feel like a million dollars. I have never spent a night in the hospital. I'm very active. At the time I started on his program, you couldn't understand me. I sounded like the godfather's godfather. In a period of about 4 months, my voice was back to normal and I've never had a sick day.

I spoke with my original diagnosing physician many, many times. I happened to know one in New York, and one in California, who are top guys in the allopathic field in otolaryngology. About two years later, I finally agreed to let them do a second in-depth biopsy on my throat, just to get them off my back, because they were friends of mine. When my right vocal cord was originally diagnosed, it was over 3/4 of an inch in diameter. They couldn't understand why all of this cleared up in such a short period of time. It was all 100 percent clear.

Arthur on Kaposi's sarcoma

I was diagnosed at the VA hospital. The doctors there suggested operating to cut out the sores on my foot. I did not agree. I had a problem with the medical professional who attended to me. He asked me if I was homosexual and I said I wasn't. He told me that those were the kinds of people who get this. He also told me I could die from this. I didn't like the approach they had there.

I decided I would try another method. Fortunately, I listened to you and learned about Dr. Revici. I began treatment with him back in 1991. I successfully overcame my condition.

Lee on breast cancer

My cancer started in 1986. I felt a lump in the right breast, and had a mammogram, which was negative. The doctor said that the lump was benign, and that I shouldn't worry. In 1988, the lump seemed bigger and harder, and I was advised to get a mammogram. This time, it showed a mass. I then had a biopsy at Beth Israel Hospital, which diagnosed a 4-cm infiltrating ductal carcinoma in my breast. I saw a number of doctors and surgeons who advised a modified, radical mastectomy, with chemotherapy and radiation.

I knew that there were other options from listening to your program and reading. I decided to try Dr. Revici's nontoxic individualized cancer therapy, even though I was warned by all the doctors that he was a quack, and that I could die without conventional treatment. I called Dr. Revici, and he told me to have a lumpectomy if I didn't want the mastectomy, and then to come for treatment. I had the lumpectomy in December 1988, and I began treatment with Dr. Revici in January 1989.

I found him to be very caring and considerate. He encouraged me to call him often to tell him how I was feeling. His own phone number was given to me.

In July 1989, I stopped the treatment because I felt that six months of it was sufficient. About nine months later, I felt another hard lump in the same breast. A mammogram revealed another mass, approximately 1.5 cm, and the tumor marker for breast cancer was high.

I returned to Dr. Revici in May 1990, and he urged me to have the lump removed. I didn't want another operation, and Dr. Revici was understanding. He said that he would try to help me anyway.

I was given a variety of Dr. Revici's medicine. At times I became discouraged, but Dr. Revici kept reassuring me that the lump would go away. Gradually, it did become softer, and after about two years I no longer felt the lump.

The last mammogram I had was negative, and the tumor marker for breast cancer was normal. I still take Dr. Revici's medicine about every two months. I also take vitamins and herbs. I changed my diet. I don't have meat or chicken, and I eat very little sugar or dairy. I drink bottled water and take exercise classes in yoga and low-impact aerobics. I am very grateful to Dr. Revici.

Fred on prostate cancer

I was given this diagnosis about three years ago. I went to see a urologist who biopsied me. It was a very unpleasant procedure. He immediately suggested that I undergo a radical prostatectomy, but the operation itself and all of its side effects were most unappealing. I went to see a radiologist who suggested radiology. Each special branch seems to have their predilection. I was somewhat turned off by what I was beginning to know were the side effects of that invasive approach also: the incontinence, the impotence, and the lowering of the immune system's abilities to take care of the body.

I finally called Dr. Revici, and decided to go with him. I've been seeing him for three years. I cannot say, unfortunately, that my tumor has completely disappeared, as has been the case for other of his patients, but it certainly seems stabilized. Furthermore, my general well-being is terrific. I feel very,

very energetic, both mentally and physically. Most of that I attribute to Dr. Revici's ministrations. I do other things to enhance my immune system, but I think that Dr. Revici's approach is key to what I hope is a stabilized situation.

Ronald on bone, lung, and kidney cancer

My experience with cancer began in 1976 when a large tumor was discovered in my pelvis just above the knee. It resulted in an amputation in 1977. In 1979, the cancer metastasized to the lung, and I had an operation on my right lung to remove a couple of nodules. To my regret, in 1980, I was diagnosed with renal cell carcinoma. At that time, they told me that I had six months to two years to live. There was no treatment available. Surgery wasn't possible. Neither was chemotherapy expected to be of any benefit.

At that point, I heard about Dr. Revici, and went to see him. I started on his therapy in October 1980. To my surprise, within about a month or so, I began to feel my energy return. My appetite began to increase, and my condition improved. I continued on his therapy for a while. Then I returned to work.

I had another episode of metastatic cancer in 1987. Again the bone cancer was active in my left hip. I went back to Dr. Revici. With his help, I went into remission. Unfortunately, in 1991, I had another episode of bone and lung cancer. I went back to Dr. Revici again and continue on his therapy until today. The tumor in the right lung was a little resistant to the treatment, but after a couple of years of treatment, it appears that the tumor is going into remission. I'm very happy about that.

I've been able to enjoy a reasonable quality of life over these years, thanks to Dr. Revici's treatment. My life certainly has been extended beyond the six months to two years that was expected by the traditional medical community.

Dr. Stanislaw Burzynski's Therapy[8]

Since 1977, Stanislaw Burzynski, M.D., Ph.D., of Houston, Texas, has helped thousands of patients recover from advanced cancer. Originally from Poland, where he was considered one of the brightest scientists and physicians, he later came to this country, and worked with Baylor University. Here he was a shining star, with over 60 articles printed in peer-reviewed journals. His amazing research showed that cancerous cells could be reprogrammed back into normal tissue.

Dr. Burzynski's treatment consists of a series of substances called antineo-

---

[8]Author interview with patients 7/13/95

plastons, which help reprogram cancer cells into normal cells. Antineoplastons are part of a larger group of chemical compounds called *peptides,* that exist in every human body. Simply stated, antineoplastons are a special class of peptides, found in the body, that combat neoplastons—abnormal cells or cancer cells. Cancer patients have a severe shortage of these cancer fighters. Antineoplastons could be the vehicle needed by the body to ward off and even reverse the development of these cancerous cells.

Dr. Burzynski put this theory into action, treating patients by reintroducing antineoplastons into the bloodstream either intravenously or orally with capsules. In many cases, tumors shrank in size or actually disappeared. Some patients even experienced a complete remission of the cancers, and years of follow-up study reveal no sign of any return.

Unfortunately, Dr. Burzynski has been targeted by the medical establishment. His clinic may be closed permanently.

Venuta on breast cancer

One week after diagnosis, I had a mastectomy. Then they wanted to give me chemotherapy but I didn't want it. I decided to go to Dr. Burzynski. He connected me to an IV for 5 months, nonstop, 24 hours a day with his antineoplaston medication. During that time, I was never sick. I had a normal life. I have a 7-year-old child. I've been going to meetings at school. I've been driving my car. I have chemotherapy, and I can drive my car. I never even lost my hair. Nobody in the whole world knew that I was having chemotherapy. After 5 years, I am talking with you.

Currently, I'm perfect. I have no cancer. I feel good and I run my own business. I go to Dr. Burzynski for check-ups, and everything looks good.

Theresa on stage 4 lymphoma

In 1984, after the birth of my daughter, I had a biopsy which showed that I had stage 4 lymphoma. My doctors said that I should go on chemotherapy right away, even though I wouldn't be able to get rid of the lymphoma. They said it was incurable.

I had a second opinion . . . and they said the same thing, but they said they could check it for awhile and not give me any chemo right away. I never did end up having chemotherapy or radiation.

Today I'm great thanks to Dr. Burzynski. He gave me the antineoplaston therapy, which means anticancer. It's a peptide that he discovered. Apparently, most peptides are growth-enhancing peptides. Peptides are the precursors to amino acids which are the precursors to proteins. The peptides that he found are peptides that inhibit the growth of certain types of cells. Rather than killing the cancer cells along with a lot of other healthy cells, peptides just keep the cancer cells from growing. They live out their lifespan and then they die off. Eventually, whatever organ is affected is turned back into a healthy organ. That's what happened with me.

While I was healing, I made a lot of changes. I realized I had a lot of anger that I wasn't dealing with. I was taught that anger is bad and hurtful, and I developed a way of suppressing my anger and not even knowing that I had it. So one part of getting well, a big part, was coming more to terms with my anger, accepting it, and expressing it appropriately, rather than stuffing it inside and turning it into cancer.

Another aspect was learning to visualize my cancer going away, and holding a more positive view of my future. I did change a lot of things. I changed my job, and I changed a lot of my relationships. I went through a lot of changes.

Today, I feel a lot different than I did then. I'm much more aware of my feelings, and physically I feel a lot better. Over the months that I worked with Dr. Burzynski's medicine, I saw my cancer gradually disappear. I was grateful to be able to deal with my healing process in a nontoxic way, and I'm really grateful to be alive.

Ellen on intestinal asbestos cancer

This is the same type of cancer that Steve McQueen died of. It was a slow-growing cancer. I was on 250 pain pills a month for ten years. Finally, Sloan Kettering gave me two years to live.

I called Dr. Burzynski and asked him if he could help me. After the first week of treatment, I was off the pain pills. I had no side effects. I was on his program for nine months and I got cured.

Tessie on lymphoma

I was advised to get chemotherapy, which I started in June 1992. In July 1993, it reappeared in my neck. My doctor said that with my condition, chemotherapy might help. But the second time that I started chemotherapy, the tumor was not getting smaller.

I had the feeling that I had to do something different. I decided to go to Dr. Burzynski because I got tired of the chemotherapy. I told my doctor that I was going to stop the chemotherapy and get a second opinion. My doctor was shocked, and he started putting pressure on me to go back on chemotherapy. He said I would lose ground, but I didn't. Today, I am free of cancer.

Actually, the chemotherapy was causing me to lose ground. I was so weak from it that I was running a fever. I had bronchitis, and I had pneumonia. My heart was also damaged from the chemotherapy. After getting well, I went back to my doctor for blood tests to send to Dr. Burzynski, and he was ignoring me.

Mary Jo on low-grade non-Hodgkin's lymphoma, stage 4

I was told that I needed a bone marrow transplant, massive chemotherapy, total body irradiation, and six weeks of total isolation in a hospital. My doctor gave me no guarantee, but he said that this was my only chance for a cure. My other option was to take chemotherapy and radiation every two years. I already had a tumor on the side of my neck, which was growing. If I didn't follow his advice, he said it would press against my organs and I would die.

I did some more research. That's when I heard about Dr. Burzynski's totally nontoxic treatment. I took the next flight to Houston, and met with him. Immediately, I had a wonderful feeling. He gave me names of other patients he treated with my condition, and I called them right away. These people were in remission from non-Hodgkin's lymphoma for over five years. I thought I would be foolish not to try it. When I called my doctor at UCLA, he was adamant that I not start Dr. Burzynski's treatment, but I did it anyway.

My medical records are open to everybody. Every CT scan I had showed a reduction. I have maintained my doctor at UCLA who says, over and over again, "I can't say it's not working, but I don't know why it's working." He calls me a spontaneous remission.

One thing that is so important about Dr. Burzynski's treatment is that it is totally nontoxic. I lived a completely normal life while I was on it. I was able to do grocery shopping, drive my kid's car pools, everything.

Dr. Lawrence Burton's Therapy[9]

I have followed Dr. Burton's work from the 1970's up until his recent death. I was always amazed at the challenges that he offered the National Cancer Institute and medicine in general. He would say, essentially, if you feel my nontoxic, noninvasive, Immuno-Augmentative Therapy (IAT), which uses the immune system to fight off cancer, is fraudulent, then what are you doing that is better? No one ever accepted his challenge. And of course, orthodox medicine can show very few successes.

The man who made such startling progress in the treatment of cancer had a long career in research. Burton decided to go into cancer research after witnessing the horrors of cancer treatment at the U.S. Navy's Cancer Center

---

[9]Author interview with patients 7/18/95

at Brooklyn Naval Hospital in the 1940's. In those days, the accepted procedure for cancer treatment was radical surgery. If you had a cancer of the foot, the leg was removed at the hip. After World War II, Burton continued his cancer studies and gradually moved up to become a senior investigator and oncologist at St. Vincent's Hospital, a noted teaching hospital in New York.

Burton's IAT has its roots in this period of his career. In 1959, Burton and a team of cancer researchers accidentally discovered a tumor-inhibiting factor that reduced or eliminated cancer in a special breed of leukemic mice. Their research progressed well enough so that, in the November 1962 issue of *Transactions of the New York Academy of Sciences*, they reported on certain substances that were capable of causing remission in over 50 percent of the leukemic mice treated.

The studies were repeated in the presence of numerous scientists and science writers, and once again the tumors almost completely disappeared. This resulted in positive publicity at first, but the findings were soon discredited by disbelieving physicians as trickery.

Despite this, Dr. Burton's team treated patients with IAT at St. Vincent's Hospital. They were working under Dr. Antonio Rottino. In 1972, Dr. Rottino announced that the IAT treatments had to cease. The treatments were considered experimental and therefore unproven and so were not appropriate to use as part of regular medical care. The actual reason for the funds being stopped was the team's refusal to give over their work to other organizations that fund cancer research, which wanted to take credit for the work. The group was forced to disband.

During this time, Long Island psychologist Martin Goldstone's wife was being treated with IAT (the Burton-Friedman technique). She had enjoyed such promising results that, when they learned that the treatments had been stopped at St. Vincent's, she and her husband and other prominent people in the Great Neck, New York community raised enough funds to establish the Immunology Research Foundation to continue the work of Doctors Burton and Friedman, Burton's associate.

The Immunology Research Center moved from Great Neck, New York to Freeport on Grand Bahama Island in 1977. Since then, over 2,500 terminal cancer patients have undergone treatment there. According to Dr. Burton, 50 to 60 percent of these patients experience tumor reduction. Many are able to resume normal lives; frequently they survive five years and more beyond the initial diagnosis of cancer (usually made by a traditional attending physician prior to Burton's involvement in the case). The five-year survival period is sufficient for the American Cancer Society and the National Cancer Institute to consider a patient cured.

Dr. John Clement, an internationally renown cancer specialist now running the Center, explains how IAT fights cancer:[10]

"IAT is a nontoxic, immune-modulation method of controlling cancers. The intellectual basis of the treatment is that many cancers can be controlled by restoring the competence of the patient's own immune system. The body's complex immune-fighting system may well be the first, best, as well as the last line of defense against many cancers. We are not dealing with toxic chemicals in any way. We are giving people solutions from the blood of healthy people, obviously screened to be completely safe and free from any type of cross-infection. We are giving humeral cytokines. Cytokines are well known by the names of various types, such as interferon and interleukin. And the substance that we are using most is called tumor necrosis factor. The method we use is similar in any type of cancer we treat. This method is recognized by some people but is completely different from most accepted types of cancer treatment.

"The way in which we use our method is that we take blood from the cancer patient and assay the blood for the factors we believe are aiding the patient's own cancer to destroy the patient. We try to correct and improve the factors in the blood by giving the patient small injections on a daily basis of the factors we are concerned with. By identifying these factors, we are able to control them, put them back into balance, and often destroy the patient's own cancer.

"The cancer patient has in their blood a system of blocking proteins. These blocking proteins prevent the patient from rejecting the cancer as a foreign body. These can be determined, defined, analyzed, and removed. If you put a kidney from some other person into a patient, the kidney will be rejected, because of these blocking proteins. These proteins have been determined. Their molecular weight is known, and they are known to be present, circulating in the blood of patients with cancer. It is our aim in our treatment to prevent these blocking proteins from preventing the patient from curing himself or herself. We measure these blocking proteins on a daily basis. We give similar proteins which, in fact, knock the blockers out, and allow the patient's own immune system to reject the patient's cancer."

Craig on lymphoma

I was originally diagnosed in 1979 with a malignant lymphoma. By the time it was diagnosed, it was already stage 4, which meant that it was in my bones.

I was given radiation and three different series of chemotherapy . . . in early 1980. When they saw how my liver was, they gave me a 10-percent chance of seeing Christmas day. I continued on more radiation and chemotherapy.

---

[10]Author interview with Dr. John Clement, 12/31/95

In the meantime, I saw a program on "60 Minutes" about Dr. Lawrence Burton in the Bahamas and how he was blackballed from the medical establishment. He was being recognized as a viable cancer researcher. I kept it in the back of my mind.

I kept getting worse and worse and worse. Finally, I went to the Bahamas as a last resort. The treatment I received was a daily injection of four different proteins . . . There were absolutely no side effects whatsoever. I began to feel better right away. Of course, I'd been through a lot of chemotherapy and I was coming out of that. It took me about a year to really start coming back, but everything has been fine. I've had a lot of check-ups ever since and there's absolutely no sign of cancer in my body.

Jill on multiple myeloma

I was diagnosed in October 1981. I was told to go on chemotherapy and radiation, which I took for three years. In March 1984, I was told by my doctor to go home and die. He said that I should make out my will, and that he would supply me with enough morphine to keep from being in too much pain.

At that point, I weighed 85 pounds. I could not lay down or sit down without a great deal of pain.

While I was waiting to die at home, I had 24-hour-a-day nurses taking care of me. During this time, I assembled quite a library of literature about cancer. One of the books I had was called *Cancer Survivors and How They Did It.* In that book is a chapter about Dr. Burton and IAT. A nurse who was taking care of me read the chapter and suggested that we call these people. We did, and we talked to a woman who survived pancreatic cancer. The nurse was terribly impressed, and we sent for the brochure. It was the end of May, and my daughter was just getting out of college. I called her and asked, "Do you want to go to the Bahamas?" Off we went. She pushed me through airports in a wheelchair.

When we reached our destination, we talked to Dr. Burton, and I started the program immediately. About six weeks into it, I turned over in bed by myself for the first time. Eventually, I was able to walk on crutches to the bathroom. The doctor in Los Angeles told me that I would never walk again. The rest is history. Here I am 14-plus years later.

Mine was not a miraculous recovery. I made progress in very small increments. When I look back on a day-to-day basis, I cannot report much change, but on a month-to-month basis, I could tell that I was definitely getting better. I began feeling a lot stronger, with less pain. Every six months, I returned to the Bahamas for a tune-up. Again, I had my blood checked daily. I got the new series of shots daily, and stayed for a month or more. Then I would once again come home, and the same sorts of things happened. I noticed that I was very gradually feeling stronger and getting better. That has continued until now.

I must interject this. At one point, I was in a very, very serious car accident, where I broke every bone in my body. Multiple myeloma is bone marrow cancer, which compromises your bones tremendously. The orthopedic doctor in the hospital put me back together. While he was in there, he said that he scraped all the old cancer cells off, but he couldn't see any new ones that developed. He didn't want to go way out on a limb and say that IAT was helpful, but he said that something had stopped the cancer growth. I think that's rather significant, and I attribute it to IAT and the good Lord above. I don't know what else I have done. It certainly wasn't the chemo and the radiation kicking in after all those years, which they like to say. Even though this accident set me back a great deal, I continue to go back to the Bahamas about every six months, and continue doing the program at home, taking shots every day.

Jesse on lymphoma

In 1980, I was diagnosed with lymphoma. I had 20 treatments of radiation, and 11 months of chemotherapy. During this time, the cancer continued to spread. It spread to both lungs, and to the bone marrow. During this two years of treatment, I had many biopsies done, which all turned out to be malignant tumors. After the two years, they told me to come back in two weeks, and they would tell me what they were going to do next, but that I had very little time left, and they were going to try to make me as comfortable as they could.

When I came home, I knew I was not going back because I had heard of this place in Freeport, Bahamas. I called a lady, and she gave me a phone number to reach the Bahamas. I called and they took me. I had to bring my records, which the doctors did not want me to have, but they couldn't hold me, so they gave me very little information to take with me.

I went to Freeport in June 1982. When I went, I really didn't go for a cure because I had been told that I had a very short time left. I could look at myself and I knew that because I had tumors all over my body and in my face. I was covered from top to bottom.

After going to Freeport, Dr. Burton told me that the lymphoma that I had, chemo would not even treat. After he told me that, I knew that he was telling the truth because it had continued to spread.

After being in Freeport for just a very few days, I had a talk with Dr. Burton, and after talking with him, I knew that he had the cure. He said to me, Mrs. Pennington, you don't have a problem. That, in itself, did so much for me because you will have a tendency to believe what a doctor tells you. There I sat, barely able to hold my head up, and Dr. Burton was telling me that I didn't have a problem.

After two weeks, all of the visible tumors were gone. After one week, I could see a great difference in the way that I felt. And after five weeks, I was sent home. It was in July 1982.

When I came back, I saw my treating physician. He said that I was cured, but that it was the chemo that cured me. He twisted his story because I had five biopsies just before leaving his care and going to the Bahamas, and they were all malignant. He did the biopsies, and he gave me the reports, telling me that he was going to make me as comfortable as he could before I died. Yet, when I came home from Freeport, he told me that I was cured.

That, in itself, makes me very bitter, knowing that a doctor will lie to you, and tell you just anything. I really don't appreciate that. To me, cancer in the United States is just a money racket. I know what they took from me, and they gave me nothing. I would love to have a refund.

INDEX

abortion, 226, 289
Abraham, Dahlia, 39,
    288-89
abrotannum, 394
abscesses, 390, 391
acanthosis, 392
accidents, 489-91, 505-6
acetaminophen, 246
acetylcarnitine, 35
acetylcholine, 32, 35, 339
acidic vs. alkaline foods,
    99-100, 140, 150,
    235, 387, 404, 414
acid indigestion, 183-84
acidophilus, 152, 259,
    274, 355-56, 358
acne, 389, 391, 392, 393,
    394
aconite, aconitum, 53,
    157-58, 167, 225
acquired immune
    deficiency
    syndrome, see AIDS
    and HIV
acupressure, 222, 352
acupuncture, 79, 147-48,
    212, 222, 229, 250,
    292, 299, 332, 402,
    421-26, 508, 539
ADD (attention deficit
    disorder), 294
adrealinum, 379
adrenal extracts, 284, 285
adrenal system, 24, 285,
    311
aerobic exercise, 263
affirmations, 352

aggression, 554-55
aging, 3-16
    antioxidant
        supplements and,
        11-12
    aromatherapy and, 14-
        15
    chelation therapy and,
        6-7
    detoxification and, 4-8
    diet and, 9-11
    juice fasting and, 4-6
    personal experiences
        with, 475
    rebuilding and, 8-16
    stress reduction and,
        15
agrimony, 190
AHT
    (autohemotherapy),
    106, 525, 526
AIDS and HIV, 59-75,
    557-58
    diet for, 60-62
    herbs for, 65-69
    supplements for, 62-65
    symptoms of, 60
    treatment of, 60-74
    what to avoid with, 74
alanine, 371
alcohol, 88, 110
    digestive disorders
        and, 194
    headaches and, 245,
        251
    heatstroke and, 267
    osteoporosis and, 332

Alcoholics Anonymous,
    17
alcoholism, 17-20
Alexander, Frederick
    Mathias, 80, 427
Alexander technique, 80,
    359, 427-28
alfalfa, 48, 238, 261, 271
algae, 10, 447
    blue-green, 399, 442
    green, 152
alkaline vs. acidic foods,
    99-100, 140, 150,
    235, 387, 404, 414
allergies, 21-31, 185-86,
    478
    arthritis and, 45, 51
    autism and, 56
    dental disorders and,
        444, 453
    diabetes and, 181
    ear infections and, 202
    environmental
        chemicals as cause
        of, 27-28
    fixed vs. cyclic, 21-22,
        185-86
    headaches and, 249-50
    learning disorders and,
        295, 297
    personal experiences
        with, 421-23, 466,
        475, 478, 479, 484,
        494, 515, 518
    protease and, 142
    respiratory illnesses
        and, 375, 377, 380

591

allergies (*cont.*)
  self-diagnosis of, 23-25
  sinusitis and, 383, 385
  supplements in
    treatment of, 28-29
  symptoms of, 24-25
  tests for, 22-23
  treatment of, 25-30
  types of, 21-22
  UTI and, 413
  what to avoid with, 30-31
allium cepa, 158
allspice, 188
aloe vera:
  for AIDS, 68
  for arthritis, 48
  for cancer, 105
  for cold and canker
    sores, 153
  for cysts, 518
  for digestive disorders, 189
  for dysmenorrhea, 198
  for fibromyalgia, 434
  for foot and leg
    problems, 233, 234, 235
  for headaches, 249
  for heatstroke, 267
  for hemorrhoids, 268
  for hepatitis, 272
  for herpes, 276
  for lupus, 298
  for skin conditions, 392
AL-721, 63-64
Altman, Nathaniel, 71
aluminum, 33
Alzheimer's disease, 13, 32-38
American Cancer Society, 97, 573-74
American ginseng, 372
Amiotte, George, 409
amphetamines, 397
anacardium, 134, 395
anchoring, 351
Anderson, Nina, 12, 294
anemia, 39-43, 357
  sickle cell, 382
angelica sinensis, 143

angina pectoris, 253, 257, 262, 458, 460
angiosarcoma, 578-79
anise, 293
ankylosing spondylitis, 44
anorexia nervosa, 205-8
antibiotics, 55-56, 109, 112, 193, 295, 303-4, 335, 413, 491, 495, 533-34
antifungals, 191
antigens, arthritis and, 51
antimonium tartaricum, 159
antineoplaston therapy, 582-84
antioxidants:
  aging and, 5, 11-12
  arthritis and, 49
  cancer and, 102-3
  digestive disorders and, 191
  for dysmenorrhea, 202
  see also specific antioxidants
aphoresis, polyatomic, 525
apis, 275, 493
apis mellifica, 167, 373, 394
apple juice, 5, 7
applied kinesiology, 23, 429-31
aqueous penicillin
  treatment, 71-72
arabinogalactan, larch, 108
arjuna, 261
Armour Thyroid, 57
arms, 506-7, 541-42
  lymphedema in, 306-9
arnica, 167, 317
aromatherapy, 14-15
  for colds and flu, 160
  crystal, 508
  description of, 432
  for dysmenorrhea, 199
  for headaches, 249
  for lupus, 299
  massage and, 505
  menopause and, 314

  for Parkinson's disease, 340
  pregnancy and, 361
  for respiratory
    illnesses, 379
  for stroke, 400
arrhythmia, cardiac, 254
arsenicum, 490
arsenicum album, 70, 135, 158, 167, 275-76
arsenicum iodadum, 70
artemesia, 191
arteriosclerosis, 239-40, 253, 255, 261, 262
  personal experiences
    with, 454, 456, 457, 458, 459-60, 462
arthritis, 12, 15, 44-54, 235-36
  allergies and, 45, 51
  causes of, 45
  gouty, 44
  osteo-, 44, 235-36, 472-73
  personal experiences
    with, 444, 460, 470-71, 473, 529-30, 543
  rheumatoid, 44, 236, 461, 521-22
  symptoms of, 45-46
  treatment of, 46-54, 146
  what to avoid with, 54
ascorbic acid, *see* vitamin C
ash:
  prickly, 49
  white, 228-29
Ashwagandha, 353
asparagus, 447
aspartame, 245, 251, 285, 326
aspirin, 46, 224, 246, 542
asthma, 375, 377, 378, 380, 494-95, 558
astragalus, 30, 66-67, 90, 105, 133, 155, 271, 284, 486
atherosclerosis, 34, 253, 461
athlete's foot, 235, 390

athletics, *see* sports
Atkins, Robert, 17
attention deficit disorder (ADD), 294
aurum metallicum, 174
aurum muriaticum, 229
autism, 55-58, 297
autohemotherapy (AHT), 106, 525, 526
autoimmune disease:
    UTI and, 413
    see also AIDS and HIV; multiple sclerosis
Ayurvedic medicine, 315, 353
    personal experiences with, 433-37, 449

back and neck pain, 76-85, 146
    personal experiences with, 428, 438-39, 464-65, 466-67, 468-69, 501-2, 505-7, 542
    preventing reoccurrence of, 82-83
    prevention of, 83-84
    professional assistance for, 78-80
    self-help for, 80-83
bad breath, 184, 443
baibu, 336
baineiting eye drops, 221
baking soda, 344, 447
balanced hormonal treatment, 52
baldness, 481-82
baptisia, 71, 225
barberry, 144, 190, 271
barley grass, 340, 406
baryta carbonica, 135
basil, 188, 314, 400, 434
Batmanghelidj, Dr., 256, 257
bee pollen, 42, 57, 152, 238, 371, 377, 399, 406
bee propolis, 152, 153, 156, 190, 274

beet juice, 5
beet leaf, 284
belladonna, 158, 167, 202-3, 225, 267, 379, 394
Bell's palsy, 467
bentonite, 7, 25, 379, 476
berberine, 144, 243, 271, 336
bergamot, 14, 276
Berwick, Ann, 330
beta carotene, 191
    aging and, 10, 11
    for AIDS, 63
    for cancer, 102
    for cold and canker sores, 152
    for ear infections, 202
    for endometriosis, 211
    for osteoporosis, 328
    for periodontal disease, 345
    for respiratory illnesses, 378
    for sinusitis, 384
    for skin conditions, 391
    for trauma, 408, 409
    for UTI, 415
Betadine, 415
beta interferon, 318
Beyerle, Stanley, 106
Bien, George, 498, 499, 500
Bifidobacterium bifidum, 192
bilberry, 220, 261
biofeedback, 148-49, 402
    description of, 438
    for eye disorders, 222
    personal experiences with, 438-39
    for trauma, 409
bioflavonoids, 11, 28, 63, 156-57, 166, 191, 228, 238, 257, 268, 280, 292, 346, 448
biological dentistry, 166, 320, 441-53
bio-oxidative therapies, 304
biotoxic reduction, 216
bitter melon, 67

blackberry, 330
black cohosh, 261, 358
black currant, 29, 49, 100, 157, 258, 313, 319, 324, 365, 371, 393
black haw (viburnum; cramp bark), 143, 199, 358, 379
black salve, 387
black walnut, 115, 298, 336
bladder, 229
    UTI and, 411-17
blisters, 232
blood:
    pH of, 387
    sickle cell anemia and, 382
    sugar, *see* hypoglycemia
    type, arthritis treatment and, 47
blood root, 387
"blue babies," 254
blueberry (huckleberry) leaves, 181, 399
blue cohosh, 358
blue-green algae, 399, 442
blue vervain, 145
Bock, Kenneth, 183
bone cancer, 567-68, 581
bones, *see* osteoporosis
boneset, 48, 159
borage, 29, 49, 100
    oil, 157, 258, 313, 319, 324, 365, 371, 393
boric acid, 27-28
boron, 50, 236, 313, 345
borrelia spirochete, 301-5
boswellia, 48, 236
bovista, 366
bowel, *see* colon; intestines
brain:
    allergies in, 24
    cancer of, 515-17
    dementia and, 32-38
    stroke and, 397-400, 461
Braly, James, 375
bran, 379
bras, 87, 308

breast cancer, 86-92, 313, 328, 477
  hormone replacement therapy and, 311
  lymphedema and, 306
  personal experiences with, 478, 528-29, 560, 565-67, 569-70, 573-74, 579-80, 582
breasts, 366
  implant reactions in, 93-94
  tenderness of, 357, 364
breathing, *see* respiratory illness
breathing exercises, 43, 307, 325
breath work, 221
bromelain, 6, 48, 142-43, 243, 377, 383
bronchitis, 375-76
bruxism, 163
Bryner, Dr., 444, 445-46, 450, 453
bryonia, 225, 314, 356
buchu, 359, 415
buckthorn, 272
Bueno, Herman, 335
bugleweed, 260
bulimia, 205-8
bunions, 236
bupleurum, 143
burdock, 8, 48, 134, 153, 271, 392, 415
Burger, Alyssa, 214
burns, 490
bursitis, 458
Burton, Lawrence, 91, 584-89
Burzynski, Stanislaw, 581-84
butcher's broom, 239, 261, 269
butyric acid, 63

cabbage juice, 5, 48
caffeine, 130, 245-46, 251, 284, 332
Calapai, Dr., 542, 543, 558
calcarea carbonica, 53
calcarea fluorica, 346-47

calcarea phosphorica, 329
calcarea sulphurica, 394
calcium:
  for allergies, 29
  for autism, 57
  for back and neck pain, 83
  for breast cancer, 90
  calcium and, 280
  for dental disorders, 165
  for foot and leg problems, 238
  heart disease and, 259, 261
  for learning disorders, 296
  menopause and, 312-13
  osteoporosis and, 327, 328
  for parasites, 336
  for periodontal disease, 345, 522
  for phobias, 353
  pregnancy and, 358
  for respiratory illnesses, 377
  for tinnitus, 404
  for TMJ, 402
calcium carbonate, 312
calcium citrate, 312, 328
calculus, 347
calendula, 167, 269, 344, 392, 395
cali chloricum, 346
calluses, 234
camphorus, 490
cancer, 95-111
  bone, 567-68, 581
  brain, 515-17
  causes of, 95-97
  cervical, 575
  colon, 532-33, 576
  colorectal, 527-28
  combination therapies for, 562-67
  Emanuel Revici's therapy for, 576-81
  Essiac tea for, 90, 106, 372, 564, 567-68

herbs and, 105-6, 486
heredity and, 96-97
Hippocrates Health Center and, 568-69
Hodgkin's disease, 530-31, 561-62, 564-65
intestinal asbestos, 583
kidney, 568-69, 581
Lawrence Burton's therapy for, 91, 584-89
leukemia, 563
liver, 489, 527-28, 566, 572, 573, 586
lung, 570, 577-78, 581
lymphatic, 547-48, 569
lymphoma, 565, 576, 582-84, 586-87, 588-89
Max Gerson's therapy for, 387, 570-76
Nicholas Gonzalez's therapy for, 569-70
ovarian, 577-78
pancreatic, 574-75
personal experiences with, 561-89
prostate, 106, 369-74, 526, 529, 563-64, 569, 580-81
psychology and, 97, 108
Reiki and, 547
714-X for, 107, 561-63, 564
skin, 386-88, 571-73, 575
Stanislaw Burzynski's therapy for, 581-84
symptoms of, 97
thyroid, 538
treatment of, 97-108, 486
what to avoid with, 108-11
see also breast cancer; chemotherapy
candida, candidiasis, 112-18, 413, 423, 558
personal experiences with, 443-44
canker sores, 152-53

cantaloupe, 408
capsaicin, 260
capsicum, 30, 336
caraway, 14
carbohydrates:
    diabetes and, 177, 179
    hypoglycemia and, 282
    intolerance of, 321, 323
    obesity and, 323
    see also complex
        carbohydrates
carcinoma, squamous
    cell, 579
cardamom, 243, 356
cardiac arrhythmia, 254
cardiomegaly, 11
cardiovascular system:
    allergies in, 24
    see also heart disease
carnivora (Venus fly
    trap), 68, 90, 107
carotenoids, 220, 326
carotid arteries, 461
carpal tunnel syndrome
    (CTS), 119-21, 457-
    58, 466, 492-93
carrot juice, 5, 391
carsinonima, 71
Carson, Rachel, 109
cartilage, torn, 469
cascara sagrada, 356
casein, 297
cassia, 143
castor oil, 238, 356
catalase, 103
cataracts, 218
caterpillar fungus, 67
catnip, 356, 379
cat's claw, 69, 90, 235, 298
cavitations, 163
cavities, 162-63
cayenne, 48-49, 134, 153,
    188, 220, 260, 280,
    378, 384, 399, 406,
    449
celandine, 284
celery, 5, 353
Centers for Disease
    Control, 59, 127
cerebral palsy, 122-23
cerebrovascular accident

(stroke), 397-400,
    461
cervical cancer, 575
cervical dysplasia, 124-26
CFS, see chronic fatigue
    syndrome
chalazions, 517-18
chamomile, chamomilla,
    14, 116, 189, 192,
    199, 203, 243, 269,
    299, 353, 392, 491
Chan, Dr., 441
Chang, R. S., 65
chaparral, 153, 336, 384,
    387
charcoal, 356
chaste berry, 313
chelate, 312
chelation therapy, 6-7, 51,
    182, 232, 239, 240,
    261-62, 374, 380,
    398, 557
    description of, 454-55
    personal experiences
        with, 455-62
chemicals,
    environmental,
    214-17
chemical sensitivity, 22,
    27-28
chemotherapy, 97-99,
    515-16, 527, 530,
    548, 561, 562, 564,
    565, 566, 567, 569,
    577, 582, 583, 586,
    587
cherry, wild, 30, 378
chestnut, horse, 239, 269
chewing, improper, 194
chickweed, 190
chimaphilia, 373
China remedy, 314
chiropractic, 553
    for arthritis, 52
    for back and neck pain,
        79
    for chronic pain, 146
    description of, 463
    for headaches, 250
    personal experiences
        with, 464-73

for TMJ, 402
chlamydia, 289
chlorella, 10, 166, 340,
    406, 447
chlorhexadine, 452
chlorophyll, 10, 48, 100,
    115, 228, 376, 377,
    391, 477
cholesterol levels, 180,
    278-81, 444
    see also heart disease
choline, 34-35, 57, 243,
    284, 319
chondroitin sulfate, 49
Chopra, Deepak, 433,
    436
chromium, 104, 132, 280,
    284, 287, 345, 371,
    392, 408, 410
chromium picolinate,
    181, 323, 356
chronic fatigue syndrome
    (CFS), 127-38, 480-
    81, 558-59
    causes of, 128-29
    symptoms of, 130
    treatment of, 131-37
chronic obstructive
    pulmonary disease
    (COPD)
    (emphysema), 376,
    552
chronic pain, see pain,
    chronic
chrysanthemums, 250
chymotrypsin, 143
cilantro, 447
cimifuga, 199
cinnamon, 143
circulatory problems:
    in feet and legs, 239-40
    personal experiences
        with, 455-62, 531-32
    UTI and, 415-16
cirrhosis of liver, 533
citrus seed extracts, 63,
    336
Clark, Norman, 454
clary sage, 15, 199, 314,
    340, 361, 400

claudication,
    intermittent, 239-
    40, 456
cleansers, 28, 214, 361-62
Clement, John, 91, 586
clothes, 84
    bras, 87, 308
    footwear, 84, 235, 236,
    240
clover, red, 8, 106, 153,
    156, 271, 477
CMV (cytomegalovirus),
    557
Coca, Dr., 23
cocaine, 397
cocculus, 317
cod liver oil, 49, 346, 415
coenzyme 1 (NADH), 11-
    12, 36, 133
coenzyme Q10, see Q10,
    coenzyme
coffea cruda, 167
coffee:
    enema of, 572, 573
    see also caffeine
Cohen, Alan, 55, 295, 321
cohosh:
    black, 261, 358
    blue, 358
Colborn, Cherie, 409
colcynthis, 198
colds and flu, 154-61
    fever and, 224-25
cold sores (fever blisters),
    152-53, 275
Coley, William, 107
Coley's toxins, 107
colitis, ulcerative, 187,
    545
colloidal silver, 156, 291-
    92
colon, 184, 192, 412
    cancer of, 532-33, 576
    see also intestines
colonics, enemas, 299,
    337, 393, 477, 478,
    480, 572, 573
colon therapy, 7, 51, 117,
    299, 325, 393
    description of, 474
    personal experiences
    with, 475-82

colorectal cancer, 527-28
combination therapies,
    562-67
comfrey, 5, 49, 153, 378,
    477
complex carbohydrates,
    189, 513
    aging and, 9-10
    AIDS and, 60
    diabetes and, 179
    heart disease and, 256
    hypoglycemia and, 283
    obesity and, 323
confidence, 499
congenital heart disease,
    254
congestive heart failure,
    253-54
conium maculatum, 373
constipation, 184, 356,
    412, 477, 479-80,
    481
contact dermatitis, 390,
    395
contraceptives, oral, 110,
    288
Cooksley, Valerie, 160,
    276
Coolmax, 235
COPD (chronic
    obstructive
    pulmonary disease)
    (emphysema), 376,
    552
copper, 251, 371, 399
coptis, 144
coriander, 15
corns, 234
corn silk, 7, 198, 372, 415
Corsello, Dr., 457
corticoid, 329
corticosteroid, 298
cortisone, 46, 52, 542
corydalis, 143, 144
coughs, 159
Coulter, Harris, 55
cramp bark (black haw;
    viburnum), 143,
    199, 358, 379
cranberry, 414
craniosacral therapy, 250,
    402

Creutzfeld-Jakob disease,
    32
Crohn's disease, 184-85,
    554
croton tiglium, 395
cryosurgery, 370
crystal aromatherapy, 508
CTS (carpal tunnel
    syndrome), 119-21,
    457-58, 466, 492-93
Culbert, Michael, 71
curcumin, 145, 271
currant, black, 29, 49,
    100, 157, 258, 313,
    319, 324, 365, 371,
    393
Cushing's disease, 423-24
cyanosis, 254
Cyclovir, 274
cyperus, 143
cyprus, 269, 314, 361
cystic bile duct, 242
cystic fibrosis, 507
cystitis, 415
    interstitial, 413
cysts, 390, 517-18
cytomegalovirus (CMV),
    557

D'Adamo, James, 47
D'Adamo, Peter, 47
dairy products, 108-9,
    186, 251, 297, 312,
    332, 345, 367
dance injuries, 506
dandelion, 8, 190, 198,
    239, 243, 329, 356,
    357
    leaf, 7
    root, 143, 181, 271, 284
daughter seed, 292
Davis, Adele, 519
DDT, 214
deer ticks, 301-5
deglycyrrhizinated
    licorice (DGL), 190
dementia, 32-38
denatured foods, 111
dental disorders, 162-69,
    491
    biological dentistry for,
    166, 320, 441-53

mercury amalgam fillings and, 163, 304, 320, 441-53, 557
personal experiences with, 441-53
see also periodontal disease
Depranil, 36
depression, 170-76, 450
chronic pain and, 147
eating disorders and, 207
homeopathy for, 174-75, 361
pregnancy and, 355, 358, 361
stroke and, 400
dermatitis, 390-91, 394
contact, 390, 395
seborrheic, 391
detoxification:
for allergies, 25-26
antiaging properties of, 4-8
for arthritis, 51
of bowel, 192
for breast cancer, 90-91
for CFS, 136-37
dental disorders and, 442
for environmental illness, 216
of respiratory system, 379
for skin conditions, 393
of specific systems, 7-8
Deutchman, Gary, 468
devil's claw, 49, 238
DGL (deglycyrrhizinated licorice), 190
DHA, 166
DHEA, 35, 103, 261, 299, 313, 329
diabetes, 177-82, 345, 423, 456-57
foot and leg problems with, 231
gestational, 356, 357
Diabinase, 179
diagaku eye drops, 220-21
diarrhea, 185, 356
diet, nutrition:

acidic vs. alkaline, 99-100, 140, 150, 235, 387, 404, 414
personal experiences with, 510-23
rotation, 26, 51
see also specific diseases, foods and drinks
Diflucan, 191
digestive disorders, 183-95
herbs for, 189-90
personal experiences with, 514-15
treatments of, 188-93
what to avoid with, 193-95
see also allergies
digestive enzymes, 29, 191, 442
digestive harmony, 116
dill, 188
dimethyl glycine, 57
dioscorea (wild yam), 143, 190, 261, 272, 313, 329, 356, 468
Dioscorides, 432
dioxin, 210, 214
dioxychlor, 63
diverticulitis, 185, 475-76
dizziness, 513-14
DLPA (dl-phenylalanine), 141, 340
DMAE, 34
DMG, 319
DMPS treatment, 444
dock, yellow, 8, 272, 357, 392
Dodson-Puziss, Sherry, 446-47
dong, 43
dong quai, 143, 144, 229, 292
Donsbach, Dr., 528, 529
dopamine, 339
dowager's hump, 330-31
Doxycycline, 431
Dramamine, 317
driving, 84
Duke, James, 65-66
dulcamara, 159, 275, 395

dysmenorrhea, 196-200
dysplasia, cervical, 124-26

ear, 536-37
infections of, 201-4, 464, 495
tinnitus in, 403-4
eating disorders, 205-8
see also obesity
echinacea:
aging and, 7, 8
for AIDS, 68-69
for allergies, 30
for cancer, 105
for CFS, 134
for cold and canker sores, 153
for colds and flu, 155, 486
for foot and leg problems, 235
for hemorrhoids, 269
for periodontal disease, 344, 449
for sinusitis, 384
for skin conditions, 392
E. coli, 411, 413
eczema, 392, 393
irritant, 390-91
EDTA (ethylene diamine tetraacetic acid), 6, 51, 261-62, 454
educational kinesiology, 352
egg lipids, 63-64
elderberry, 384
electromagnetic radiation (EMR), 87-88, 110, 150
elm, slippery, 144, 156, 186, 269, 357, 378, 415
emphysema (chronic obstructive pulmonary disease), 376, 552
EMR (electromagnetic radiation), 87-88, 110, 150
encephalitis, 295
endometriosis, 209-13, 483

endorphins, 140-41, 145
enemas, colonics, 299,
    337, 393, 477, 478,
    480
  coffee, 572, 573
Energetics, 287
environmental illness,
    214-17, 429-30
Environmental
    Protection Agency,
    109
enzymes, 107, 357, 371
  aging and, 12
  arthritis and, 51
  cancer and, 103-4
  digestive, 29, 191, 442
enzyme therapy, 483-85
EPA fatty acid, 166
ephedra, 397
ephedra vulgaris, 379
epinephrine, 494
episiotomy problems, 357
Epsom salts, 269, 447
Epstein, Paul, 283, 285
Epstein-Barr virus, 273,
    436-37, 441, 457,
    557, 559-60
essential fatty acids, see
    fatty acids, essential
essential oils, 276, 432
    see also aromatherapy;
    specific oils
Essiac, 90, 106, 372, 564,
    567-68
estradiol, 313
estriol, 313
estrogen, 86, 88, 214, 329
  fibroids and, 226, 228,
    229
  headaches and, 246
  infertility and, 288
  plant, 312
  PMS and, 363, 364,
    365, 367
  UTI and, 411, 412
estrogen replacement
    therapy, 328
estrone, 313
ethylene diamine
    tetraacetic acid
    (EDTA), 6, 51, 261-
    62, 454

eucalyptus, 330, 361, 379,
    384, 392
Eupatorium perfoliatum,
    159
euphrasia, 158
Euphytose, 402
evening primrose oil:
  for allergies, 29
  for arthritis, 49
  for athlete's foot, 235
  for colds and flu, 157
  for dysmenorrhea, 197
  for headaches, 250
  for heart disease, 258
  for hepatitis, 271
  menopause and, 313
  for MS, 319
  for obesity, 324
  for periodontal
    disease, 346
  for PMS, 365
  for prostate conditions,
    371
  for skin conditions, 393
exercise:
  aerobic, 263
  for arthritis, 53
  for back and neck pain,
    81-82
  for breast cancer, 90-91
  for CFS, 136
  cholesterol and, 281
  for chronic pain, 145-
    46
  for depression, 172
  for diabetes, 180-81
  for dysmenorrhea, 199
  for eye disorders, 221-
    22
  for fibroids, 228
  for foot and leg
    problems, 232, 236,
    237
  for heart disease, 262-
    63
  lungs and, 7-8
  for lupus, 299
  menopause and, 314-
    15
  for obesity, 324-25
  for osteoporosis, 329-
    32

  for PMS, 365
  pregnancy and, 359
  Rolfing and, 550
  for UTI, 415-16
  weight, 263
eyebright, 181
eye problems, 218-23
  diabetes and, 179, 456
  eye crossing, 221
  personal experiences
    with, 481, 517-18,
    535-36

false unicorn root, 229
Fargelin, 268-69
farsightedness, 219
fasting:
  aging and, 4-6
  for allergies, 25
fat, dietary, 86, 92, 229,
    256, 279, 319, 323
fatty acids, essential, 271
  for AIDS, 64
  in alcoholism
    treatment, 18
  for allergies, 29
  for candidiasis, 115
  for dental disorders,
    166
  for depression, 173
  DLPA, 141, 340
  for heart disease, 258
  menopause and, 312
  for obesity, 323-24
  for PMS, 365
  for skin conditions, 393
    see also omega-3 fatty
    acid
Feldman, Martin, 302
fennel, 14, 189, 293, 314,
    356, 415
fenugreek, 378
ferrum phosphoricum,
    158, 167, 203, 493
ferrum picricum, 373
fever, 224-25
  flu and, 154-61
fever blisters (cold sores),
    152-53, 275
feverfew, 144, 249, 250
fiber, 100, 188, 211, 279,

283-84, 312, 328, 356
fibrocystic conditions, 313
fibroids, 226-30
fibromyalgia, 246, 431, 433-34
fibromyoma uteri, 226
fibrosis:
    cystic, 507
    idiopathic pulmonary, 433-34
figwort, 379
Finman-Nahman, Tova, 117
fish oil, 50, 192, 220, 251, 256, 258, 312, 365
Flagyl, 336, 558
flatulence, 185, 356
flavonoids, 102
flaxseed, 7, 415
    oil, 29, 35-36, 50, 100, 202, 243, 298, 312, 323, 365, 371, 377, 478
Floradix, 42
flu and colds, 154-61
    fever and, 224-25
Fludamide, 370
fluoridation, 165
fluoride, 171
folic acid:
    anemia and, 40, 42
    cancer and, 104
    depression and, 171
    heart disease and, 258
    infertility and, 291
    menopause and, 312
    pregnancy and, 358
folliculinum, 366
food coloring, 380
food poisoning, 490
foot and leg problems, 146, 231-41
    circulatory problems, 239-40
    external, 232-35
    internal, 238-39
    joint pain, 235-36, 536-37, 542-43
    lymphedema, 306-9
    osteoporosis and, 329

personal experiences with, 456, 464-65, 467-69, 509, 531-32, 533-34, 541-43
footwear, 84, 235, 236, 240
fo-ti tieng, 13
Frank, Mark, 202
frankincense, 15
Fredericks, Carlton, 442, 513
fructo-oligosaccharides, 192, 259
fructose litchi, 292
fruits, 189, 323
FSH, 312
Fulton, Susan, 120
fungal infections, 235
fungal rashes, 390
fungus, caterpillar, 67

GABA, 353
gallbladder, 271
gallstones, 242-44
gamma linoleic acid (GLA), 29, 49, 64, 100, 157, 166, 313, 319, 323-24, 365, 371
ganoderma (reishi) mushrooms, 134, 271, 280, 291
gardenia, 198
garlic, 220
    aging and, 8, 10, 13
    for AIDS, 61
    for allergies, 29
    for cancer, 105
    for candidiasis, 115-16
    for CFS, 134
    cholesterol and, 280
    for cold and canker sores, 153
    for dental disorders, 166
    for digestive disorders, 191
    for ear infections, 204
    for heart disease, 260
    for hepatitis, 272
    for lymphedema, 307, 308

for MS, 319
for parasites, 336
for periodontal disease, 344, 346
for respiratory illnesses, 379
for stroke, 399
for trauma, 408
for UTI, 415
gastric reflex, 186
gastrointestinal system:
    allergies in, 24
    bladder and, 229, 411-17
    indigestion and, 14, 183-84
    parasites in, 334-38
    PMS and, 366
    pregnancy and, 356-57, 358
    see also colon; digestive disorders; intestines
gelsemium, 69, 135, 159, 225
general practitioners, 78
genistein, 104
geranium, 400
German chamomile, 116
Gerson, Max, 387, 570-76
Gestalt therapy, 502
gestational diabetes, 356, 357
Giardia lamblia, 336
ginger, 105, 144, 220
    cholesterol and, 280
    for colds and flu, 155-56
    for digestive disorders, 190
    for fibromyalgia, 433, 434
    for heart disease, 260
    for motion sickness, 317
    for osteoporosis, 330
    pregnancy and, 358
    for respiratory illnesses, 378
    for sinusitis, 384
    for trauma, 408
    for TSS, 406

ginger, wild, 143, 144
gingivitis, 163, 342, 346, 347
ginkgo biloba:
  aging and, 13
  for Alzheimer's and dementia, 37-38
  for autism, 57
  cancer and, 105
  for diabetes, 181
  for eye disorders, 220
  for headaches, 250-51
  for heart disease, 260
  for infertility, 293
  for Parkinson's disease, 340
  for respiratory illnesses, 378
  for stroke, 399
ginseng, 13, 30, 292, 406
  American, 372
  cancer and, 105
  panax, 67, 134, 486
  Siberian, 19, 67, 134, 284, 285, 372
GLA (gamma linoleic acid), 29, 49, 64, 100, 157, 166, 313, 319, 323-24, 365, 371
glaucoma, 218, 456
glucosamine, 49-50
glucosamine sulfate, 236
glucose tolerance factor, 284
glutamic acid, 18, 371
glutamine, L-glutamine, 18, 57, 191, 284, 303-4
glutathione, 191, 220, 271, 559
glutathione peroxidase, 64, 103, 377
gluten, 297
glycine, 371
glycyrrhizin (licorice root), 69, 134, 144, 153, 156, 191, 372, 378, 559
Godall, Elmira, 443
Gofman, John, 87
goldenrod, 415

goldenseal:
  for cold and canker sores, 153
  for colds and flu, 155, 486
  for foot and leg problems, 235
  for gallstones, 243
  for hepatitis, 271
  for hypoglycemia, 284
  for parasites, 336
  for periodontal disease, 344, 449
  pregnancy and, 359
  for sinusitis, 384
  for UTI, 144, 415
Goldstone, Martin, 585
Gonzalez, Nicholas, 569-70
Goodheart, George, 429
Gordon, Pat, 40
gotu kola, 13, 220, 239, 298
gout, 236
gouty arthritis, 44
grapefruit seed extract, 63, 191
grape seed extract, 50, 103, 220, 340
grasses, 208
gravel root, 243
green algae, 152
greens:
  aging and, 10
  AIDS and, 61
  cancer and, 100
  eating disorders and, 208
green tea, 101, 156, 198
Gregory, Dick, 510, 521
grinding of teeth, 163
Grout, Pam, 325
Gulf War syndrome, 129
gum disease, see periodontal disease
gynecologists, 79

Hahnemann, Samuel, 488
Haldol, 340
halibut oil, 415
han man chow, 229

haw, black (viburnum; cramp bark), 143, 199, 358, 379
hawthorn, 340, 399, 406
  berry, 220, 260
hay fever, 21
HCA (hydroxy citric acid), 324
HDL's (high-density lipoproteins), 278, 280, 281
headaches, 144, 245-52
  biofeedback for, 148
  herbs for, 143-44, 249
  mercury fillings and, 447-48, 453
  personal experiences with, 439, 447-48, 453, 465, 470, 491, 520, 523
  sinus, 248
  treatment of, 247-51
hearing, 536-37
  tinnitus and, 403-4
heart attacks, 458, 460, 478-79
  stroke vs., 397
heartburn, 357
heart disease, 253-65
  diabetes and, 178-79
  eating disorders and, 206
  herbs for, 260-61
  mercury and, 449-50
  personal experiences with, 455-62, 553
  power of the mind with, 264
  symptoms of, 255
  treatment of, 255-64
  types of, 253-55
heat exhaustion, 266-67
heat stress detoxification, 216
heatstroke, 266-67
heavy metal toxicity, 56, 232, 297, 340, 457-58
heel imbalances, 238
Hellerwork, 212
hemorrhoids, 268-69, 361

hepar sulphuris, 116, 158-59, 168
hepar sulphuris calcareum, 203, 373, 394, 491
hepatitis, 231, 270-72, 426
   personal experiences with, 510-11, 528, 532, 533
herbastatin, 116
herbs, 12
   for AIDS, 65-69
   in alcoholism treatment, 19
   for allergies, 29-30
   for Alzheimer's and dementia, 37-38
   for anemia, 43
   for arthritis, 48-49
   for breast cancer, 90
   for cancer, 90, 105-6, 387
   for candidiasis, 115-16
   for CFS, 133-34
   for cholesterol, 280
   for chronic pain, 143-45
   for cold and canker sores, 153
   for colds and flu, 155-56
   for depression, 173
   description of therapy with, 486-87
   for diabetes, 181
   for digestive disorders, 189-90
   for dysmenorrhea, 198
   for endometriosis, 212
   for eye disorders, 220-21
   for fibroids, 228-29
   for fibromyalgia, 434
   for foot and leg problems, 235
   for headaches, 143-44, 249
   for heart disease, 260-61
   for heat stroke, 267
   for hemorrhoids, 268-69

   for hypoglycemia, 284
   for infertility, 293
   for insomnia, 539
   for lupus, 298
   for lymphedema, 307
   menopause and, 313
   for osteoporosis, 329
   for parasites, 336
   for Parkinson's disease, 340
   for phobias, 353-54
   pregnancy and, 357, 358-59
   for prostate conditions, 371-72
   for sinusitis, 384
   for skin cancer, 387
   for skin conditions, 391-92
   for stroke, 399
   for TMJ, 402
   for TSS, 406
   for UTI, 415
heredity, 96-97, 350, 390
hernias, 424, 493
herpes, 152-53, 273-77, 557
high blood pressure (hypertension), 254, 255-56, 438-39, 456, 459, 461, 552
high-density lipoproteins (HDL's), 278, 280, 281
Hildebrand, Gar, 387
Hippocrates, 474, 486
Hippocrates Health Center, 568-69
HIV, see AIDS and HIV
Hodgkin's disease, 530-31, 561-62, 564-65
Hoffer, Abram, 17
homeopathy, 19
   for AIDS, 69-71
   for arthritis, 52-53
   for candidiasis, 116-17
   for CFS, 134-36
   for colds and flu, 157-59
   for dental disorders, 167-68

   for depression, 174-75, 361
   description of, 488-89
   for diabetes, 182
   for dysmenorrhea, 198-99
   for ear infections, 202-3
   for fever, 224-25
   for heatstroke, 267
   for herpes, 275-76
   menopause and, 313-14
   for motion sickness, 317
   for osteoporosis, 329, 332
   for periodontal disease, 346
   personal experiences with, 430, 489-95
   for PMS, 366
   pregnancy and, 356, 361
   for prostate conditions, 373
   for respiratory illnesses, 379
   sequential, 493-94
   for skin conditions, 394-95
homocysteine, 332
honey, 190, 276, 377
hops, 340, 353
horehound, 30, 379
hormonal imbalance, 468-69
hormonal treatment, balanced, 52
hormone replacement therapy, 110, 311
horse chestnut, 239, 269
horseradish, 188, 336, 378, 384
horsetail, 329, 359
hoxsey herbs, 106
HPV (human papilloma virus), 124
huckleberry (blueberry) leaves, 181, 399
Hudson, Tori, 125, 212
Hufnagel, Vicki, 93, 357

Hugger, Heel, 238
Huggins, Dr., 441
human papilloma virus (HPV), 124
Hydergine, 36-37
hydrangea root, 372
hydrastinum muriaticum, 229
hydrazine sulfate, 107
hydrochloric acid, 42, 243, 377
Hydrofloss, 452
hydrogen peroxide, 337, 344, 380, 524, 534
hydrotherapy, 25, 292-93
hydroxy citric acid (HCA), 324
Hydroxyurea, 382
hygiene products, 27, 214, 234
hyperbaric oxygen therapy, 398, 524
hypercholesterolemia, 279, 286-87
hypericum, 168, 204, 490
hypericum perforatum, 276
hyperopia, 219
hypertension (high blood pressure), 254, 255-56, 438-39, 456, 459, 461, 552
hyperthermia, 566
hyperthyroidism, 512
hypnotherapy, 496-504
    description of, 496-97
    personal experiences with, 497-504
hypoglycemia, 282-85, 345, 357, 512-13, 518-19
hypothyroidism, 33, 56, 57, 129-30, 254, 321-22
    treatment of, 286-87
hyssop, 379
hysterectomy, 210-11, 226-27, 357, 577

IAT (Immuno-Augmentative Therapy), 91, 584-89

ibuprofen, 142, 197, 247
idiopathic pulmonary fibrosis, 433-34
IgG ELISA, 375
ignatia, 69, 159, 174
imagery, 351
immunizations, see vaccinations
Immuno-Augmentative Therapy (IAT), 91, 584-89
immunotherapy, neutralization, 27
Indian snakeroot, 261
indigestion, 183-84
    aromatherapy for, 14
indomethacin, 145
indosin, 107
infections, 233
    arthritis and, 45
    ear, 201-4, 464, 495
    personal experiences with, 491, 526-27, 533-34
    UTI, 144, 411-17
    yeast, 413-14, 425, 483-85
    see also specific infections
infertility, 288-93
inflammatory bowel disease, 191
influenza and colds, 154-61
ingrown toenails, 237
injuries, 142, 237-38, 506, 509
inositol, 35, 57, 243, 319, 353
insomnia, 129, 508, 538-39
    aromatherapy for, 14
insulin, 177-82
interferon, 107, 533
intermittent claudication, 239-40, 456
internists, 78
interstitial cystitis, 413
intestinal flora, 64
intestines:
    cancer of, 583-84
    detoxification of, 7

twisted, 476-77
    see also colon
intravenous peroxide therapy, 524
intrinsic factor, 42
iodadum, 70
iodine, 206, 287
ipecacuanha, 379
iron, 42, 228, 291
    pregnancy and, 358
irritable bowel syndrome, 186, 189
irritant eczema, 390-91
iscador, 107
ischemic optic neuropathy, 535-36
isoflavones, 365

jamaica weed, 271-72
jasmine, 361
jelly, royal, 285, 406
Jensen, Bernard, 476
jet lag, 317
jock itch, 390
joint pain, 235-36, 536-37, 542-43
    see also arthritis
Jones, Kenneth, 115-16
Joseph, John, 410
juice, 11
    aging and, 4-6
    for AIDS, 61
    for arthritis, 47-48
    for cancer, 101
    for CFS, 131
    for chronic pain, 140
    for lymphedema, 307
    for respiratory illnesses, 376
    for sinusitis, 383
    for skin conditions, 391
    for tinnitus, 403
juniper, 15, 359, 415
juvenile rheumatoid arthritis, 44

kali bichromicum, 159
kali muriaticum, 203
kali phosphoricum, 135
Kaplan, Robert Michael, 221
Kaposi's sarcoma, 579

kava kava, 144, 353-54
kelp, 10, 261, 292
Keuneke, Robin, 484
Keyes, Dr., 451
kidneys, 231, 236
    cancer of, 568-69, 581
    chelation therapy and,
        454, 456
    detoxification of, 7
    diabetes and, 179, 180
    skin conditions and,
        389, 391, 392, 393
    UTI and, 412, 413
kinesiology, 250
    applied, 23, 429-31
    educational, 352
kola nut, 324
Konlee, Mark, 62
Korins, Kevin, 69
kreosotum, 116
Krieger, Dolores, 149
ku shen, 116, 336

laccaninum, 366
lachasis, 366
lactobacillus, 152, 274
Lactobacillus
    acidophilus, 192
lady's slipper, 340, 353
larch arabinogalactan,
    108
l-arginine, 258
lavender, 14, 199, 249,
    264, 276, 299, 340,
    379, 392, 400, 505
laxatives, 184
l-carnitine, 258, 284, 291,
    324
l-cysteine, 319, 377
LDL's (low-density
    lipoproteins), 278-
    79, 281
lead poisoning, 457-58
leaky gut syndrome, 22
learning disorders, 294-
    97
lecithin, 18, 34-35, 243,
    258, 280, 324, 393,
    399
leg problems, see foot and
    leg problems
legustrum, 67

leiomyoma uteri, 226
lei wan, 336
lemon, 14, 63, 269, 361,
    400, 414
lentinan, 106
leptotania, 67-68
leukemia, 563
Levin, Dr., 458
l-glutamine, glutamine,
    18, 57, 191, 284,
    303-4
LH, 312
licorice, 186, 190, 378,
    434, 486
    root (glycyrrhizin), 69,
        134, 144, 153, 156,
        191, 372, 378, 559
Liefman, Robert, 52
life plant (phyllantius),
    69, 271
light therapy, 174
lilac, 299
lily of the valley, 260
lime seed extract, 63
linoleic acid, 279
linseed oil, 238
lipids, egg, 63-64
lipoma, 518-19
lipoproteins, 278
live cell therapy, 72
liver, 19, 87, 102, 173,
    190, 211, 229, 231,
    239, 243, 280
    beet juice and, 5
    cancer and, 489, 527-
        28, 566, 572, 573,
        586
    cirrhosis of, 533
    dental disorders and,
        446, 447, 449
    detoxification of, 7
    hypoglycemia and, 284
    personal experiences
        with problems of,
        465-66, 489
    skin conditions and,
        389, 391, 393
    see also hepatitis
liver concentrate, 287
l-lysine, 152, 274
l-methionine, methione,

18, 243, 284, 332,
    377
lobelia, 271, 378
lomacium, 134
Lombardi, Susan, 6
lotus root, 384
low-density lipoproteins
    (LDL's), 278-79,
    281
l-tryptophane,
    tryptophane, 36,
    353
Lucidril, 37
lungs:
    cancer of, 570, 577-78,
        581
    detoxification of, 7-8
Lungtanxieganwan, 249,
    365
lungwort, 378, 379
Lupron, 227, 370
lupus, 298-300, 570
    see also allergies;
        arthritis
Lycium rehmannia, 221
lycopene, 10
lycopodium, 135, 356
Lyme disease, 301-5, 431,
    457
lymphatic system, 87, 508
    cancer of, 547-48, 569
    detoxification of, 8
    manual drainage of,
        306
lymphedema, 306-9
lymphoma, 565, 576, 582-
    84, 586-87, 588-89

McCabe, Ed, 526
McDonagh, Dr., 462
McQueen, Steve, 583
macrobiotic foods, 101
macular degeneration,
    219
Magidson, Elaine, 350
magnesia phosphorica,
    198-99
magnesium:
    for Alzheimer's and
        dementia, 35
    for autism, 57

magnesium (*cont.*)
for back and neck pain, 83
for CFS, 132-33
cholesterol and, 280
for dental disorders, 165
depression and, 171, 173
for diabetes, 181
for digestive disorders, 188, 191
for dysmenorrhea, 197
for foot and leg problems, 238
for headaches, 246, 250-51
for heart disease, 259
for hemorrhoids, 268
for learning disorders, 295-96
menopause and, 312
for MS, 319
for osteoporosis, 328
for parasites, 336
for periodontal disease, 345, 522
for phobias, 353
for PMS, 364
for prostate conditions, 371
for respiratory illnesses, 377
for stroke, 398
for tinnitus, 404
for TMJ, 402
for trauma, 408, 409
magnetic healing:
for chronic pain, 149
for dental disorders, 451
for foot and leg problems, 235
for lymphedema, 307
for MS, 319
for respiratory illnesses, 380
for skin conditions, 393
ma huang, 359
malabsorption syndrome, 186
malaria, 520-21

malic acid, 250
mallow, 190
Mandell, Marshall, 296
manganese, 83, 165, 345
manual lymphatic drainage, 306
margarine, 264-65
marigolds, 344
marjoram, 14, 199, 220, 264, 340
marshmallow, 269
root, 278, 415
Martin, William, 307
massage therapy, 80, 237-38, 402
description of, 505
for headaches, 248
for lupus, 299
lymphatic, 8
personal experiences with, 505-9
pregnancy and, 360
see also reflexology
maxepa, 259
meat, 229, 337
cancer and, 108
meditation, 91-92, 136, 553-55
medorrhinum, 70
melanoma, 571-73, 575
melatonin, 36, 91-92, 103, 317
melia, 143
Mellaril, 340
melon, bitter, 67
melon juices, 6
memory loss, 15, 548
menopause, 310-16, 450
candidiasis and, 113
depression and, 174-75
UTI and, 411, 412
menstrual pain, 196-200, 481
herbs for, 143
personal experiences with, 436-37
menstruation, 480
endometriosis and, 210
headaches and, 246
hypothyroidism and, 286
infertility and, 292

see also menopause; premenstrual syndrome
mercurius, 70, 203, 491
mercurius solubilis, 168, 346
mercurius vivus, 158
mercury, 33
in fillings, 163, 304, 320, 441-53, 557
methionine, l-methione, 18, 243, 284, 332, 377
migraine headaches, *see* headaches
milk thistle, 7, 19, 190, 239, 243, 271, 533
minerals:
aging and, 12
in alcoholism treatment, 18
allergies and, 29
Alzheimer's, dementia and, 33
arthritis and, 50
autism and, 56
diabetes and, 181
eating disorders and, 207-8
ming mu, 221
mint, 144
mistletoe, 90, 260
molasses, unsulfured, 406
monosodium glutamate (MSG), 245, 251, 380
morning sickness, 355-56, 358
Moss, Ralph, 98
motherwort, 260
motion sickness, 317
Motrin, 46, 542
MS (multiple sclerosis), 318-20, 411, 471-72, 491-92, 495, 497
MSG (monosodium glutamate), 245, 251, 380
Mucokehl, 182
mullein, 190, 379
oil, 204
mullein leaf, 30

multiple myeloma, 587-88

multiple sclerosis (MS), 318-20, 411, 471-72, 491-92, 495, 497

muriaticum acid, 135

muscle tightness, chronic, 508-9

mushrooms:
AIDS and, 61
cancer and, 101

myeloma, multiple, 587-88

myelosis, 227

myocarditis, 254

myoma coagulation, 227

myomectomy, 226

myopia, 219

myrrh, 235, 276, 344, 378

n-acetyl-cysteine, 36, 104, 377

NADH (nicotinamide adenine dinucleotide), 11-12, 36, 133

Naltrexone, 72

naoili, 15

Naprosyn, 542

National Cancer Institute, 105, 584

natmur, 314, 366, 494

natrum muriaticum, 158, 174, 275

natrum sulphuricum, 379

naturopathy, 125

nearsightedness, 219

neck pain, see back and neck pain

neroli, 299

nervines, 340, 353, 379

nervous system balance, 437

nettles, 49, 190, 269, 329, 357, 378, 392
stinging, 30, 134

neural tube defects, 358

neurolinguistic programming, 351-52

neurologists, 79

neuromuscular therapy, 53

neuropathy:
ischemic optic, 535-36
peripheral, 231-32

neurosurgeons, 78-79

neutralization immunotherapy, 27

Newman, Lynn, 392

niacin (vitamin B3), 173, 220, 251, 259, 280, 319

niacinamide (vitamin B3), 50, 132, 287

nickel, 390

nicotinamide adenine dinucleotide (NADH), 11-12, 36, 133

nitric acid, 314

nitricium acidum, 346

Norden, Michael, 174

Norman, Laura, 366, 545

nose:
fractured, 556-57
runny, 523

Null, Gary, 513-14, 517, 518, 519

nutrition, see diet, nutrition; specific diseases, foods and drinks

nux vomica, 19, 135, 159, 356

Nystatin, 191

oats, 134, 190, 392

obesity, 207, 321-26, 498, 501, 511-12

obstetricians, 79

Olestra, 326

olive oil, 100, 204

Olson, Sharon, 276

omega-3 fatty acid:
for Alzheimer's and dementia, 36
for arthritis, 50
for depression, 173
for digestive disorders, 192
for ear infections, 202
for eye disorders, 220

for gallstones, 243

for headaches, 251

for heart disease, 256, 258

for lupus, 298

menopause and, 312

obesity and, 323-24

for phobias, 353

for prostate conditions, 371

for respiratory illnesses, 376

omega 6 fatty acid, 100, 173, 220, 256, 258, 312, 323, 324

onions, 10, 336

opium, 494

orange seed extract, 63

Oregon grape, 116, 243
root, 144, 271, 392

origanum, 190

Orinase, 179

Ornish, Dean, 256

orthopedic doctors, 78

orthotics, 236

osha root, 67-68, 359

osteoarthritis, 44, 235-36, 472-73

osteocalcin, 328

osteopathic physicians, 119-20, 402

osteoporosis, 12, 312, 327-33, 455

ovarian cancer, 577-78

oxygen therapy, 524-34
hyperbaric, 398, 524
see also ozone therapy

ozone therapy, 71, 232
for cancer, 106
for foot and leg problems, 233, 236, 238, 239-40
for Lyme disease, 304
personal experiences with, 510-11, 526-34, 560, 566
for sickle cell anemia, 382

PACT, 370

Page, Linda Rector, 243, 406

pain, chronic, 139-51
  acupuncture for, 147-48
  biofeedback for, 148-49
  causes of, 139
  chiropractic for, 146, 469-70
  exercises for, 145-46
  herbs for, 143-45
  home remedies for, 146-47
  magnetic healing for, 149
  personal experiences with, 426, 431, 469-70, 493-94
  psychology and, 147
  therapeutic touch for, 149-50
  treatment of, 140-50
  what to avoid with, 150
  see also back and neck pain; joint pain
Palmar, B. J., 463
palmetto, saw, 372
palmitate, 392
panax ginseng, 67, 134, 486
pancreas, 177, 285
  cancer of, 574-75
pancreatic enzymes, 107
pantothenic acid (vitamin B5), 18, 29, 50, 285, 312, 408, 409
papain, 143, 243
papayas, 143, 357
parasites, 194, 334-38
parathyroid gland, 327
parathyroids, 329
Parkinson's disease, 339-41, 391
parsley, 7, 415
passionflower, 353
pau d'arco, 115-16, 191, 272, 298, 387
PCO's, 340
pectin, 279
pennyroyal, 359
Pepper, Claude, 571

peppermint, 15, 276, 356, 358, 384, 400, 505
  oil of, 192, 249, 264, 314, 356, 357, 384
peptic ulcers, 186-87
periodontal disease, 141, 163, 342-48
  personal experiences with, 443, 448-49, 451-53, 522
peripheral neuropathy, 231-32
peristalsis, 356
Perry, Dolores, 511, 515, 518
personal hygiene products, 27, 214, 234
pesticides, 27-28, 109, 340
petroleum, 275
pets, 337-38, 494
phenylalanine, 36
philodendron, 198
phlebitis, 239
phobias, 349-54
phosphatidylcholine, 243
phosphatidylserine, 36, 340
phosphoric acid, 70, 135
phosphorus, 89-90, 239, 275, 314, 327, 371
phyllanthius (life plant), 69, 271
physiatrists, 79
physical therapists, 79-80
phytoestrogens, 89, 315, 365
phytoprogesterones, 315
phytosterols, 372
piles (hemorrhoids), 268-69, 361
pine:
  bark extract, 220
  white, 340, 378
pineapple, 142-43, 377
  juice of, 6, 48, 383
Piracetam, 37
Pitoway, Ken, 492
Pittman, John, 526
pituitary tumors, 423-24
Pixley, Charles, 561
Pizzorno, John, 292-93

plantain, 190
plantar warts, 392
plants, household, 249
pleurisy, 445-46
PMS (premenstrual syndrome), 143, 363-68, 401
pneumonia, 445-46, 480
poison ivy, 390, 392, 395
poison oak, 390, 392
polio, 512-13, 519
pollen, bee, 42, 57, 152, 238, 371, 377, 399, 406
polyatomic aphoresis, 525
poplar bark, tulip, 133
poria cocos, 134
pork, 54
post-polio syndrome, 512-13
post-traumatic stress disorder, 409-10
posture, 84, 146
potassium, 35, 181, 206, 259, 324, 404, 408, 409
potato juice, 48
Prednisone, 46, 298, 318
pregnancy, 209
  anemia and, 40-41
  candidiasis and, 113
  depression and, 355, 358, 361
  fibroids and, 227
  personal experiences with, 466, 493
  problems with, 355-62
  TMJ and, 401
  UTI and, 415
Premarin, 311
premenstrual syndrome (PMS), 143, 363-68, 401
Pressman, Allen, 82
pressure point therapy, 119, 137, 247-48, 367
Price, Shirley, 14
prickly ash bark, 49
primrose oil, 100

see also evening
primrose oil
probiotics, 192
Proffman, Dr., 469
progesterone, 86, 88, 313,
329, 361, 363-64,
365, 411
progressive relaxation
training, 402
promiscuity, 110
propolis, 344
bee, 152, 153, 156, 190,
274
Proscar, 370
prostaglandins, 196, 197,
365, 372, 395
prostate, 206
cancer of, 106, 369-74,
526, 529, 563-64,
569, 580-81
conditions of, 369-74
prostate glandulars, 371
protease, 142-43
proteins:
digestive disorders
and, 194-95
obesity and, 322
pregnancy and, 358
proteolytic enzymes, 371
protozoa, 334, 336
Prozac, 363
psoriasis, 389-90, 391,
392, 393, 435, 464
psoriatic arthritis, 44
psychodrama, 502
psychological factors:
Alzheimer's disease
and, 13, 32-38
autism and, 55-58, 297
cancer and, 97, 108
chronic pain and, 147
hypnotherapy and,
497-99, 502-4
hypothyroidism and,
286
parasites and, 335
phobias and, 349-54
PMS and, 363-68
qi gong and, 537-38,
539-40
tai chi and, 554-55
trauma and, 408-10

see also depression
psychoneuroimmunology,
91-92
psychotherapy, 172
psyllium, 7, 117, 192, 324,
356, 379, 476, 478
puirogenium, 491
pulsatilla, 116, 159, 175,
199, 203, 366, 394
pumpkin, 312, 336, 371,
372
purification lodge, 409-10
pycnogenol, 28, 152, 191,
399
pygeum africanum, 372
pyridoxine, *see* vitamin B6
Pyrogenium, 71

qi gong, 535-40
Q10, coenzyme:
for Alzheimer's and
dementia, 34
for autism, 57
for cancer, 103
for CFS, 133
for cold and canker
sores, 153
for dental disorders,
166, 442
for digestive disorders,
191
for heart disease, 257-
58
for MS, 319
for periodontal
disease, 345-46,
448, 449, 522
for respiratory
illnesses, 378
for stroke, 399
quar gum, 324
quercetin, 18, 28, 152,
191, 271, 280, 377

radiation, 87, 110, 362,
515, 530, 561, 565,
566, 567, 586, 587
ragweed, 21
Rapp, Doris, 296
rashes, 234-35, 301, 390,
423, 444
raspberry leaf, 358

red, 293
reconstruction, 227
reconstructive therapy,
53, 119-21, 541-43
red clover, 8, 106, 153,
156, 271, 477
red raspberry leaf, 293
reflexology:
for colds and flu, 160
colon therapy and, 474
for eye disorders, 222
for headaches, 248-49
personal experiences
with, 544-45
for PMS, 366-67
for prostate conditions,
373
for sinusitis, 384-85
for skin conditions, 393
regression, 502
Reich's technology, 563
Reiki, 15, 546-48
reishi (ganoderma)
mushrooms, 134,
271, 280, 291
relaxation, 402
for CFS, 136
for phobias, 351
resentment, 498-99
Resnik, Dr., 451
respiratory illness, 375-81
asthma, 375, 377, 378,
380, 494-95, 558
respiratory system:
allergies in, 24
detoxification of, 379
Revici, Emanuel, 72-75,
140, 576-81
Reye's syndrome, 224
rheumatic fever, 254
rheumatic heart disease,
254
rheumatoid arthritis, 44,
236, 461, 521-22
rheumatologists, 79, 431
rhododendron, 52
rhumex crispus, 159
rhus toxicodendron, 52,
395, 492
riboflavin, 11, 251
ringworm, 390
Ritalin, 295

Robbins, Dr., 469, 556
Rogers, Sherry, 444
Rolfing, 80, 549-50
Roman chamomile, 14
Rooney, Diane, 384-85
root canal therapy, 165
rose, 15, 199, 400
rosemary, 15, 144-45, 188, 238, 276, 330, 400
rotation diet, 26, 51
Rottino, Antonio, 585
royal jelly, 285, 406
runny nose, 523
rutin, 280

sabal serrulata, 373
sabina, 314
SAD (seasonal affective disorder), 174
safflower oil, 312
sage, 238, 276, 330, 505
clary, 15, 199, 314, 340, 361, 400
St. John's wort, 69, 173
salvia, 143
sandalwood, 199
sanguinaria, 387
sarcoma, Kaposi's, 579
sarsaparilla, 14, 198
sauna, 8
saw palmetto, 372
Scarchilli, Dr., 459
Schachter, Michael, 302, 303, 460, 565, 566
Schauss, Alex, 296
Schwank, Dr., 472
Schweitzer, Albert, 575
sciatica, 145, 466, 467-68, 470-71
sea sickness, 317
seasonal affective disorder (SAD), 174
sea vegetables, 10, 207-8, 323
seaweed, 101
seborrheic dermatitis, 391
secale, 314
Seidman, Barry, 499, 501, 502, 503
selenium, 11, 35, 57, 103,

212, 220, 259, 271, 291, 295-96, 371, 399
self-hypnosis, 503
senna, 356
sepia, 174-75, 314, 356
sequential homeopathy, 493-94
sesame oil, 312, 328
Sessions, Dr., 455, 456
714-X, 107, 561-63, 564
sexual relations, 110
hypothyroidism and, 286
infertility and, 288-93
menopause and, 311
UTI and, 411, 416
sexual transmitted diseases, see AIDS and HIV; herpes
shark cartilage, 64, 104, 238
shark liver oil, 104
shepherd's purse, 228
shiatsu, 80, 508, 551-52
shi hu, 220-21
shingles, 273, 275-76
Shinitksy, Meier, 64
showers, warm and cold, 43
Siberian ginseng, 19, 67, 134, 284, 285, 372
sickle cell anemia, 382
Siebert, Marjorie, 112
silica, 116, 165, 168, 327
silver, colloidal, 156, 291-92
Silverman, Dr., 431
silymarin, 19, 243, 271
Simonton, Carl, 91, 108
Sinclair, Thomas, 383-84
sinus problems, 159, 248, 361, 383-85, 444
see also allergies; headaches
sitz baths, 416
skin:
brushing of, 8, 43
detoxification of, 8
skin conditions, 389-96
acne, 389, 391, 392, 393, 394
allergies, 24

athlete's foot, 235, 390
cancer, 386-88, 571-73, 575
dermatitis, 390-91, 394, 395
dry skin, 233-34
personal experiences with, 423, 424-25, 466
psoriasis, 389-90, 391, 392, 393, 435, 464
rashes, 234-35, 301, 390, 423, 444
skullcap, 143, 340, 353, 379
slippery elm, 144, 156, 186, 269, 357, 378, 415
Smith, Lyndon, 296
snakeroot, Indian, 261
SOD (superoxide dismutase), 10, 50, 103
sodium, 5
sodium nitrate, 245, 251
sodium selenite, 319
soidago virgaurea, 379
solar plexus, 193
Solu-Medrol, 318
soybean products, 101
menopause and, 310, 312
spasmodic torticollis, 506
spirulina, 10, 42, 324, 340, 406
spleen, UTI and, 412-13
spondylitis, ankylosing, 44
spongia tosta, 379
sports, 523
injuries in, 142, 237-38, 506, 509
medicine specialists, 79
spruce, 278
squamous cell carcinoma, 579
Staphylococcus aureus, 405-7
staphysagria, 168, 373, 494
star fruit juice, 48
Stelazine, 340

Stern, Eli, 557
steroids, 298, 318
stinging nettles, 30, 134
stomach problems, 5
  pain, 144, 537-38
Strauss, Charlotte
    Gerson, 571, 572
strawberry leaves, 392
stress, 512
  aging and, 15
  asthma and, 375
  cholesterol and, 281
  dental disorders and,
    163-64
  digestive disorders
    and, 192-93, 194
  dysmenorrhea and,
    199
  eating disorders and,
    206
  headaches and, 247
  lupus and, 299
  massage and, 507, 509
  personal experiences
    with, 536, 540, 552
  pregnancy and, 362
  respiratory illnesses
    and, 379
  skin conditions and,
    390, 395
  TMJ and, 401
  trauma and, 408-10
stretching, 145-46, 199,
  238
stroke, 397-400, 461
  heart attacks vs., 397
sugar, 347
  addiction to, 502-3
  candidiasis and, 114
  hypoglycemia and, 283
  PMS and, 367
  pregnancy and, 356
sulfites, 380
sulphur, 19, 394
sulphur amino acids, 296
sunflower seeds, 371
sunstroke, 266-67
superoxide dismutase
    (SOD), 10, 50, 103
Superskin, 232
supplements, *see specific*

diseases and
supplements
Swank, Dr., 318
sweat lodge, 409-10
sweet fennel, 14
Swiss irrigator, 451-52
syphilinum, 70

Tacrin, 37
tai chi chuan, 553-55
tansy, 260-61
taste, loss of, 206
taurine, 36, 243, 259
TB (tuberculosis), 424
tea tree oil, 117, 235, 276,
    302, 344
teeth, *see* dental disorders
temporomandibular
    joint (TMJ)
    dysfunction, 401-2
tetracycline, 392
therapeutic touch, 149-50
Thermax, 235
Thermostat, 235
thistle, milk, 7, 19, 190,
    239, 243, 271, 533
Thorazine, 340, 470
thuja, 70, 373
thyme, 378, 379, 384, 392
thymus glandulars, 104
thyroid, 27, 206, 231, 286-
    87, 468, 512
  cancer of, 538
  hypothyroidism and,
    33, 56, 57, 129-30,
    254, 286-87, 321-22
thyroid supplements, 9
ticitum acid, 135-36
ticks, deer, 301-5
tinea cruris, 390
tinea versicolor, 390
tinnitus, 403-4
TMJ
    (temporomandibular
    joint) dysfunction,
    401-2
tobacco products, 88,
    109, 126, 284, 332
tobaccum, 317
toenails, ingrown, 237
tofu, 197, 256
Tolinase, 179

torticollis, spasmodic,
    506
toxemia, 493
toxic shock syndrome
    (TSS), 405-7
TPA, 398
Trahan, Christopher,
    143, 487
trauma, 408-10, 493-94,
    549-50, 556-57
tremors, 339
triglycerides, 278, 280
Triple Estrogen, 313
trypsin, 143
tryptophane, l-
    tryptophane, 36,
    353
TSS (toxic shock
    syndrome), 405-7
tuberculosis (TB), 424
tulip poplar bark, 133
tumors, 499-500
  see also cancer
turmeric, 105, 260, 271
tyramine, 245, 251
tyrosine, 36, 133, 287

ukrain, 107
ulcerative colitis, 187, 545
ulcers, 531-32
  peptic, 186-87
  varicose, 239
uncaria tomensoa, 372
urinary tract infection
    (UTI), 144, 411-17
urine therapy, 72
usnea, 134
uterus, 209-13
  bleeding in, 226-30
  cancer of, 328
UTI (urinary tract
    infection), 144,
    411-17
utica urens, 395
uva ursi, 372, 415

vaccinations, 55, 295
  CFS and, 128-29
  individualized, 106-7
valerian, 19, 143-44, 249,
    261, 340, 353, 379
Valium, 363, 471

vanadium, 345
vanadyl sulfate, 181
varicose ulcers, 239
varicose veins, 239, 361
varicosities, 531
vegetables, 188, 283, 328
   AIDS and, 60-61
   cruciferous, 100
   menopause and, 312
   sea, 10, 207-8, 323
Venus fly trap
   (carnivora), 68, 90,
   107
Vergara, Nilsa, 546-48
vervain, blue, 145
Veterans Administration,
   409
viburnum (black haw;
   cramp bark), 143,
   199, 358, 379
viburnum opulus, 143
Vietnam War, 409-10,
   470-71
vision problems, *see* eye
   problems
vision therapy, 221
vitamins:
   Alzheimer's, dementia
   and, 33
   autism and, 56
   personal experiences
   with, 556-60
   stroke and, 399
vitamin A:
   aging and, 11
   for arthritis, 49
   for back and neck pain,
   83
   for cancer, 102
   for CFS, 559
   for cold and canker
   sores, 152-53
   for dental disorders,
   165
   for eye disorders, 220
   for fibroids, 228
   for foot and leg
   problems, 233
   obesity and, 323, 326
   for periodontal
   disease, 345, 346

for prostate conditions,
   371
   for skin conditions,
   391, 392, 393
   for tinnitus, 404
   for UTI, 415
vitamin B complex, 517,
   556
   in alcoholism
   treatment, 18
   for allergies, 29
   for arthritis, 50
   for back and neck pain,
   83
   for candidiasis, 115
   for CFS, 132
   for chronic pain, 141
   for cold and canker
   sores, 152
   for depression, 171,
   173
   for digestive disorders,
   191
   for ear infections, 202
   endometriosis and, 211
   for eye disorders, 220
   for hepatitis, 271
   for herpes, 274
   hypoglycemia and,
   283, 284
   infertility and, 288
   menopause and, 312
   for periodontal
   disease, 448
   for phobias, 353
   for PMS, 364
   for respiratory
   illnesses, 377
   for stroke, 399
   for TMJ, 402
   for trauma, 408-9
vitamin B1, 141
vitamin B2, 287
vitamin B3:
   niacin, 173, 220, 251,
   259, 280, 319
   niacinamide, 50, 132,
   287
vitamin B5 (pantothenic
   acid), 18, 29, 50,
   285, 312, 408, 409
vitamin B6 (pyridoxine):

for acne, 393
   for AIDS, 63, 64-65
   for autism, 57
   for CFS, 132
   cholesterol and, 280
   for headaches, 250
   for hypoglycemia, 284
   for infertility, 291
   for learning disorders,
   296
   menopause and, 312
   for MS, 319
   for PMS, 364
   pregnancy and, 355,
   358
   for prostate conditions,
   371
vitamin B12:
   for anemia, 39-40, 42
   for chronic pain, 141
   for heart disease, 258
   for hepatitis, 271
   for infertility, 291
   for MS, 319
   for parasites, 336
   pregnancy and, 358
vitamin C (ascorbic acid),
   271, 556
   aging and, 9, 11
   for AIDS, 62
   in alcoholism
   treatment, 18
   for allergies, 28
   for Alzheimer's and
   dementia, 35
   for arthritis, 49
   for autism, 57
   for back and neck pain,
   83
   for cancer, 102
   for candidiasis, 115
   for CFS, 132, 559
   cholesterol and, 280
   for cold and canker
   sores, 152, 153
   for colds and flu, 156
   for dental disorders,
   141, 165, 442, 443,
   444, 451
   for depression, 173
   for digestive disorders,
   191

for ear infections, 202
for endometriosis, 211
for eye disorders, 220
for fibroids, 228
for foot and leg
  problems, 232, 235,
  236, 238, 239
for gallstones, 243
for heart disease, 257
for hemorrhoids, 268
for hepatitis, 528
hypoglycemia and,
  284, 285
for infection, 527
for infertility, 292
menopause and, 312
for MS, 319
for obesity, 324
for osteoporosis, 328
for Parkinson's disease,
  340
for periodontal
  disease, 345, 346,
  448, 449, 522
for PMS, 364
pregnancy and, 358
for prostate conditions,
  371
for respiratory
  illnesses, 377, 378
for sinusitis, 383-84
for skin conditions, 391
for stroke, 399
for trauma, 408, 409,
  556
for UTI, 414, 415
vitamin D, 89-90, 165,
  220, 233, 291, 312,
  319, 326, 329, 393,
  404
vitamin E:
  aging and, 11
  for allergies, 29
  for Alzheimer's and
    dementia, 35
  for arthritis, 49
  for autism, 57
  for cancer, 103
  for CFS, 132
  cholesterol and, 280
  for cold and canker
    sores, 153

for dental disorders,
  165
for digestive disorders,
  191
for endometriosis, 212
for eye disorders, 220
for fibroids, 228
for foot and leg
  problems, 233, 236,
  239
for heart disease, 257,
  260
for hemorrhoids, 269
for hepatitis, 271
for hypoglycemia, 284
for infertility, 291
menopause and, 312
for MS, 319
obesity and, 323, 326
for periodontal
  disease, 345, 449,
  522
for PMS, 364
pregnancy and, 358
for respiratory
  illnesses, 378
for skin conditions, 393
for stroke, 399
for tinnitus, 404
vitamin K, 271, 326, 328,
  355
Vitex, 313
Vogeler, Sara, 53, 506,
  507

walnut, black, 115, 298,
  336
warrior's grass, 229
warts, 233
  plantar, 392
water, 11, 256-57, 265,
  337
  pregnancy and, 356,
    358
  skin conditions and,
    391
  UTI and, 414, 416
Watts, Dr., 451
We Care Health Center,
  6
weight exercises, 263
wheat bran, 192

wheat germ, 406
wheatgrass, 340, 406
wheat products, 186, 518,
  520
white ash, 228-29
white pine, 340, 378
white willow bark, 49,
  144, 212
wild cherry, 30, 378
wild ginger, 143, 144
wild yam (dioscorea),
  143, 190, 261, 272,
  313, 329, 356, 468
Williams, Michael, 99
willow bark, white, 49,
  144, 212
windflower, 203
wintergreen, 372, 392
witch hazel, 269, 392
women:
  anemia in, 40-41
  hypnotherapy for, 496
  osteoporosis in, 327-33
  parasites in, 335
  phobias in, 349
  TMJ in, 401
  UTI in, 411-17
  see also menopause;
    menstruation;
    pregnancy;
    premenstrual
    syndrome
Women's Harmony, 365
wood betony, 144, 272
worms, 334
wormwood, 292
wounds, 233
wrinkles, 10

xenoestrogens, 87, 214
Xiao Yao Wan, 90, 198,
  249, 365
X-rays, 87

yam, wild (dioscorea),
  143, 190, 261, 272,
  313, 329, 356, 468
yam extract, 313
yeast:
  brewer's, 406
  candidiasis and, 114

yeast infections, 413-14, 425
    personal experiences with, 483-85
yellow dock, 8, 272, 357, 392
yellow dye #5, 380
yerba mate, 324
ylang ylang, 14, 264
yoga, 80, 263, 330-31, 379
yogurt, 152, 274, 345
yucca, 49, 238
yudaiwan, 116
Yunnan Pai Yao, 198
Yurkovsky, Dr., 461

zhang yan, 221
zinc:
    aging and, 11

for allergies, 29
for Alzheimer's and dementia, 35
for back and neck pain, 83
for cancer, 104
for CFS, 132
for cholesterol, 280
for cold and canker sores, 152
for dental disorders, 165
for diabetes, 181
for ear infections, 202
eating disorders and, 205-6, 207
for hypoglycemia, 284, 285
for hypothyroidism, 287

infertility and, 289, 291, 292
for learning disorders, 296
menopause and, 312
for periodontal disease, 448
for PMS, 364
pregnancy and, 358
for prostate conditions, 370-71
for sinusitis, 384
for skin conditions, 392
for tinnitus, 404
for trauma, 408, 409
for UTI, 415
zinc picolinate, 57, 384
Zovirax, 274

NEW YORK TIMES BESTSELLING AUTHOR

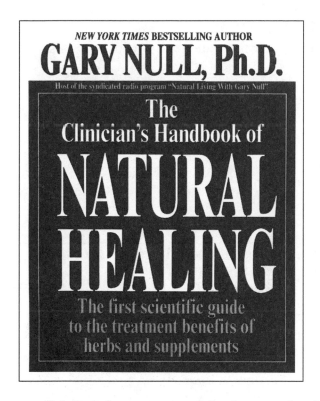

The Clinician's Handbook of Natural Healing
By Gary Null, Ph.D.
$25.00
880 pages

The companion reference to *The Complete Encyclopedia of Natural Healing,* is based on ten years of painstaking analysis of 1.3 million scientific peer review studies done by qualified researchers and published in major journals. For the first time ever, alternative and traditional doctors, nutritionists, and other health professionals have easy access to the solid scientific research justifying the use of natural supplements in the treatment of illness. Nutritionist, author, and national radio host Dr. Gary Null combines for the first time in one volume all of the important peer-review scientific studies that explore the impact of nutrients on major medical conditions to bring you the evidence that alternative healing can prevent and treat major diseases. This authoritative handbook is written in an accessible manner so both laymen and professionals can easily use it.

ISBN#: 1-57566-720-7

Turn to the next page to place an order…

To Order *The Clinician's Handbook of Natural Healing*

The Clinician's Handbook of Natural Healing
ISBN #: 1-57566-720-7   Price: $25.00

(If ordering via mail please complete this order form and mail it with remittance to the address provided below):

Quantity of Books	Unit Price	Total

Subtotal	$
8.25 % Sales Tax (NY only)	$
8.25 % Sales Tax (TN only)	$
*Shipping & Handling	$
Total Order	$

---

*Shipping & Handling depend on the number of books bought—see below:
1 Book–$5.95   2-5 Books–$9.95   6-10 Books–$13.95

For orders over 10 books, please call customer service at the phone number below.

To Order By Telephone (Call Toll-Free):
With MC or Visa, call 888-345-BOOK (2665) Mon.-Fri., 9:00-5:00 Eastern Standard Time
http://www.kensingtonbooks.com

To Order By Mail:
Just fill out the information below and send this page with your remittance to:
> **Order Dept.**
> **Kensington Publishing Corp.**
> **850 Third Avenue**
> **New York, NY 10022**

- -

Name

Address

City   State   Zip

MC/Visa #   Exp. Date

Signature (cannot process without signature)

Check/Money Order enclosed for $ Payable to Kensington Publishing Corp.

Daytime Phone

*GNCG98